Proceedings of the Fourth International Symposium

RECENT ADVANCES IN OTITIS MEDIA

June 1–4, 1987
Bal Harbour, Florida

Proceedings of the Fourth International Symposium

RECENT ADVANCES IN OTITIS MEDIA

June 1–4, 1987
Bal Harbour, Florida

Editorial Committee
David J. Lim, M.D., *Editor-in-Chief*
Charles D. Bluestone, M.D.
Jerome O. Klein, M.D.
John D. Nelson, M.D.

Associate Editors
Thomas F. DeMaria, Ph.D.
Lauren O. Bakaletz, Ph.D.

Presented by
Department of Otolaryngology
Ohio State University College of Medicine

Sponsored by
The Center for Continuing Medical Education
Ohio State University College of Medicine

and
The Deafness Research Foundation

1988
B.C. Decker Inc • Toronto • Philadelphia

Publisher	B.C. Decker Inc 3228 South Service Road Burlington, Ontario L7N 3H8		B.C. Decker Inc 320 Walnut Street Suite 400 Philadelphia, Pennsylvania 19106	

Sales and Distribution

United States
and Possessions — The C.V. Mosby Company
11830 Westline Industrial Drive
Saint Louis, Missouri   63146

Asia — **Info-Med Ltd.**
802–3 Ruttonjee House
11 Duddell Street
Central Hong Kong

Canada — The C.V. Mosby Company, Ltd.
5240 Finch Avenue East, Unit No. 1
Scarborough, Ontario   M1S 5P2

South Africa — **Libriger Book Distributors**
Warehouse Number 8
"Die Ou Looiery"
Tannery Road
Hamilton, Bloemfontein 9300

United Kingdom,
Europe and the
Middle East — **Blackwell Scientific Publications, Ltd.**
Osney Mead, Oxford OX2 OEL, England

South
America — **Inter-Book Marketing Services**
Rua das Palmeriras, 32
Apto. 701
222–70 Rio de Janeiro
RJ, Brazil

Australia and
New Zealand — **Harcourt Brace Jovanovich Group
(Australia) Pty Limited**
30–52 Smidmore Street
Marrickville, N.S.W. 2204
Australia

Japan — **Igaku-Shoin Ltd.**
Tokyo International P.O. Box 5063
1–28–36 Hongo, Bunkyo-ku, Tokyo 113,
Japan

NOTICE

The authors and publisher have made every effort to ensure that the patient care recommended herein, including choice of drugs and drug dosages, is in accord with the accepted standards and practice at the time of publication. However, since research and regulation constantly change clinical standards, the reader is urged to check the product information sheet included in the package of each drug, which includes recommended doses, warnings, and contraindications. This is particularly important with new or infrequently used drugs.

Recent Advances in Otitis Media

ISBN 1-55664-087-0

Library of Congress catalog card number: 83–72419

10 9 8 7 6 5 4 3 2 1

CONTRIBUTORS

SUDHIR P. AGARWAL, M.D.

Medical Fellow, Department of Otolaryngology, University of Minnesota Medical School, Minneapolis, Minnesota

JACK W. ALAND Jr., M.D.

Resident, Division of Otolaryngology, University of Alabama School of Medicine, Birmingham, Alabama

DAVID M. ALBERT, F.R.C.S.

Registrar, King's College Hospital, London, United Kingdom

TOMAS ALBREKTSSON, M.D., Ph.D.

Professor and Chairman, Department of Handicap Research, University of Göteborg, Göteborg, Sweden

CAROLE ALLEN, M.D.

Staff Pediatrician, East Boston Neighborhood Health Center; Assistant Visiting Physician, Boston City Hospital and Associate Physician, Beth Israel Hospital, Boston, Massachusetts

BERNDT ALM, M.D.

Specialist, Department of Pediatrics, University of Göteborg, Göteborg, Sweden

RENNER S. ANDERSON, M.D.

Assistant Clinical Professor of Pediatrics, University of Minnesota Medical School, Minneapolis; General Pediatrician, Park Nicollet Medical Center and Vice-Chairman, Research, Park Nicollet Medical Foundation, St. Louis Park, Minnesota

BENGT ANDERSSON, M.D., Ph.D.

Resident, Clinical Immunology, University of Göteborg, Göteborg, Sweden

U.K. ANDREASSEN, M.D.

ENT Department, Gentofte University Hospital, Hellerup, Denmark

GUSTAV ANIANSSON, M.D.

Graduate Medical Student, Department of Clinical Immunology, University of Göteborg, Göteborg, Sweden

MATTI ANNIKO, M.D., Ph.D.

Professor, Department of Otolaryngology–Head and Neck Surgery, Umeå University Hospital, Umeå, Sweden

C.L.M. APPELMAN, M.D.

Resident in Research, Department of General Practice, University of Utrecht, Utrecht, The Netherlands

EDWARD L. APPLEBAUM, M.D.

Lederer Professor and Head, Department of Otolaryngology–Head and Neck Surgery, University of Illinois College of Medicine, Chicago, Illinois

AKIO ARAKI, M.D.

Department of Otolaryngology, Tokai University Tokyo Hospital, Tokyo, Japan

MIKKO AROLA, M.D.

Clinical Research Fellow, Department of Pediatrics, Turku University Hospital, Turku, Finland

DAN BAGGER-SJÖBÄCK, M.D., Ph.D.

Associate Professor, Department of Otolaryngology, Karolinska Hospital, Stockholm, Sweden

LAUREN O. BAKALETZ, Ph.D.

Assistant Professor, Department of Otolaryngology, Otologic Research Laboratories, Ohio State University College of Medicine, Columbus, Ohio

ROBERT L. BALDWIN, M.D.

Clinical Professor in Otolaryngology, University of Alabama School of Medicine; Chief of Otolaryngology, St. Vincent's Hospital, Birmingham, Alabama

VIGGO BALLE, M.D.

ENT Department, Gentofte University Hospital, Hellerup, Denmark

EUNICE BAND, R.N.

Research Nurse, Department of Nursing, St. Boniface General Hospital, Winnipeg, Manitoba, Canada

STEPHEN J. BARENKAMP, M.D.

Assistant Professor, Department of Pediatrics, Washington University School of Medicine; Staff Pediatrician, Division of Infectious Diseases, Children's Hospital at Washington University Medical Center, St. Louis, Missouri

LOREN J. BARTELS, M.D.

Associate Professor of Surgery, Department of Surgery, University of South Florida College of Medicine, Tampa, Florida

MAHA BASSILA, M.D.

Assistant Professor, Department of Otolaryngology, Albert Einstein College of Medicine, Bronx, New York

PAUL B. BATALDEN, M.D.

Vice President for Medical Care, Hospital Corporation of America, Nashville, Tennessee

SHARON BATCHER, B.S.

Staff Research Associate, Division of Otolaryngology, University of California, San Diego, School of Medicine, La Jolla, California

EDWIN H. BEACHEY, M.D.

Professor of Medicine, Microbiology, and Immunology, University of Tennessee College of Medicine; Chief, Division of Infectious Diseases and Associate Chief of Staff for Research, Veterans Administration Medical Center, Memphis, Tennessee

LUISA BELLUSSI, M.D.Ch.

Researcher I, ENT Clinic, University of Rome, La Sapienza, School of Medicine, Rome, Italy

JOEL M. BERNSTEIN, M.D., Ph.D.

Clinical Associate Professor of Pediatrics and Otolaryngology, State University of New York, Buffalo, New York

RICHARD S. BERNSTEIN, Ph.D.

Assistant Professor of Otorhinolaryngology, Albert Einstein College of Medicine, Bronx, New York

LUCIA BIGALLI, M.D.

Pediatric Department 4, University of Milan, Milan, Italy

MARK M. BLATTER, M.D.

Clinical Instructor, University of Pittsburgh School of Medicine, Pittsburgh, Pennsylvania

CHARLES D. BLUESTONE, M.D.

Professor of Otolaryngology, University of Pittsburgh School of Medicine; Director, Department of Pediatric Otolaryngology, Children's Hospital, Pittsburgh, Pennsylvania

FRANK F. BODOR, M.D.

Staff Pediatrician, Fairview Hospital Physicians Center, Cleveland, Ohio

SHARON BOEHM, B.S.

Laboratory Technician, Children's Hospital, Pittsburgh, Pennsylvania

BARRY D. BOONE, B.A.

EEG and Evoked Potential Laboratory, University of Texas Medical Branch, Galveston, Texas

VINCENT M. BOUTON, M.D.

Ancien Interne des Hopitaux Privés de Paris; Specialiste ORL et Chirurgie Maxillo-Faciale, Paris, France

CAROLINE E. BRAIN, M.R.C.P.

Community Medical Officer, North Southwark and Lewisham Health District, London, United Kingdom

LORNA BRATTON, M.B., Ch.B.

Director of Maternal Child Health, East Boston Neighborhood Health Center; Assistant Visiting Physician, Boston City Hospital and Associate Physician, Beth Israel Hospital, Boston, Massachusetts

LINDA BRODSKY, M.D.

Associate Professor of Otolaryngology, State University of New York; Staff, Childrens' Hospital, Buffalo, New York

LEON M. BROSTOFF, M.D.

Clinical Instructor of Pediatrics, University of Pittsburgh School of Medicine; Pediatrician, Health America Corporation, Pittsburgh, Pennsylvania

KAREN C. BROWN, M.S.

Audiologist, University of Texas, Callier Center for Communication Disorders, Dallas, Texas

ORVAL E. BROWN, M.D.

Assistant Professor of Otorhinolaryngology, University of Texas Southwestern Medical School; Attending Physician, Children's Medical Center and Parkland Memorial Hospital, Dallas, Texas

DAVID J. BURAN, M.D.

Associate Clinical Professor of Otolaryngology, University of Minnesota Medical School, Minneapolis; Chair, Department of Otolaryngology–Head and Neck Surgery, Park Nicollet Medical Center, St. Louis Park, Minnesota

MARGARET R. BURCHINAL, Ph.D.

Psychometrician and Investigator, Frank Porter Graham Child Development Center, University of North Carolina School of Medicine, Chapel Hill, North Carolina

DANIEL M. CANAFAX, Pharm.D.

Associate Professor of Pharmacy, Department of Pharmacy Practice, College of Pharmacy, University of Minnesota Medical School, Minneapolis, Minnesota

ERDEM I. CANTEKIN, Ph.D.

Professor of Otolaryngology, University of Pittsburgh School of Medicine, Pittsburgh, Pennsylvania

JAMES R. CARLSON, M.D.

Assistant Clinical Professor, University of Connecticut Health Center, Farmington; Staff, Stamford Hospital and St. Joseph Medical Center, Stamford, Connecticut

BRITT CARLSSON-NORDLANDER, M.D., Ph.D.

Assistant Professor, University of Stockholm; Staff, Department of Otolaryngology, Södersjukhuset, Stockholm, Sweden

ANNA-MARY CARPENTER, M.D., Ph.D.

Professor Emerita, Department of Anatomy, University of Minnesota, Minneapolis, Minnesota; Professor of Pathology, Indiana University, Northwestern Section, Indianapolis, Indiana

MARGARETHA L. CASSELBRANT, M.D., Ph.D.

Research Assistant Professor of Otolaryngology, University of Pittsburgh School of Medicine; Director, Clinical Research, Department of Pediatric Otolaryngology, Children's Hospital, Pittsburgh, Pennsylvania

ANTONINO CATANZARO, M.D.

Associate Professor of Medicine, University of California, San Diego, School of Medicine, La Jolla, California

KENNY H. CHAN, M.D.

Assistant Professor of Otolarngology, University of Pittsburgh School of Medicine; Staff Otolaryngologist, Children's Hospital, Pittsburgh, Pennsylvania

CYNTHIA CHASE, Ph.D.

Psychologist, Boston University School of Medicine and Boston City Hospital, Boston, Massachusetts

MYUNG-HYUN CHUNG, M.D.

Assistant Professor, Department of Otorhinolaryngology, Yonsei University College of Medicine, Seoul, Korea; Post-Professional Researcher, Department of Otolaryngology, Ohio State University College of Medicine, Columbus, Ohio

ROBERT J. CIPOLLE, Pharm.D., F.C.C.P.

Associate Dean and Associate Professor of Pharmacy, College of Pharmacy, University of Minnesota School of Medicine, Minneapolis, Minnesota

ALBERT M. COLLIER, M.D.

Professor of Pediatrics and Chief, Pediatric Infectious Disease Division, Department of Pediatrics, University of North Carolina School of Medicine, Chapel Hill, North Carolina

MAUREEN COLLISON, M.D., F.R.C.P.

Assistant Professor, Department of Pediatrics, University of Manitoba Faculty of Medicine; Staff Physician, Emergency Department, Children's Hospital, Winnipeg, Manitoba, Canada

HARRY S. COURTNEY, Ph.D.

Research Associate, University of Tennessee College of Medicine; Research Microbiologist at Veterans Administration Medical Center, Memphis, Tennessee

YOSHIHIRO DAKE, M.D.

Lecturer, Otorhinolaryngology, Wakayama Medical College, Wakayama, Japan

KATHY DALY, M.P.H.

Assistant Scientist, Department of Otolaryngology, University of Minnesota School of Medicine; Epidemiologist, Minnesota Department of Health, Minneapolis, Minnesota

GERDA G. De LANGE, Ph.D.

Department of Immunohaematology, Central Laboratory of The Netherlands, Red Cross Blood Transfusion Service, Amsterdam, The Netherlands

THOMAS F. DeMARIA, Ph.D.

Assistant Professor, Otologic Research Laboratories, Department of Otolaryngology, Ohio State University College of Medicine, Columbus, Ohio

R.A. De MELKER, M.D.

Professor, General Practice, University of Utrecht, Utrecht, The Netherlands

ELLEN E. DEMPSEY, M.Sc.

Manager of Cardiovascular Research, Nordic Laboratories, Montreal, Quebec, Canada

MAGDA De SMEDT

Technical Engineer, University Hospital, Ghent, Belgium

ALAN DESPINS, B.S.

Research Assistant, Department of Pathology, University of Connecticut Health Center, Farmington, Connecticut

DENNIS C. DIRKMAAT, B.A.

Research Technician, Otitis Media Research Center, Children's Hospital, Pittsburgh, Pennsylvania

WARREN F. DIVEN, Ph.D.

Associate Professor of Pathology and Biochemistry, University of Pittsburgh School of Medicine, Pittsburgh, Pennsylvania

MARION P. DOWNS, M.A., D.H.S.

Professor Emerita, Department of Otolaryngology, University of Colorado Health Sciences Center, Denver, Colorado

WILLIAM J. DOYLE, Ph.D.

Associate Professor of Otolaryngology, University of Pittsburgh School of Medicine; Director, Laboratory Research, Department of Pediatric Otolaryngology, Children's Hospital, Pittsburgh, Pennsylvania

DIANE M. DRYJA, B.S.

Clinical Instructor, Medical Technology, Departments of Pediatrics and Immunology, State University of New York, Buffalo, New York

LAWRENCE DUSSACK, B.S.

EEG and Evoked Potential Laboratory, University of Texas Medical Branch, Galveston, Texas

JAMES EDLIN, B.S.

Research Assistant, Department of Otolaryngology, University of Minnesota Medical School, Minneapolis, Minnesota

RONEL ENRIQUE, M.D.

Resident, Department of Otolaryngology, Henry Ford Hospital, Detroit, Michigan

GARY R. ERDMANN, Ph.D.

Assistant Professor of Pharmacy, College of Pharmacy, University of Minnesota Medical School, Minneapolis, Minnesota

YUSUKE ESAKI, M.D.

Resident, Department of Otolaryngology, Osaka City University Medical School, Osaka, Japan

HOWARD FADEN, M.D.

Professor of Pediatrics, State University of New York; Attending Physician, Division of Infectious Diseases, Children's Hospital, Buffalo, New York

PATRICIA FALL, R.N., B.S.N., C.P.N.P.

Certified Pediatric Nurse Practicioner, Children's Hospital, Pittsburgh, Pennsylvania

JOY FEHRIBACH, B.S.

Research Assistant in Pediatrics, Cleveland Metropolitan General Hospital, Cleveland, Ohio

JENS U. FELDING, M.D.

Assistant Professor and Senior Registrar, ENT Department, University Hospital, Århus, Denmark

MOGENS FIELLAU-NIKOLAJSEN, M.D.

Medical Candidate, Århus University, Århus; Staff, ENT Clinic, Odense, Denmark

TERESE FINITZO, Ph.D.

Associate Professor, University of Texas, Callier Center for Communication Disorders, Dallas, Texas

PHILIP FIREMAN, M.D.

Professor of Pediatrics, University of Pittsburgh School of Medicine; Director, Allergy and Immunology, Children's Hospital of Pittsburgh, Pittsburgh, Pennsylvania

GILBERT FISCH, M.D.

Associate Clinical Professor of Pediatrics, Boston University School of Medicine, Boston; Attending Pediatrician, Framingham Union Hospital, Framingham, Massachusetts

KATHLEEN FLAHERTY, B.S.

Research Assistant, Department of Pathology, University of Connecticut Health Center, Farmington, Connecticut

ELLEN FORMBY, M.A.

Speech-Language Pathologist, University of Texas, Callier Center for Communication Disorders, Dallas, Texas

DOUGLAS FREEMAN, M.D.

Chief, Department of Otolaryngology, Kaiser Foundation Hospital, Sacramento, California

ANDERS FREIJD, M.D.

Associate Professor, Karolinska Institute, Huddinge University Hospital, Huddinge, Sweden

SANDY FRIEL-PATTI, Ph.D.

Associate Professor, University of Texas, Callier Center for Communication Disorders, Dallas, Texas

ULLA FRYKSMARK, M.D., Ph.D.

Assistant Professor, University of Lund; Staff, Department of Otolaryngology, Malmö General Hospital, Malmö, Sweden

TATSUYA FUJIYOSHI, M.D.

Assistant Professor, Department of Otolaryngology, University Hospitals of the Medical College of Oita, Oita, Japan

ROBERT S. FULGHUM, Ph.D.

Associate Professor, Department of Microbiology and Immunology, East Carolina University School of Medicine, Greenville, North Carolina

ILANA GELERNTER, M.Sc.

Statistician, Statistical Laboratory, Tel Aviv University, Tel Aviv, Israel

SEZELLE A. GEREAU, M.D.

Resident in Otolaryngology, Montefiore Medical Center, Bronx, New York

MELANIE GERO, M.D.

Chief Resident of Pathology, Long Island Jewish Medical Center, New Hyde Park, New York

G. SCOTT GIEBINK, M.D.

Professor, Departments of Pediatrics and Otolaryngology, University of Minnesota Medical School, Minneapolis, Minnesota

PETER H. GILLIGAN, Ph.D.

Assistant Professor of Microbiology, Immunology, and Pathology, University of North Carolina School of Medicine; Associate Director, Clinical Microbiology-Immunology Laboratories, The North Carolina Memorial Hospital, Chapel Hill, North Carolina

MONIKA GINZEL, B.S.

Institute for General and Experimental Pathology, University of Innsbruck Medical School, Innsbruck, Austria

JEAN B. GLEASON, Ph.D.

Professor and Chair, Department of Psychology, Boston University; Research Associate, Aphasia Research Center, Boston University School of Medicine, Boston, Massachusetts

PAMELA GOLDIE, M.D.

Department of Anatomy, University of Umeå, Umeå, Sweden

YOKO GOTODA, M.D.

Department of Otolaryngology, Tokyo Women's Medical College, Tokyo, Japan

MARCOS V. GOYCOOLEA, M.D., M.S., Ph.D.

Staff Physician, Minnesota Ear, Head, and Neck Clinic, Minneapolis, Minnesota; Director, Otology and Research Departments, Audia Chile, Santiago, Chile.

MICHAEL G.A. GRACE, Ph.D., P.Eng.

Adjunct Professor of Surgery, Clinical Professor of Medicine, University of Alberta Faculty of Medicine, Edmonton, Alberta, Canada

ROBERTO GRADINI, M.D.

Research Associate, Pathology, Loyola University Medical Center, Chicago, Illinois

PER G.B. GRANSTRÖM, M.D., D.D.S., Ph.D.

Honorary Associate Professor, Göteborg University; Fellow, ENT Department, Sahlgren's Hospital, Göteborg, Sweden

JUDITH S. GRAVEL, Ph.D.

Assistant Professor of Otolaryngology, Rose F. Kennedy Center, Albert Einstein College of Medicine, Bronx, New York

STEPHEN R. GRIFFITH, M.D.

Resident, Department of Otolaryngology, Ohio State University, Columbus, Ohio

TORSTEN GRUNDITZ, M.D.

Associate Professor, Malmö General Hospital, Malmö, Sweden

SUSAN GUGENHEIM, M.S., CCC-Sp.

Speech Pathologist, Denver, Colorado

JACK M. GWALTNEY Jr., M.D.

Professor of Medicine, University of Virginia School of Medicine, Charlottesville, Virginia

PEKKA HALONEN, M.D.

Professor and Director, Department of Virology, Turku University, Turku, Finland

YUKIYOSHI HAMAGUCHI, M.D.

Chief Assistant, Department of Otorhinolaryngology, Mie University School of Medicine, Mie, Japan

TAKEHIRO HANADA, M.D.

Department of Otolaryngology, Faculty of Medicine, Kagoshima University, Kagoshima, Japan

YUTAKA HANAMURE, M.D.

Faculty Lecturer, Department of Otolaryngology, Faculty of Medicine, Kagoshima University, Kagoshima, Japan

DAVID M. HARRIS, Ph.D.

Medical Staff, Department of Psychiatry, Ravenswood Hospital Medical Center; Associate Director, Education, Wenske Laser Center and Ravenswood Hospital Medical Center, Chicago, Illinois

JEFFREY P. HARRIS, M.D., Ph.D.

Associate Professor of Surgery, Otolaryngology, University of California, San Diego, School of Medicine; Chief of Otolaryngology, University of California San Diego Medical Center, La Jolla, California

GÖRAN HARSTEN, M.D.

Department of Otorhinolaryngology, University of Lund, Lund, Sweden

FREDERICK G. HAYDEN, M.D.

Assistant Professor of Medicine, Department of Internal Medicine, University of Virginia School of Medicine, Charlottesville, Virginia

ANTHONY R. HAYWARD, M.D., Ph.D.

Professor of Pediatrics, Microbiology, and Immunology, University of Colorado School of Medicine, Denver, Colorado

JESPER HELDRUP, M.D.

Department of Pediatrics, University Hospital, Lund, Sweden

STEN O.M. HELLSTRÖM, M.D., Ph.D.

Associate Professor, Department of Anatomy, University of Umeå; Staff, Department of Otorhinolaryngology–Head and Neck Surgery, Umeå University Hospital, Umeå, Sweden

FREDERICK W. HENDERSON, M.D.

Associate Professor of Pediatrics, University of North Carolina School of Medicine; Attending Pediatrician, The North Carolina Memorial Hospital, Chapel Hill, North Carolina

WILLIAM A. HENDRICKSE, M.D., M.R.C.P.

Resident, Psychiatry Division, University of Texas Southwestern Medical Center, Dallas, Texas

ANN HERMANSSON, M.D.

Department of Otorhinolaryngology, Lund University Hospital, Lund, Sweden

J. PATRICK HIEBER, M.D.

Clinical Associate Professor, The University of Texas Health Science Center, Dallas, Texas

TONI M. HOEPF, M.S.

Research Assistant, Otologic Research Laboratories, Department of Otolaryngology, Ohio State University College of Medicine, Columbus, Ohio

JÖRGEN HOLMQUIST, M.D., Ph.D.

Associate Professor, ENT Department, University of Göteborg and Sahlgren's Hospital, Göteborg, Sweden

LEIF HOLMQUIST, Ph.D.

Associate Professor, King Gustav V Research Institute, Karolinska Hospital, Stockholm, Sweden

KEIJI HONDA, M.D.

Assistant Professor, Department of Otolaryngology, Kansai Medical University, Osaka, Japan

JUNG J. HONG, B.S.

Division of Infectious Diseases, Children's Hospital, Buffalo, New York

IWAO HONJO, M.D.

Professor and Chairman, Department of Otolaryngology, Faculty of Medicine, Kyoto University, Kyoto, Japan

G.J. HORDIJK, M.D.

Professor, ENT Department, University of Utrecht; Surgeon, Department of Otorhinolaryngology, University Hospital, Utrecht, The Netherlands

FUMIHIKO HORI, M.D.

Associate, Department of Otolaryngology, University Hospitals of the Medical College of Oita, Oita, Japan

YOSHIRO HORI

Department of Otolaryngology, Kansai Medical University, Osaka, Japan

KAZUMASA HOSHINO, M.D.

Professor and Chairman, Department of Anatomy, Faculty of Medicine, Kyoto University, Kyoto, Japan

VIRGIL M. HOWIE, M.D.

Professor, Department of Pediatrics, University of Texas Medical Branch, Galveston, Texas

KOJI HOZAWA, M.D.

Associate, Department of Otolaryngology, Tohoku University School of Medicine, Sendai, Japan

TI HSIEH, M.D.

Professor and Chairman, Department of Otolaryngology, National Taiwan University Hospital, Taipei, Taiwan

JAMES R. HUMBERT, M.D.

Professor of Medicine, Tulane University School of Medicine, New Orleans, Louisiana

BURKHARD HUSSL, M.D.

University of Innsbruck Medical School, Innsbruck, Austria

G. HVID, M.D.

ENT Department, Frederiksberg Hospital,
Copenhagen, Denmark

SOON-JAE HWANG, M.D.

Associate Professor, Department of Otolaryngology, Korea
University College of Medicine, Seoul, Korea

ISSEI ICHIMIYA, M.D.

Postgraduate Student, Medical College of Oita; Staff,
Department of Otolaryngology, University Hospitals of the
Medical College of Oita, Oita, Japan

HIROSHI IKEOKA, M.D.

Resident, Department of Otolaryngology, Osaka City University
Medical School, Osaka, Japan

CARL F. ILARDI, M.D.

Assistant Professor of Pathology, School of Medicine, Health
Sciences Center, State University of New York at Stony Brook;
Staff Pathologist, Long Island Jewish Medical Center,
New Hyde Park, New York

MASASHI INAGAKI, M.D.

Head, Department of Otorhinolaryngology, Yokkaichi City
Hospital, Japan

NAOKI INAMURA, M.D.

Associate, Department of Otolaryngology, Tohoku University
School of Medicine, Sendai, Japan

LEIF INGVARSSON, M.D., Ph.D.

Department of Otorhinolaryngology, Malmö General Hospital,
University of Lund, Malmö, Sweden

CHIYONORI INO, M.D.

Department of Otolaryngology, Kansai Medical University,
Osaka, Japan

MASAKO ISHIDOYA, M.D.

Associate, Department of Otolaryngology, Tohoku University
School of Medicine, Sendai, Japan

TETSUO ISHII, M.D.

Department of Otolaryngology, Tokyo Women's Medical
College, Tokyo, Japan

JUICHI ITO, M.D.

Assistant Professor, Department of Otolaryngology, Faculty of
Medicine, Kyoto University, Kyoto, Japan

PAUL H.K. JAP, M.D.

Department of Cell Biology, University of Nijmegen,
Nijmegen, The Netherlands

ANDERS M. JENSEN, M.Sc.

Consultant Statistician, Birkerød, Denmark

ANNA LISE JEPPESEN, M.A.

Psychology Candidate, Hjørring, Denmark

ULF JOHANSSON, M.D.

Department of Otorhinolaryngology–Head and Neck Surgery,
Umeå University Hospital, Umeå, Sweden

CANDICE E. JOHNSON, M.D., Ph.D.

Assistant Professor of Pediatrics, Case Western University
School of Medicine; Staff Pediatrician, Cleveland Metropolitan
General Hospital, Cleveland, Ohio

FINN JÖRGENSEN, M.D.

ENT Department, University of Göteborg, Göteborg; ENT
Specialist, County Hospital, Borås, Sweden

K. JOZAKI, M.D.

Department of Pediatrics, Keio University, Tokyo, Japan

LUIS F. JUAREZ, M.D.

Resident, Department of Otolaryngology, Children's Hospital,
Mexico City, Mexico

STEVEN K. JUHN, M.D.

Professor of Otolaryngology, University of Minnesota Medical
School, Minneapolis, Minnesota

TIMOTHY T.K. JUNG, M.D., Ph.D.

Associate Professor, Division of Otolaryngology–Head and Neck
Surgery, Department of Surgery, Loma Linda University School
of Medicine, Loma Linda, California

HIROMU KAKIUCHI, M.D.

Assistant, Otorhinolaryngology, Wakayama Medical College,
Wakayama, Japan

PHILLIP H. KALEIDA, M.D.

Assistant Professor of Pediatrics, University of Pittsburgh School
of Medicine; Staff Pediatrician, Children's Hospital and Clinical
Research Pediatrician, Otitis Media Research Center,
Department of Pediatric Otolaryngology, Children's Hospital,
Pittsburgh, Pennsylvania

OLOF KALM, M.D., Ph.D.

Associate Professor of Otorhinolaryngology, University of Lund;
Senior Physician, Department of Otorhinolaryngology,
University Hospital, Lund, Sweden

HEINO KARJALAINEN, M.D.

Departments of Otolaryngology and Medical Microbiology,
University of Oulu, Oulu, Finland

NILS G. KARLSSON, M.D., Ph.D.

Honorary Associate Professor, Göteborg University; Consultant,
ENT Department, Sahlgren's Hospital, Göteborg, Sweden

PEKKA H. KARMA, M.D.

Professor of Otolaryngology, University of Tampere; Head,
Department of Otolaryngology, Tampere University Central
Hospital, Tampere, Finland

**COLLIN S. KARMODY, M.D., F.R.C.S. (Edin),
F.A.C.S.**

Professor of Otolaryngology, Tufts University School of
Medicine; Senior Surgeon, New England Medical Center,
Boston, Massachusetts

HIROFUMI KATO, M.D.

Department of Otolaryngology, Medical College of Oita,
Oita, Japan

SHOKO KATO, M.D.

Resident, Department of Otolaryngology, Osaka City University
Medical School, Osaka, Japan

MIRIAM KAUFSTEIN, B.Sc.

Director, Laboratory of Bacteriology, Hillel-Jaffe Memorial
Hospital, Hadera, Israel

NOBUKO KAWASHIRO, M.D.

Department of Otolaryngology, Tokai University Tokyo
Hospital, Tokyo, Japan

HIDEYUKI KAWAUCHI, M.D.

Assistant Professor, Department of Otolaryngology, University
Hospitals of the Medical College of Oita, Oita, Japan

WILLIAM J. KEITH, Ph.D.

Acting Director, National Audiology Center,
Auckland, New Zealand

ELIZABETH M. KEITHLEY, Ph.D.

Assistant Professor of Otolaryngology, University of California,
San Diego, School of Medicine, La Jolla, California

GEORG KELETI, Ph.D.

Adjunct Associate Professor of Microbiology, Industrial
Environmental Health Science, Graduate School of Public
Health, University of Pittsburgh School of Medicine,
Pittsburgh, Pennsylvania

MARGARET A. KENNA, M.D.

Assistant Professor, Surgery and Pediatrics, Yale University
School of Medicine, New Haven, Connecticut

THOMAS L. KENNEDY, M.D.

Associate Clinical Professor, Department of Pediatrics,
University of Connecticut Health Center,
Farmington, Connecticut

HEE NAM KIM, M.D.

Department of Otolaryngology, Yonsei University College of
Medicine, Seoul, Korea

ETSUKO KIMURA, M.D.

Department of Otolaryngology, Tokyo Women's Medical
College, Tokyo, Japan

RYUZI KIYOTA, M.D.

Department of Otolaryngology, Faculty of Medicine, Kagoshima
University, Kagoshima, Japan

JEROME O. KLEIN, M.D.

Professor of Pediatrics, Boston University School of Medicine
and Boston City Hospital, Boston, Massachusetts

JOANN K. KNOX

Community Program Specialist, Otitis Media Program,
University of Minnesota Medical School,
Minneapolis, Minnesota

MATTHEW A. KOCH, M.D.

Biostatistician, Frank Porter Graham Child Development Center,
University of North Carolina School of Medicine,
Chapel Hill, North Carolina

KEIJIRO KOGA, M.D.

Department of Otolaryngology, National Children's Hospital,
Tokyo, Japan

RAGNHILD KORNFÄLT, M.D.

Associate Professor of Pediatrics, University of Lund,
Lund, Sweden

HIROYUKI KOSHIMO, M.D.

Resident, Department of Otolaryngology, Osaka City University
Medical School, Osaka, Japan

MARKKU KOSKELA, M.D.

Departments of Otolaryngology and Medical Microbiology,
University of Oulu, Oulu, Finland

MIRJANA KOSTICH, M.D.

Staff Pediatrician, East Boston Neighborhood Health Center;
Assistant Visiting Physician, Boston City Hospital and Associate
Physician, Beth Israel Hospital, Boston, Massachusetts

DONALD L. KREUTZER, Ph.D.

Associate Professor of Pathology, University of Connecticut
Health Center, Farmington, Connecticut

DEBORAH A. KRYSTOFIK, R.N.

Division of Infectious Diseases, Children's Hospital,
Buffalo, New York

NOBUO KUBO, M.D.

Assistant, Department of Otolaryngology, Kansai Medical
University, Osaka, Japan

WIM KUIJPERS, Ph.D.

Department of Otolaryngology, University of Nijmegen,
Nijmegen, The Netherlands

TADAMI KUMAZAWA, M.D.

Professor, Department of Otolaryngology, Kansai Medical
University, Osaka, Japan

KYOSUKE KURATA, M.D.

Division of Otolaryngology, Shizuoka General Hospital,
Shizuoka, Japan

ATSUSHI KURIHARA, Ph.D.

Associate, Department of Otolaryngology, Tohoku University
School of Medicine, Sendai, Japan

YUICHI KURONO, M.D.

Department of Otolaryngology, Medical College of Oita,
Oita, Japan

MARCIA KURS-LASKY, M.S.

Department of Statistics, University of Pittsburgh School of
Medicine, Pittsburgh, Pennsylvania

HELEN KUSMIESZ, R.N.

Research Nurse, Department of Pediatric Infectious Diseases, University of Texas Southwestern Medical Center, Dallas, Texas

PER L. LARSEN, M.D.

ENT Department, Gentofte University Hospital, Hellerup, Denmark

AMY LARSSON, M.D.

Department of Otolaryngology, Malmö General Hospital, Malmö, Sweden

PETER LARSSON

Associate Professor and Senior Clinical Bacteriologist, University of Göteborg, Göteborg, Sweden

LEONARD J. LASCOLEA, M.D.

Professor of Pediatrics, State University of New York; Chief, Bacteriology Laboratory, Children's Hospital, Buffalo, New York

CLAUDE LAURENT, M.D.

Department of Otorhinolaryngology, Central Hospital, Falun, Sweden

MARIA LAURIELLO, M.D.

ENT Clinic, University of L'Aquila, Rome, Italy

CHAP T. LE, Ph.D.

Associate Professor of Biometry, University of Minnesota School of Public Health, Minneapolis, Minnesota

CHINH T. LE, M.D.

Associate Clinical Professor, Department of Pediatrics, University of California School of Medicine, Davis; Chief, Pediatric Infectious Disease, Kaiser Foundation Hospital, Sacramento, California

JAE-SUNG LEE, M.D.

Resident, Division of Otolaryngology, Department of Surgery, Loma Linda University School of Medicine, Loma Linda, California

MIREILLE LEMAY, M.D.

Fellow in Pediatric Infectious Disease, Boston University School of Medicine, Boston, Massachusetts

GERALD LEONARD, M.D.

Assistant Professor of Surgery and Chief, Division of Otolaryngology, University of Connecticut Health Center, Farmington, Connecticut

G.J. LEPPINK, Ph.D.

Professor in Mathematical Statistics, University of Utrecht, Urecht, The Netherlands

TORBEN LILDHOLDT, M.D., Ph.D.

Department of Otolaryngology, Vejle Hospital, Vejle, Denmark

KARIN LILJA

Lab Technician, Department of Otorhinolaryngology, Central Hospital, Falun, Sweden

DAVID J. LIM, M.D.

Professor, Department of Otolaryngology and Anatomy and Director, Otological Research Laboratories, Ohio State University College of Medicine, Columbus, Ohio

L. LIND, M.D.

Institute of Microbiology, Sahlgren's Hospital, Göteborg, Sweden

BRUCE LINDGREN, M.S.

Research Fellow, Biometry Division School of Public Health, University of Minnesota Medical School, Minneapolis, Minnesota

JØRGEN LOUS, M.D.

Medical Candidate and Lecturer, Århus University, General Practitioner and Director, Otitis Media Study Group, Hjørring, Denmark

KAJ LUNDGREN, M.D., Ph.D.

Department of Otolaryngology, Malmö General Hospital, University of Lund, Malmö, Sweden

LARS LUNDMAN, M.D.

Clinical Fellow, Department of Otolaryngology, Karolinska Hospital, Stockholm, Sweden

MICHAL LUNTZ, M.D.

Staff, Kupat-Holim, Sapir Medical Center, Meir General Hospital, Kfar Saba, Israel

JUKKA LUOTONEN, M.D.

Departments of Otolaryngology and Medical Microbiology, University of Oulu, Oulu, Finland

KENJI MACHIKI, M.D.

Assistant, Department of Otolaryngology, Institute of Clinical Medicine, The University of Tsukuba, Tsukuba-Shi, Japan

NORIO MAEDA, M.D.

Assistant, Department of Otolaryngology, Kansai Medical University, Osaka, Japan

YUICHI MAJIMA, M.D.

Assistant Professor, Department of Otorhinolaryngology, Mie University School of Medicine, Mie, Japan

HENRIK MALMBERG, M.D.

Department of Otolaryngology, Helsinki University Hospital, Helsinki, Finland

ELLEN M. MANDEL, M.D.

Assistant Professor of Pediatrics, University of Pittsburgh School of Medicine, Pittsburgh, Pennsylvania

COLIN D. MARCHANT, M.D.

Associate Professor, Department of Pediatrics, Tufts University School of Medicine; Attending Staff Physician, Department of Infectious Disease (Pediatrics), Boston Floating Hospital, Boston, Massachusetts

PAOLA MARCHISIO, M.D.

Pediatric Department 4, University of Milan, Milan, Italy

HENRY G. MARROW, M.D.

Assistant Professor, Department of Clinical Pathology and Diagnostic Medicine, East Carolina University School of Medicine, Greenville, North Carolina

MASAMI MASAKI, M.D.

Department of Otorhinolaryngology, University of Texas Southwestern Medical Center, Dallas, Texas

EMILIA MASSIRONI, M.D.

Pediatric Department 4, University of Milan, Milan, Italy

A. RICHARD MAW, M.S., F.R.C.S.

Clinical Lecturer and Head, Department of Otolaryngology, University of Bristol; Consultant Otolaryngologist, Bristol Royal Infirmary and the Bristol Royal Hospital for Sick Children, Bristol, United Kingdom.

TIMOTHY P. McBRIDE, M.D.

Assistant Professor of Otolaryngology, University of Pittsburgh School of Medicine; Staff Otolaryngologist, Department of Pediatric Otolaryngology, Pittsburgh, Pennsylvania

CECELIA M. McCARTON, M.D.

Associate Professor of Medicine and Director, Low Birth Weight Infant Follow-Up and Evaluation (LIFE) Program, Rose F. Kennedy Center, Albert Einstein College of Medicine, Bronx, New York

TREVOR J. McGILL, M.D.

Associate Professor of Otolaryngology, Harvard Medical School; Associate in Chief, Department of Otolaryngology, The Children's Hospital, Boston, Massachusetts

LILLIAN McMAHON, M.D.

Assistant Professor in Pediatrics, Boston University School of Medicine; Pediatric Hematologist, Boston City Hospital and Program Director, Boston Sickle Cell Center, Boston, Massachusetts

PAULA MENYUK, Ph.D.

Professor, Boston University School of Medicine, Boston, Massachusetts

MARTHA MERROW, B.S.

Research Associate, Department of Pediatrics, University of Connecticut Health Center, Farmington, Connecticut

YUSSI MERTSOLA, M.D.

Clinical Research Fellow, Department of Pediatrics, Turku University Hospital, Turku, Finland

OLLI MEURMAN, M.D.

Consulting Virologist, Department of Virology, Turku University, Turku, Finland

WILLIAM L. MEYERHOFF, M.D., Ph.D.

Professor and Chairman, Department of Otorhinolaryngology, University of Texas Southwestern Medical Center, Dallas, Texas

STANLEY K. MILLER, B.S.

Research Assistant, Division of Otolaryngology, Department of Surgery, Loma Linda University School of Medicine, Loma Linda, California

ROBERT P. MILLS, M.Phil., F.R.C.S.

Senior Registrar, King's College Hospital, London, United Kingdom

TOYOHIKO MINAMI, M.D.

Assistant, Department of Otolaryngology, Kansai Medical University, Osaka, Japan

GORO MOGI, M.D.

Professor and Head, Department of Otolaryngology, University Hospitals of the Medical College of Oita, Oita, Japan

JACOB G. MOL, M.D.

Surgeon, Department of Otolaryngology, University Hospital, Utrecht, The Netherlands

TIMOTHY B. MOLONY, M.D.

Resident in Otolaryngology, University of South Florida College of Medicine, Tampa, Florida

LINDA MOORE, Ph.D.

Instructor in Medicine, Tulane University School of Medicine, New Orleans, Louisiana

MAXINE MORGAN, M.D.

Resident in Surgery, Bronx Municipal Hospital Center, Bronx, New York

YUKIHIKO MORIKAWA, M.D.

Department of Pathology, National Children's Hospital, Tokyo, Japan

TETSUO MORIZONO, M.D., D.M.S., M.S.

Associate Professor, Department of Otolaryngology, University of Minnesota Medical School, Minneapolis, Minnesota

THOMAS MORLEDGE, M.D.

Resident in Pediatrics, Cleveland Metropolitan General Hospital, Cleveland, Ohio

DAVID MUCHOW

Otopathology Laboratory, Department of Otolaryngology, University of Minnesota Medical School, Minneapolis, Minnesota; Co-Director, Research Department, Audia Chile, Santiago, Chile

KENZOU MURANO, M.D.

Department of Otolaryngology, Faculty of Medicine, Kagoshima University, Kagoshima, Japan

TIMOTHY F. MURPHY, M.D.

Assistant Professor of Medicine, Erie County Medical Center and Tissue Typing Laboratory, State University of New York, Buffalo, New York

YASUSHI NAITO, M.D.

Postgraduate Student, Department of Otolaryngology, Faculty of Medicine, Kyoto University, Kyoto, Japan

YOSHIAKI NAKAI, M.D.

Professor and Chairman, Department of Otolaryngology, Osaka City University Medical School, Osaka, Japan

JOHN D. NELSON, M.D.

Professor of Pediatrics, Department of Pediatric Infectious Diseases, University of Texas Southwestern Medical Center, Dallas, Texas

LARS K. NIELSEN, M.D.

Department of Clinical Chemistry, Ålborg Hospital, Ålborg, Denmark

KAZUMASA NISHIMURA, M.D.

Department of Radiology and Nuclear Medicine, Faculty of Medicine, Kyoto University, Kyoto, Japan

TAKUO NOBORI, M.D.

Associate Professor, Department of Otolaryngology, Faculty of Medicine, Kagoshima University, Kagoshima, Japan

KARYL NORCROSS, M.D., Ph.D.

Associate Professor, Neurology Department, University of Texas Medical Branch, Galveston, Texas

ÅSA NORDLING, B.M.

Department of Anatomy, University of Umeå, Umeå, Sweden

JERRY L. NORTHERN, Ph.D.

Professor of Otolaryngology, University of Colorado Health Sciences Center, Denver, Colorado

ROBERT J. NOZZA, Ph.D.

Assistant Professor, Department of Otolaryngology, University of Pittsburgh School of Medicine; Director of Audiology, Children's Hospital, Pittsburgh, Pennsylvania

OLLE NYLÉN, M.D., Ph.D.

Associate Professor and Senior Otorhinolaryngologist, Department of Otorhinolaryngology, University of Göteborg, Göteborg, Sweden

ETSUROU OBATA, M.D.

Department of Otolaryngology, Faculty of Medicine, Kagoshima University, Kagoshima, Japan

PEARAY L. OGRA, M.D.

Professor, Departments of Pediatrics and Microbiology, State University of New York; Chief, Division of Infectious Diseases and Microbiology Laboratories, Children's Hospital, Buffalo, New York

YOSHIHIRO OHASHI, M.D.

Assistant Professor, Department of Otolaryngology, Osaka City University Medical School, Osaka, Japan; Post-Professional Researcher, Department of Otolaryngology, Ohio State University College of Medicine, Columbus, Ohio

KJELL OHLSSON, M.D., Ph.D.

Professor, University of Lund; Staff, Department of Surgical Pathophysiology, Malmö General Hospital, Malmö, Sweden

FUMIO OHNO, M.D.

Department of Otolaryngology, Faculty of Medicine, Kagoshima University, Kagoshima, Japan

MASARU OHYAMA, M.D.

Professor and Chairman, Department of Otolaryngology, Faculty of Medicine, Kagoshima University, Kagoshima, Japan

SEISHI OKA, D.D.S., Ph.D.

Lancaster Cleft Palate Clinic, Lancaster, Pennsylvania

TAKUJI OKITSU, M.D.

Chief, Department of Otolaryngology, Tohoku Teishin Hospital, Sendai, Japan

SVEN A.S. OLLING, M.D.

Honorary Associate Professor, Göteborg University; Consultant, Department of Pathology, Sahlgren's Hospital, Göteborg, Sweden

BERTIL OLOFSSON, M.D., Ph.D.

Department of Otolaryngology, Malmö General Hospital, University of Lund, Malmö, Sweden

DAVID OLSON, B.S.

Research Assistant, Division of Otolaryngology, Loma Linda University School of Medicine, Loma Linda, California

ERVIN OSTFELD, M.D., M.Sc.

Senior Lecturer, Otolaryngology, Sackler School of Medicine, Tel Aviv University, Tel Aviv and Scientific Adviser, Department of Polymer Research, Weizmann Institute of Science, Rehovot; Head, Department of Otolaryngology, Hillel-Jaffe Memorial Hospital, Hadera, Israel

MARY JEAN OWEN, M.D.

Fellow, Department of Pediatrics, University of Texas Medical Branch, Galveston, Texas

DENISE PAGE, M.D.

Assistant Professor in Pathology, Boston University School of Medicine; Pathologist, Boston City Hospital, Boston, Massachusetts

TAUNO PALVA, M.D.

Professor and Chairman, Department of Otorhinolaryngology, Helsinki University Hospital, Helsinki, Finland

MICHAEL M. PAPARELLA, M.D.

Clinical Professor and Chairman Emeritus, Department of Otolaryngology, University of Minnesota Medical School; Secretary of the International Hearing Foundation, Minnesota Ear, Head, and Neck Clinic, Minneapolis, Minnesota

JACK L. PARADISE, M.D.

Professor of Pediatrics and Community Medicine, University of Pittsburgh School of Medicine; Medical Director, Ambulatory Care Center, Children's Hospital, Pittsburgh, Pennsylvania

IN YONG PARK, M.D.

Department of Otolaryngology, Yonsei University College of Medicine, Seoul, Korea

KEE HYUN PARK, M.D.

Department of Otolaryngology, Yonsei University College of Medicine, Seoul, Korea

DESIDERIO PASSALI, M.D.

Professor and Chairman, ENT Clinic, University of L'Aquila, Rome, Italy

STEPHEN I. PELTON, M.D.

Associate Professor of Pediatrics, Boston University School of Medicine; Associate Visiting Physician, Boston City Hospital, Boston, Massachusetts

MATTI A. PENTTILÄ, M.D.

Instructor in Otolaryngology, University of Tampere; Senior Otolaryngologist, Department of Otolaryngology, Tampere University Central Hospital, Tampere, Finland

HANS PETERSON, M.D.

Senior Pediatrician, Outpatient Organization, Göteborg, Sweden

JEAN PLUM, M.D., Ph.D.

Senior Lecturer, State University; Senior Staff Member, Department of Bacteriology and Virology, University Hospital, Ghent, Belgium

DAVID POOLE, M.D.

Resident, Division of Otolaryngology, Department of Surgery, Loma Linda University School of Medicine, Loma Linda, California

KARIN PRELLNER, M.D., Ph.D.

Associate Professor of Otorhinolaryngology, Lund University Hospital, Lund, Sweden

NICOLA PRINCIPI, M.D.

Pediatric Department 4, University of Milan, Milan, Italy

DAVID PROOPS, F.R.C.S.

Department of Otolaryngology, Children's Hospital, Birmingham, United Kingdom

JUHANI S. PUKANDER, M.D.

Assistant Professor of Otolaryngology, University of Tampere; Senior Otolaryngologist, Department of Otolaryngology, University Hospital of Tampere, Tampere, Finland

ANNE PUTTO-LAURILA, M.D.

Resident, Department of Pediatrics, Turku University Hospital, Turku, Finland

YRJÖ QVARNBERG, M.D.

Chief, Otolaryngological Department, Central Hospital, Jyväskylä, Finland

GEROLD H. RACH, M.D.

Otolaryngologist, Willemstad, Curaçao, Netherlands Antilles

JORMA RAHNASTO, M.D.

Chief, Otolaryngological Department, Central Hospital, Vaasa, Finland

SIMO RÄISÄNEN, M.D., Ph.D.

Departments of Otolaryngology and Clinical Laboratory, Central Hospital of Keski-Pohjanmaa, Kokkola, Finland

ANDREW P. REID, F.R.C.S.(Edin)

Department of Otolaryngology, Children's Hospital, Birmingham, United Kingdom

ÅKE REIMER, M.D.

Assistant Professor, University of Lund; Staff, Department of Otolaryngology, Malmö General Hospital, Malmö, Sweden

CHARLES B. REIMER, M.D.

Chief of Immunochemistry, Division of Host Factors, Centers for Disease Control, Atlanta, Georgia

KEITH S. REISINGER, M.D.

Clinical Instructor, University of Pittsburgh School of Medicine, Pittsburgh, Pennsylvania

ULF E.J. RENVALL, M.D., Ph.D.

Honorary Associate Professor, Göteborg University; Chief Physician, ENT Department, Sahlgren's Hospital, Göteborg, Sweden

PETER RIGNÉR, M.D.

Attending Physician, ENT Outpatient Unit, Department of Otorhinolaryngology, University of Göteborg, Göteborg, Sweden

MARY LOU RIPLEY-PETZOLDT, B.A.

Junior Scientist, Department of Laboratory Medicine and Pathology, University of Minnesota Medical School, Minneapolis, Minnesota

ELLEN RISHIKOF, M.Sc.

Audiologist, Montreal Children's Hospital, Montreal, Quebec, Canada

JOHN B. ROBBINS, M.D.

Chief, Laboratory of Developmental and Molecular Immunity, National Institutes of Child Health and Human Development, National Institutes of Health, Bethesda, Maryland

JOANNE E. ROBERTS, Ph.D.

Clinical Assistant Professor of Speech and Hearing Sciences, University of North Carolina; Investigator, Frank Porter Graham Child Development Center, Chapel Hill, North Carolina

HOWARD E. ROCKETTE, Ph.D.

Professor of Biostatistics, Graduate School of Public Health, University of Pittsburgh School of Medicine; Director of Biostatistics, Otitis Media Research Center, Children's Hospital, Pittsburgh, Pennsylvania

TIMOTHY J. ROCKLEY, F.R.C.S.

Queen Elizabeth Hospital, Birmingham, United Kingdom

PETER ROLAND, M.D.

Assistant Professor, University of Texas Southwestern Medical School, Dallas, Texas

KRISTIAN P.L. ROOS, M.D., Ph.D.

Chief Physician, ENT Department, Sahlgren's Hospital, Göteborg, Sweden

BERNARD A. ROSNER, Ph.D.

Associate Professor of Preventive Medicine and Clinical Epidemiology (Biostatistics), Harvard Medical School; Statistician, Channing Laboratory, Boston, Massachusetts

ROBERT J. RUBEN, M.D.

Professor and Chairman, Department of Otolaryngology and Professor of Pediatrics, Albert Einstein College of Medicine and Montefiore Medical Center, Bronx, New York

JOYCE N. RUSS, R.N.

Staff Nurse, Park Nicollet Medical Center, St. Louis Park, Minnesota

OLLI RUUSKANEN, M.D.

Assistant Professor, Department of Pediatrics, Turku University Hospital, Turku, Finland

ALLEN F. RYAN, Ph.D.

Professor of Otolaryngology, University of California, San Diego, School of Medicine, La Jolla, California

BRITTA RYNNEL-DAGÖÖ, M.D., Ph.D.

Associate Professor, Karolinska Institute, Huddinge University Hospital, Huddinge, Sweden

JACOB SADÉ, M.D.

Professor, Department of Otolaryngology, Meir General Hospital, Kfar Saba, Israel

DEBORAH SADLER-KIMES, Ph.D.

Research Associate, Department of Anthropology, University of Pittsburgh, Pittsburgh, Pennsylvania

MAKOTO SAKAI, M.D., F.A.C.S

Department of Otolaryngology, Tokai University School of Medicine, Tokyo, Japan

KENJI SAKAKURA, M.D.

Assistant, Department of Otorhinolaryngology, Mie University School of Medicine, Mie, Japan

YASUO SAKAKURA, M.D.

Professor and Chairman, Department of Otorhinolaryngology, Mie University School of Medicine, Mie, Japan

ISAMU SANDO, M.D., D.M.S.

Professor of Otolaryngology and Pathology, University of Pittsburgh School of Medicine, Pittsburgh, Pennsylvania

CARMELO SARACENO, M.D.

Clinical Associate Professor, University of South Florida College of Medicine, Tampa, Florida

YUTAKA SASAKI, M.D.

Associate, Department of Otolaryngology, Tohoku University School of Medicine, Sendai, Japan

HIROAKI SATO, M.D.

Department of Otolaryngology, Faculty of Medicine, Kyoto University, Kyoto, Japan

PATRICIA A. SCHACHERN, B.S.

Scientist, Otopathology Laboratory, Department of Otolaryngology, University of Minnesota Medical School, Minneapolis, Minnesota

MELVIN D. SCHLOSS, M.D., F.R.C.S.(C)

Associate Professor of Otolaryngology, McGill University Faculty of Medicine; Director, Division of Otolaryngology, Montreal Children's Hospital, Montreal, Quebec, Canada

STEN-HERMANN SCHMIDT, M.D.

Department of Otorhinolaryngology–Head and Neck Surgery, Umeå University Hospital, Umeå, Sweden

RACHEL SCHNEERSON, M.D.

Medical Officer, Laboratory of Developmental and Molecular Immunity, National Institute of Child Health and Human Development, National Institutes of Health, Bethesda, Maryland

ELINOR SCHOENFELD, Ph.D.

Cancer Research Scientist II, Roswell Park Memorial Institute, Buffalo, New York

ALIX E. SEDERBERG-OLSEN, M.D.

Medical Assistant, ENT Clinic, Elsinore, Denmark

JØRGEN F. SEDERBERG-OLSEN, M.D.

Assistant Professor, University of Copenhagen, Copenhagen; Staff, ENT Clinic, Elsinore, Denmark

JACOB SEGAL, M.D., D.M.D.

Otolaryngologic Specialist, Department of Otolaryngology, Hillel-Jaffe Memorial Hospital, Hadera, Israel

ANNE E. SELTZ, M.A., CCC-A.

Director of Audiology, Park Nicollet Medical Center, St. Louis Park, Minnesota

LINDA L. SETTLE, M.D.

Resident Physician, Pediatrics, Emory University School of Medicine; Staff, Scottish Rite Children's Hospital, Atlanta, Georgia

PATRICIA SHARP, B.S.

Staff Research Associate, Division of Otolaryngology, University of California, San Diego, School of Medicine, La Jolla, California

SHARON SHELTON, B.S.

Clinical Microbiologist, Department of Pediatric Infectious Diseases, University of Texas Southwestern Medical Center, Dallas, Texas

AARON E. SHER, M.D.

Department of Otolaryngology, State University of New York Medical Center, Albany, New York

YOSHIHIRO SHIBAHARA, M.D., D.M.S.

Assistant Professor of Otolaryngology, Tohoku University School of Medicine, Sendai, Japan

MAMORU SHIBUYA, M.D.

Associate, Department of Otolaryngology, Tohoku University School of Medicine, Sendai, Japan

MARK J. SHIKOWITZ, M.D.

Assistant Professor of Otolaryngology, School of Medicine, Health Sciences Center, State University of New York at Stony Brook; Attending Surgeon, Department of Otolaryngology, Long Island Jewish Medical Center and Schneider Childrens Hospital, New Hyde Park, New York

TETSUYA SHIMA, M.D.

Department of Otolaryngology, Faculty of Medicine, Kagoshima University, Kagoshima, Japan

HIROYUKI SHIMIZU, M.D.

Associate Professor, Department of Public Health, Tokoku University School of Medicine, Sendai, Japan

HIDEICHI SHINKAWA, M.D.

Assistant Professor, Department of Otolaryngology, Tohoku University School of Medicine, Sendai, Japan

DAVID SHIPP, M.A.

Audiologist, Department of Communication Disorders, St. Boniface General Hospital, Winnipeg, Manitoba, Canada

ROBERT J. SHPRINTZEN, Ph.D.

Professor, Departments of Plastic Surgery and Otolaryngology, Montefiore Medical Center, Bronx, New York

ISAAC SHUBICH, M.D.

Professor of Otolaryngology, National University of Mexico; Head, Otolaryngology Department, Children's Hospital, Mexico City, Mexico

PAUL A. SHURIN, M.D.

Associate Director, Clinical Investigation, Medical Research Division, Lederle Laboratories, Pearl River, New York

GEORGE R. SIBER, M.D.

Associate Professor of Medicine, Harvard Medical School; Associate Physician, Dana-Farber Cancer Institute and Director, Biologic Laboratories, Massachusetts Department of Public Health, Boston, Massachusetts

EUGENE J. SIDOTI Jr., M.D.

Associate Clinical Professor of Pediatrics, Montefiore Medical Center, Bronx, New York

MICHAEL I. SIEGAL, Ph.D.

Professor of Physical Anthropology, Department of Anthropology, University of Pittsburgh, Pittsburgh, Pennsylvania

ANNE S. SIMPSON, M.B., Ch.B., D.Com.H., D.O., MCC.M.

Medical Superintendent, Middlemore Hospital, Auckland, New Zealand

MARKKU M. SIPILÄ, M.D.

Instructor in Otolaryngology, University of Tampere; Senior Otolaryngologist, Department of Otolaryngology, Tampere University Central Hospital, Tampere, Finland

PEKKA SIPILÄ, M.D.

Department of Otolaryngology, University of Oulu, Oulu, Finland

DAVID P. SKONER, M.D.

Assistant Professor of Pediatrics, University of Pittsburgh School of Medicine; Director of Laboratory Services, Division of Allergy and Immunology, Children's Hospital, Pittsburgh, Pennsylvania

LESLEY SMALLMAN, F.R.C.Path.

Department of Otolaryngology, Children's Hospital, Birmingham, United Kingdom

ROBERT SMITH, M.D.

Medical Fellow, Department of Otolaryngology, University of Minnesota Medical School, Minneapolis, Minnesota

OVE SÖDERBERG, M.D., Ph.D.

Department of Otorhinolaryngology, University of Umeå, Umeå, Sweden

MARK SOLFELT, M.D.

Postgraduate Level II Resident, Butterworth General Surgery Residency, Michigan State University College of Human Medicine, East Lansing, Michigan

CHRISTINA H. SØRENSEN, M.D.

Department of Otorhinolaryngology, University Clinic, Gentofte Hospital, Hellerup, Denmark

SIMON SORGER

Lab Technician, Montreal Children's Hospital, Montreal, Quebec, Canada

SVEN-ERIC STANGERUP, M.D.

ENT Department, Gentofte University Hospital, Hellerup, Denmark

JOHN STANIEVICH, M.D.

Associate Professor of Pediatrics and Otolaryngology, State University of New York, Buffalo, New York

DAVID R. STAPELLS, Ph.D.

Assistant Professor of Otorhinolaryngology and Neuroscience, Albert Einstein College of Medicine, Bronx, New York

SIDNEY STAROBIN, M.D.

Associate Clinical Professor of Pediatrics, Boston University School of Medicine, Boston; Attending Pediatrician, Framingham Union Hospital, Framingham, Massachusetts

LARS-ERIC STENFORS, M.D., Ph.D.

Department of Otolaryngology, Central Hospital of
Keski-Pohjanmaa, Kokkola, Finland

CECILIA STENSTRÖM, M.D.

Department of Otorhinolaryngology, Malmö General Hospital,
University of Lund, Malmö, Sweden

JANET S. STEPHENSON, B.S., R.M.

Supervisor, Department of Otolaryngology, Microbiology
Research Laboratory, Children's Hospital,
Pittsburgh, Pennsylvania

DAVID STEVENS, D.D.S.

Assistant Professor of Pediatrics, Albert Einstein
College of Medicine, Bronx, New York

IAN A. STEWART, M.B., Ch.B., F.R.C.S.(Edin)

Senior Lecturer, Otolaryngology–Head and Neck Surgery,
University of Otago; Head, Department of Otolaryngology–Head
and Neck Surgery, Dunedin Hospital, Dunedin, New Zealand

TORGNY STIGBRAND, M.D.

Departments of Anatomy and Physiological Chemistry,
University of Umeå, Umeå, Sweden

PETER STRINGHAM, M.D.

Staff Pediatrician, East Boston Neighborhood Health Center;
Assistant Visiting Physician, Boston City Hospital and Associate
Physician, Beth Israel Hospital, Boston, Massachusetts

MITSUKO SUETAKE, M.D.

Associate, Department of Otolaryngology, Tohoku University
School of Medicine, Sendai, Japan

FRANK SUNDLER, M.D., Ph.D.

Associate Professor, Department of Medical Cell Research,
University of Lund, Lund, Sweden

HIDEAKI SUZUKI, M.D.

Associate, Department of Otolaryngology, Tohoku University
School of Medicine, Sendai, Japan

MASASHI SUZUKI, M.D.

Postgraduate Student, Medical College of Oita; Staff,
Department of Otolaryngology, University Hospitals of the
Medical College of Oita, Oita, Japan

CATHARINA SVANBORG-EDEN, M.D., Ph.D.

Professor, Clinical Bacteriology, Department of Clinical
Immunology, University of Göteborg, Göteborg, Sweden

J. DOUGLAS SWARTS, B.S.

Laboratory Supervisor, Department of Otolaryngology,
Children's Hospital, Pittsburgh, Pennsylvania

SHOUSUN C. SZU, Ph.D.

Senior Staff Fellow, Laboratory of Developmental and
Molecular Immunity, National Institute of Child Health and
Human Development, National Institutes of Health,
Bethesda, Maryland

TOSHIHIDE TABATA, M.D.

Professor of Otorhinolaryngology, Wakayama Medical College,
Wakayama, Japan

TOMONORI TAKASAKA, M.D.

Professor and Chairman, Department of Otolaryngology, Tohoku
University School of Medicine, Sendai, Japan

MIKIKO TAKAYAMA, M.D.

Department of Otolaryngology, Tokyo Women's Medical
College, Tokyo, Japan

KAZUHIKO TAKEUCHI, M.D.

Assistant, Department of Otorhinolaryngology, Mie University
School of Medicine, Mie, Japan

BARBARA TALLAN, M.S.

Research Associate, Otologic Research Laboratories, Department
of Otolaryngology, Ohio State University College of Medicine,
Columbus, Ohio

MASAHITO TANKE, M.D.

Department of Otolaryngology, Kansai Medical University,
Osaka, Japan

LLOYD TARLIN, M.D.

Assistant Professor of Pediatrics, Boston University School of
Medicine, Boston; Attending Pediatrician, Framingham Union
Hospital, Framingham, Massachusetts

DAVID W. TEELE, M.D.

Professor of Pediatrics, Boston University School of Medicine;
Associate Visiting Physician in Pediatrics, Boston City Hospital,
Boston, Massachusetts

ANDERS TENGBLAD, Ph.D.

Department of Otorhinolaryngology, Central Hospital,
Falun, Sweden

JENS THOMSEN, M.D., Ph.D.

Associate Professor and Co-Chairman, ENT Department,
Gentofte University Hospital, Hellerup, Denmark

MATTI S. TIMONEN, M.D.

Head, Department of Pediatrics, Hyvinkää Regional Hospital,
Hyvinkää, Finland,

RUPERT TIMPL, Ph.D.

Max Planck Institute for Biochemistry, Munich, Germany

ANDERS TJELLSTRÖM, M.D., Ph.D.

Associate Professor, ENT Department, University of
Göteborg, Göteborg, Sweden

N. WENDELL TODD, M.D., F.A.C.S.

Assistant Professor of Surgery, Otolaryngology, Emory
University School of Medicine; Staff, Henrietta Egleston
Hospital for Children, Grady Memorial and Emory University
Hospitals, Atlanta, Georgia

JOHN S. TODHUNTER, Ph.D.

Research Assistant Professor, Electrical Engineering, University of Pittsburgh, Pittsburgh, Pennsylvania

KOICHI TOMODA, M.D., Ph.D.

Associate Professor, Department of Otolaryngology, Kansai Medical University, Osaka, Japan

KAZUHIRO TOMONAGA, M.D.

Department of Otolaryngology, Medical College of Oita, Oita, Japan

EDITH TONNAER, M.D.

Department of Otolaryngology, University of Nijmegen, Nijmegen, The Netherlands

MIRKO TOS, M.D.

Professor and Chairman, ENT Department, Gentofte University Hospital, University of Copenhagen, Hellerup, Denmark

F.W.M.M. TOUW-OTTEN, Ph.D.

Assistant Professor in Research in General Practice, University of Utrecht, Utrecht, The Netherlands

YUJI TOYAMA, M.D.

Department of Otolaryngology, Kansai Medical University, Osaka, Japan

AUSTIN TRINIDADE, M.B., Ch.B., F.R.C.S.(Edin)

Senior Registrar, Department of Otolaryngology, San Fernando General Hospital, Trinidad and Tobago, West Indies

HIROYUKI TSUJI, M.D.

Assistant, Department of Otolaryngology, Kansai Medical University, Osaka, Japan

HIROSHI TSURUMARU, M.D.

Department of Otolaryngology, Faculty of Medicine, Kagoshima University, Kagoshima, Japan

ABRAHAM TZADIK, M.D.

Assistant Professor, Division of Otolaryngology, University of Connecticut Health Center, Farmington, Connecticut

ROLF UDDMAN, M.D.

Associate Professor, University of Lund; Staff, Department of Otolaryngology, Malmö General Hospital, Malmö, Sweden

SHIGEHIRO UEYAMA, M.D.

Postgraduate Student, Medical College of Oita; Staff, Department of Otolaryngology, University Hospitals of the Medical College of Oita, Oita, Japan

KOTARO UKAI, M.D.

Associate Professor, Department of Otorhinolaryngology, Mie University School of Medicine, Mie, Japan

PAUL van CAUWENBERGE, M.D.

Senior Lecturer, State University; Senior Otolaryngologist, University Hospital, Ghent, Belgium

PAUL van den BROEK, M.D., Ph.D.

Professor of Otolaryngology and Chairman, Department of Otolaryngology, University of Nijmegen, Nijmegen, The Netherlands

LUCA VASSALLI, M.D.

Instructor, Department of Otolaryngology–Head and Neck Surgery, University of Illinois College of Medicine, Chicago, Illinois

RENÉ VEJLSGAARD, M.D.

Chairman, Department of Clinical Microbiology, Herlev University Hospital, Herlev, Denmark

BARBARA VIETMEIER, B.S.

Medical Technician, Otitis Media Research Center, Children's Hospital, Pittsburgh, Pennsylvania

MATTI K. VILJANEN, M.D.

Consulting Microbiologist, Department of Medical Microbiology, Turku University, Turku, Finland

BENJAMIN VOLOVITZ, M.D.

Associate Professor, Pediatric Department, Hasharon Hospital, Petah Tiqwa, Israel

DEWEY D. WALKER, M.D.

Assistant Clinical Professor, Department of Pediatrics, University of Colorado Health Sciences Center, Denver, Colorado

INA F. WALLACE, Ph.D.

Assistant Professor of Pediatrics and Psychiatry, Albert Einstein College of Medicine, Bronx, New York

NORITAKE WATANABE, M.D.

Department of Otolaryngology, Medical College of Oita, Oita, Japan

DARA WEGMAN, B.S.

Research Assistant in Pediatrics, Cleveland Metropolitan General Hospital, Cleveland, Ohio

ROBERT C. WELLIVER, M.D.

Professor of Pediatrics, State University of New York; Attending Pediatrician, Children's Hospital, Buffalo, New York

DANIEL WHITLEY Jr., M.D.

Division of Otolaryngology, Department of Surgery, Duke University Medical Center, Durham, North Carolina

GEORG G. WICK, M.D.

Professor, Institute for General and Experimental Pathology, University of Innsbruck, Innsbruck, Austria

LOUISE WIDEMAR, M.D., Ph.D.

Department of Audiology, Karolinslea Institute; Staff, Department of Audiology, Södersjukhuset, Stockholm, Sweden

EIZE WIELINGA, M.D.

Department of Otolaryngology, University of Nijmegen, Nijmegen, The Netherlands

MARK E. WILSON, Ph.D.

Assistant Professor of Oral Biology, State University of New York, Buffalo, New York

CHARLES G. WRIGHT, Ph.D.

Assistant Professor of Otorhinolaryngology, University of Texas Southwestern Medical School, Dallas, Texas

PETER F. WRIGHT, M.D.

Associate Professor of Pediatrics, Division of Infectious Diseases, Vanderbilt University School of Medicine, Nashville, Tennessee

FREDERICK P. WUCHER, M.D.

Assistant Clinical Professor, University of Pittsburgh School of Medicine, Pittsburgh, Pennsylvania

NOBUYA YAGI, M.D.

Associate Professor, Department of Otolaryngology, Faculty of Medicine, Kyoto University, Kyoto, Japan

TATSUJI YAMAGUCHI, M.D.

Department of Otorhinolaryngology, The Jikei University School of Medicine, Tokyo, Japan

TOSHIO YAMASHITA, M.D.

Associate Professor, Department of Otolaryngology, Kansai Medical University, Osaka, Japan

EITAN YANIV, M.D.

Sackler School of Medicine, Tel-Aviv, Israel

YI-HSIEN YEN, M.D.

Division of Otolaryngology, Shizuoka City Hospital, Shizuoka, Japan

SANG BIN YIM, M.D.

Department of Otolaryngology, Yonsei University College of Medicine, Seoul, Korea

RIITTA YLITALO, M.D.

Departments of Otolaryngology and Clinical Laboratory, Central Hospital of Keski-Pohjanmaa, Kokkola, Finland

TAE-HYUN YOON, M.D.

Research Fellow, Department of Otolaryngology, University of Minnesota Medical School, Minneapolis, Minnesota

NOBUO YOSHIE, M.D.

Professor, Department of Otolaryngology, Institute of Clinical Medicine, The University of Tsukuba, Tsukuba-Shi, Japan

HIROYUKI YOSHIMURA, M.D.

Department of Otolaryngology, Medical College of Oita, Oita, Japan

YI-HO YOUNG, M.D.

Department of Otolaryngology, National Taiwan University Hospital, Taipei, Taiwan

GERHARD A. ZIELHUIS, M.Sc., Ph.D.

Senior Lecturer in Epidemiology and Acting Director, Department of Epidemiology, University of Nijmegen, Nijmegen, The Netherlands

PREFACE

It is hard to believe that we have already had our fourth symposium. The first two meetings took place in 1975 and 1979 in Columbus, Ohio, while the third was held in 1983 in Fort Lauderdale, Florida. The first symposium came about as a result of a discussion between David Lim and Charley Bluestone in 1973 at the annual meeting of the American Otological Society. Although research on otitis media was in its infancy and limited primarily to clinical studies, there were a few of us engaged in basic scientific research into otitis media. Even among clinicians, there were otolaryngologists and pediatricians studying otitis media from quite different perspectives. The time seemed right for an international symposium on otitis media with effusion. We discussed the idea with Ben Senturia, who was skeptical at first because he felt a scientific symposium would not appeal to clinicians and would attract few attendees. We reviewed various strategies and concluded that although a clinical meeting would draw a larger crowd, a scientific meeting would be more valuable. Though the attendance might be small, we would have a true forum for researchers.

When European and Japanese investigators were asked whether they would be interested in such a meeting, key researchers responded enthusiastically. We invited 50 speakers to the first meeting and were comforted by the thought that at least 50 people would be present at the meeting. To our delight, the meeting was attended by 120 people. Although it was small, enthusiasm and excitement were in the air. The mixture of basic and clinical papers proved to be an excellent way to promote interaction among investigators from different disciplines.

At the end of the first symposium we were convinced that a second should be held. The goal again was to provide a forum for researchers, at which only new data would be presented and where all could freely exchange ideas. We apppointed the national advisors, who could alert us to new studies being conducted in their countries and recommend new investigators. Papers were accepted on the basis of the scientific merit of the abstracts submitted.

At the second symposium, 90 papers were presented and about 250 researchers were in attendance. For the third symposium, 11 state-of-knowledge papers, two panel discussions, 107 free papers, and 30 posters were presented. The fourth symposium was bigger and better than ever, with six special lectures, 158 paper presentations in two parallel sessions, and 51 poster presentations. There were a total of 93 presenters, with 300 attendees representing 22 countries. This continued success does not come by itself, but is due largely to the many faithful who have given unselfish support. Without their support, the symposia could not have grown as they have.

The proceedings of the first meeting were printed as a supplement to *Annals of Otology, Rhinology and Laryngology* (Suppl. 25, 299 pages), and 25,000 copies were distributed—5,000 to *Annals* subscribers and 20,000 as complimentary copies by Dow Pharmaceutical Company. The second proceedings were also published as an *Annals* supplement (Suppl. 68, 362 pages), and 20,000 complimentary copies were distributed by Eli Lilly and Company. The 371-page proceedings of the third symposium were published as a book by B.C. Decker Inc. Eli Lilly again distributed 20,000 complimentary copies in the United States. These proceedings became valuable references for researchers and clinicians alike.

We have held a research conference after each symposium. Because so many renowned researchers on otitis media were gathered, we decided to capitalize on the opportunity for them to discuss the current status of research and to recommend future directions. The first conference was funded by the Deafness Research Foundation and the next three by the National Institute of Neurological and Communicative Disorders and Stroke of the National Institutes of Health. For the third and fourth symposia, the National Institute of Allergy and Infectious Diseases was also a co-sponsor.

The conference reports have been published as supplements to *Annals* (Suppls. 26, 69, and 116) to promote world-wide dissemination.

The first extraordinary meeting of this symposium took place in Kyoto, Japan, in January 1985, under the direction of Professors Tadami Kumazawa and Kazutomo Kawamoto. The proceedings of this meeting were published as Suppl. 1 to *Auris Nasus Larynx* (Tokyo). Research interest among Japanese scientists was heightened by this meeting, evidenced by the increase in high-quality research papers from Japan presented at the fourth symposium. Another symposium on otitis media was organized in Jerusalem in November 1985, under the direction of Professor Jacob Sadé.

Co-chairman Charley Bluestone gets the major credit for obtaining support from the pharmaceutical industry. The other members of the program committee, Jerry Klein and John Nelson, spent many hours reviewing abstracts, soliciting support, and carrying out numerous chores related to the organization of this symposium. Although Ray Ogra and Scott Giebink were not program committee members, their advice was invaluable. We are also indebted to the program advisors who brought our attention to new areas of research and to young investigators throughout the world.

We are grateful to the Deafness Research Foundation for co-sponsoring this symposium, and in particular to Walter Petryshyn, Medical Director of the DRF, for his support. We are greatly indebted to the National Institute of Neurological and Communicative Disorders and Stroke for supporting the symposium research conference. We also acknowledge Beecham Laboratories, Eli Lilly, Glaxo Inc., Lederle International, Norwich Eaton Pharmaceuticals, Inc., and Ross Laboratories for their generous support of this meeting. Finally, we are grateful for the support of the following important people: David Schuller, Chairman of the Department of Otolaryngology at The Ohio State University; Jon Hollett, Director of the CCME and his staff; and particularly the dedicated staff of the Otological Research Laboratories at The Ohio State University, who helped with the many nuts and bolts of this symposium. Among those who deserve special mention are Thomas DeMaria, Lauren Bakaletz, Toni Hoepf, Barbara Tallan, Ilija Karanfilov, Katherine Adamson, Valerie Jones, Hyuk Soo Jang, Susan Girgis, Gene Fu, Jodie Marmon, Winnie Don, and Melanie Peoples. Thomas DeMaria and Lauren Bakaletz also provided valuable editorial support for this book. Ray Ogra, of the University of Rochester, also provided an invaluable contribution in reviewing many papers for the proceedings.

We are also grateful to Eli Lilly for supporting the publication of the proceedings of this meeting and to the editorial and production staff of B.C. Decker Inc who helped to put this book together.

May 12, 1988

David J. Lim, M.D.
Charles D. Bluestone, M.D.
Jerome O. Klein, M.D.
John D. Nelson, M.D.

CONTENTS

EPIDEMIOLOGY

SCREENING AND DIAGNOSIS

Eustachian Tube Function

Eustachian Tube Physiology

ANATOMY AND MORPHOLOGY

IMMUNOLOGY

PREVENTION AND MEDICAL MANAGEMENT

SURGICAL MANAGEMENT

PATHOGENESIS

MICROBIOLOGY

BIOCHEMISTRY

Sequelae

PATHOLOGY

ANIMAL MODELS

EPIDEMIOLOGY

RISK FACTORS FOR OTITIS MEDIA WITH EFFUSION

MASAKO ISHIDOYA, M.D., TOMONORI TAKASAKA, M.D., and HIROYUKI SHIMIZU, M.D.

Otitis media with effusion, one of the most common middle ear diseases among children, is characterized by middle ear effusion, impaired mobility of the eardrum, and conductive hearing loss. Despite language and learning problems caused by hearing loss due to otitis media with effusion and its sequelae,[1,2] the etiopathogeneses are not yet understood.

Although there have been many epidemiologic studies of the risk factors for otitis media with effusion, such as age, season, upper respiratory infection, and acute otitis media,[3,4] only a few have published, especially case control studies. We report here the risk factors for otitis media with effusion in Japanese elementary school children based on a strictly matched case control study.

MATERIALS AND METHODS

Tympanometric screening was performed in 7,040 children in the first, second, and third grades of 21 elementary schools in the suburbs of Sendai from January to March 1986. The children with type C_2 and B tympanograms were advised to have further otologic examinations by otolaryngologists, who sent us the results of their examinations and diagnoses. The examinations were performed within 2 months after the initial tympanometric screening at the schools.[5]

In July 1986 we sent the parents questionnaires concerning such factors as the children's care during infancy, history of infectious or allergic diseases, and exposure to swimming. One hundred fifty-four children were selected as case subjects from 220 children who were diagnosed as having otitis media with effusion by otolaryngologists. Then two classmates were selected as controls for each case, a total of 308 control children; they were matched by sex and age and confirmed to be free from otitis media.

The odds ratio, an estimated relative risk, was computed by the logistic regression method.[7]

RESULTS

Of the 14,080 ears in which tympanometric screening was performed, 451 (3.2 percent) and 311 (2.2 percent) showed type C_2 and B tympanographic findings, respectively. The distributions of the tympanogram types in boys and girls are given in Table 1. Although types C_2 and B were more common in boys than in girls, there were no significant differences statistically. The distribution of the tympanogram types in each grade is shown in Table 2. There were no significant differences among the grades, but abnormal tympanograms tended to decrease with increasing age.

Five hundred ninety-four children (8.4 percent) had abnormal tympanograms and were advised to

TABLE 1 Distribution of Tympanogram Types in 14,080 Ears in Boys and Girls

	A and C_1		C_2		B		Others*		Total	
	No.	%	No.	%	No.	%	No.	%	No.	%
Boys	6,857	93.7	267	3.6	173	2.4	19	0.3	7,316	100
Girls	6,434	95.1	184	2.7	138	2.1	8	0.1	6,764	100
Total	13,219	94.4	451	3.2	311	2.2	27	0.2	14,080	100

* Cases with perforation, ventilation tubes, and ear wax.

TABLE 2 Distribution of Tympanogram Types by School Grade

	Tympanogram Types										
	A and C_1		C_2		B		Others		Total	
	No.	%	No.	%	No.	%	No.	%	No.	%
1st grade	4,284	92.7	182	3.9	139	3.0	15	0.3	4,620	100
2nd grade	4,376	94.2	154	3.3	109	2.3	5	0.1	4,644	100
3rd grade	4,631	96.2	115	2.4	63	1.3	7	0.1	4,816	100
Total	13,391	94.4	451	3.2	311	2.2	27	0.2	14,080	100

undergo further otologic examination. Of these, 434 consulted ENT specialists, and 220 (3.1 percent) were diagnosed as having otitis media with effusion. The number of boys with abnormal tympanograms was 1.2 times that of girls (Table 3). Furthermore, the prevalence of otitis media in boys was 1.7 times greater than in girls. The percentages of the children with otitis media in the first, second, and third grades were 4.2, 2.8, and 2.4 percent, respectively. The prevalence follows the same trend as the proportion of abnormal tympanograms.

The results of our case control study of 154 pairs are presented in Table 4. The relative risk of chronic sinusitis was calculated to be 2.1, which was statistically significant ($p < 0.05$). The relative risk of tonsillar hypertrophy and adenoid vegetation was 2.9 ($p < 0.01$) and that of acute otitis media was 3.2 ($p < 0.01$). A history of more than two episodes of acute otitis media during the previous year remarkably increased the risk of otitis media with effusion. There were no significant differences in allergic manifestations, such as nasal allergy, bronchial asthma, and atopic dermatitis. Furthermore, we found no significant differences related to bottle feeding during infancy, repeated episodes of gastroenteritis and upper respiratory infection, exposure to pets or swimming, and the use of carpets in homes.

DISCUSSION

The proportions of type C_2 and B tympanograms in our study tended to decrease with increasing age. A higher percentage of abnormal tympanograms has been reported in preschool children than in our study.[2,6] Although the peak incidence of otitis media with effusion has been reported to occur between ages 5 and 7 years,[7] abnormal tympanograms were found frequently in younger children. Therefore further investigations are necessary to clarify the relationship between abnormal tympanograms and otitis media, especially in younger children. The incidence of children with abnormal tympanograms was 8.4 percent and that of otitis media was 3.1 percent. Nineteen percent of the boys and 39 percent of the girls with abnormal tympanograms had not undergone otologic examination. If all of them had consulted ENT specialists, the prevalence of otitis media might have been greater than 3.1 percent. In a study in Finland the prevalence of otitis media in 7 to 8 year old school children was 2.8 percent.[8]

We carefully matched our 154 cases with 308 controls and found that chronic sinusitis, hypertrophy of tonsils and adenoids, and acute otitis media were statistically significant risks for the development of otitis media. Many studies have reported that acute otitis media plays an important role in predisposing to otitis media.[4,5,9] We found that the children with otitis media with effusion had had frequent episodes of acute otitis media within the previous year. The episodes of acute otitis may have a close relationship to the occurrence of otitis media with effusion, and the latter may be one of the factors inducing acute otitis media. It is widely accepted that adenotonsillectomy alone has little impact on otitis media, but in our study hypertrophy of tonsils and adenoids increased the risk of otitis

TABLE 3 Children with Abnormal Tympanograms and Otitis Media with Effusion

	Children with Types C_2 and B		Children Undergoing Examinations	Children Diagnosed with Otitis Media		Total	
	No.	%	No.	No.	%	No.	%
Boys	339	9.3	276	142	3.9	3658	100
Girls	255	7.5	158	78	2.3	3382	100
Total	594	8.4	434	220	3.1	7040	100

TABLE 4   Factors Related to Otitis Media with Effusion

Factors	Relative Risk	Percentage in Control Group
Bottle feeding	0.9	76
Gastroenteritis	0.6	4
Upper respiratory infection	1.4	17
Chronic sinusitis	2.1*	10
Nasal allergy	1.4	14
Asthma	0.5	11
Atopic dermatitis	0.8	31
Hypertrophy of tonsils and adenoids	2.9[+]	7
Acute otitis media	3.2[+]	27
Number of episodes of acute otitis media during previous year		
0	1.0	82
1	3.9[+]	17
More than 2	11.5[+]	1
Exposure to pets	1.1	36
Exposure to swimming	1.0	23
Use of carpets in home	1.2	72

* $p < 0.05$.
[+] $p < 0.01$.

media nearly three times and may participate in the pathogenesis of otitis media in some way.

Although there have been various studies of the relationship between otitis media and allergy, no significant differences were found in our study. Further studies along this line are required. Recently the number of the children who go to swimming school has increased in our region, and some are concerned about the effect of swimming on otitis media and other diseases. The relative risk of exposure in swimming schools was not high in this study, but it is possible that some children diagnosed as having otitis media had stopped swimming before the questionnaires were sent out 4 months after the tympanometric screenings.

REFERENCES

1. Menyuk P. Effect of persistent otitis media on language development. Ann Otol Rhinol Laryngol 1980; 89(Suppl 69):257.
2. Tos M, et al. Spontaneous course of secretory otitis and change of the ear drum. Arch Otolaryngol 1984; 110:281–289.
3. Draper WL. Secretory otitis media in children: a study of 540 children. Laryngoscope 1967; 77:636–653.
4. Schutte PK, et al. Secretory otitis media—a retrospective general practice survey. J Laryngol Otol 1981; 95:17–22.
5. Breslow NE, et al. Statistical methods in cancer research. Lyon: International Agency for Research on Cancer, 1980.
6. Tos M, et al. Tympanometry in 2 year old children. ORL 1978; 40:77–85.
7. Kokko E. Chronic secretory otitis media in children. Acta Otolaryngol (Suppl) 1975; 327:1–47.
8. Virolainen E, et al. Prevalence of secretory otitis media in seven to eight year old school children. Ann Otol Rhinol Laryngol 1980; 89 (Suppl 68):7–10.
9. Kraemer MJ, et al. Risk factors for persistent middle-ear effusions. JAMA 1983; 249:1022–1025.

RISK FACTORS FOR PERSISTING OTITIS MEDIA WITH EFFUSION IN CHILDREN

PAOLA MARCHISIO, M.D., LUCIA BIGALLI, M.D., EMILIA MASSIRONI, M.D., and NICOLA PRINCIPI, M.D.

Acute otitis media is one of the most common problems in infants and children.[1] In most of the cases acute symptoms resolve in a short time, usually with the help of antimicrobial drugs, but effusion may persist for a long time in the middle ear cavity. Many authors in recent years have associated persistence of effusion with hearing loss and with possible language, behavioral, and learning deficits.[2,3]

The aim in our study was to evaluate factors predisposing to the development of chronic otitis media with effusion after an acute episode of middle ear infection in a population of urban children in Italy.

MATERIALS AND METHODS

The patient material consisted of 196 children, aged 5 months to 12 years, selected consecutively, who visited the Pediatric Department of the University of Milan because of acute otitis media. The diagnosis of acute otitis media was based on clinical data (fever or earache or both), pneumatic otoscopic findings (hyperemia, opacity accompanied by immobility, and fullness or bulging of the tympanic membrane), and tympanometric findings (a flat type B curve). All children were treated with a 10 day course of amoxicillin (50 mg per kg per day in three divided doses). Clinical, otoscopic, and tympanometric findings were evaluated at midtreatment and at days 15, 30, 60, and 90 after the acute episode in all children. No other treatment was given during the follow-up period.

Chronic otitis media with effusion was defined as the unilateral or bilateral persistence of effusion demonstrated by pneumatic otoscopy (an abnormal appearance of the tympanic membrane—immobile, opaque, or with the presence of air-fluid levels) and tympanometry (type B curve) for at least 12 weeks after the acute episode.

The children were divided into two groups: one with chronic otitis media with effusion and one in which the effusion cleared up (nonchronic effusion). Epidemiologic data were obtained by means of a questionnaire filled out by the parents of all the children. Statistical differences between the groups were evaluated by the chi square test in regard to several factors: duration of acute otitis, sex, age at the first episode of acute otitis, history of acute otitis media, season of onset of the acute episode, day care attendance, parental smoking, birth order, family history of middle ear disease, and atopic disease.

RESULTS

One hundred ninety-six children were enrolled in the study: 24 were excluded from final analysis (13 in the chronic group and 11 in the nonchronic one) because of recurrent acute otitis media during the follow-up period. Thus 172 children were finally analyzed. Ninety-six (55.8 percent) were boys. The mean age was 41.7 months (range, 5 to 146 months). Eighty-one children (47.1 percent) were considered to have chronic otitis media with effusion.

No significant correlation was found between the occurrence of chronic effusion and sex, birth order, family history of middle ear disease, number of previous episodes of acute otitis media, atopic disease, parental smoking, day care attendance, and history of recurrent upper respiratory tract infections.

In regard to the age at the time of the acute episode of acute otitis media, we found that children with chronic effusion were significantly younger than those in whom the effusion cleared up. The mean age in the chronic group was 25.4 months, compared with 47.3 months in the nonchronic group ($p < 0.05$). Moreover, we found that the younger the child, the greater the possibility of developing chronic effusion. Seventy-seven percent of the children younger than 1 year of age had chronic effusion after the acute episode, compared with 53.8 percent of those aged 1 to 3 years and 36.7 percent of those older than 3 years ($p < 0.05$).

Home crowding, defined as the ratio between the number of persons living in an apartment and the number of rooms in the apartment, was significantly correlated with chronic effusion: only 24.7 percent of the children with chronic otitis media lived in an ideal situation (that is, less than or one person per room), whereas 45.7 percent lived in very

TABLE 1   Home Crowding and Development of Chronic Otitis Media with Effusion

Person Per Room	All Ages*		<3 Years+	
	Chronic Otitis Media (N=81)	Nonchronic Otitis Media (N=91)	Chronic Otitis Media (N=45)	Nonchronic Otitis Media (N=29)
≤1	24.7	36.2	22.2	24.1
1–2	29.6	39.6	35.5	44.8
≥2	45.7	24.6	42.3	31.1

* $p < 0.05$.
+ $p > 0.05$.

TABLE 2   Season of Onset of Acute Otitis Media and Development of Chronic Otitis Media with Effusion

| Season | All Ages* | | <3 Years[+] | |
	Chronic Otitis Media (N=81)	Nonchronic Otitis Media (N=91)	Chronic Otitis Media (N=45)	Nonchronic Otitis Media (N=29)
Winter	39.5	32.9	33.3	34.5
Spring	28.4	45.0	24.4	37.9
Summer	3.7	5.6	6.7	3.5
Autumn	28.4	16.5	35.6	24.1

* $p < 0.05$.
[+] $p > 0.05$.

crowded apartments. The difference between the incidences of chronic and nonchronic effusion at different stages of home crowding is statistically significant. However, when we consider the children younger than 3 years of age as a separate group, we observe that even if the upward trend is still present, the difference between the two groups is no longer statistically significant (Table 1).

Likewise, the occurrence of acute otitis media in winter (that is, from December to February) and in autumn (September to November) leads to significantly more persisting effusions compared with spring and summer, but only when the overall study population is evaluated; in children younger than 3 years the difference is no longer significant. In fact, in every season the majority of younger children tend to develop chronic effusion (Table 2).

DISCUSSION

The roles of various factors in determining the persistence of effusion are still controversial. Many authors have stressed the importance of sex, age, season, parental smoking, living conditions, atopic disease, and a history of acute otitis media, whereas others have found contrary data.[4-6] However, most of those studies have dealt with children with secretory otitis media without any strict correlation with a recent acute infectious episode and with patients older than 2 years of age.

In our population, that is, an urban population, in a very crowded and polluted area, age is the most important single factor predisposing to chronic persistence of effusion after an acute episode of otitis media. What seems more important to us is the fact that, in young children, no other single factor was significantly associated with the development of

chronic effusion after acute otitis media. It appears that young children in some way have an "intrinsic" tendency to develop chronic effusion. Other factors, such as home crowding, may exert an influence only where they persist for years in the life of the child.

Our data suggest that a program of prevention of risk factors should consider the characteristics of the population that would benefit from it. At least in Italy, no specific effort to reduce the frequency of risk factors for chronic effusion reported by other authors would be of any value in children younger than 3 years of age. Instead our efforts should be directed to prevent the acute episode if possible.

REFERENCES

1. Paradise JL. Otitis media in infants and children. Pediatrics 1980; 65:917–943.
2. Teele DW, et al. Otitis media with effusion during the first three years of life and development of speech and language. Pediatrics 1984; 74:282–287.
3. Paradise JL. Long term effects of short-term hearing loss: menace or myth? In: Bluestone CD, Klein JO, Paradise JL. Workshop on the effects of otitis media on the child. Pediatrics 1983; 72:647–648.
4. Kraemer MJ, Richardson MA, Weiss NS, Furukawa CT, Shapiro GG, Pierson WE, Bierman W. Risk factors for persistent middle-ear effusions. JAMA 1983; 249:1022–1025.
5. Stewart IA, Kirkland C, Simpson A, Silva P, Williams S. Some developmental characteristics associated with otitis media with effusion. In: Lim DJ, Bluestone CD, Klein JO, Nelson JD, eds. Recent advances in otitis media with effusion. Proceedings of the Third International Symposium. Toronto: BC Decker, 1984:25–27.
6. van Cauwenberge PB. Relevant and irrelevant predisposing factors in secretory otitis media. Acta Otolaryngol (Stockh) 1984; 414 Suppl:147–153.

INCIDENCE AND RISK FACTORS OF ACUTE OTITIS MEDIA IN CHILDREN: LONGITUDINAL COHORT STUDIES IN AN URBAN POPULATION

LEIF INGVARSSON, M.D., Ph.D., KAJ LUNDGREN, M.D., Ph.D., and BERTIL OLOFSSON, M.D., Ph.D.

Acute otitis media is one of the most common complications of upper respiratory tract infections in preschool children, and so far there is no sign that the quantitative importance of middle ear disease is diminishing. Children with repeated episodes of acute otitis media pose special medical and socioeconomic problems.

Interest in epidemiologic studies of acute otitis media in children has been increasing in recent years among otolaryngologists and pediatricians.[1-4] Different prospective epidemiologic studies have added greatly to our understanding of the incidence and risk factors of acute otitis media in children. Studies in Sweden, Finland, and the United States have confirmed earlier studies indicating that the highest incidence of otitis media is in children less than 2 years of age.[5-7]

The city of Malmö, Sweden, offers unique conditions for epidemiologic studies with a well defined population in a restricted geographic area. From 1977 to 1986 we conducted a prospective epidemiologic study of the occurrence of acute otitis media among the children born and living in the city. The aim in this article is to present some results from the 10 year investigation of the incidence and risk factors associated with acute otitis media among the children in Malmö.

METHOD AND MATERIAL

Since 1977 all cases of acute otitis media (reddened bulging eardrum with or without spontaneous perforation and otorrhea) among children living in Malmö have been registered. That is, all children born in 1977 or later and diagnosed as having acute otitis media by a doctor in the city are registered. The patient's birth date and the date and place of diagnosis are obtained from official computerized data files containing information about the patient's dwelling in the city, the type of housing, and the type of day care at the time of diagnosis.

The investigation began in 1977 and continued for 10 years, that is, until 1986. Preliminary results from the cohort studies were published earlier.[5, 8-10] This presentation includes results from the completed investigation (1977–1986), and in these years 25,206 children were diagnosed, a total of 34,197 episodes of acute otitis media. Five hundred to 600 episodes diagnosed from October to December 1986 have not yet been computerized and are thus not included in this presentation.

RESULTS

Incidence

The annual incidence was highest for children aged 1 year, and boys had the highest incidence—45 episodes of acute otitis media per 100 at risk compared to 38 per 100 at risk in girls. Fifty-four percent of all episodes were diagnosed in boys. The difference in incidence between boys and girls was more pronounced among children who had six or more episodes of acute otitis media before the age of 2 years. In this group of "otitis prone" children, 61 percent were boys and 39 percent were girls.

Seasonal Variations

Seasonal and annual variations in incidence were registered during the 10 years. In 1977, 1978, and 1980 the highest figures were found in December, whereas most episodes were registered during the first three to four months of the year in some years (1983 and 1984). Viral disease epidemi (for instance, epidemics of influenza) or weather variations from one year to another are possible causes for these variations.

Cumulative Incidence

At 3 years of age among the boys and at 3 years and 7 months among the girls, 50 percent of the children born in Malmö had been diagnosed as having had at least one episode of acute otitis media; this is illustrated in Figure 1. At the age of 7 years

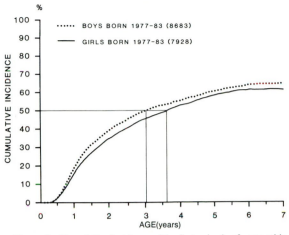

Figure 1 Cumulative incidence of the first episode of acute otitis media in relation to sex.

65 to 70 percent of all the children had had at least one episode. The cumulative incidence values for the first episode of acute otitis media differs among children living in different districts of Malmö and in different types of housing in the districts. However, this does not mean that otitis prone children are more frequently found in districts with the highest cumulative incidence values.

Type of Day Care and Occurrence of Acute Otitis Media

In Sweden, preschool children are cared for at home or in other private or public day care centers or in family day care homes. The relationship be-

tween these 3 main types of care has changed drastically during the 1980s so that an increasing number of children, especially the youngest (less than 3 years of age), are cared for in public day care centers. This development is directed by the present Swedish government.

Our investigations have shown that children entering public day care centers very early in life (before the age of 3 years) are subject to significantly more episodes of acute otitis media than those cared for at home during the first 4 years of life. The investigation from 1980 to 1985 also showed than an increasing number of all registered episodes of acute otitis media were diagnosed in the youngest age groups; this is illustrated in Figure 2. In 1980 to 1981, 39 percent of all registered episodes were diagnosed in children less than 2 years of age, and 13 percent were diagnosed in children 6 to 7 years of age. Corresponding figures in 1984–1985 were 44 percent in children less than 2 years and 8 percent in those between 6 and 7 years of age.

Age at the First Episode of Acute Otitis Media

Children suffering from the first episode of acute otitis media very early in life have a greater risk of becoming "otitis prone." In our study 2978 children were followed during their first 4 years of life. Among 1055 children in whom the first episode of acute otitis media occurred before the age of 1 year, 130 (12 percent) were diagnosed as having had at least six episodes before the age of 4 years. Corresponding figures for children aged 1 year and

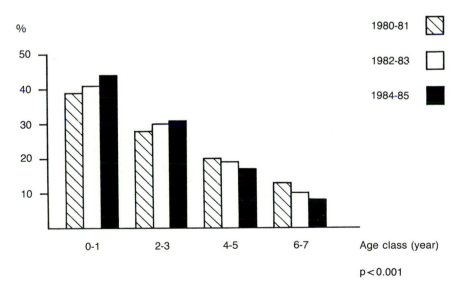

Figure 2 Relation of diagnosed episodes of acute otitis media to age classes.

2 years or more before the first episode was diagnosed were 35 (4 percent) and 5 (0.5 percent) respectively.

CONCLUSIONS

Sixty-five to 70 percent of all preschool children (less than 7 years of age) have at least one episode of acute otitis media. The highest incidence in our study was found in 1 year old boys. At the age of 3 years about 50 percent of all children in Malmö are diagnosed as having had at least one episode. An early occurrence increases the risk of becoming otitis prone, and boys have a greater risk than girls of becoming otitis prone.

Seasonal variations in incidence are generally very consistent from one year to another. However, differences are registered, and they may be influenced by outbreaks of viral illness epidemics, such as influenza, or weather variations between different years.

The cumulative incidence differs in children living in different districts and different types of housing in the city. These variations could not be explained by differences in the type of day care provided for the children in these districts.

Day care in large groups—mostly in public day care centers during the first years of life (less than 3 years of age)—seems to be one of the most important reasons that children get upper respiratory tract infections and, as a complication of these viral infections, also acute bacterial infections like acute otitis media. Children attending public day care centers early in life are also more apt to have recurrent episodes of the disease than those cared for at home or in private care centers.

Four to 5 percent of all children in Malmö can be regarded as being otitis prone. Since these children need the most effort and help both medically and socially, our main interest has been focused on studies of these children in recent years.

These studies were supported by grants from the Swedish Medical Research Council (B 86-27X-6279-05A and B 86-27P-6741-03).

REFERENCES

1. Kudrjavcev T, Schoenberg BS. Otitis media and developmental disability. Epidemiologic considerations. Ann Otol Rhinol Laryngol 1979; Suppl 60:88-98.
2. Hinchcliffe R. Epidemiological aspects of otitis media. In: Glorig A, Gervin K, eds. Otitis media. Proceedings of the national conference. Springfield, Illinois: Charles C Thomas, 1972: 36-43.
3. Teele DW, Klein JO, Rosner BA. Epidemiology of otitis media in children. Ann Otol Rhinol Laryngol 1980; 89 (Suppl 68):5-7.
4. Giebink GS. Epidemiology and natural history of otitis media. In: Lim DJ, Bluestone CD, Klein JO, Nelson JD, eds. Recent advances in otitis media with effusion. Proceedings of the Third International Symposium. Toronto: BC Decker, 1984: 5-9.
5. Ingvarsson L, Lundgren K, Olofsson B, Wall S. Epidemiology of acute otitis media. Acta Otolaryngol 1982; 388 Suppl:3-52.
6. Pukander H, Sipilä M, Karma P. Occurrence of and risk factors in acute otitis media. In: Lim DJ, Bluestone CD, Klein JO, Nelson JD, eds. Recent advances in otitis media with effusion. Proceedings of the Third International Symposium. Toronto: BC Decker, 1984: 9-13.
7. Teele DW, et al. Middle ear disease and the practice of pediatrics. JAMA 1983; 249:1026-1029.
8. Ingvarsson L, Lundgren K, Olofsson B. Epidemiology of acute otitis media in children—a cohort study in an urban population. In: Lim DJ, Bluestone CD, Klein JO, Nelson JD, eds. Recent advances in otitis media with effusion. Proceedings of the Third International Symposium. Toronto: BC Decker, 1984: 19-22.
9. Lundgren K, Ingvarsson L, Olofsson B. Epidemiologic aspects in children with recurrent acute otitis media. In: Lim DJ, Bluestone CD, Klein JO, Nelson JD, eds. Recent advances in otitis media with effusion. Proceedings of the Third International Symposium. Toronto: BC Decker, 1984: 22-25.
10. Ingvarsson L, Lundgren K, Stenström C, Olofsson B, Wall S. The epidemiology of acute otitis media. In: Sadé J, ed. Acute and secretory otitis media. Amsterdam: Kugler Publications, 1986: 125-128.

PERSISTENCE OF MIDDLE EAR EFFUSION AND ITS RISK FACTORS AFTER AN ACUTE ATTACK OF OTITIS MEDIA WITH EFFUSION

JUHANI S. PUKANDER, M.D. and PEKKA H. KARMA, M.D.

Middle ear diseases are becoming increasingly important health problems among pediatric populations. Although their acute seriousness has dramatically decreased during recent decades, prolonged effusion inside the middle ear is regarded as an increasingly frequent disorder in association with an acute attack of otitis media with effusion (AOME).[1,2] This effusion may impair the child's hearing at an age critical for the acquisition of linguistic skills, leading to disturbances in language development.[3] The aim of this work was to study the occurrence of middle ear effusions after acute otitis media and to evaluate the risk factors affecting the persistence of middle ear effusions for 2 months or longer.

MATERIAL AND METHODS

The study population consisted of 753 children with acute otitis media with effusion in three Finnish urban areas. The mean age of the children was 11.6 months (range, 7 to 29 months); 53.5 percent were boys. Attacks of acute otitis media with effusion were diagnosed in every case by definite criteria, including at least one of the following acute symptoms: fever, otalgia, irritability, tugging or rubbing of ears, or the simultaneous pressure of other respiratory infection or gastrointestinal symptoms, as well as evidence of middle ear effusion determined by pneumatic otoscopy or acute otorrhea not caused by external otitis. The otoscopic evidence of middle ear effusion was confirmed in 94.6 percent of the acute cases by myringotomy. In addition to aspiration of the middle ear effusions, all acute attacks were treated with antibiotics, primarily penicillin V, 25 to 35 mg per kilogram twice daily for 10 days. After the first visit all the children were followed mainly by the same physician at 2 to 3 week intervals until the ear(s) was healthy and free of effusion. Also during these follow-up visits, myringotomy and aspiration were performed if an effusion was suspected. Epidemiologic data for the risk analyses were collected by repeated questionnaires filled out by the parents of the children.

Statistical risk analyses were calculated using the chi square test, the t test, and the correlation coefficient.

RESULTS

The resolution of the middle ear effusion was very rapid during the first weeks of follow-up (Fig. 1). At the first 2 week follow-up visit, 55.8 percent of the children were free of effusion. Effusions were present only at 4 and 8 weeks in 21.1 and 7.4 percent.

Girls recovered significantly ($p < 0.05$) more quickly than boys, the mean duration of the effusion being 13.4 days among girls and 18.0 days among boys ($p < 0.001$). The seasonal factor affected strikingly the persistence of the effusion. The risk of a prolonged effusion (≥ 2 months) was greater ($p < 0.025$) if acute otitis media was contracted during the winter (December through March) compared to attacks encountered in the summer (May through August; Fig. 2).

Atopic allergy was found to predispose the child ($p < 0.001$) to a prolonged duration of middle ear effusion (Table 1), whereas atopy of the parent(s) did not affect this risk. Other significant risk indicators were the history of previous otitis attack(s) ($p < 0.01$) and attending day care centers ($p < 0.05$; Table 2). A negative correlation ($p < 0.05$) was found between the duration of breast feeding and the duration of the effusion. On the other hand, smoking habits of the parent(s), night-time bottles, the type of housing, or the place of residence did not affect the risk of prolonged effusion formation.

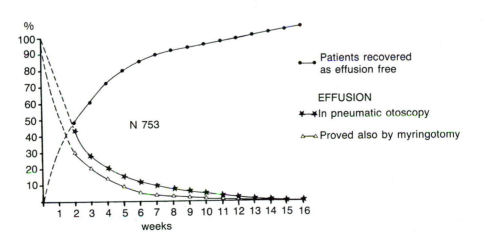

Figure 1   Recovery rate in children and persistence of effusion in the ear(s) judged by pneumatic otoscopy and by myringotomy.

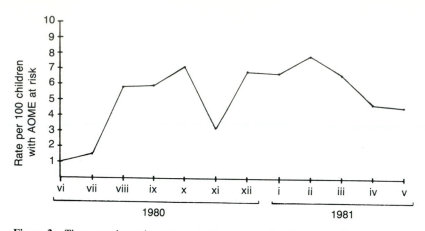

Figure 2   Three month moving average incidence rate of prolongation of effusion over 2 months among children with acute otitis media with effusion, by season.

DISCUSSION

The clinical behavior and treatment of acute otitis media have changed considerably from that of earlier decades. For example, in the 1950s as many as 40 percent of the attacks of acute otitis media were expressed as spontaneous perforation and discharge.[4] Myringotomy was carried out more often than nowadays.[5] At the moment the long lasting nonsymptomatic middle ear effusion is becoming the main sequela of acute otitis media among children. Increasing numbers of children spend more of their infant life with middle ear effusion.[2] Although the significance of this disturbance is still not fully comprehended and many factors may affect the impact of otitis media on language development,[6] there is also evidence that impaired hearing due to middle ear effusions is associated with inferior verbal ability in a child.[3]

The present study is one of the very few in recent years in which myringotomy and aspiration were almost always performed when effusion was suspected in the middle ear. The active drainage of the middle ear may be the reason for more rapid clearance of effusions in this study than in studies

in which children were treated only with antibiotics.[7]

The risk indicators affecting the occurrence of acute otitis media are well known.[8,9] These factors also seem often to predispose to the prolongation of effusion after acute otitis media with effusion.

Boys are know to be more susceptible than girls to many infectious diseases, otitis media included.[10,11] The male predominance in some reports is striking.[1,12] In the present study the persistence of middle ear effusions after acute otitis media was also significantly longer among boys than among girls.

Opinions regarding the role of atopic allergy in otitis media are contradictory. Some reports oppose the view that allergy plays a role in the pathogenesis of otitis media with effusion.[7,12] However, in the present study, consistent with some other reports,[1] a positive correlation was found between allergy and persistent middle ear effusion. However, we could not confirm the predisposing role of a positive family history of allergy.

Environmental factors enhancing the spread of respiratory viruses seem to be of some importance.[13] Prolongation of effusion was found to be more prevalent during the winter months when viral

TABLE 1   Atopy of the Child and Prolongation of Effusion

	Persistence of Effusion			
	<2 Months		≥2 Months	
Atopic Manifestations	N	(%)	N	(%)
No	642	(90.8)	30	(65.2)
Yes	65	(9.2)	16	(34.8)
$X^2 = 29.459$, DF = 1, p = <0.001				

TABLE 2   Day Care and Prolongation of Effusion

	Persistence of Effusion			
	<2 Months		≥2 Months	
Attending Day Care at Time of Acute Otitis Media with Effusion	N	(%)	N	(%)
No	536	(83.9)	24	(70.6)
Yes	103	(16.1)	10	(29.4)
$X^2 = 4.08$, DF = 1, p = 0.043				

respiratory diseases are also more common. People also spend more time indoors in winter, which creates favorable conditions for respiratory diseases to spread. These facts especially apply to children attending day care centers, who accordingly, in the present study, suffered more often from persistent middle ear effusions than home cared children, an observation also made previously.[16] On the other hand, the impact of day care was not so prominent in this study as it was in our respective findings concerning acute otitis media.[8] One explanation for this might be that the children in the present study were reasonably young (mean age, 11.6 months) and thus their attendance at day care centers was remarkably shorter in duration.

Prolonged breast feeding may cover the transient immunoglobulin gap of an infant during the first year of life,[14] thus preventing the baby from contracting acute otitis media as well as persistence of middle ear effusion during this period with a relative immunoglobulin deficiency. Accordingly an almost significant negative correlation between the duration of breast feeding and the duration of middle ear effusions was found in our study.

In one of our earlier reports tobacco smoking by parent(s) was a significant risk factor in acute otitis media.[8] When we analyzed acute attacks in the children in the present study, the mother's smoking increased the risk of acute otitis media in the child.[15] However, smoking did not have an effect on the prolongation of otitis media in these children. Thus it seems that a parent's smoking may predispose to acute otitis media, but it is no longer a cause of prolongation of the disease.

This study showed that the epidemiologic risk factors affecting the prolongation of effusion in the middle ear(s) are mainly the same as those that also predispose a child to acute otitis media. Thus, the same health educational and environmental factors should be taken into consideration when attempting to prevent this increasingly frequent condition from impairing hearing among young children.

REFERENCES

1. Draper WL. Secretory otitis media in children: a study of 540 children. Laryngoscope 1967; 77:636–653.
2. Bluestone CD, Klein JO. Otitis media with effusion atelectasis and eustachian tube dysfunction. In: Bluestone CD, Stool SE, eds. Pediatr Otolaryngol 1983; 1:356–364.
3. Klein JO. Otitis media with effusion and development of speech and language. In: Bluestone CD, Doyle WJ, eds. Eustachian tube function: physiology and role in otitis media. Workshop report. Ann Otol Rhinol Laryngol 1985; 95 (Suppl 120):53–54.
4. Medical Research Council's working-party for research in general practice. Acute otitis media in general practice. Lancet 1957; ii:510–514.
5. Heller G. A statistical study of otitis media in children. J Pediatr 1940; 17:322–330.
6. Hall DM, Hill P. When does secretory otitis media affect language development? Arch Dis Child 1986; 61:42–47.
7. Barritt PW, Darbyshire PJ. Deafness after otitis media in general practice. J Roy Coll Gen Pract 1984; 34:92–94.
8. Pukander J, Luotonen J, Timonen M, Karma P. Risk factors affecting the occurrence of acute otitis media among 23-year-old urban children. Acta Otolaryngol (Stockh) 1985; 100:119–123.
9. Strangert K. Otitis media in young children in different types of daycare. Scand J Infect Dis 1977; 9:119–123.
10. Perrin JM, Charney E, MacWitney JB Jr, McInery TK, Miller RL, Nazarian LF. Sulfisoxazole as chemoprophylaxis for recurrent otitis media. A doubleblind crossover study in pediatric practice. N Engl J Med 1974; 291:664–667.
11. Ingvarsson L. Acute otitis media in children. Studies on epidemiology, diagnosis and treatment. Malmö: University of Lund, Sweden 1982 (dissertation).
12. Habib MA. Non-suppurative otitis media in children. A retrospective study of 100 cases. J Laryngol 1979; 93:129–133.
13. Hinchcliffe R. Epidemiology and otolaryngology. In: Hinchcliffe R, Harrison D, eds. Scientific foundations of otolaryngology. London: William Heinemann, 1976:133–138.
14. Saarinen UM. Prolonged breast feeding as prophylaxis for recurrent otitis media. Acta Paediatr Scand 1982; 71:567–71.
15. Sipilä M, Pukander J, Kataja M, Timonen M, Karma P. The Bayesian approach to the evaluation of risk factors in acute and recurrent acute otitis media. Acta Otolaryngol Stockh 1988 (in press.)
16. Fiellau-Nikolajsen M. Tympanometry in 3-year old children. Type of care as an epidemiologic factor in secretory otitis media and tubal dysfunction in unselected populations of 3-year-old children. ORL 1979; 41:193–205.

GENERAL ILLNESS AMONG OTITIS PRONE AND ORDINARY CHILDREN

CECILIA STENSTRÖM, M.D. and LEIF INGVARSSON, M.D., Ph.D.

Recurrent episodes of acute otitis media are common in preschool children. Children with recurrent episodes of acute otitis media also seem to be more susceptible to secretory otitis media. The question whether otitis prone children are generally more susceptible to other infections and diseases has not yet been studied systematically and remains to be answered. Our aim in this investigation was to study the number of cases of middle ear disease and other types of infections and diseases in a group of otitis prone children and a control group.

MATERIAL AND METHODS

In the city of Malmö, Sweden, all cases of acute otitis media in children diagnosed by a doctor have been recorded since 1977. This study of the incidence of acute otitis media includes all children born in 1977 or later and living in Malmö.[1-3] From this registry, 252 children born between 1977 and 1981 had been recorded as having had six or more episodes of acute otitis media and were defined as being otitis prone. Two hundred fifty-two children randomly chosen from the population in Malmö and matched for age and sex with the otitis prone children constituted the control group. The study period extended from 1977 to 1983. The oldest children were thus followed for 6 to 7 years and the youngest for 2 to 3 years. Sixty-one percent were boys and 39 percent girls.

The medical records from the ENT and pediatric departments were studied for all the 504 children. In Malmö about 75 percent of all medical care to children is provided in the ENT and pediatric departments. Visits to general practitioners and private ENT or pediatric physicians were not included in this study.

RESULTS

For all parameters studied there were no differences between boys and girls, and thus the results are not separated according to sex in this presentation.

The numbers of ambulatory visits and hospital admittances to the ENT and pediatric departments

are illustrated in Table 1. In otitis prone children there was a total of 39 visits per child to both departments compared with nine visits per child in the control group. Sixty-four percent of the visits took place before the age of 3 years. The otitis prone children had been admitted three times more often than the control group to the ENT department and twice as often to the pediatric department.

The total number of diagnosed episodes of acute otitis media in the ENT and pediatric departments were recorded. In the control group, 112 (44 percent) had never been diagnosed for acute otitis media and 95 (38 percent) had one to two episodes. In the otitis prone group, 170 (68 percent) were recorded as having had six to 11 episodes; 46 (18 percent) had 12 or more episodes.

Diagnosed episodes of secretory otitis media were recorded from the medical records in the ENT department. In the control group, 154 (61 percent) had never been diagnosed for secretory otitis media, and 81 (32 percent) had had one to two episodes. In the otitis prone group 96 percent of the children had been diagnosed as having had at least one episode of secretory otitis media, 125 (50 percent) for three to five episodes, and 33 (13 percent) for six to 11 episodes. Chronic secretory otitis media (i.e., a duration longer than 3 months) had been diagnosed at least once in 44 percent of the otitis prone children but in only 9 percent of the control children.

Rhinopharyngitis, bacterial rhinitis and sinusitis, tonsillitis, and other ENT diagnoses were registered in the medical records from the ENT department. The otitis prone children were diagnosed as having these diseases two to four times more often than the control children.

The ENT operations performed in the children included myringotomy, intubation, adenoidectomy, and tonsillectomy. The first three operations were performed three to eight times more often in the otitis prone children than in the control group. No difference was found in the tonsillectomy frequency,

TABLE 1 Ambulatory Visits and Hospital Admittances in the ENT and Pediatric Departments for Otitis Prone Children and a Control Group

| Children Born in 1977–1981 | Total No. | Mean Number of Visits per Child | | | Hospital Admittances | |
		ENT Dept.	Ped. Dept.	Total	ENT Dept. (No., %)	Ped. Dept (No., %)
Otitis prone children	252	28	11	39	83(33)	155(63)
Control group	252	5	4	9	28(11)	92(37)

TABLE 2 Bronchopulmonary, Gastrointestinal and Allergic Diseases Diagnosed at Least Once in the ENT and Pediatric Departments

Children Born in 1977–1981	Total No.	Bronchopulmonary Diseases		Gastrointestinal Diseases		Allergic Diseases	
		No.	%	No.	%	No.	%
Otitis prone children	252	134	53	112	44	92	37
Control group	252	80	32	82	33	43	17
		$p < 0.001$		$0.01 > p > 0.001$		$p < 0.001$	

which was very low in both groups (3 and 2 percent, respectively).

The registration of bronchopulmonary, gastrointestinal, and allergic diseases diagnosed in the ENT and pediatric departments is given in Table 2. There were twice as many children in the otitis prone group with allergic diseases; also for the other diseases there were statistically significant differences between the two groups.

DISCUSSION

In 1975 Howie et al[4] defined the "otitis prone" condition in children diagnosed in six or more episodes of acute otitis media before the age of 6 years. The children in this study were chosen according to this definition.

The mean number of ambulatory visits in the ENT and pediatric departments was more than four times greater for the otitis prone children than for the children in the control group. Sixty-four percent of the visits were made in patients as young as 2 years of age, and in the following years the additional visits took place. Thus the majority of ambulatory visits were made before the age of 3 years.

Great differences between otitis prone and ordinary children were found in the amount, recurrence, and duration of secretory otitis media. The otitis prone children were also found to have had other ENT diseases (rhinopharyngitis, bacterial rhinitis and sinusitis, and tonsillitis) more frequently than the control group, and this difference was also

found in bronchopulmonary, gastrointestinal, and allergic diseases.

The otitis prone children proved to be great consumers of medical care, and their total amount of illness results in a great many ambulatory visits, operations, and admittances to hospital.

It is of great importance to try to explain why some children have recurrent episodes of acute otitis media and to study the factors increasing the susceptibility to different diseases and infections. The present study is a part of a large case control study of otitis prone children in which environmental, socioeconomic, and demographic factors are being further analyzed.

REFERENCES

1. Ingvarsson L, Lundgren K, Olofsson B, Wall S. Epidemiology of acute otitis media in children. Acta Otolaryngol (Stockh) 1982; (Suppl 388):3–52.
2. Ingvarsson L, Lundgren K, Olofsson B. Epidemiology of acute otitis media in children—a cohort study in an urban population. In: Lim DJ, Bluestone CD, Klein JO, Nelson JD, eds. Recent advances in otitis media with effusion. Proceedings of the Third International Symposium. Toronto: BC Decker, 1984:19.
3. Lundgren K, Ingvarsson L, Olofsson B. Epidemiologic aspects in children with recurrent acute otitis media. In: Lim DJ, Bluestone CD, Klein JO, Nelson JD, eds. Recent advances in otitis media with effusion. Proceedings of the Third International Symposium. Toronto: BC Decker, 1984:22.
4. Howie VM, Ploussard JH, Sloyer J. The "otitis prone" condition. Am J Dis Child 1975; 129:676–678.

EPIDEMIOLOGY OF ACUTE OTITIS MEDIA IN BOSTON CHILDREN FROM BIRTH TO SEVEN YEARS OF AGE

JEROME O. KLEIN, M.D., DAVID W. TEELE, M.D., BERNARD A. ROSNER, Ph.D., and the Greater Boston Otitis Media Study Group: LLOYD TARLIN, M.D., PETER STRINGHAM, M.D., SIDNEY STAROBIN, M.D., LILLIAN McMAHON, M.D., MIRJANA KOSTICH, M.D., GILBERT FISCH, M.D., LORNA BRATTON, M.B., Ch.B., and CAROLE ALLEN, M.D.

To determine the epidemiology of acute otitis media in infants and children, we studied 498 children from birth to the seventh birthday. The children were enrolled and observed in two Greater Boston clinics: a private practice in the suburbs, Holliston and Framingham, and a neighborhood health center in East Boston. The parents of children in the private practice were in higher socioeconomic groups than the parents of children who were cared for in the neighborhood health center. For the purposes of this presentation we include only children who remained active in the practice to age 7 years.

We defined acute otitis media as effusion in the middle ear of a child with one or more acute signs of illness—e.g., a specific sign of ear infection (ear pain, ear tugging, or otorrhea) or a systemic sign (fever, irritability, anorexia, vomiting, or diarrhea). A new episode was defined only after 21 days following initial observations of a prior episode. We diagnosed middle ear effusion by pneumatic otoscopy; the diagnostic ability of the participating pediatricians in the two clinics was verified by dual examinations with one of the authors (JOK or DWT). During the child's years 4 to 7, oto-admittance was used regularly to supplement pneumatic otoscopy. Children were examined regularly (mean, 33 examinations); six pediatricians performed 82.33 percent of the 16,427 examinations.

Selected results from the epidemiologic data are presented here in brief; a complete report is in preparation for publication elsewhere.

AGE SPECIFIC INCIDENCE OF ACUTE OTITIS MEDIA

In the first year of life 62 percent of the children had at least one episode of acute otitis media and 17 percent had three or more episodes. Each year thereafter the episodes of acute otitis media diminished: in the third year of life 41 percent of the children had had one or more episodes and 7 percent had had three or more episodes, and in the seventh year of life 30 percent had had at least one episode and 4 percent had had three or more episodes.

By seven years of age 93 percent of the children had had at least one episode of acute otitis media and 74 percent had had three or more episodes. The mean number of episodes was 1.2 in the first year of life, decreasing to 0.4 in the seventh year.

AGE AT FIRST EPISODE OF ACUTE OTITIS MEDIA

If a child did not have otitis media by 2 years of age, he was unlikely to have problems with middle ear infections. Of the children who had acute otitis media during the first seven years of life, in 66 percent the initial episode occurred in the first year of life and in 17 percent the first episode occurred in the second year of life. In only 14 percent of the children did the first episode occur in the third year or after.

The age at the time of the first episode was significantly and inversely associated with an increased risk of recurrent acute otitis media. For this analysis we determined the number of new episodes that occurred in the 24 months after the first diagnosis of acute otitis media. Of the children who had an episode in the first 3 months of life, 51 percent had three or more episodes in the next 24 months, whereas of the children whose first episode occurred after age 12 months, only 13 percent had three or more episodes in the next 24 months. These results suggest that children who are likely to have recurrent middle ear infections may be identified by an initial episode of acute otitis media early in life.

BREAST FEEDING AND RECURRENT ACUTE OTITIS MEDIA

Children who were breast fed had fewer episodes of acute otitis media during the first year of

TABLE 1   Duration of Breast Feeding and Risk of Acute Otitis Media During First Year of Life

Duration of Breast Feeding	No.	≥ 3 Episodes of Acute Otitis Media (%)
Never breast fed	433	76 (18)
≤ 3 mo	43	4 (9)
4–6 mo	46	5 (11)
7–9 mo	46	4 (9)
>10 mo	70	6 (9)

life than children who were bottle fed (Table 1). This apparent protective effect was approximately equivalent for children who were breast fed for 3 months or for more than 10 months. Conversely, being bottle fed was significantly associated with an increased risk of recurrent acute otitis media by 1 year of age.

CONCLUSIONS

1. The highest age specific incidence of acute otitis media occurred in the first year of life.

2. By seven years of age more than 90 percent of the children observed from birth had had at least one episode of acute otitis media, and approximately three quarters had had three or more episodes.
3. The age at the first episode of acute otitis media was an important predictor for recurrent middle ear infections.
4. Breast feeding was associated with a decreased risk of recurrent acute otitis media during the first year of life.

REFERENCES

1. Howie VM, Ploussard JH, Sloyer J. The "otitis-prone" condition. Am J Dis Child 1975; 129:676–678.
2. Teele DW, Klein JO, Rosner BA. Epidemiology of otitis media in children. Ann Otol Rhinol Laryngol 1980; 89(68):5–6.
3. Teele DW, Klein JO, Rosner B, et al. Burden and practice of pediatrics: middle ear disease during the first five years of life. JAMA 1983; 249:1026–1029.

INCIDENCE, PREVALENCE, AND DURATION OF OTITIS MEDIA IN INFANTS

TERESE FINITZO, Ph.D., PETER ROLAND, M.D., SANDY FRIEL-PATTI, Ph.D., J. PATRICK HIEBER, M.D., KAREN C. BROWN, M.S., and ELLEN FORMBY, M.A.

The Dallas Cooperative Project began to enroll infants in a longitudinal investigation of speech-language learning and early middle ear disease in April 1984. To date, 437 infants from a single Dallas pediatric practice have been enrolled prior to age 6 months. All infants meet the enrollment criteria shown in Table 1.

Although our major question deals with speech-language learning and conductive hearing loss, to address it effectively we must be able to identify otitis media and track its course in our young study subjects. Two hundred eighty-eight infants were followed for 1 year—from the first "official" visit at 6 months through the 18 month old check-up. Contact was made in a variety of settings—regular well visits and sick visits at the pediatrician's office dur-

TABLE 1   Enrollment Criteria

Normal newborn examination
Apgar score at least 7/8
Birth weight greater than 2,400 grams
Pregnancy 37 weeks or longer
English as the only language in the home—including live-ins
Attendance at all well baby checks—prior to the cut-off for enrollment, which is 6 months
Normally developing at time of enrollment (no neurologic problems or major physical defects)
No multiple births

Goal: A minimum of 250 children. Reached statistically by studying drop-out records in pediatricians' offices

ing which immittance, pneumatic otoscopy, and some language screening were undertaken, twice yearly Callier visits in which extensive assessments included pneumatic otoscopy, immittance, as well as audiologic and language assessments, and home or day care visits in which immittance and some language assessments were carried out. Home visits were employed to identify unrecognized asymptomatic otitis media in otherwise well children who did not visit the pediatrician's office between well visits.

In 288 children, 3,072 contacts were made in 1 year. Four hundred forty-six (14.5 percent) of these were Callier visits, 678 (22.1 percent) were regular well check-ups, 1,208 (39.3 percent) were sick visits, and 632 (20.6 percent) were home visits. Thus we averaged 11 contacts per subject for this 12 month period, between the 6 month and 18 month visits. Our goal was to contact a child every 8 weeks, a minimum of six contacts per year.

Otitis media is identified by combining otoscopic results and immittance into codes, similar to those described by Castlebrant et al.[1] We are interested in how the codes relate to hearing loss rather than to effusion per se. In Table 2, we describe these codes.

In 32.8 percent of these 3,072 visits, a code 4 classification—presumptively otitis media—was identified in at least one ear. In 1 year of data collection, 77.4 percent of the 288 infants had one episode of code 4. Thus 22.6 percent of infants between 6 and 18 months of age had never had effusion that we identified. In 49 percent of the cases, the effusions were bilateral. One must remember that we are not talking about acute infection in our youngsters but rather simply the presence of fluid.

Of the 1,886 well or sick visits that took place in the pediatrician's office, a code 4 classification (effusion) was identified in 38 percent of the cases in one or both ears. Classifying by visit types, 77.5 percent of all visits in patients with otitis media identified were sick visits, while 22.5 percent were well visits. Moreover, the incidence of effusion at Callier visits, also presumptively well visits, was 27 percent.

Although it is tempting to conclude that as many as 25 percent of the infants between 6 and 18 months of age have asymptomatic otitis media with effusion, the pediatrician (JPH) on our project cautioned us about overstating the case. At the well checks, parents often report the well known symptoms of irritability, wakefulness, and stuffy nose in a child without acute infection but with effusion. Consequently it is perhaps more accurate to state that 25 percent of our study subjects had effusion during this period that would not be recognized without close surveillance and attention at well child check-ups.

The duration of effusion is clearly of importance to those interested in the potential impact of otitis media with effusion on speech-language learning. Presumptively, the longer otitis media persists, the more likely it is that the associated conductive hearing loss will adversely affect language. To track our infants' experience with otitis media over time, we developed a series of indexes to allow us to examine any duration of interest. We made an a priori decision at the project's onset that assumed that better ear codes would be more closely linked to language learning than worse ear codes. Theoretically, if hearing in at least one ear is relatively unaffected by otitis media, language learning should not be delayed. At least, we hypothesized, it should be less affected in the child with unilateral rather than bilateral disease. The basis for this decision rested on a preliminary investigation in which we did see a significant correlation between hearing loss averaged in the better ear over time and speech-language learning.[2]

For reasons that are beyond the scope of this article, following some early analyses we discovered that unilateral disease may indeed be of critical importance to language learning. Therefore, we instituted the use of otitis media indexes that applied to mean and duration weighted mean codes for the worse ear as well as the better ear.

We are also tracking the total number of days

TABLE 2   Codes

Code 1: Normal
  Normal otoscopic examination results with no air-fluid level
  Type A or A' tympanogram except when otitis media with effusion is identified during otoscopic examination

Code 2: Abnormal middle ear status
  Normal otoscopic examination results with type As, A+, C1, C2, or C3 tympanogram
  Abnormal otoscopic examination results confirming otitis media with effusion with types A or A' tympanogram

Code 3: Tympanostomy tube
  All ears with tympanostomy tubes reported in place in tympanic membrane

Code 4: Otitis media with effusion
  Type B tympanogram
  Abnormal tympanogram A+, As, C1, C2, or C3 with otoscopic confirmation of otitis media with effusion
  Type A or A1 with otoscopic examination revealing visible air-fluid level

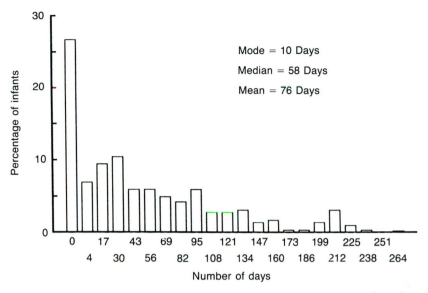

Figure 1   Total days with code 4 disorders, either ear, in 288 infants aged 6 through 18 months.

with otitis media with effusion. In Figure 1 we examine the distribution of total days with otitis media for 288 children 6 to 18 months of age. This curve is definitely a skewed and bimodal distribution. Forty-three percent of our young subjects experienced less than 2 weeks of effusion in 1 year. The mode for this distribution is 10 days. Fifty-three percent of the group had less than 30 days of effusion. The median value is 58 days, while the mean of 75 days of effusion per year is clearly skewed by the distribution. Eight percent of our sample experienced effusion for 6 months or longer in 1 year. Although these numbers were initially surprising, one must remember that 25 percent of our subjects were identified as having effusion at the well child checks; 25 percent of 365 days is 91 days.

It is the data base on effusion obtained in multiple settings that we will relate to hearing and speech-language learning. The 18 month old youngsters who are language delayed have more severe otitis media histories, as defined by our mean indexes, than their playmates with normal language. However, the opposite is not true. Although our numbers are small at this age, as a group the children with histories of severe otitis media are not language delayed at 18 months. This population is also bimodal, with one group appearing to be resilient to the effects of early otitis media and the second group faltering. The project's goal in the coming years is to identify the factors that are important in normal language learning in children with and without otitis media with effusion.

The authors of this paper wish to acknowledge the contributions of study team members William Meyerhoff, M.D., Ph.D., Terri Henderson, M.S., Debbie Muffly, M.S., Cathy Balay, M.S., and Lisa Williams.

Research for this work was supported by NIH grant RO1 NS 1967503 and the American Hearing Research Foundation.

REFERENCES

1. Castlebrant ML, Brostoff LM, Cantekin EI, Doyle W, Fria T. Otitis media with effusion in preschool children. Laryngoscope 1985; 95:428–436.
2. Friel-Patti S, Finitzo-Hieber T, Conti G, Brown KC. Language delay in infants associated with middle ear disease and mild, fluctuating hearing impairment. Pediatr Infect Dis 1982; 1:104–109.

INCIDENCE OF OTITIS MEDIA IN VERY LOW BIRTH WEIGHT INFANTS

JUDITH S. GRAVEL, Ph.D., CECELIA M. McCARTON, M.D., and
ROBERT J. RUBEN, M.D.

The infant born at a very low birth weight (VLBW ≤ 1500 g) is at neurodevelopmental risk owing to the immaturity of numerous biologic systems. Premature infants may spend 2 to 3 months in a neonatal intensive care unit. A high incidence of otitis media with effusion has been reported among infants cared for in neonatal intensive care units.[1] Some researchers suggest that early episodes of otitis media experienced in the intensive care unit could affect the long term otologic course in VLBW neonatal intensive care unit survivors.[2,3] The present investigation prospectively examined the middle ear status in a group of VLBW babies whose neonatal period was spent in an intensive care unit. The purpose of the study was to determine whether a group of very low birth weight infants who received intensive care during the neonatal period had a greater incidence of otitis media than a group of normal full term (FT) babies who had routine hospital stays in a well baby nursery.

METHODS

Sixty-seven infants were regularly followed through our facility for 1 year. Forty-six (22 males and 24 females) very low birth weight and 21 full term babies (11 males and 10 females) composed the sample. The VLBW infants were cared for in a neonatal intensive care unit for various periods of time during the neonatal course. The average length of stay for infants in the unit was 57 days (SD = 26). The mean birth weight for the VLBW group was 1225.3 g (SD = 213.2). The mean gestational age estimated by the Ballard examination administered shortly after birth was 30.6 weeks (SD = 1.9).[4] The FT infants averaged 39.9 weeks gestational age (SD = 0.4), and the mean birth weight for the group was 3281.2 g (SD = 262.5). The FT infants were recruited from the well baby nursery at the same facility.

The 67 infants composing this cohort were enrolled in the Low Birthweight Infant Follow-up and Evaluation (LIFE) Program of the Rose F. Kennedy Center for Mental Retardation and Human Development, Bronx, New York. Infants enrolled in this program receive all their medical, neurologic, and developmental follow-up through the facility. All babies were born to families living in low socioeconomic urban neighborhoods.

Pediatric nurse practitioners carried out all the routine medical examinations of the babies. The nurse practitioners were trained and supervised in the use of pneumatic otoscopy by a pediatric otolaryngologist. The training included instruction in the technique, otoscopic inspections in the operating room before and after myringotomies, and tandem otoscopic examinations by physicians and nurse practitioners in regularly scheduled pediatric ENT clinics. Agreement between the examiners was determined for a small subset of LIFE Program participants. Concordance was better than 90 percent between observers.

During each infant's visit the pediatric nurse practitioner was required to examine the ears and complete a nine item check list, which queried tympanic membrane characteristics such as position, appearance, color, and mobility. On the basis of the examination the pediatric nurse practitioner judged each ear as normal, suspicious, or positive for otitis media with effusion. On the same form the infant was designated as either clinically symptomatic or asymptomatic with regard to overall well-being. Presenting symptoms, if any, were recorded and therapy plans were indicated.

The majority of infants were scheduled for routine medical and auditory assessment visits beginning at 40 weeks postconceptional age. The otoscopy records for the VLBW and FT infants were examined for a 1 year period. For the purpose of this study the maximal number of otoscopic inspections considered for any infant was set at 13 for the time period spanning 40 weeks postconceptional age to 12 months, or one otoscopic examination per month. Only otoscopic inspections that were separated by an approximate 30 day interval were considered. Thus, if an infant underwent otoscopy twice during a particular month, only a single examination was registered for that period. As an example of these calculations, if an infant was examined at eight monthly visits during the year and experienced judgments positive for otitis media in both ears at two visits, that infant was regarded as having bilateral otitis media in 25 percent of the first year visits.

RESULTS

On the average each baby received 8.5 (SD = 1.9) otoscopic examinations over the 1 year period; the range was 5 to 13 inspections. VLBW infants received an average of 8.9 (SD = 2.0) inspections; the FT infants averaged 7.6 (SD = 1.5).

A review of the completed otoscopic rating forms revealed that when an ear was judged as having otitis media with effusion, most often the tympanic membrane was observed to be pink or red and opaque and had reduced mobility or absence of mobility to positive or negative pressure. The tympanic membrane position was usually neutral or convex. Less frequently some ears with positive otitis media ratings were observed to be translucent and of normal color. On such occasions fluid levels behind the eardrum were reported. In most cases positive otitis media judgments were applied to infants who concomitantly displayed medical symptoms—most frequently nasal discharge or an erythematous pharynx. To a much lesser extent, other symptoms (such as fever, cough, or irritability) were also noted.

VLBW and FT infants had similar otologic courses during the first year. Significance testing revealed no difference between the VLBW (M = 68.6, SD = 21.3) and FT (M = 67.7, SD = 20.6) groups for either the percentage of visits at which middle ears were considered normal bilaterally (t_{65} = 0.15, n.s.), or the percentage of visits at which the VLBW infants (M = 25.9, SD = 17.3) and the FT (M = 27.4, SD = 17.1) infants were judged to have otitis media in one or both ears (t_{65} = − 0.35, n.s.). Only seven (15.2 percent) of the VLBW infants were free of otitis media at all first year visits. Similarly, three (14.3 percent) of the FT group never had a positive otoscopy rating during the first year. Therefore the percentages of infants experiencing at least one episode of otitis media during the first year were 84.8 percent and 85.7 percent for the VLBW and FT infants, respectively. No relationship was found between the birth weight of the VLBW infants and their percentage visits with either normal middle ears bilaterally (r = − 0.14) or middle ear effusions (r = 0.26). Further, there was no relationship between days spent in the neonatal intensive care unit and normal (r = 0.11) or

positive otitis media visits (r = − 0.22) during the first year.

Significance testing revealed no difference between the groups in the mean age of infants at the time of the initial otoscopy rating consistent with otitis media. The corrected age (chronologic age minus the number of weeks the infant was premature) of the VLBW infants was used for these calculations; VLBW infants were 5.9 months old and FT babies were 6.4 months of age (t_{65} = − 0.80, n.s.).

Socioeconomic status was not a factor in this cohort. All infants in this study were born to families living in low socioeconomic urban neighborhoods. The Hollingshead four factor index of social status was used to assess socioeconomic status.[5] There was no difference between the VLBW (M = 25.9, SD = 10.2) and FT (M = 28.1, SD = 11.1) infants' scores on the socioeconomic status index (t_{65} = − 0.79, n.s.). On the average, cohort families fell within the two lowest strata (scores ≤ 30) of the scale (ceiling score = 66).

DISCUSSION

This investigation found no difference in the percentage of visits at which VLBW neonatal intensive care unit graduates were judged to have otitis media when compared to full term control subjects. This was true for at least the first year of life when infants' corrected ages were considered. Further, no relationship was found between birth weight or days spent in the neonatal intensive care unit and the otologic outcome in the VLBW infants.

Published studies suggest that there is a high incidence of otitis media in neonatal intensive care units.[1] One factor implicated in the high incidence of middle ear disease in the neonatal intensive care unit is the use of mechanical ventilation provided through nasotracheal intubation.[1,6] The tube reportedly introduces a physical inhibitor of normal eustachian tube function. Further, its presence within the nasopharynx may cause edema and infection, resulting in an increased risk of middle ear disease.

None of the VLBW infants in this cohort, however, underwent nasotracheal intubation. Infants requiring mechanical ventilation in our neonatal intensive care unit undergo endotracheal intubation (through the oral pharynx) with an infant pressure ventilator (BP200). This practice may contribute to the otologic similarity of this group of VLBW infants to the FT infants sampled. However, we do not know the otologic status of the VLBW infants prior to their achieving 40 weeks postconceptional age or while they were in intensive care.

Overall, both VLBW and FT infants had a high incidence of otitis media during the 1 year observation period; 85 percent of the infants had at least one episode of otitis media during the first year. This figure likely reflects the regular otoscopic examinations completed in infants during their frequent visits to the LIFE Program. Episodes of middle ear disease were not always clinically symptomatic; that is, many of the infants judged to have otitis media were not in acute distress. In addition, all infants were considered of low socioeconomic status and thus were representative of similar socioeconomic levels. Thus, no relationship between otitis media and socioeconomic status could be determined owing to the homogeneity of the present sample on this variable.

During the first year of life (based on corrected age), VLBW infants who were cared for in our neonatal intensive care unit were not considered a group at greater risk for otitis media than infants who received normal, well baby care. Although these results may be representative of only this sample of babies, we now consider otitis media to be more common in the infants followed by our program than previously suspected.

We wish to thank Anne Hogan, Wilma Spinner, Mary Ellen Lynch, and Maureen McElhinney of the LIFE Program for their invaluable contributions to this research.

This study was supported by Clinical Research Center Grant (NS 19748) from the National Institute of Neurological and Communicative Disorders and Stroke.

REFERENCES

1. Balkany T, Berman S, Simmons M, et al. Middle ear effusion in neonates. Laryngoscope 1978; 88:398–405.
2. DeSa DJ. Mucosal metaplasia and chronic inflammation in the middle ear of infants receiving intensive care in the neonatal period. Arch Dis Child 1983; 58:24–28.
3. McCormick MC. The contribution of low birth weight to infant mortality and childhood morbidity. N Engl J Med 1985; 312:82–90.
4. Ballard JL, Novak KK, Driver MA. A simplified score for assessment of fetal maturation of newly born infants. J Pediatr 1979; 95:769–774.
5. Hollingshead AB. Four factor index of social status. Unpublished manuscript. New Haven: Yale University, 1975.
6. Persico M, Barker GA, Mitchell DP. Purulent otitis media—a "silent" source of sepsis in the pediatric intensive care unit. Otolaryngol Head Neck Surg 1985; 93:330–334.

TYMPANOMETRIC DETERMINATION OF THE OUTCOME OF ACUTE OTITIS MEDIA

PAUL A. SHURIN, M.D., COLIN D. MARCHANT, M.D., CANDICE E. JOHNSON, M.D., Ph.D., THOMAS MORLEDGE, M.D., DARA WEGMAN, B.S., and JOY FEHRIBACH, B.S.

Successful management of acute otitis media may be defined by a decrease in clinical signs and symptoms such as earache and fever, by resolution of the middle ear effusion,[1] by the pattern of recurrent infections occurring during the convalescent period,[2] by improvement in conductive hearing,[3] or by a beneficial effect on such potential long term effects as language development.[4] Prolonged middle ear effusion is the most frequent sequela of acute otitis media and is the probable pathologic cause of other delayed effects of the disease. Clinical trials are now providing criteria for more refined use of medical and surgical therapy. Objective diagnostic methods will be required for these advances to have maximal benefit. Improved diagnostic methods must also be applicable to the testing of young infants. We have shown susceptance tympanometry and measurement of stapedius reflex thresholds to have many of the requirements for such testing when applied in selected patients in research trials.[5,6] We have now evaluated these methods in children who have recovered clinically from acute middle ear infection.

METHODS

Seventy-four children visited a general pediatric clinic for acute otitis media and were admitted to the study after parental consent was obtained. The initial diagnosis was confirmed otoscopically by the investigators and by tympanocentesis of each affected ear. Antimicrobial therapy was given for 10 days. Otoscopy by trained observers and susceptance tympanometry with acoustic reflex threshold measurement were performed 1 month after presentation and the findings analyzed using our published criteria.[6]

RESULTS

Of 112 ears tested at 1 month, 57 (51 percent) were judged otoscopically to have middle ear effusion and 55 (49 percent) to be free of effusion. Otoscopy and tympanometry gave concordant results in 95 of these ears (85 percent; Table 1). The two major findings in effusion free ears of young infants are the presence of a measurable peak in the tympano-

TABLE 1   Otoscopic and Tympanometric Findings at 1 Month (Number of Ears)

Tympanogram Peak Susceptance	Otoscopic Diagnosis	
	Middle Ear Effusion	No Effusion
Present	16	54
Absent	41	1
	p < 0.0005	

gram tracing and the presence of a detectable acoustic reflex threshold with an ipsilateral stimulus of <100 db HL.[6] These findings were concordant in 35 of 43 otoscopically normal ears (81 percent); the comparable figure was 93 percent in a previous study (Table 2). Otoscopic and tympanometric findings were also more frequently discordant in this than in previous studies (Table 3).

DISCUSSION

From the present results and our published findings with these tympanometric methods we conclude the following:

1. Susceptance tympanograms with peaks greater than 0 mmho provide objective evidence of resolution of acute otitis media.
2. The correlation of tympanometric and otoscopic findings is less in children studied 1 month after acute otitis media than previously reported for highly selected populations.
3. Susceptance tympanograms with a probe tone of 660 Hz are more accurate in infants than tympanograms obtained at 220 Hz.
4. The standards used are applicable to infants as young as 2 weeks of age.

We believe the lower concordance of tympanometric peak and normal otoscopic diagnosis found

TABLE 2   Present Study and Published Results in Otoscopically Normal Ears: the Presence of a Tympanogram Peak and the Presence of the Acoustic Reflex (Number of Ears)

Susceptance Peak	Present Detectable Reflex Threshold	
	+	−
Study 1*	63 (93%)	5
Present study	35 (81%)	8

* Study 1: Data from Marchant CD, McMillan PM, Shurin PA, Johnson CE, Turcyzk VA, Feinstein JC, Murdell-Panek D. Objective diagnosis of otitis media in early infancy by tympanometry and ipsilateral acoustic reflex thresholds. J Pediatr 1986; 109:590.

TABLE 3   Present Study and Published Results: Otoscopic Diagnosis and Presence of Tympanogram Peak (Number of Ears)

Susceptance Peak Present	Otoscopic Diagnosis	
	Middle Ear Effusion	No Effusion
Study 1*	1 (1%)	113 (99%)
Study 2	4 (6%)	64 (94%)
Present study	16 (23%)	54 (77%)

* Study 1: Data from Shurin PA, Pelton SI, Finkelstein J. Tympanometry in the diagnosis of middle ear effusion. N Engl J Med 1977; 296:412.
   2: Data from Marchant CD, McMillan PM, Shurin PA, Johnson CE, Turcyzk VA, Feinstein JC, Murdell-Panek D. Objective diagnosis of otitis media in early infancy by tympanometry and ipsilateral acoustic reflex thresholds. J Pediatr 1986; 109:590.

in the present study to be a reflection of the dynamic state of resolution of middle ear disease in the present study group as compared with the highly selected groups studied previously. However, it has been shown in each of our three studies using this procedure with tympanograms obtained with the Grason-Stadler otoadmittance meter that the presence of a detectable tympanometric peak provides strong evidence for absence of a middle ear effusion. This criterion for the resolution of otitis media with effusion may be applied both to clinical research and to pediatric practice.

REFERENCES

1. Shurin PA, Pelton SI, Donner A, Klein JO. Persistence of middle ear effusion after acute otitis media in children. N Engl J Med 1979; 300:1121.
2. Carlin SA, Marchant CD, Shurin PA, Johnson CE, Murdell-Panek D. Early recurrences of otitis media: reinfection or relapse? J Pediatr 1987; 110:20.
3. Fria TJ, Paradise JL, Sabo DL, Elster BA. Conductive hearing loss in infants and young children with cleft palate. J Pediatr 1987; 111:84.
4. Teele DW, et al. Otitis media with effusion during the first three years of life and development of speech and language. Pediatr 1984; 74:282.
5. Shurin PA, Pelton SI, Finkelstein J. Tympanometry in the diagnosis of middle ear effusion. N Engl J Med 1977; 296:412.
6. Marchant CD, McMillan PM, Shurin PA, Johnson CE, Turcyzk VA, Feinstein JC, Murdell-Panek D. Objective diagnosis of otitis media in early infancy by tympanometry and ipsilateral acoustic reflex thresholds. J Pediatr 1986; 109:590.

FAMILY STUDIES IN SEROUS OTITIS MEDIA

TIMOTHY J. ROCKLEY, F.R.C.S.

Prompted by a clinical impression of family case clustering of serous otitis media in children, this study was undertaken to determine whether there is an increased frequency of middle ear disease in the families of children with serous otitis media and also whether social and economic factors might play a part in causing any observed familial influence.

METHODS

A study group and a control group were selected from children in the hospital, and their parents were interviewed and examined.

Study Group

Seventy-eight children with persistent symptomatic serous otitis media composed the study group. These children, aged 4 to 14 years, were admitted to the hospital for surgical treatment of serous otitis media; all had been symptomatic for at least 6 months.

Control Group

Thirty-nine children were selected from in patients of the same age group, admitted for nonotologic surgery. None had a history of deafness or otalgia either in the child or in siblings, and in all cases the tympanic membranes had a normal appearance on otoscopy. All subjects in both groups were of caucasian origin, with no cases of cleft palate or Down's syndrome.

For each child in the study, both parents were interviewed and questioned about the following topics: age and occupation of parents, size of family, smoking habits, and whether any otologic symptoms (deafness, otalgia, or otorrhea) or operations were recalled from childhood. All the parents' ears were then examined to look for tympanic membrane abnormalities representing the long term sequelae of serous otitis media—tympanosclerosis, segmental atrophy, or perforation of the pars tensa, retraction of the pars flaccida or posterior segment of the pars tensa, or the presence of cholesteatoma or previous radical mastoid surgery.[1] Both parents of each child were examined; there were thus 156 subjects in the study group and 78 controls.

The significance of any differences between the study and control groups was tested using the chi square test with Yates' correction.

RESULTS

Questionnaire

No differences were observed between study and control groups with respect to socioeconomic status, size of family, or parental smoking habits. Fifteen children with serous otitis media 20 percent had a sibling who was treated surgically for the same condition.

Otoscopy

Seventy-four parents were identified as having abnormalities of the tympanic membrane. These abnormalities were significantly more frequent among parents in the study group (Table 1).

Distribution of specific tympanic membrane abnormalities in the two groups is shown in Table 2 (23 subjects had more than one abnormality). Each abnormality was observed more frequently in the study group, but individually none of these differences is statistically significant.

Table 3 compares the 74 parents who had abnormal tympanic membranes with the 160 in whom no abnormality was seen, relating otoscopic tympanic membrane abnormality to what the parents remembered of childhood otologic symptoms. Apart from a significantly increased history of recurrent otalgia, there was little difference in childhood symptoms between the two groups, especially in regard to hearing impairment. Sixteen of the parents (22 percent) with abnormal tympanic membranes recalled no otologic symptoms.

DISCUSSION

These findings confirm the clinical impression of a familial influence in serous otitis media and its sequelae. Bearing in mind that there is no effect demonstrable due to smoking habits, family size, or social class (in agreement with most published epidemiologic data[2]) and considering that the parents and their children are separated by a generation in which there has been tremendous change in social circumstance and the pattern of ear disease in the United Kingdom, this evidence suggests a genetic component in the etiology of serous otitis media. Further research would be necessary to identify a mode of inheritance (e.g., single gene effect or multifactorial) or to identify a specific abnormality (perhaps anatomic or immunologic) that might be inherited.

The presence of marked racial differences in the incidence of serous otitis media[3] and an observed association with certain ABO blood groups[4] suggest a genetic component in its etiology, but population based epidemiologic studies fail to support the notion that parental disposition is a significant etiologic factor.[5] However, this conclusion was reached on the basis of otologic history alone. The present

TABLE 1 Results of Otoscopy

	Study $n = 156$	Control $n = 78$
Parents with tympanic membrane abnormalities	60 (38%)	14 (18%)

$$X^2 = 9.2; p < 0.005$$

TABLE 2 Distribution of Specific Tympanic Membrane Abnormalities

	Study $n = 156$		Control $n = 78$	
	No.	%	No.	%
Pars tensa				
Segmental atrophy	19	12	4	5
Segmental retraction	12	7	1	1
Perforation	3	2	1	1
Tympanosclerosis	17	11	6	8
Pars flaccida				
Retraction	23	15	6	8
Atticoantral disease	4	3	1	1

TABLE 3 History of Childhood Ear Symptoms

	Parents with Abnormal Tympanic Membrane (n = 74)	%	Normal Tympanic Membrane (n = 160)	%
Never had any symptoms	16	22	98	61
Otalgia, one or two occasions	19	26	32	20
Recurrent troublesome otalgia	34	46	26	16*
Deafness	4	5	6	4
Otorrhea	11	15	2	1
Deafness with otorrhea	6	8	1	1

* $X^2 = 21.8$; $p < 0.001$.

study suggests that an otologic history is an unreliable guide to the individual's disposition to childhood serous otitis media (see Table 3) and that careful otoscopy yields more information.

REFERENCES

1. Tos M, Stangerup S-E, Holm-Jensen S, Sørensen CH. Spontaneous course of secretory otitis and changes in the eardrum. Arch Otolaryngol 1984; 110:281–289.
2. van Cauwenberge PB. Relevant and irrelevant predisposing factors in secretory otitis media. Arch Otolaryngol (Stockh) 1984; Suppl 414:147–153.
3. Klein JO. Epidemiology of otitis media. In: Harford ER, Bess FH, Bluestone CD, Klein JO, eds. Impedance screening for middle ear disease in children: proceedings of a symposium in Nashville. New York: Grune & Stratton, 1978.
4. Mortenson EH, Lildholt T, Gammelgard NP, Christensen PH. Distribution of ABO blood groups in secretory otitis media and cholesteatoma. Clin Otolaryngol 1983; 8:263–265.
5. Tos M, Poulson G, Borch J. Etiologic factors in secretory otitis. Arch Otolaryngol 1979; 105:582–588.

EPIDEMIOLOGY OF OTITIS MEDIA IN AN ETHNICALLY MIXED ISLAND POPULATION

COLLIN S. KARMODY, M.D., F.R.C.S. (Edin), F.A.C.S.
and AUSTIN TRINIDADE, M.B., Ch.B., F.R.C.S. (Edin)

The comparative incidence of otitis media among racial groups has long been difficult to ascertain. To date almost all epidemiologic studies of otitis media have concentrated on assessing various factors in a comparatively homogeneous ethnic population. In ethnically mixed populations, socioeconomic factors that affect the various groups have prevented the making of valid comparisons.

Kessner et al,[1] in a comparative study of deprived urban populations, found the frequency of otorrhea and hearing impairment to be almost twice as high in white subjects as in blacks. Conversely, Okafor[2] reported a very high incidence of chronic otorrhea in Nigeria, a predominantly black population.

In an attempt to answer the question of racial variations in the incidence of otitis media, a study was undertaken on the island of Trinidad. Trinidad and Tobago are the most southerly of the West Indian islands and together form a twin island independent state. They enjoy a tropical climate with a 6 month rainy season and a 6 month dry season. The population is 1.2 million (Table 1).[3] The ethnic mix of the population is 40 percent black (African origin, ancestral home West Africa), 40 percent East Indian (ancestral home India), and 20 percent a

TABLE 1   Trinidad and Tobago: Demographic and Climatic Statistics

Population: 1.2 million (1984)
Area: 5,128 sq. km.
Population density: 228/sq. km.
Average temp.: max. 92° F, min. 71° F
Average rainfall: 200 mm

mixture of European stock with a liberal sprinkling of Chinese, Middle Eastern, and mixed races (Table 2).[4] Although there is some mixture of the races, the two predominant racial groups for the most part have kept their ethnic heritages but have the same socioeconomic status. Their diets differ slightly.

MATERIALS AND METHODS

We studied 400 patients with otitis media who visited the Department of Otolaryngology, San Fernando General Hospital, San Fernando, South Trinidad, in the 6 month period from September 1986 to February 1987. Patients with acute otitis were seen both on an emergency basis and in the clinics by appointment. They were either self-referred or referred by the primary physician.

Hospital care in Trinidad and Tobago is free to the general population, but otolaryngology services are available only at the two major hospitals in the capital city, Port of Spain, and in the town of San Fernando. Each hospital therefore provides otolaryngologic care for roughly half the island's population. The otolaryngology clinics at the San Fernando General Hospital handle over 8,000 patient visits per year, and the department sees an average of 12 emergencies daily.

All patients diagnosed by the staff of the department as having otitis media, either acute or chronic, were entered into the study. Excluded were those with significant associated problems such as neoplasms and cleft palates. Patients were matched for age, sex, socioeconomic level, demographics (rural versus urban), and living conditions (e.g., running

water, plumbing, toilet facilities). All the patients were examined by one of the authors (AT). Demographic data were collected by a questionnaire completed by the patient but checked by the physician.

The population is so evenly distributed that in such a wide regional survey, local clustering of races was not considered to be statistically significant. We believe that the cohort is representative of the general population. This report is concerned only with the ethnics of the patient population, but at a later date other factors will be discussed.

RESULTS

Of the 400 patients studied, there were 352 Indians (88 percent), 43 blacks (10.75 percent), 5 of mixed races, and no whites or Chinese (Table 3). One hundred eighteen patients (29.5 percent) had acute otitis media and 282 patients (70.5 percent), chronic otitis. About 75 percent of the patients were from middle and lower income families; a few were from upper income families and the rest were unemployed. Surprisingly there were no Chinese patients; this is contrary to what would be expected on the basis of other epidemiologic studies, which generally suggest a high prevalence of otitis media in Orientals. Climate seemed to have no effect on otitis media, as there was no difference in incidence during the 4 months of rainy season and 2 months of dry season that the study spanned.

DISCUSSION

The results of this study demonstrate an overwhelming predominance of Indians with otitis media. This can be taken to indicate that Indians have an abnormally high incidence of otitis media per se. During the same period of this study, 12 white patients with otitis media were seen in the private offices of one of the authors (AT). By extrapolation, considering the number of whites in the general

TABLE 2   Population of Trinidad and Tobago by Ethnic Origin (1984)

Ethnic Group	Numbers	%
Black	430,864	40.8
East Indian	429,187	40.7
Mixed	172,285	16.3
White	9,946	0.9
Chinese	5,562	0.5
Others	7,019	0.7

TABLE 3   Ethnic Distribution of 400 Patients with Otitis Media

East Indian	352 (88%)
Black	43 (10.75%)
White	0
Chinese	0
Mixed	5 (1.25%)
Total	400

population, it seems as though the incidence of otitis media is the same in Indians and whites.

We therefore consider the raw data to indicate a low frequency of otitis media in blacks when compared to Indians and whites. The Oriental segment of the population is too small for significant comparison. Although this study is preliminary and still to be subjected to statistical analysis, the difference between racial groups in terms of the raw data is so impressive that it would be a great surprise if a formal analysis concluded differently.

Okafor [2] has discussed his experience in a teaching hospital in Nigeria, reporting 386 new cases of chronic suppurative otitis media seen over a 2 year period. He concluded there was a high "prevalence" of chronic otitis media in Nigeria.

Comparison between our study and Okafor's is difficult. The impression, however, is that Okafor's data were collected from a much larger, overwhelmingly black population and that his total number of cases, although slightly smaller than ours, took four times as long to collect (6 months versus 2 years).

A number of other authors have reported high incidences of otitis media in various ethnic groups. Baxter and Ling [5] found a high prevalence in the Eskimos of Baffin Island. Camben et al [6] reported a high incidence in native Indians in British Columbia. Martin (quoted by Hinchcliffe [7]), working in Uganda, observed that cholesteatoma was less frequent in the native population than in the English. Eagles et al [8] studied ear disease in 5,748 school children in Pittsburgh over a 6 year period. Although 70 percent of their subjects were white, no reference was made about racial differences in their report.

A number of investigators have tried to explain the cause of racial differences in otitis media. Most have concentrated on the structure and function of the eustachian tube. Ratnesar [9] studied luminal diameters of eustachian tubes in three ethnic groups— Eskimos, North American Indians, and Caucasians—and concluded that Caucasians have narrow eustachian tubes. He attributed the high incidence of cholesteatoma in Caucasians to the lesser aeration of the tympanomastoid complex. This concept, of course, does not explain the higher incidence of chronic otitis media without cholesteatoma in the other groups.

Our study has shown that in general blacks have a lower incidence of otitis media than other racial groups. It is obvious that racial differences in the incidence are not explicable by purely anatomic factors. The more plausible explanation might be in the subtle (or not so subtle) immunologic variations that to date have been only marginally explored. The results show an overwhelmingly higher incidence in East Indians and a comparatively low incidence of otitis media in blacks.

REFERENCES

1. Kessner D, Snow CK, Singer T. Assessment of medical care for children: contrasts in health care status. Vol. 3. Washington, D.C.: Institute of Medicine, National Academy of Sciences, 1974.
2. Okafor BC. The chronic discharging ear in Nigeria. J Laryngol Otol 1984; 98:113–119.
3. Population census. Central Statistical Office, Ministry of Information, Trinidad and Tobago, 1984.
4. Trinidad and Tobago Statistical Pocket Digest. Central Statistical Office, Trinidad and Tobago, 1985.
5. Baxter JD, Ling D. Ear disease and hearing loss among the Eskimo population of the Baffin Zone. Can J Otolaryngol 1974; 3:110–122.
6. Camben K, Galbraith JD, Kong G. Middle ear disease in Indians of the Mount Currie Reservation, British Columbia. Can Med Assoc J 1965; 93:1301.
7. Hinchcliffe R. Cholesteatoma: epidemiological and quantitative aspects. In: McCabe BF, Sadé J, Abramson M, eds. Cholesteatoma. First international conference. Birmingham, AL: Aesculapius, 1977:277.
8. Eagles EL, Wishik SM, Doefler LG. Hearing sensitivity and ear disease in children: a prospective study. Laryngoscope 1967.
9. Ratnesar P. Chronic ear disease along the coasts of Labrador and northern Newfoundland. J Otolaryngol 1976; 5(2):122–130.

FAMILIAL PREDISPOSITION FOR OTITIS MEDIA IN PAROCHIAL SCHOOL CHILDREN

N. WENDELL TODD, M.D., F.A.C.S. and LINDA L. SETTLE, M.D.

Otitis media is common, yet there is no accepted explanation for why it affects only some children and why some of these have life-long disease. Typically otitis media begins in infancy, is a bilateral phenomenon, leaves residual tympanic membrane scarring, and is associated with minimal mastoid pneumatization. The racial variations in otitis media incidence (a high incidence in native Americans and Australian aborigines and a comparatively low incidence in blacks) may be regarded, in a sense, as a form of familial predisposition. A familial occurrence has been suggested for otitis media in infants[1] and children[2] and in Apache Indians[3] and for mastoid size[4] and cholesteatoma[5] in adults. However, each of these studies was relatively limited. An additional query about a familial aggregation of otitis media seemed appropriate.

This report addresses the point prevalence of tympanoscopic abnormalities in sibling children at a parochial school. The children were seen during routine screening for visual and auditory acuity.

SUBJECTS AND METHODS

On October 8, 1985, 233 of the 307 children enrolled in kindergarten through the fifth grade of the Immaculate Heart of Mary School, Atlanta, participated in health screening. Almost all the children were Caucasian.

Tympanoscopy was done by two physicians, an otolaryngologist and a third year pediatric resident, using a Seigel tympanoscope with headlight illumination (NWT) and a Welch-Allyn tympanoscope with its incorporated illumination (LLS). No attempt was made to retrieve or rearrange cerumen. Pneumatic tympanoscopy was utilized sporadically. Each ear of each child was assessed independently by each examiner. Each examiner was blind as to whether a given child had a sibling in the school. The findings were independently recorded on separate roster sheets. All the children were seen during one morning, over a 4 hour period. The children were seen sequentially by classroom.

The tympanic membrane findings were categorized as normal, scarred, or clinical otitis. Scarring was classified as fibrotic, atrophic, or sclerotic changes. The "scarred" and "clinical otitis" categories subsequently were grouped and considered "abnormal" for data analysis. Each case was classified according to the abnormality found in either ear.

Five children were excluded from data analysis: four with both tympanic membranes obscured by cerumen to each examiner's view and one with an obvious craniofacial syndrome (cleft lip and palate). In 15 children both tympanic membranes were obscured by cerumen to one examiner. For the analyses requiring congruous interexaminer data, we excluded seven who mistakenly were evaluated by only one examiner and 62 in whom the ear status was labeled differently by the two examiners (Table 1).

TABLE 1   Each Observer's Categorization of Each Child's Tympanoscopically Worse Ear*

| Pediatrician | Otolaryngologist | | | |
	Obscured by Cerumen	Normal	Abnormal	Total
Obscured	4	7	8	19
Normal	0	90	49	139
Abnormal	0	13	54	67
Total	4	110	111	225

* Omitted from this table are the seven children seen by only one examiner and the one child with obvious craniofacial syndrome.

The school's directory of students was used to identify presumptive siblings defined as persons sharing a surname and listed as living in a household of the same surname. Forty-five sibling pairs were available for data analysis. There were seven families each with three siblings seen during the screening. In each of these seven sibships at least one child had been excluded already from data analysis; the remaining sibling pairs were used in assessing the distribution of the ear status. Two sets of twins were listed; however, one set was absent from school that day and the other set was not usable (because one child's ear status was incongruously labeled by the two examiners). Thus, each of the analyzed sibling pairs was independent; that is, no child was involved in more than one sibling pair for data analysis.

The kappa index was used to express the extent of agreement between the two observer's findings.[6] The data from the siblings were sorted into normal-normal, normal-abnormal, and abnormal-abnormal pairs. The comparison of the observed and the expected binomial distributions of the pairs was done with the chi square test for goodness of fit, with one degree of freedom.[7]

RESULTS

Clinical otitis media was uncommonly identified: one child had tympanotomy tubes and one had serous otitis media. The strength of interobserver agreement was fair (kappa = 0.39). Abnormal tympanic membranes were found in seemingly similar incidences among boys and girls, among each of the grades and classes within each grade, by each examiner. The children of the last class examined had incidences of abnormality similar to those in the children of classes examined earlier. By the otolaryngologist's assessment, about half the children were categorized as having abnormal findings; by the pediatrician's assessment, about one-third had abnormal findings (see Table 1).

It is unlikely that the distribution of normal-normal, normal-abnormal, and abnormal-abnormal pairs among siblings was due to chance alone (Table 2). This was apparent for each examiner's data ($p < 0.05$ and $p < 0.10$) and for the grouped data ($p < 0.02$). A relative excess of normal-normal and abnormal-abnormal sibships and a relative deficiency of normal-abnormal sibships were evident in each examiner's data and in the grouped data.

DISCUSSION

These sibling data may suggest that otitis has a familial aggregation in these parochial school children in Atlanta. The relative excess of sibling pairs whose otitis status was labeled as normal-normal and abnormal-abnormal, compared to that expected by chance alone, is similar to that of Apache Indian first degree relative pairs.[3] Thus the data of these separate studies would complement the argument for a familial aggregation of otitis media. The number of brother-brother, brother-sister, and sister-sister pairs in each study was too few for statistical analysis of a sex linked familial aggregation.

The "fair" strength of interobserver agreement does not negate the inferences made. However, the study involves four assumptions that should be considered:

1. The assumption that tympanic membrane

TABLE 2 Distribution of Tympanoscopic Findings in the Worse Ear in Sibling Pairs

Sibling Pair	Examiners Agreed		Otolaryngologist		Pediatrician	
	Observed	Expected*	Observed	Expected*	Observed	Expected*
Normal-normal	5	2.64	15	10.27	19	16.02
Normal-abnormal	3	7.72	17	22.46	10	15.98
Abnormal-abnormal	8	5.64	13	12.27	7	4.00
Total	16	16.00	45	45.00	36	36.00
Chi square	5.997 $p < 0.02$		3.541 $p < 0.10$		5.041 $p < 0.05$	

* Expected under the assumption of no association of tympanoscopic findings in the sibling pairs.

scarring is indicative of otitis media at least having occurred in the past in that person. Tos et al[8] report that "long-lasting negative pressure and the inflammatory changes of the eardrum in secretory otitis are probably the main causes of all kinds of eardrum abnormality." However, eardrum findings are not static over time and are known to change to better or worse.

2. The assumption that scarring and clinical otitis can be grouped as "abnormal" rather than being ranked in order of severity of the otitis media condition. The Apache point prevalence study, by not suggesting an association of severity of otitis media in first degree relatives, would endorse this grouping.[3]

3. The assumption that the sociocultural kinship as defined in this study was indicative of biologic facts.

4. The assumption that the not-examined bias does not negate the inferences made: that is, that the school children who did not participate in the screening did not have a counterbalancing distribution of normal-abnormal ears in sibling pairs. Since 75.9 percent participated in the study, this assumption seems safe.

Whether the familial aggregation of otitis media is due to genetic or environmental effects is speculative. The results reported here seem compatible with a hypothesis previously offered: that a person's genetically determined "different" eustachian tubes (different in musculoskeletal anatomy[9] and differ-

ent in ventilatory function[10]) are the crucial factor that allows other potential insults to contribute to the occurrence of otitis media. The list of potential contributing insults would at least include upper respiratory infections, inhalant allergy and irritants, feeding practice, and large adenoids.

REFERENCES

1. Klein JO. Persistent middle ear effusions: natural history and morbidity. Pediatr Infect Dis 1982; Suppl. 1:S4–S10.
2. Tos M, Poulsen G, Borch J. Etiologic factors in secretory otitis. Arch Otolaryngol 1979; 106:582–588.
3. Todd NW. Familial predisposition for otitis media in Apache Indians at Canyon Day, Arizona. Genet Epidemiol 1987; 4:25–31.
4. Dahlberg G, Diamant M. Hereditary character of the cellular system in the mastoid process. Acta Otolaryngol (Stockh) 1945; 33:378–389.
5. Plester D. Hereditary factors in chronic otitis with cholesteatoma. Acta Otorhinolaryngol Belg 1980; 34:51–55.
6. Feinstein A. Clinical epidemiology: the architecture of clinical research. Philadelphia: WB Saunders, 1985:184.
7. Bliss CI. Statistics in biology: statistical methods for research in the natural sciences. Vol 1. New York: McGraw-Hill, 1967.
8. Tos M, Stangerup S-E, Holm-Jensen S, Sørensen CH. Spontaneous course of secretory otitis media and changes of the eardrum. Arch Otolaryngol 1984; 110:281–289.
9. Todd NW, Martin WS. Relationship of eustachian bony landmarks and temporal bone pneumatization. Ann Otol Rhinol Laryngol 1988; 97(3), in press.
10. Magnuson B, Falk B. Diagnosis and management of eustachian tube malfunction. Otolaryngol Clin North Am 1984; 17:659–671.

EPIDEMIOLOGY AND NATURAL HISTORY OF SECRETORY OTITIS

MIRKO TOS, M.D., SVEN-ERIC STANGERUP, M.D., G. HVID, M.D., and U. K. ANDREASSEN, M.D.

We wish to present an up to date report on the point prevalence, incidence, period prevalence, and spontaneous remission of secretory otitis, as determined by tympanometric screening in healthy children. Since 1977 we performed a total of 36 screenings in three randomized cohorts of healthy

children. The first cohort was observed from birth to the age of 8 years, the second from ages 2 to 9 years, and the third from ages 4 to 10 years.

The epidemiologic results in the first tympanometric screenings have been published previously for each cohort.[1-6] These results are dealt with here in summary form. The results of the most recent screenings have not been published previously nor have the calculations of the period prevalences.

Tympanometry as a diagnostic tool for screening children was introduced by Brooks[7] and has since been employed mainly in Scandinavia. In Göteborg, Sweden the prevalence of type B tympanograms was 2 percent among 7 year old children and 0.5 percent among 10 year old children.[8] In Denmark the point prevalence of type B tympanograms was 9 percent at age 3 years, 8 percent at age 6 years, and 3 percent at age 11 years.[9]

Owing to considerations of space, only the most conspicuous figures are presented here; some of them have already been discussed elsewhere.[1-6]

MATERIAL AND METHOD

Cohort I

This cohort originally comprised 150 newborn children who were born in the maternity ward of the Gentofte Hospital from January to April 1977.[1,5,6] During the first 2 years we performed screenings every third month and later once every year. At the fifteenth trial in 1985 the children were 8 years of age, but by this time the cohort had been reduced by 50 percent.

Cohort II

This cohort originally consisted of 278 otherwise healthy 2 year old children, born during the first 10 days of every month in 1976 in two municipalities of Copenhagen County (Gentofte and Ballerup), comprising 120,000 inhabitants.[2,3,5,6]

At the first examination in November 1977 the oldest children were almost 2 years of age; the youngest (born in November and December 1976) were just under 1 year old. The first four screenings were performed at 3 month intervals, the fifth screening took place 6 months later, and thereafter tympanometry was repeated annually until the eleventh screening when the children were 9 years old.

Cohort III

This cohort originally comprised 373 otherwise healthy children born during the first 10 days of every month in 1975 in two other municipalities of Copenhagen County (Gentofte and Gladsaxe), comprising 130,000 inhabitants.[4-6] At the first trial in February 1979 the youngest children of the cohort, born in December 1975, were just over 3 years old, whereas those born in January 1975 were almost 4 years old. The first five screenings were performed at 3 month intervals; since then the screenings were performed annually. At the tenth screening in 1985 the children were 10 years old and 63 percent of the original cohort attended this examination.

Each examination included tympanometry, using a Madsen ZO 70 tympanometer at a frequency of 220 Hz; otoscopy, using Siegle's speculum when necessary; and, at the annual examinations, otomicroscopy.

For practical reasons the middle ear pressures were divided into type A (0 to -99 mm H_2O), type C_1 (-100 to -199 mm H_2O), type C_2 (-200 to -350 mm H_2O), and type B (a flat curve without an impedance minimum).

RESULTS

Point Prevalence of Secretory Otitis

The point prevalence is the percentage of ears with a type B tympanogram in a given cohort at a given point in time. In cohort I normal typanmanometric conditions were found at birth; thus, only one ear showed a pressure of -125 mm H_2O.[1] Later the tympanometric conditions gradually deteriorated, and at 12 months secretory otitis was demonstrated in 13 percent of the ears (Table 1). The main reasons for the deterioration of the tympanometric conditions during the first year of life are catarrh and upper respiratory tract infections. At ages 2, 3 (cohorts I and II), and 4 years (cohort III) the point prevalence ranged from 7 to 19 percent. At ages 5 and 6 the point prevalence was still high, whereas at age 7 years it dropped to about 7 percent and to 2 to 4 percent at ages 8 to 10 years. This age dependent improvement of the tympanometric conditions after the age of 7 years is also illustrated by the increasing percentage of ears with a type A tympanogram, which did not exceed 50 percent before the age of 7 years (Table 1).

Spontaneous Remission of Secretory Otitis

About 50 percent of the ears changed tympanometric type between each of the examinations per-

TABLE 1 Point Prevalence of Secretory Otitis and Distribution of Tympanogram Types in Three Different Cohorts of Randomized, Otherwise Healthy Children

Cohort No	Screening No	Age	Time of Tympanometry		No of Ears	A	C_1	C_2	B	X^2 Test
I	1	2–4 days	January–February	1977	300	90	10	—	—	
	2	3 months	May	1977	252	82	17	1	—	$p<0.001$
	2	6 months	August	1977	238	62	27	10	1	
	2	9 months	November	1977	236	47	38	11	4	
	5	12 months	February	1978	206	40	28	19	13	$p<0.001$
	6	15 months	May	1978	132	43	24	19	14	
	7	18 months	August	1978	132	45	28	15	12	
	8	21 months	November	1978	132	42	20	19	19	
	9	24 months	February	1979	132	39	26	21	14	
	10	3 years	February	1980	170	26	28	38	9	$p<0.001$
	11	4 years	February	1981	144	20	35	27	17	
	12	5 years	February	1982	124	40	28	19	13	
	13	6 years	February	1983	106	37	26	34	3	$p<0.001$
	14	7 years	February	1984	154	61	27	8	4	
	15	8 years	February	1985	148	65	28	10	3	
II	1	2 years	November	1977	556	50	19	20	11	
	2		February	1978	508	47	18	20	14	$p<0.001$
	3		May	1978	480	52	22	15	11	
	4		August	1978	440	64	19	11	7	$p<0.001$
	5	3 years	February	1979	404	47	24	18	11	
	6	4 years	February	1980	368	37	22	27	14	
	7	5 years	February	1981	280	37	22	29	11	
	8	6 years	February	1982	254	43	24	24	9	
	9	7 years	February	1983	230	51	26	17	7	$p<0.001$
	10	8 years	February	1984	250	78	16	4	2	
	11	9 years	February	1985	262	63	27	8	2	
III	1	4 years	February	1979	746	36	21	29	14	$p<0.001$
	2		May	1979	670	41	25	23	11	
	3		August	1979	666	38	29	23	10	
	4		November	1979	576	32	31	23	14	$p<0.001$
	5	5 years	February	1980	628	27	25	31	18	
	6	6 years	February	1981	538	30	27	28	14	$p<0.001$
	7	7 years	February	1982	590	43	23	27	7	
	8	8 years	February	1983	412	50	28	18	4	
	9	9 years	February	1984	406	61	22	15	3	$p<0.001$
	10	10 years	February	1985	470	67	19	12	2	

formed every 3 months (Table 2); in some ears the type improved and in others it deteriorated.

As part of the general improvement of the tympanometric conditions, the type B tympanograms improved in about 50 percent of the ears during a period of 3 months (see Table 2). The extent of improvement was dependent upon the season of the year and the age of the child. During the first year of life, however, there was improvement in the tympanometric type in only 20 to 30 percent of the ears. More common at this age was a deterioration in the tympanometric type; e.g., type C deteriorated to type B and did not improve before the end of the second year of life. In cohort II spontaneous remission was demonstrated in a considerable number of ears from February to May and from May to August in 1978, when improvement was demonstrated in 76 percent of ears with a type B tympanogram. In cohorts II and III, 50 percent of the type B tympanograms improved during the winter months, i.e., from the examination in November to the one in February.

Spontaneous remission was common among children aged 6 to 10 years, at times reaching 80 percent. However, at these ages the interval between trials was 1 year (see Table 2). Spontaneous improvement in a type B tympanogram usually occurred via type C_2 or C_1, but recurrence of type B did occur.

TABLE 2 Improvement to a Better Type and Deterioration to a Worse Type in Different Evaluations of the Three Series in Table 1

Cohort and Time of Evaluation	Period	All Types			Type B Only Improved
		Improved (%)	Deteriorated (%)	Unchanged (%)	
I. February to May 77	3 months	1	23	76	—
May to August 77	3 months	12	32	56	—
August to November 77	3 months	17	33	51	25
November 77 to February 78	3 months	17	35	48	18
February to May 78	3 months	23	30	47	27
May to August 78	3 months	23	19	58	38
August to November 78	3 months	17	33	50	19
November 78 to February 79	3 months	21	23	56	44
February 79 to February 80	1 year	19	34	47	58
February 80 to February 81	1 year	27	27	46	47
February 81 to February 82	1 year	53	19	28	78
February 82 to February 83	1 year	34	35	31	90
February 83 to February 84	1 year	40	10	49	67
February 84 to February 85	1 year	22	18	59	50
II. November 77 to February 78	3 months	26	26	48	50
February 78 to May 78	3 months	30	18	52	63
May 78 to August 78	3 months	30	18	52	76
August 78 to February 79	6 months	16	35	50	48
February 79 to February 80	1 year	20	36	44	58
February 80 to February 81	1 year	24	26	50	59
February 81 to February 82	1 year	35	24	40	58
February 82 to February 83	1 year	32	21	47	63
February 83 to February 84	1 year	49	6	46	100
February 84 to February 85	1 year	12	33	55	40
III. February 79 to May 79	3 months	32	21	47	59
May 79 to August 79	3 months	25	27	48	39
August 79 to November 79	3 months	20	32	49	27
November 79 to February 80	3 months	23	36	41	46
February 80 to February 81	1 year	42	22	36	55
February 81 to February 82	1 year	46	17	38	84
February 82 to February 83	1 year	35	22	43	75
February 83 to February 84	1 year	32	22	46	77
February 84 to February 85	1 year	26	19	55	67

The relatively high point prevalence incidences of secretory otitis included ears that were type B for an extended period of time (i.e., already type B at the preceding trial), "new" ears in which the condition recently deteriorated to type B, and finally ears with recurrence of a type B tympanogram (see Table 1).

Period Prevalence

The period prevalence incidence indicates the percentage of ears with secretory otitis during a given period of time. The calculation of the period prevalence was based on the children who attended all trials. In cohort I, 14 percent of the ears had type B curves at the five screenings performed during the first year of life (Table 3), 44 percent of the ears had type B curves at the 11 screenings performed during the first 4 years, and 44 percent of the ears had type B curves at the 15 trials performed during the entire period of 8 years.

In cohort II, in children aged 2 years, the period prevalence incidence was 28.6 percent for a period of 9 months, covering four screenings at 3 month intervals. At six screenings from ages 2 to 4 years the period prevalence was 39 percent, and at 11 screenings from ages 2 to 7 years it was 42.5 percent (see Table 3).

The calculation of the period prevalence was valid only for the periods during which tympanometry was performed every third month. For the

TABLE 3 Prevalence of Type B in Different Evaluations in Three Cohorts of Children

Type B at Number of Screenings	Cohort and Number of Screenings and Age Period							
	I 1–5 0–1 No = 180 %	I 1–11 0–4 No = 132 %	I 1–15 0–8 No = 100 %	II 1–4 2–3 No = 444 %	II 1–6 2–4 No = 368 %	II 1–11 2–9 No = 212 %	III 1–5 5–6 No = 576 %	III 1–10 4–10 No = 382 %
B at one	11.1	22.7	25.0	18.2	21.7	18.9	16.7	18.9
B at two	2.0	6.8	9.0	5.4	7.1	10.4	5.5	6.8
B at three	1.3	3.8	6.0	3.4	4.1	6.1	2.3	2.9
B at four		3.0	2.0	1.6	3.8	2.8	4.5	3.4
B at five		2.3	0.0		1.9	2.4	3.1	2.4
B at six		3.0	1.0		0.3	1.4		2.4
B at seven		0.8	1.0			0.0		1.1
B at eight						0.0		0.3
B at nine		1.5				0.5		0.3
B at ten						0.0		0.0
At at least one	14.4	43.9	44.0	28.6	38.9	42.5	32.1	38.5

children of the older age groups who were subjected to annual trials, only the point prevalence for the individual age group could be calculated (Table 1). In view of the fact that most cases of type B curves in the older age groups were recurrent cases, the period prevalence incidence was not markedly affected by the number of annual screenings in children aged 6 to 10 years (Table 3). However, the actual number of ears showing a type B tympanogram at more than one trial increased (Table 3).

Although many children suffered from secretory otitis, only relatively few ears were associated with prolonged disease. In all three cohorts the majority of ears had type B tympanograms at less than four screenings (Table 3).

When we evaluated the cohorts on the basis of the period prevalence incidences of type B or C_2 (Table 4), matters appeared more serious. In all three cohorts almost 80 percent of all the ears had type B or C_2 curves at least once and 20 to 30 percent had type B or C_2 curves at more than five trials. These protracted cases represent ears with type B tympanograms that improved to type C_2 only to deteriorate again to type B, or ears with type C_2 for an extended period of time without demonstration of type B.

TABLE 4 Prevalence of Type B or C at Different Screenings in Three Cohorts of Children

Type B at Number of Screenings	Cohort and Number of Screenings and Age Period					
	I 1–11 0–14 No = 132 %	I 1–15 0–8 No = 100 %	II 1–6 2–4 No = 368 %	II 1–11 2–9 No = 212 %	III 1–5 4–5 No = 576 %	III 1–10 4–10 No = 382 %
B or C_2 at one	20.5	18.0	23.6	24.1	24.1	15.7
B or C_2 at two	12.1	22.0	14.1	13.2	14.2	13.1
B or C_2 at three	17.4	15.0	12.2	14.2	11.5	11.8
B or C_2 at four	10.6	16.0	11.1	9.4	10.4	9.7
B or C_2 at five	5.3	8.0	5.2	8.0	13.2	9.4
B or C_2 at six	5.3	4.0	3.3	4.7		6.3
B or C_2 at seven	4.5	3.0		3.8		6.0
B or C_2 at eight	1.5	1.0		2.8		5.2
B or C_2 at nine	1.5	0.0		1.4		3.7
B or C_2 at 10	0.0	0.0		0.0		1.6
B or C_2 at 11	0.0	0.0		0.5		0.0
At at least one	78.7	87.0	69.5	82.1	73.4	82.5

REFERENCES

1. Tos M, Poulsen G, Hancke AB. Screening tympanometry during the first year of life. Acta Otolaryngol 1979; 88:388–394.
2. Tos M, Poulsen G, Borch J. Tympanometry in two-year-old children. ORL J Otorhinolaryngol Relat Spec 1978; 40:77–85.
3. Tos M. Spontaneous improvement of secretory otitis and impedance screening. Arch Otolaryngol 1980; 106:345–349.
4. Tos M, Holm-Jensen S, Sørensen CH, Mogensen C. Spontaneous course and frequency of secretory otitis in four-year-old children. Arch Otolaryngol 1982; 108:4–10.
5. Tos M. Epidemiology and spontaneous improvement of secretory otitis. Acta Otorhinolaryngol Belg 1983; 37:31–43.
6. Tos M, Stangerup S-E, Hvid G, Andreassen UK,Thomsen J. Epidemiology of natural history of secretory otitis. In: Sade J, ed. Acute and secretory otitis media. Amsterdam: Kugler, 1986:95.
7. Brooks DN. An objective method of detecting fluid in the middle ear. Int Audiol 1968; 7:280–286.
8. Renvall U, Liden G, Jungert S, Nilsson E. Impedance audiometry in the detection of secretory otitis media. Scand Audiol 1975;4:119–124.
9. Fiellau-Nikolajsen M, Lous J, Pedersen SV, Schousboe HH. Tympanometry in the three-year-old children (I). Scand Audiol 1977; 6:199–204.

PROGRESSION OF DRUM PATHOLOGY FOLLOWING SECRETORY OTITIS MEDIA

PER L. LARSEN, M.D., MIRKO TOS, M.D., and SVEN-ERIC STANGERUP, M.D.

Epidemiologic studies with repetitive tympanometry in otherwise healthy Danish children aged 1 to 10 years showed that about 80 percent of the children had had at least one episode of secretory otitis media. About 30 percent had protracted episodes (exceeding 3 months), and approximately 10 percent experienced a prolonged course of disease (1 to 4 years).[1] Repetitive otomicroscopy in the same children revealed changes of the tympanic membrane in about one third of the cases.[2] These changes were particularly frequent in children who sustained long lasting or recurrent episodes of secretory otitis media. Several studies have shown that tympanic membrane changes develop in 25 to 60 percent of the children treated for secretory otitis media. The changes derive partly from treatment of the disease and partly from protracted episodes of secretory otitis media.[3-7]

Much knowledge has been gathered about tympanic membrane changes and their progression in children. Their further development, however, and identification of the cases that may result in chronic otitis media in adults are not fully understood. To elucidate these matters, we performed follow-up examinations in children who had been treated for secretory otitis from 1967 to 1974. The first re-evaluation was carried out in 1974 and the second in 1985, i.e., 11 to 18 years after treatment. The median ages of the children at the follow-up examinations were 4 and 20 years, respectively. The tympanic membrane changes were observed over a period of 16 years. This long observation period exceeds that of most studies hitherto performed.

PATIENTS AND METHODS

The present series consisted of 220 children (372 ears) who were treated by the insertion of grommets and adenoidectomy for secretory otitis media during the period 1967 to 1974. Follow-up was conducted in 1974 and again in 1985. A total of 103 patients (47 percent) attended the last follow-up. Of the 117 nonattenders, 55 could not be traced, 48 did not appear for examination, 11 had moved abroad, and 3 had died. Tympanometry and otomicroscopy were performed at both follow-up examinations, and all alterations of the tympanic membranes were thoroughly recorded. The nonattenders did not differ from those attending in regard to attic retractions, tensa disease, and tympanometric findings (McNemar's test). The median observation time was 5 years at the first follow-up (range, 0.5 to 7 years) and 16 years at the second (range, 11 to 18 years).

RESULTS

Comparison of eardrum changes recorded at the first and second follow-up examinations revealed a statistically significant deterioration (p <0.01, X^2 test). Eardrum disease was demonstrated in 47 percent of the children at the first examination and in 63 percent at the second. Comparison with the randomized cohorts of otherwise healthy children also revealed statistically significant differences (p<0.001, X^2 test; Table 1). Tympanosclerosis and atrophy accounted for the most frequent alterations of the tympanic membrane, a finding in accord with previous studies.[8] Further types of change included those in the attic and the pars tensa.

Attic Retractions

Attic retractions were divided into four types:[9] A type I retraction denoted a slight retraction with air still present between Shrapnell's membrane and the neck of the malleus. A type II retraction indicated that the retraction had reached the neck of the malleus and might be adherent to it. A type III retraction reached behind the bony annulus, which might be slightly resorbed. Type IV indicated a large retraction; the membrane lay against the neck of the malleus and a part of the malleus head. The bottom of the retraction pocket was still visible. There was extensive resorption of the bony annulus.

In attic cholesteatoma the retraction pocket is filled with a whitish mass. The bottom of the retraction cannot be surveyed, even after thorough cleaning. An attic retraction was found in 36 percent of the ears at the second follow-up. This is significantly different from findings in cohort studies of otherwise healthy children (p <0.001, Mann-Whitney test; Table 2). Severe retractions, i.e., types III and

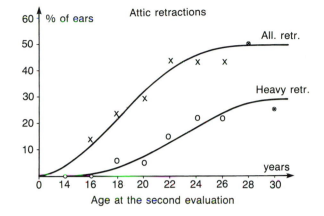

Figure 1 Relation between number of attic retractions and the age of the patient at the second follow-up.

IV with resorption of the bony annulus, were demonstrated in 6 percent of the ears. Attic cholesteatoma occurred in three patients (1.7 percent of the ears), and the diagnosis was confirmed at surgery. A correlation analysis of retraction type and age at the second follow-up showed the fewest and slightest retractions among the youngest patients, aged 14 to 20 years (Fig. 1); compared with the results in other age groups, 21 to 25 years and 26 to 30 years, a significant difference was found between the youngest and oldest groups of patients (p <0.005, Mann-Whitney test).

Changes in the Pars Tensa

Changes in the pars tensa included tympanosclerosis and atrophy.[10] In tympanosclerotic ears there was hyalin degeneration of the fibrous and elastic fibers, and the tympanic membrane was whitish, thickened, and rigid. In atrophic ears the lamina propria contained a reduced number of fibrous and

TABLE 1 Eardrum Disease in Secretory Otitis Media 11 to 18 Years After Treatment with Grommets and Adenoidectomy, Compared with a Randomized Cohort of Otherwise Healthy Children

		Cohort Age	
Eardrum Disease	Treated Secretory Otitis media, 11–18 Years Postop. (n = 178) %	5 Years (n = 444) %	10 Years (n = 470) %
Attic only (8)	4.5	14.9	14.7
Attic and tensa (56)	31.5	3.1	11.7
Tensa only (48)	27.0	5.7	6.4
Total cases (112)	63.0	23.7	32.8
X^2 test	p < 0.001	p < 0.01	

TABLE 2 Types of Retraction in Secretory Otitis Media 11 to 18 Years After Treatment with Grommets and Adenoidectomy, Compared with a Randomized Cohort of Otherwise Healthy Children

Type of Retraction	Treated Secretory Otitis Media 11–18 Years Postop. (n = 178) %	Randomized Cohort Age	
		5 Years (n = 444) %	10 Years (n = 470) %
I	13.5	9.2	10.6
II	14.6	7.1	11.1
III	4.5	1.1	4.3
IV	1.7	0.7	0.4
Attic cholesteatoma	1.7	-	-
Total	36.0	18.0	26.4
Mann-Whitney test	$p < 0.001$	$p < 0.01$	

elastic fibers, and the eardrum was pellucid, thin, and slack. Often a combination of tympanosclerosis and atrophy occurred, and there were varying degrees of retraction of atrophic eardrums, such as myringoincudopexy, in which the eardrum lay against the incudostapedial joint, and myringostapediopexy, with resorption of the long leg of the incus and adhesion of the eardrum to the stapes (Fig. 2A). Adhesive otitis was characterized by an atrophic retracted eardrum adhering to the medial wall; in most cases the posterior part was adherent. Other findings included perforations (Fig. 2B), sinus cholesteatoma, and tensa retraction cholesteatoma.

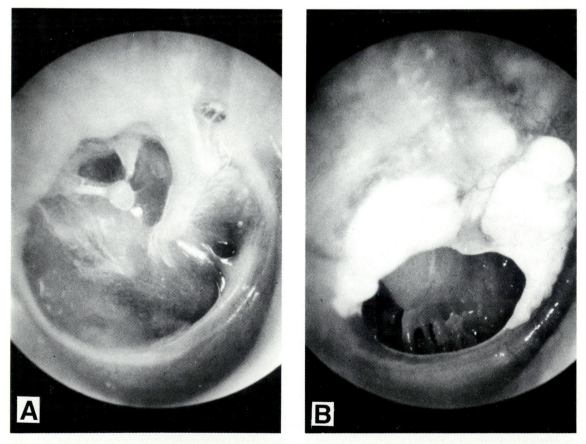

Figure 2 Changes in pars tensa. *A*, Myringostapediopexy. The long leg of the incus is resorbed and the eardrum adheres to the stapes. *B*, Perforation of a strongly tympanosclerotic eardrum.

There was a significant incidence of deterioration of the pars tensa, from 47.2 percent at the first follow-up visit to 58.4 percent at the second ($p < 0.05$, Mann-Whitney test; Table 3). The most conspicuous changes occurred in the ears with atrophy (Fig. 3), which relatively often at the second follow-up visit showed a deterioration to fixation, adhesive otitis, and perforation. The number of ears with atrophy and fixation as well as adhesive otitis (i.e., the most severe changes) increased markedly between the first and second follow-up examinations. However, even in these severely afflicted groups, improvement did occur—in one case, even normalization (see Fig. 3). Perforations were demonstrated

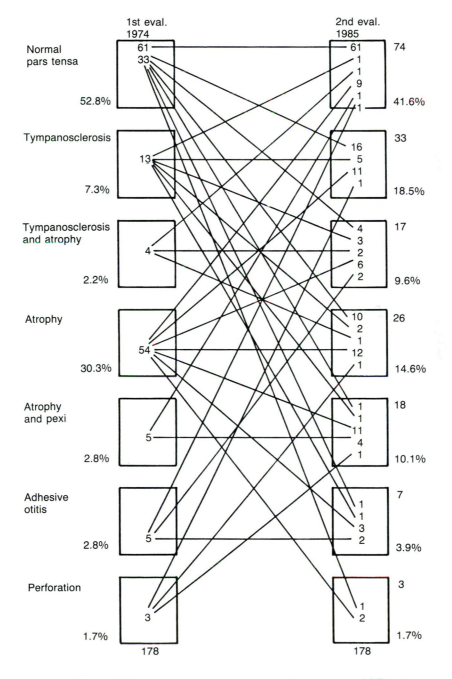

Figure 3 Changes in the pars tensa from the first to the second follow-up.

TABLE 3 Pathologic Changes in the Pars Tensa 6 Months to 7 Years and 11 to 18 Years After Treatment for Secretory Otitis Media, Compared with a Randomized Cohort of Children Ages 5 and 10 Years

	Treated Secretory Otitis		*Randomized Cohort*	
	0.6—7 Years	*11—18 Years*		
	After Surgery	*After Surgery*	*5 Years*	*10 Years*
Disease of Pars Tensa	*(n = 178), %*	*(N = 178), %*	*(n = 444), %*	*(n = 470), %*
Tympanosclerosis	7.3	18.5	5.6	5.1
Tympanosclerosis and atrophy	2.2	9.6	2.0	2.3
Atrophy	30.3	14.6	2.5	8.1
Atrophy and fixation	2.8	10.1	0.7	2.3
Adhesive otitis	2.8	3.9	-	-
Perforation	1.7*	1.7	0.2	0.2
Abnormal pars tensa	47.2	58.4	8.8	18.0
Mann-Whitney test	$p < 0.05$			
		$p < 0.001$		$p < 0.01$

* All three perforations closed by tympanoplasty.

in three ears at the first follow-up (see Table 3), and tympanoplasty was performed in all three cases. At the second follow-up, perforations were found in three other ears. Two of these showed atrophy at the first follow-up, whereas a normal pars tensa was found in the last case (see Fig. 3).

DISCUSSION

The present series showed a considerably higher incidence of tensa changes and attic retractions than that found in studies of randomized cohorts of otherwise healthy children ($p < 0.01$, Mann-Whitney test; see Table 3), although the latter did show a considerable progression of changes of the pars tensa from age 5 to 10 years ($p < 0.01$, Mann-Whitney test). This was particularly pronounced in the group with atrophy and in the group with atrophy and fixation (see Table 3).

It has been shown that the slightest eardrum changes, such as local patches of tympanosclerosis and atrophy, may heal spontaneously.[8] However, in case of the smallest changes, the evaluation may be influenced by interobserver variability as well as by intraobserver variability.

Although normalization appears to be possible in a few ears with severe changes of the pars tensa (see Fig. 3), the general finding in our study was progression of the condition from the first to the se-

cond follow-up examination. The longer the observation time, the higher the incidence of eardrum changes.

The changes described herein resemble those seen in patients with chronic otitis media, and secretory otitis media thus appears to be an important predisposing factor in chronic otitis media.

REFERENCES

1. Tos M. Epidemiology and natural history of secretory otitis. Am J Otol 1984; 5:459–462.
2. Tos M, Hvid G, Stangerup S-E, Andreassen UK. Prevalence and progression of sequelae after secretory otitis. Ann Otol Rhinol (in press).
3. Kokko E. Chronic secretory otitis media in children. Acta Otolaryngol (Suppl) 1975; 327:7–44.
4. Kilby D, Richards SH, Hart G. Grommets and glue ears. Two-years results. J Laryngol 1972; 86:881–888.
5. Bonding P, Lorenzen E. Cicatricial changes of the eardrum after treatment with grommets. Acta Otolaryngol 1973; 75:275–276.
6. Barfoed C, Rosborg J. Secretory otitis media. Arch Otolaryngol 1980; 106:553–556.
7. Lildholdt T. Ventilation tubes in secretory otitis media. Acta Otolaryngol (Suppl) 1983; 398:1–30.
8. Tos M, Stangerup S-E, Holm-Jensen S, Sørensen CH. Spontaneous course of secretory otitis and changes of the eardrum. Arch Otolaryngol 1984; 110:281–289.
9. Tos M, Poulsen G. Attic retractions following secretory otitis. Acta Otolaryngol 1980; 89:217–222.
10. Tos M, Poulsen G. Changes of pars tensa after secretory otitis. ORL J Otorhinolaryngol Relat Spec 1979; 41:313–328.

LONG TERM FOLLOW-UP OF CHILDREN WITH OTITIS MEDIA WITH EFFUSION

MAKOTO SAKAI, M.D., F.A.C.S., KEIJIRO KOGA, M.D., NOBUKO KAWASHIRO, M.D., AKIO ARAKI, M.D., and YUKIHIKO MORIKAWA, M.D.

The course of otitis media with effusion varies greatly among individual children. A short minor episode of hearing impairment is hardly enough to bring a child to an otolaryngologist, but some patients seek otologic treatment because of a protracted course or recurrent episodes throughout childhood. Our aims in this study were to define the important prognostic variables in regard to the outcome of the disease and to identify signs, symptoms, duration of disease, tympanographic patterns, and other factors affecting the severity of the disease during the course of treatment. We also studied appropriate modalities of treatment, including myringotomy with and without insertion of a tympanostomy tube, in children with otitis media with effusion.

MATERIALS AND METHODS

This study comprised 87 children (59 boys and 28 girls between the ages of 3 and 8 at the initial visit) who had symptoms and clinical findings of otitis media with effusion. All had been treated only by myringotomy followed by 4 days' administration of oral doses of amoxicillin; they or their parents had refused other procedures such as insertion of a tympanostomy tube or adenoidectomy. Seven improved before myringotomy was performed, and seven others failed to appear for follow-up examinations for more than 6 months. The remaining 73 eligible cases were divided into two groups according to the duration of the disease from the initial visit to the time of cure.

In the early cure group patients were cured within 2 years; the late cure or intractable group required more than 2 years of treatment (Table 1). Cure was defined as one winter season without any symptoms, abnormal otoscopic findings, or type B tympanographic findings after the initiation of treatment.

All patients were examined once every 1 or 2 months at outpatient clinic visits when otoscopic examination, pure tone audiometry, and tympanometry were carried out. Diagnostic myringotomy was performed if it was necessary to confirm the presence of effusion in the middle ear cavity.

Computer analysis of the clinical data was performed to correlate the duration of the disease with symptoms and test findings. The early cure group comprised 82 ears in 43 children and the late cure group, 54 ears in 30 children. Multivariable statistical analysis was performed by entering the data regarding clinical features for the following: age at the initial visit, hearing level at the initial visit, the time required for tympanographic findings to improve from type B to type A or C, and the frequency of myringotomy throughout treatment.

RESULTS

The age at the initial visit in the majority of children with otitis media with effusion was 4 years. The ages at the time of cure, on the other hand, ranged from 2 to 14 years, mostly at ages 6 to 10. There was no difference in age distribution between the early and late cure groups.

The mean air conduction hearing level at the initial visit was compared in the early and late cure groups, and the hearing level was 5 db higher at 1,000 and 2,000 Hz and 5 db lower at 4,000 Hz in the early cure group than in the late cure group.

TABLE 1 Number of Children and Duration of Disease

Male	59	67.8%
Female	28	32.2%
Total	87	
	7	Not followed
	7	Cured without myringotomy
Eligible	73	
	43	Cured within 2 years (early cure group)
	30	Cured after 2 years (late cure group)

However, there was no difference in mean hearing levels at the other frequencies, and no statistical difference was found between the groups.

In the early cure group 106 myringotomies were performed, and the average frequency was 1.2 times per ear. In the late cure group 272 myringotomies were performed, and the average was 3.7 times per ear. A higher frequency of myringotomy in 1 treatment year was found in the early cure group. However, the frequency of myringotomy in the late cure group was greater than that in the early cure group; this finding was not statistically significant.

In 82 ears in the early cure group, 46 myringotomy procedures 1½ months after the initial visit disclosed the presence of middle ear effusion. Of the 46 ears, 14 showed effusion in the following 1½ months, and myringotomy at the end of 5 months of treatment showed only four ears to be positive for effusion. Thus almost 90 percent of the ears with effusion at the initial visit and in the following 1½ months showed no further effusion 5 months after the initiation of treatment. In 54 ears in the late cure group, 89 myringotomies were performed at the initial visit, and in the following 6 months middle ear effusion developed. However, 38 ears were positive for effusion after 6 months; then the number of ears positive for middle ear effusion gradually decreased. Thus, even in the late cure group, almost 90 percent of the ears had no effusion within 3 years after the initial visit.

In studying improvement in the tympanogram from type B to type A or C in the early cure group of 82 ears, 49 cases were analyzed. Improvement in the tympanogram was found in 36 ears, or 73.5 percent of the cases, within 4 months of treatment (Fig. 1). On the other hand, in 48 of the 54 ears of the late cure group, there were only 27 ears (56.6 percent) in which tympanographic evidence of improvement was found within 6 months of treatment (Fig. 2).

A relative increase in the number of ears showing tympanographic evidence of improvement was found within 3 months after the initial visit in the early cure group, but such an increase was noted only after 2 to 3 years of treatment in the late cure group. This tendency coincided with a decrease in middle ear effusion.

DISCUSSION

Otitis media with effusion is the greatest health problem among young children. There have been numerous publications regarding the natural history and risk factors in this disease, and over the last decade we have become increasingly familiar with the epidemiology of otitis media with effusion. However, there are still many unsolved problems, particularly in regard to management of the disease. If we could foresee the results of treatment in the early stage of the disease, the appropriate modality of treatment could be selected in individual cases. We have been trying to elucidate the important diagnostic variables contributing to the prognosis of the disease.

Gates et al[1] conducted a randomized clinical trial with four treatment modalities: myringotomy with and without adenoidectomy and use of a tympanostomy tube with and without adenoidectomy. Then he analyzed the major independent variables

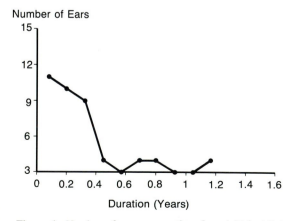

Figure 1 Number of ears versus time from initial visit to tympanographic evidence of improvement (from type B to type A or C) in the early cure group.

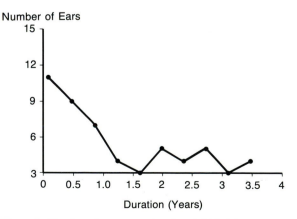

Figure 2 Number of ears versus time from initial visit to tympanographic evidence of improvement (from type B to type A or C) in the late cure group.

such as age, sex, race, family history of otitis media, allergy, and type of middle ear effusion to predict whether a patient might fall into the groups not requiring further surgery after myringotomy. They failed to find any variables showing a statistical relationship with the clinical outcome. However, this study did not incorporate changes in tympanographic pattern as a variable.

Tos et al[2] performed a cohort study of otitis media with effusion and investigated the natural history of the disease in terms of changes in tympanogram types over the course of the disease. They concluded that short but recurring episodes of 1 to 6 months' duration occurred in about 25 percent of the ears, and the prognosis in this group was satisfactory.

In our study 73.5 percent of the children in the early cure group showed improvement in tympanographic patterns within 4 months of treatment, and 56.6 percent of those in the late cure group improved within 6 months of treatment. Both groups were treated with myringotomy with antibiotics, but no further surgical intervention was required during the course of the disease. Therefore, when there is improvement in the tympanographic pattern from type B to type A or C within 4 months of treatment, the patient can be treated by myringotomy and antibiotics. The prognosis is most likely to be favorable and the disease most likely will be cured within 2 years after the initiation of treatment.

CONCLUSION

If a patient with otitis media with effusion shows improvement in tympanogram type B to type A or C within 4 months of treatment, he can be treated only with myringotomy and antibiotics and most likely will be cured within 2 years of the initial visit.

The age at the initial visit, the hearing level at the initial visit, and the frequency of myringotomy have no correlation with the prognosis of the disease.

The age at the time of cure in this study was usually about 10 years.

REFERENCES

1. Gates GA, Wachtendorf C, Hearne EM, Holt GR. Treatment of chronic otitis media with effusion: results of myringotomy. Auris Nasus Larynx 1985; 12(Suppl 1):262-264.
2. Tos M, Stangerup S-E, Andreassen UK, Hvid G, Thomsen J, Holm-Jensen S. Natural history of secretory otitis media. In: Lim DJ, Bluestone CD, Klein JO, Nelson JD, eds. Recent advances in otitis media with effusion. Proceedings of the Third International Symposium. Toronto: BC Decker, 1984: 36-40.

SCREENING AND DIAGNOSIS

METHODOLOGIC ISSUES IN SCREENING FOR OTITIS MEDIA

HOWARD E. ROCKETTE, Ph.D. and MARGARETHA L. CASSELBRANT, M.D., Ph.D.

There has been extensive discussion in the literature in regard to screening for otitis media with effusion.[1-3] Our objective here is to discuss methodologic issues in screening, emphasizing aspects that are different in otitis media with effusion from those that occur in screening for other diseases. Also, some problems that have been discussed previously in general terms will be quantified.

Among the problems of screening for any disease are variations in methods of diagnosis, identification of a high risk group, control of an excessive number of false positive responses, determination of whether early diagnosis is beneficial to the patient, and evaluation of cost versus benefit. Methods of diagnosis suggested for screening for otitis media with effusion include tympanometry, acoustic reflex testing, pure tone audiometry, pneumatoscopy, and a combination of these methods.[3-5] Although this aspect of screening is important and each method has differing accuracy and cost, a comparison of the benefits of different methods of diagnosis will not be addressed in this discussion. Instead we will discuss methodologic issues of screening that are relevant regardless of which of these diagnostic methods one decides to use.

The identification of a high risk group is desirable in a screening program, since it is more efficient to concentrate resources on groups that are most likely to have disease. However, it is often not recognized that screening for a disease with a low prevalence may result in an unacceptably high number of people that are falsely identified as having the disease. The percentage of false positive cases that are identified is a function of the prevalence of the disease and the accuracy of the diagnostic technique. Accuracy is usually determined by the sensitivity and specificity. Sensitivity is defined to be the probability of correctly diagnosing an individual with the disease, and specificity is the probability of correctly diagnosing an individual without the disease.

Table 1 summarizes the percentage of false posi-

TABLE 1 Percentage of False Positive Results as a Function of Prevalence*

Prevalence (%)	False Positive (%)
1	94
5	75
10	59
15	47
20	39
50	14

* Sensitivity = 0.95; specificity = 0.85.

tive cases as a function of the prevalence, assuming that a diagnostic technique has a 0.95 sensitivity and a 0.85 specificity. Even though these values of sensitivity and specificity are probably optimistic as indicators of diagnostic accuracy in screening for otitis media with effusion,[1,6,7] if the prevalence were 15 percent, approximately half the patients diagnosed as positive would not have the disease.

One of the problems that has been ignored in discussions of screening programs for otitis media with effusion is that the sensitivity and specificity of diagnostic techniques have been determined by ear and not by child. Table 2 summarizes the sensitivity and specificity in diagnosing a child for selected sensitivities and specificities for an ear, assuming that the incidences of error in the two ears are independent. If at least one ear were required to be positive in order to classify the child as positive, the sensitivity for the child would increase but the specificity would decrease. This decreased specificity would increase the percentage of false positive cases beyond those shown in Table 1.

For example, an ear diagnosis that has a 0.95 sensitivity and a 0.85 specificity would have a 0.998 sensitivity and a 0.72 specificity for the child, and a disease prevalence of 20 percent would result in 53 percent false positives. One way to overcome such a lowering of the specificity is to require both ears to be positive before one considers the child to be

TABLE 2 Sensitivity and Specificity of Diagnosing Otitis Media with Effusion in a Child with Bilateral or Unilateral Disease Given Accuracy of Diagnosis by Ear

Ear		Child		
Sensitivity	Specificity	Sensitivity (Bilateral)	Sensitivity (Unilateral)	Specificity
0.90	0.75	0.99	0.92	0.56
0.90	0.80	0.99	0.92	0.64
0.90	0.85	0.99	0.92	0.72
0.95	0.75	0.99+	0.96	0.56
0.95	0.80	0.99+	0.96	0.64
0.95	0.85	0.99+	0.96	0.72

TABLE 3 Estimated Accuracy of Multiple Testing Assuming Effusion 50% of the Time*

No. Tests	No. Required Positive	Sensitivity	Specificity
1	1	0.55	0.85
2	1	0.80	0.72
	2	0.30	0.98
3	1	0.91	0.61
	2	0.57	0.94
	3	0.17	0.99+

* Sensitivity = 0.95; specificity = 0.85.

positive. Thus one is attempting to identify only bilaterally affected children. Assuming a 0.95 sensitivity and a 0.85 specificity by ear, requiring both ears to test positive lowers the sensitivity to 0.90 for a child with bilateral disease but the specificity for a child with no disease is 0.98. With such a strategy a disease prevalence of 20 percent would result in 8 percent false positives.

A second problem associated with the diagnosis of otitis media with effusion relates to the recurrent nature of the disease. During a specified period a child may not have the disease all the time. Thus, it may be desirable for the screening program to identify children who have disease a large percentage of the time. Several investigators have discussed screening in the context of multiple tests.[8–10] Unfortunately the accuracy of any diagnostic procedure in identifying such children is greatly reduced because of the possibility of screening when there is no disease.

For example, if one attempts to identify a child who has otitis media with effusion 50 percent of the time, assuming a 0.5 probability of screening the child when the disease is present, with a single test the sensitivity would be lowered from 95 to 55 percent. Although a low sensitivity can be improved by increasing the number of tests performed and requiring only one of several tests to be positive, such a strategy would result in a decrease in specificity. Table 3 summarizes the effect of various strategies of multiple screening on sensitivity and specificity.

The effect of the variability in the presence of fluid on the accuracy of diagnosis could be decreased from the magnitude indicated in Table 3 if additional information regarding the occurrence of otitis media with effusion were considered. For example, strategies that consider the effect of season on the disease or the pattern of disease occurrence in given populations would enable development of a strate-

gy that is more efficient in identifying individuals satisfying the definition of the disease.[10] However, such strategies might not be optimal or as efficient in a population different from the one in which the strategy was derived.

A major issue in determining whether a patient benefits by early diagnosis is the existence of an effective treatment. The extent to which earlier treatment affects the course of otitis media with effusion is still unclear. Furthermore, assessment of the benefit of treatment requires one to define benefit and leads naturally to the concept of a cost-benefit analysis. One of the aspects of otitis media that makes it different from many other diseases for which screening has been considered, is the lack of clarity in regard to measuring the benefit. One might evaluate the cost to the patient in money, the avoidance of more treatment later, earlier improvement in function (such as less time with impaired hearing loss), or the possibility of a long term effect on social development or IQ. In any cost-benefit analysis, false negative ascertainments (children who are falsely identified as disease free) as well as false positive identifications must be taken into account. Although the impact of otitis media with effusion on each of these measures of benefit is still subject to debate, even if agreement existed about the effect of otitis media on these parameters, it is unlikely that a single index could be accepted as the sole indicator of patient benefit. This is unlike the situation in screening for many chronic diseases in which improved survival of the patient is usually acknowledged as the primary patient benefit.

No positive statements can be made in regard to the complex problem of whether screening should or should not be done at this time. However, sufficient information exists about the relative efficacies of differing methods of treatment from large scale clinical trials and about the prevalence of disease from epidemiologic studies so that evaluations of various strategies could be made relative to the different measures of benefit. In cases in which no precise estimates are available, it is possible to estimate some range of factors, and a formal evaluation could probably eliminate certain screening strategies from consideration. For example, although one might not be able to decide whether screening is efficacious, one could eliminate certain procedures as being less advantageous than others under a wide range of possible scenarios, and thus make progress toward better understanding of the cost-benefit of screening programs.

This study was funded by the Otitis Media Research Center (NS 16337), Children's Hospital of Pittsburgh.

REFERENCES

1. Paradise JL, Smith CG. Impedance screening for preschool children—state of the art. Ann Otol Rhinol Laryngol 1979; 88:56–65.
2. Bluestone CD, Fria TJ, Arjona SK, Casselbrant ML, Schwartz DM, Ruben RJ, Gates GA, Downs MP, Northern JL, Jerger JF, Paradise JL, Bess FH, Kenworthy OT, Rogers KD. Controversies in screening for middle ear disease and hearing loss in children. Pediatrics 1986; 77:57–70.
3. Wachtendorf CA, Lopez LL, Cooper JC, Hearne EM, Gates GA. The efficacy of school screening for otitis media. In: Lim DJ, Bluestone CD, Klein JO, Nelson JD, eds. Recent advances in otitis media with effusion. Proceedings of the Third International Symposium. Toronto: BC Decker, 1984:242.
4. Liden G, Renwall V. Impedance and tone screening of school children. Scand Audiol 1980; 9:121–126.
5. Grosso P, Rupp RR. Pure tone and tympanometric screening: an ideal pair in identification audiometry. J Am Aud Soc 1978; 4:11–15.
6. Brooks DN. Acoustic impedance studies on otitis media with effusion. Int J Pediatr Otorhinolaryngol 1982; 4:142–147.
7. Hoover KM, Chermak GD, Doyle CS. A comparative study of immittance screening procedures with preschool aged children. Am J Otol 1982; 4:142–147.
8. Poulsen G, Tos M. Repetitive tympanometric screenings of two-year-old children. Scand Audiol 1978; 9:21–28.
9. Fiellau-Nikolajsen M. Serial tympanometry and middle ear status in 3-year-old children. ORL J Otorhinolaryngol Relat Spec 1980; 42:220–232.
10. Casselbrant ML, Fuchs C, Bostoff LM, Cantekin EI. Strategies in screening for otitis media. Poster, 4th International Symposium on Recent Advances in Otitis Media, Bal Harbour, Florida, June 1987.

DIAGNOSTIC VALUE OF OTOSCOPIC SIGNS IN ACUTE OTITIS MEDIA

PEKKA H. KARMA, M.D., MATTI A. PENTTILÄ, M.D., MARKKU M. SIPILÄ, M.D., and MATTI S. TIMONEN, M.D.

To diagnose acute otitis media, signs of middle ear effusion must be present, together with acute ear related symptoms.[1,2] In clinical practice the correct diagnosis depends mainly upon the ability of the otoscopist to detect the presence or absence of acute middle ear effusion. However, the otoscopic criteria of acute otitis media (and its middle ear effusion) vary greatly among clinicians as well as in different studies.[3] Redness, bulging, or impaired mobility of the tympanic membrane are suggested as indicative of the condition.[1,4–6] However, opinions about the consistency of these findings differ,[1,7,8] and they all also can result from causes other than middle ear suppuration.

In this study we tried to determine the value of various otoscopic findings in detecting the middle ear effusion of acute otitis media in two large unselected groups of small children of the same age but living in different geographic areas. Each group was examined by a single study doctor—an otolaryngologist or a pediatrician. The otoscopic findings were compared with those from myringotomy. Interobserver or intergroup variations in otoscopic findings and their effects on the clinical diagnosis of acute otitis media were also studied.

MATERIAL AND METHODS

Altogether 2,911 children ages ½ to 2½ years were followed for 1 to 2 years for otitis episodes in the cities of Tampere and Oulu in Finland. There was a total of 11,804 ear related visits; of these, visits with a tympanostomy tube in one or both ears (271) and visits with incomplete data (990) were excluded. In Tampere, in 5,949 visits 1,688 children were examined by an otolaryngologist (group I), and in Oulu, in 5,855 visits 1,223 children were examined by a pediatrician (group II). The age distribution at the visits was similar in both groups. Of all the visits, 75.1 percent were due to acute symptoms. Myringotomy was performed in 61.7 percent of the "acute" visits and a middle ear effusion was obtained in 83.5 percent of these. Tympanic membrane perforation was found in one or both ears in 4.2 percent of the acute visits; these visits were also excluded from further analyses.

Each visit was classified according to the ear with the more severe tympanic membrane findings. An order of severity of the findings was established for color (distinctly red, cloudy, slightly red, and normal), for position (bulging, retracted, and normal), and for mobility (distinctly impaired, slightly impaired, and normal).

The diagnostic usefulness of different otoscopic findings in detecting middle ear effusions in acute otitis media was evaluated by certain variables calculated as percentages from the original figures: (1) sensitivity (the presence of certain otoscopic findings in the presence of a middle ear effusion), (2) specificity (the absence of certain otoscopic findings in the absence of a middle ear effusion), (3) false positive cases (the absence of a middle ear effusion in the presence of certain otoscopic findings), and (4) false negative cases (the presence of a middle ear effusion in the absence of certain otoscopic findings). Because the diagnostic value of a finding is also dependent on the frequency of acute otitis media in the study population, we also analyzed the predictability of the findings by using the odds. From the total incidence figures of acute otitis media in each group (F), we calculated the corresponding prior odds (OPr; odds before otoscopy) and

posterior (postexamination) odds (OPo; odds for the positive otoscopic findings).[9]

RESULTS

Myringotomy confirmed acute otitis media in 56.2 percent of 4,234 visits with otoscopic tympanic membrane data in patients with acute symptoms in Tampere and in 38.1 percent of 3,718 acute visits in Oulu (p < 0.001). However, in acute visits a middle ear effusion was found during myringotomy, when done, with about the same frequency (86.3 and 81.7 percent) and the total incidence of acute otitis media per 100 children was almost the same (1.56 and 1.58) in the two groups of children in the two areas.

The occurrence of different otoscopic findings (sensitivity) in acute ear related visits with middle ear effusion is presented in Table 1. Tympanic membrane redness of varying degrees was seen in only 17.5 percent (Tampere, group I) and 26.9 percent (Oulu, group II) of these visits; the percentages did not vary much regardless of whether middle ear effusion was present in acute visits or not. Cloudiness of the tympanic membrane was a common finding in acute otitis media. Bulging of the tympanic membrane was found in 61.2 and 41.3 percent of acute visits with middle ear effusion but very rarely if there was no middle ear effusion. Retraction of the tympanic membrane was infrequent in both groups. If there was a middle ear effusion, the mobility of the tympanic membrane was almost always impaired, in most cases distinctly. In cases with acute otitis media the tympanic membranes were normal in color in 1.1 and 6.0 percent, normal in mobility in 1.7 and 5.6 percent, but normal in position in 32.3 and 39.3 percent.

TABLE 1 The Value of Tympanic Membrane Findings in Diagnosing Middle Ear Effusion in Patients with Acute Symptoms

Tympanic Membrane Findings	Sensitivity		Specificity		False Positives		False Negatives	
	Group I (%)	Group II (%)	Group I (%)	Group II (%)	Group I (%)	Group II (%)	Group I (%)	Group II (%)
Red	17.5	26.9	84.5	84.0	40.4	48.6	56.1	35.2
Cloudy	81.4	67.1	95.3	89.5	4.3	20.2	20.2	18.8
Abnormal color	98.9	94.0	79.8	73.5	13.5	29.6	1.7	4.9
Bulging	61.2	41.3	96.8	96.9	4.0	11.0	33.9	27.1
Retracted	6.5	19.4	90.6	87.9	53.2	50.4	57.0	36.0
Abnormal position	67.7	60.7	87.3	84.8	12.7	29.0	32.1	22.2
Impaired mobility	98.3	94.4	79.4	71.9	13.9	31.9	2.7	4.8

A battery of variables to describe the value of different otoscopic findings in diagnosing acute otitis media are also calculated in Table 1. The table suggests the specificity of tympanic membrane redness to be good in acute otitis media. However, the incidence of false positive and false negative findings in regard to the presence of middle ear effusion was unacceptably high. In regard to cloudiness all the variables showed rather good values. The same was true for distinctly impaired mobility of the tympanic membrane, but in cases with only slightly impaired tympanic membrane mobility the specificity was poor and the proportion of false positive findings was high. Bulging showed poor sensitivity, very good specificity, very few false positive findings, but many false negative findings. The value of retraction of the tympanic membrane diagnosing acute otitis media was very poor with most variables measured.

The posterior odds with different otoscopic findings in detecting middle ear effusion during an acute ear related visit (Table 2) depicts the probability of finding an effusion behind a cloudy, bulging, or distinctly hypomobile tympanic membrane to be high, but that for tympanic membrane redness to be very poor. There was also a distinct difference in the frequency of acute otitis media (prior odds) in the two groups of patient visits involving acute symptomatology, which is reflected in the posterior odds figures presented for single tympanic membrane findings in group I and II.

There were some interobserver-intergroup vari-

ations in the frequencies of the findings and in the variables calculated. In acute otitis media the tympanic membrane was found to be red or retracted more frequently in group II than in group I (see Table 1), and cloudy or bulging tympanic membranes were more frequent in group I. These differences were statistically significant (p < 0.001). The specificities of the different findings were about the same in both groups, but the predictive value of cloudiness as an indicator of acute middle ear effusion was higher (i.e., fewer false positive findings) in group I. On the other hand, different false negative tympanic membrane findings were more frequently recorded in group I.

DISCUSSION

Frequent myringotomies and the remarkable numbers (13.7 to 18.3 percent) of negative aspirations suggest that all the ears with effusions were probably found and myringotomy performed. Therefore we can reliably relate ear symptoms and otoscopic findings to the presence of middle ear effusion found during myringotomy and the absence of middle ear effusion not found during myringotomy or not even suspected during pneumatic otoscopy.

All the parameters and variables in the present study indicated that redness of the tympanic membrane is an inconsistent finding in acute otitis media[1,7] and cannot be regarded as a reliable indicator of the disease. On the other hand, cloudiness of the tympanic membrane showed high sensitivity and specificity, a low incidence of false findings, and high odds for the presence of middle ear effusion. Thus its diagnostic importance seems to be great in acute otitis media. For distinctly impaired mobility of the tympanic membrane, the variables had about the same value in diagnosing acute otitis media as cloudiness. The value of slightly impaired mobility was less. The diagnostic usefulness of tympanic membrane bulging was decreased by poor sensitivity and the large number of false negative findings.

It appears that cloudiness, distinctly impaired mobility, and bulging of the tympanic membrane, if present, rather reliably indicated the middle ear effusion of acute otitis media, but redness, retraction, and slightly impaired mobility of the tympanic membrane were not of much use in detecting acute effusion. In acute otitis media the incidences of normal tympanic membrane findings were very low except for position, and the predictive value of the normal looking tympanic membrane was good in indicating the absence of a middle ear effusion.

There were variations in the incidences of

TABLE 2 The Odds with Different Tympanic Membrane Findings in Detecting Middle Ear Effusions in Patients with Acute Symptoms

	Group I	Group II
Without otoscopy (prior odds, OPr*)	1.3	0.6
Otoscopic tympanic membrane findings (posterior odds, OPo*)		
Distinctly red	2.3	1.2
Slightly red	0.6	0.2
Cloudy	22.3	4.0
Normal color	0.01	0.05
Bulging	24.6	8.4
Retracted	0.9	1.0
Normal position	0.5	0.3
Distinctly impaired mobility	15.5	3.7
Slightly impaired mobility	1.4	0.5
Normal mobility	0.03	0.05

* OPr = F/(1−F), where F = incidence of acute otitis media. OPo = (OPr) × (sensitivity / [1− specificity]).

different otoscopic findings between the two groups. In addition to the clinical differences between the acute visits in the two areas, there might have been observer related differences in interpreting the otoscopic findings. However, the two doctors found a similar frequency of acute otitis media among those suspected as well as in the two child populations that were followed. This suggests that pneumatic otoscopy as performed and interpreted by the two representatives of the two specialties taking care of children with ear problems has an equally high diagnostic value.

REFERENCES

1. Bluestone C. State of the art: definitions and classifications. In: Lim DJ, Bluestone CD, Klein JO, Nelson JD, eds. Recent advances in otitis media with effusion. Proceedings of the Third International Symposium. Toronto: BC Decker, 1984:1–4.

2. Karma P, Palva T, Kouvalainen K, Kärjä J, Mäkelä PH, Prinssi VP, Ruuskanen O, Launiala K. Finnish approach to the treatment of acute otitis media. Report of the Finnish consensus conference. Ann Otol Rhinol Laryngol 1987; 96(Suppl 129):1–19.

3. Hayden G. Acute suppurative otitis media in children. Diversity of clinical diagnostic criteria. Clin Pediatr 1981; 20:99–104.

4. Paparella MM, Bluestone CD, Arnold W, Bradley WH, Hussl B, Münker G, Naunton RF, Sadé J, Tos M, van Cauwenberge P. Panel report: definition and classification. Recent advances in otitis media with effusion. Report of research conference. Ann Otol Rhinol Laryngol 1985; 94(Suppl 116):8–9.

5. Mortimer E. Suppurative otitis media: a pediatric view. Otolaryngol Clin North Am 1978; 9:679–687.

6. Gates GA. Differential otomanometry. Am J Otolaryngol 1986; 7:147–150.

7. Pukander J. Clinical features of acute otitis media among children. Acta Otolaryngol (Stockh) 1983; 95:117–122.

8. Hayden G, Schwartz R. Characteristics of earache among children with acute otitis media. Am J Dis Child 1985; 139:721–723.

9. Sackett DL, Haynes RB, Tuqwell P. Clinical epidemiology. A basic science for clinical medicine. Vol. 1. Boston: Little, Brown, 1985:3–155.

OBSERVER INVARIANT DIAGNOSIS OF MIDDLE EAR EFFUSIONS

LEON M. BROSTOFF, M.D. and ERDEM I. CANTEKIN, Ph.D.

When doing studies on otitis media with effusion (OME) it is desirable to have a noninvasive diagnostic test that is simple, accurate, and objective so that the results will be reproducible. We present an attempt to simplify a "current" algorithm[1] used to combine otoscopy with tympanometry for the diagnosis of otitis media with effusion (Fig. 1).

MATERIALS AND METHODS

We studied tympanograms and otoscopic findings in 22,403 ears in children aged 7 months to 12 years. The data were recorded in various clinical studies conducted between 1978 and 1984 at the Otitis Media Research Center at the Children's Hospital of Pittsburgh. Trained audiologists conducted tympanometry in a standard way using acoustic impedance bridges (Madsen model Z073) coupled to XY plotters. Each tympanogram was classified into one of 15 types according to a previously described scheme.[2] For each tympanogram type T_n, a likelihood ratio LR_n was calculated:

$$LR = \frac{P(T_n/OME)}{P(T_n/NO\ OME)}$$

where $P(T_n/OME)$ is the probability of tympanogram type n given positive otoscopic findings and $P(T_n/NO\ OME)$ is the probability of tympanogram type n given negative otoscopic findings. Although myringotomy ideally would be used as the gold standard, tympanometry was initially compared to otoscopy as a provisional gold standard in order to provide estimates of its diagnostic reliability, and the accuracy of each otoscopist was validated with respect to findings on myringotomy. Tympanogram types were clustered according to this likelihood ratio and combined with otoscopy results in an al-

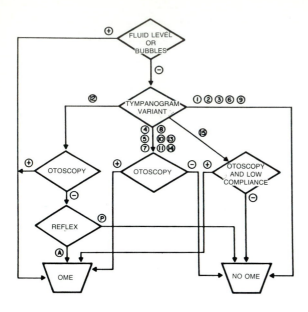

Figure 1 "Current" algorithm for identification of otitis media with effusion (OME). Otoscopic observation of fluid level or bubbles overrides decision tree, classifying given ear in otitis media present category. Low compliance indicates values less than five arbitrary units used by Madsen electroacoustic impedance bridge.

TABLE 1 Logarithm of Likelihood Ratios (LR_n) of Tympanogram Types (T_n) for a Combined Data Set (n = 22,403 Ears)

	T_n	Log LR_n	n
Group I	3	−1.28	171
	1	−1.17	4,426
	9	−0.89	1,072
	6	−0.86	227
	4	−0.61	3,284
	10	−0.41	216
Group II	7	−0.14	1,253
	15	−0.13	464
	11	−0.04	120
	14	+0.02	2,379
	5	+0.24	297
	8	+0.39	711
Group III	12	+0.85	5,889
	13	+1.10	1,894

gorithmic scheme. Finally, the algorithm was externally validated on a separate data set (n = 507 ears) by comparing its results to myringotomy findings/the gold standard.

RESULTS

The likelihood ratios (LR_n) for 14 of the 15 tympanogram types are shown in Table 1 (type 2 is no longer used). LR_n had a range from 0.05 to 12, a change of more than two orders of magnitude. The tympanogram types cluster into three groups, as illustrated in Figure 2. These groups are somewhat reminiscent of Jerger's original classification of tympanograms[3] into types A, B, and C, but with different boundary conditions.[2] Group I consists of types 1, 3, 4, 6, 9, and 10, which are most likely to occur in the absence of effusion. Tympanograms in group II have likelihood ratios close to 1 (log LR_n is close to 0) and are indeterminate; they provide little information about the probability of an effusion.

The "new" algorithm, depicted in Figure 3, is based on this clustering. If the otoscopist observes gas bubbles or a liquid meniscus behind the tympanic membrane, however, the decision will be oti-

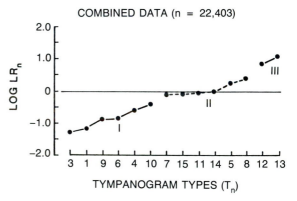

Figure 2 Clustering of tympanogram types by logarithm of likelihood ratios (LR_n) shown in Table 1.

tis media with effusion regardless of the tympanogram type.

By using a previous data set of myringotomy findings, tympanometry findings, and validated otoscopy findings, the accuracy and otoscopic share of the "new" algorithm were compared to those of the "current" algorithm (Table 2). The sensitivity of the "new" algorithm was 6 percentage points higher than that of the "current" algorithm, and the specificity was 4 percentage points higher, giving an error incidence of 10 percent as opposed to 16 percent. Furthermore, in the "new" algorithm, the decision was based on otoscopic observation in less than 15 percent of the cases, whereas the "current" algorithm relies on otoscopy over 90 percent of the time.

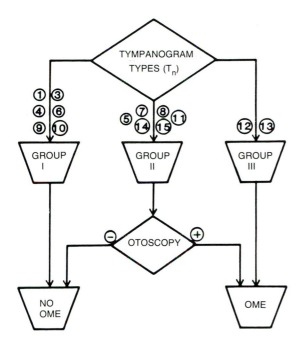

Figure 3 "New" algorithm for identification of otitis media with effusion (OME). The tympanogram variants shown in Figure 2 are clustered into three groups. In the contradictory condition of effusion-free (no otitis media with effusion) by the algorithm and the otoscopic observation of liquid meniscus or gas bubbles, the decision will be reversed to otitis media with effusion.

TABLE 2 Performance of the Diagnostic Algorithms for the Identification of Middle Ear Effusions (n = 507 Ears)

Algorithm	Sensitivity (%)	Specificity (%)	Error Incidence (%)	Otoscopic Share (%)
"Current"	87	80	16	93
"New"	93	84	10	14

final word, it is a step toward decreasing the disadvantages of otoscopy or tympanometry alone in studies of otitis media with effusion. It remains dependent on a validated otoscopist, but less so than the "current" algorithm. Both algorithms are based on a particular bridge and tympanogram classification scheme. Although the sensitivity and specificity are independent of the effusion prevalence in the population, extrapolation to another possibly more diverse population must be with caution.

Study supported in part by the National Institute of Neurological and Communicative Disorders and Stroke, National Institutes of Health (grant NS16337).

REFERENCES

1. Cantekin EI. Algorithm for diagnosis of otitis media with effusion. Ann Otol Rhinol Laryngol 1983; 92 (Suppl 107):6.
2. Cantekin EI, Bluestone CD, Fria TJ, et al. Identification of otitis media with effusion in children. Ann Otol Rhinol Laryngol 1980; 89 (Suppl 68):190–195.
3. Jerger J. Clinical experience with impedance audiometry. Arch Otolaryngol 1970; 92:311–324.

DISCUSSION

This simplified algorithm represents an improvement over the current one. Though not the

PILOT IMPEDANCE SCREENING PROGRAM IN THE SOUTH ISLAND OF NEW ZEALAND

IAN A. STEWART, M.B., Ch.B., F.R.C.S. (Edin), WILLIAM J. KEITH, Ph.D., and ANNE S. SIMPSON, M.B., Ch.B., D.Com.H., D.O., MCC.M.

In early 1983 an impedance screening program was introduced in the cities of Christchurch, Timaru, and Dunedin in the South Island of New Zealand. The purpose was to evaluate impedance screening as a possible replacement of or addition to pure tone screening. This report presents and discusses results from the Dunedin study, because more detail was

available relative to this study and the screening criteria varied to a small degree in other cities. Similar trends are evident in the other cities compared to Dunedin. In addition, information about the therapeutic approach of primary care physicians is available for the Dunedin district. To simplify discussion, results are presented for children screened as

TABLE 1 Bilateral Failure at First Test

Age	1983		1984		1985	
	%	No. Screened	%	No. Screened	%	No. Screened
3	8.1	2010	3.7	1418	3.7	1373
5	8.6	2385	5.1	2110	2.9	2210
7	4.3	2220	2.6	2220	Not available	

having possible disease in both ears, because screening criteria for unilateral disease varied over the period.

MAIN STUDY

Subjects and Methods

The attempt was made to include as many as possible of 3, 5, and 7 year old children in the districts. Coverage of the 5 and 7 years olds at school was relatively simple, because children in New Zealand enter school immediately following their fifth birthday. Although precise figures cannot be given owing to variation in school rolls through the year, it is likely that coverage approached 100 percent and certainly exceeded 95 percent. The precise 3 year old population of the district is not known, but on the basis of birth data for 3 years previously, and in a slightly falling overall population, coverage for the impedance screening program is estimated at 80 percent for 3 year olds in 1983. This relatively high figure was achieved because a high proportion of children attend kindergarten or other preschool groups.

Screening was carried out at the school or at a preschool center by a Department of Health vision-hearing screening technician, using a Macromatics screening tympanometer. Vision-hearing testers operate within the community; their education is to the secondary school level, with a short training course in testing.

Ears were regarded as "abnormal" when they showed a compliance of less than 0.30 cc and a middle ear pressure more negative than -200 daPa.

All children showing bilateral "abnormalities" were retested after approximately 3 months. In 1983, the children failing the second test were referred to the ENT Clinic at Dunedin Hospital where they were evaluated by the principal author. In 1984 and 1985 children failing the second test were referred to the family physician (in New Zealand otolaryngologists and pediatricians are not primary care physicians). Thus in 1983 treatment was usually initiated by an otolaryngologist and in 1984 and 1985 by the family physician.

Results

The results are shown in Table 1. The decline in prevalence for children showing bilateral otitis media with effusion between 1983 and 1985 is apparent. Although numbers have been well maintained for the 5 and 7 year olds, there has been a definite fall-off in the number of 3 year old children reached by the program. These figures relate to children failing initial testing.

Table 2 shows the number of children who failed the initial screening test bilaterally and also failed the test bilaterally 3 months later. There is again a drop between 1983 and 1985.

SECONDARY STUDY

These results suggested a marked decline in the prevalence of otitis media with effusion in this community between 1983 and 1985, as evidenced by children failing initial impedance screening tests.

There was also a decline in children failing screening tests bilaterally who also failed bilaterally 3 months later. It was at about the time of introduction of the impedance screening program that extended (3 week) antimicrobial courses were first routinely used by otolaryngologists in Dunedin in the treatment of otitis media with effusion. Because all children with persistent effusions were referred to the hospital clinic, family doctors received letters

TABLE 2 Children Failing Bilaterally at First Test

	% Still Failing Bilaterally at Second Test 3 Months Later		
	Age 3	Age 5	Age 7
	%	%	%
1983	38	45	39
1984	19	24	19
1985	10	17	Not available

about their patients, recommending extended antimicrobial therapy courses. It is possible that more widespread prescribing of extended antibiotic courses by family doctors had reduced the overall prevalence of otitis media with effusion in the screened population. To test this hypothesis, family physicians in practice in the Dunedin district as of March 1987 were sent a retrospective questionnaire about prescribing habits.

Methods

Seventy-five family physicians were asked the following questions:

Were you in family practice in this district in 1982? If not, when did you commence practice?

What was your usual treatment for a child with a chronic middle ear effusion in 1982?

If your usual treatment changed between 1982 and 1985, what was your treatment in 1985?

Results

Forty-seven replies were obtained (62 percent): three of these were from physicians who did not normally treat otitis media with effusion and five were from newcomers to family practice over the period. Of the remaining 39 physicians, 21 responded that they had changed their prescribing habits to longer (14 to 28 day) antibiotic courses between 1982 and 1985. A further eight replied that they had prescribed long antibiotic courses for otitis media with effusion prior to 1983, four said that they prescribed 5 to 10 day courses, five made no mention of duration of course, and one did not consider that the disorder should be treated. One had changed to ketotifen as the primary treatment of otitis media with effusion.

Including the newcomers to family medicine, 31 of the 46 (67 percent) regarded antibiotic courses of 14 days or longer as the standard treatment of otitis media with effusion in 1987. The therapeutic choices of these family physicians are shown in Table 3. Five practitioners spontaneously commented that they had

TABLE 3   Therapeutic Choice for Otitis Media with Effusion by 43 Family Physicians

Antimicrobial therapy	
Trimethoprim-sulfonamide	29
Amoxicillin	20
Cefaclor	7
Amoxicillin-clavulanic acid	5
Erythromycin	3
Penicillin	2
Nonantimicrobial therapy	
Pseudoephedrine	12
Decongestant nose drops	5
Ketotifen	2
Intranasal steroid spray	1
Antihistamine	1
No treatment	1

discontinued pseudoephedrine therapy for otitis media with effusion between 1982 and 1985.

DISCUSSION

There can be little doubt that the screening program produced a greatly heightened awareness of the problem in the local community: it is now rare to encounter a parent who does not have some knowledge of otitis media. Because parents are informed of initial screening failures, it is likely that children would present to family doctors and have treatment prescribed before the second screening test was carried out, particularly after the initial year when the scheme was established. This may well explain the drop in numbers of children failing bilaterally on the second screening test.

Although precise figures are not available, there has also been a marked decline in the numbers of children undergoing surgery for the placement of tympanostomy tubes, and reduced pressure for clinic appointments when only patients with persistent problems unresponsive to antibiotic therapy tend to be referred.

We acknowledge the contributions of the vision hearing testers of the New Zealand Department of Health, and also the services of Jan McLeod and Elizabeth Greig in collating data.

DIAGNOSTIC RELIABILITY OF IMPEDANCE AUDIOMETRY IN CASE OF OTITIS MEDIA WITH EFFUSION

IN YONG PARK, M.D., HEE NAM KIM, M.D., MYUNG-HYUN CHUNG, M.D., KEE HYUN PARK, M.D., and SANG BIN YIM, M.D.

Otitis media with or without effusion is a worldwide child health problem, and therefore accurate detection of middle ear effusion is important for the proper diagnosis and management of these diseases. Impedance audiometry combined with pneumatic otoscopy is the most accurate diagnostic test for detecting otitis media with effusion.[1,2]

Recently Teele and Teele[3] developed an acoustic reflectometer, which has displayed a high degree of sensitivity (94.4 percent) and a high degree of specificity (79.2 percent). However, we have found that it is not easy to apply these impedance audiometric findings directly to clinical practice, because the normal range of compliance in Korean children seems to be different from those of other races. Moreover, systems for classifying impedance audiometric data differ from laboratory to laboratory.

In this study we developed a new classification of tympanograms according to tympanometric values in Korean children and investigated its diagnostic reliability.

MATERIALS AND METHODS

To derive data in normal subjects, the tympanometric peak pressure and the compliance were measured in 126 ears in 79 healthy children, who showed less than a 10 db air-bone gap and in whom findings in physical examinations were normal.

From 1981 to 1986 myringotomies with and without ventilation tubes were performed in 290 patients (528 ears) aged 2 to 15 years under general anesthesia without nitrous oxide or local anesthesia. These patients were diagnosed as having otitis media with effusion by physical examination and impedance audiometry. The impedance tests were done with a Teledyne Avionics instrument (type TA-3D) and a Grason-Stadler instrument (1723 middle ear analyzer). The viscosity of the fluid was judged by naked eye examination. The cases were analyzed in regard to the diagnostic reliability of impedance audiometry on the basis of age, sex, and fluid characteristics.

RESULTS

The normal values of the tympanometric peak pressure and compliance in Korean children were determined as a 2 SD range as seen in Table 1. The normal range of the tympanometric peak pressure was -62.5 to 43.6 mm H_2O, and the normal range of compliance was 0.20 to 0.73 cc.

The tympanograms were arbitrarily classified according to tympanometric peak pressure and compliance, as in Figure 1. Area A was defined as an area between 0.2 and 0.75 cc in compliance and between -100 mm H_2O and 100 mm H_2O in tympanometric peak pressure. Area B was defined as an area less than 0.2 cc in compliance and less than -100 mm H_2O in tympanometric peak pressure. Area C was defined as an area greater or equal to 0.2 cc in compliance and less than -100 mm H_2O in tympanometric peak pressure (Fig. 1).

Table 2 shows the sensitivity, specificity, and probability of fluid in each area. The sensitivity of the test of fluid presence was higher in area B than in area C, but the specificity of the test of fluid presence was higher in area C than in area B. The probability of the presence of fluid in area B was 90.0 percent and in area C, 77.8 percent (Table 2).

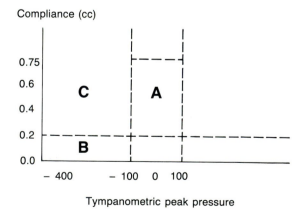

Figure 1   Classification of tympanograms.

52

TABLE 1   Normal Values of Tympanometric Peak Pressure and Compliance in Korean Children

	Mean	SD	Range (± 2 SD)
Tympanometric peak pressure (mm H_2O)	−9.4	26.5	− 62.5–43.6
Compliance (cc)	0.41	0.16	0.20–0.73*

* Lowest value in normal child.

TABLE 2   Diagnostic Reliability of the Presence of the Fluid in Each Area

	Area B	Area C
Sensitivity	73.7%	17.0%
Specificity	50.7%	70.7%
Probability	90.0%	77.8%

The sensitivity and specificity of the test of fluid presence in each area were similar, but the probabilities of fluid presence in each area were different statistically (Table 3).

The findings in myringotomies were not correlated with areas of the tympanogram.

There was no statistical difference in the distribution of otitis media with effusion in each area between the two age groups (Table 4).

There was no statistical difference in fluid detectability in each area in males and females (Table 5).

DISCUSSION

The present study provides new information concerning the validity of tympanometric testing in Korean pediatric patients. The normal range of compliance in Korean children seems to be different

TABLE 3   Diagnostic Reliability of Serous and Mucoid Fluid in the Presence of Fluid in Each Area

	Area B		Area C	
	Serous	Mucoid	Serous	Mucoid
Sensitivity	75.0%	76.8%	17.0%	15.9%
Specificity	26.7%	33.1%	83.0%	80.6%
Probability	90.0%*	72.2%*	24.7%*	64.9%*

* p value < 0.05.

TABLE 4   Area of Tympanogram and Fluid Presence in Two Age Groups

Area of Tympanogram	Total	Age	
		Less Than 6 Years*	7 to 15 Years*
A	40	26	14
B	371	190	181
C	99	59	40

* p value > 0.05.

TABLE 5   Area of Tympanogram and Fluid Presence in Males and Females

Area of Tympanogram	Male*			Female*		
	Total	Fluid	No Fluid	Total	Fluid	No Fluid
A	25	20	5	15	10	5
B	205	182	23	166	152	14
C	56	46	10	43	31	12

* p value > 0.05.

from those in other races, as seen in Table 1, and requires further study. We suggest that the difference in compliance is related to the size of the eardrum and the middle ear space in the Korean child.

The sensitivity and specificity of the presence of fluid in each area of our own classification are similar to those found in other studies in spite of the differences in classification and testing methods.

This study demonstrates that impedance audiometry affects the high probability of the presence of fluid in areas B and C but is not influenced by age, sex, or fluid characteristics.

REFERENCES

1. Paradise JL, Smith CG, Bluestone CD. Tympanometric detection of middle ear effusion in infants and young children. Pediatrics 1976; 58:198–210.
2. Cantekin EI, Bluestone CD, Fria TG, et al. Identification of otitis media with effusion in children. Ann Otol Rhinol Laryngol 1980; 89(Suppl 68):190–195.
3. Teele DW, Teele J. Detection of middle ear effusion by acoustic refectometry. J Pediatr 1984; 104(6):832–838.
4. Fiellau-Nikolajsen M. Tympanometry and secretory otitis media. Acta Otolaryngol 1983; Suppl 394:1–73.
5. Margolis RH, Shanks JE. Tympanometry. In: Katz J, ed. Handbook of clinical audiology. 3rd ed. Baltimore: Williams & Wilkins, 1985: 438.

RELATIONSHIPS AND CORRELATIONS AMONG AUDITORY BRAINSTEM RESPONSE (ELECTROPHYSIOLOGY), OTOSCOPY, AND TYMPANOMETRY IN SIX AND TWELVE MONTHS OF INFANTS WITH AND WITHOUT OTITIS MEDIA

PETER ROLAND, M.D., TERESE FINITZO, Ph.D., SANDY FRIEL-PATTI, Ph.D., KAREN C. BROWN, M.S., and WILLIAM L. MEYERHOFF, M.D., Ph.D.

The Dallas Cooperative Project on early hearing development is a 3-year prospective longitudinal study designed to determine whether the conductive hearing loss associated with middle ear effusion leads to a demonstrable delay in the acquisition of both expressive and receptive language skills. To date, 437 6-month-old infants have been enrolled. Two hundred eighty-eight infants have been followed from age 6 months past the eighteenth month evaluations. A total of 3,072 separate evaluations are included, with an average of 11 evaluations of each child during the first year. Every 6 months the children are seen at the Callier Center at which time immittance, otoscopy, and measurement of the hearing threshold are performed at the same visit. At 6 months all threshold evaluations are done by auditory brainstem response audiometry. At 12 months some children have undergone auditory brainstem response audiometry (ABR), but all children undergo visual reinforced audiometry.

Otoscopy performed at the Callier Center is done by one of three otolaryngologists, two of whom are otologists and one of whom is a pediatric otolaryngologist (Fig. 1). The results of the otoscopic examination are recorded on a single form. A number of different characteristics are recorded, but ultimately the examiner must decide between the presence or absence of effusion. The examiner performs the otoscopic evaluation without benefit of either immittance or ABR data.

An immittance examination is performed at the same visit. Subsequent to performance of the examination the tympanogram is "scored" by a certified audiologist who records the results according to the tympanogram "type." So far, statistical examination of our data has not revealed any significant differences between the subtypes of A or C tympanograms. The numbers, however, are small, and when larger numbers are available, we shall attempt a more rigorous statistical analysis.

With the otoscopic and immittance data, "ear codes" are developed as described by Cantekin and Casselbrant.[1] The codes tend to favor immittance data unless bubbles are seen otoscopically (Table 1).

OTOSCOPIC EXAMINATION FORM

NAME _____ DATE _____

SUBJECT NUMBER _____ PROCEDURE CODE _____

EXAMINER _____

1 Condition of the external auditory canal

Right	Left
1 Patent	1 Patent
2 Occluded	2 Occluded
3 Partially Occluded	3 Partially Occluded

2 Tympanic membrane perforation
  1 Right ear only
  2 Left ear only
  3 Both ears
  4 Intact TM's

3 Condition of tympanic membrane

Right	Left
1 Retracted	1 Retracted
2 Bulging	2 Bulging
3 Opaque	3 Opaque
4 Tympanosclerosis	4 Tympanosclerosis
5 Air-fluid level	5 Air-fluid level

4 Color of tympanic mmbrane

Right	Left
1 Red	1 Red
2 Blue/gray	2 Blue/gray
3 Silver	3 Silver

5 Tubes inserted
  1 Right ear only
  2 Left ear only
  3 Both ears
  4 Intact TM's

6 Tubes are in place
  1 Right ear only
  2 Left ear only
  3 Both ears
  4 Out in both ears
  5 Not applicable

7 Pneumo otoscopy completed
  1 Right ear only
  2 Left ear only
  3 Both ears
  4 Not done

8 Movement present
  1 Right ear only
  2 Left ear only
  3 Both ears
  4 Not present
  5 Not applicable

9 Middle ear tissue present
  1 Right ear only
  2 Left ear only
  3 Both ears
  4 Not present
  5 Not applicable

10 Middle ear effusion
  1 Right ear only
  2 Left ear only
  3 Both ears
  4 Not present
  5 Not applicable

Comments _____

_____

_____

Checked	Entered	Copy Checked
( )	( )	( )

Figure 1 Results of otoscopy are recorded on this form. The normal color is considered to be silver. "Middle ear tissue" in item 9 refers to the presence or absence of cholesteatoma.

TABLE 1   Codes

Code 1: Normal
  Normal findings on otoscopic examination
  with no air-fluid level present
  Type A or A' tympanogram except when
  otitis media with effusion is identified
  during otoscopic examination

Code 2: Abnormal middle ear status
  Normal findings on otoscopic examination
  with type As, A+, C1, C2, or C3
  tympanogram
  Abnormal findings on otoscopic examination
  confirming otitis media with effusion with
  type A or A' tympanogram

Code 3: Tympanogram tube
  All ears with tympanotomy tubes reported in
  place in tympanic membrane

Code 4: Otitis media with effusion
  Type B tympanogram
  Abnormal tympanogram A+, As, C1, C2,
  or C3 with otoscopic confirmation of otitis
  media with effusion
  Type A or A' tympanogram and otoscopic
  examination revealing visible air-fluid level

RESULTS

The use of ear codes was evaluated early in our study and has been reported elsewhere on several occasions. Our most recent data relating to 430 ears evaluated at 6 months reveal statistically significant differences (p < 0.00001) for both ABR thresholds and latency at 60 db and ear codes 1, 2, and 4. Discrimination is quite good in that 94 percent of code 1 (normal) ears had a 20 db threshold, whereas only 40.2 percent of code 4 (effusion) ears had a 20 db threshold. No code 1 ear had a threshold lower than 30 db, and all thresholds of 60 db were code 4. There is a significant positive correlation (R=0.54; p < 0.0001) between ABR, threshold, and ear code (Fig. 2). There were similar differences for latency at 60 db, with a mean latency of 7.3 msec for code 4 ears compared with 6.67 msec for code 1 ears (Fig. 3). Moreover, there is a statistically significant positive correlation (R=0.56; p < 0.0001) between ABR and visual reinforced audiometry at 12 months with 2,000 kHz stronger than 500 Hz. The ear code is better correlated with the minimal response of 500 Hz than with 2 kHz. This is con-

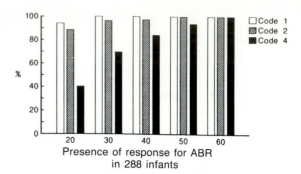

Figure 2 The horizontal axis represents the presence of a V wave on the ABR examination at a given decibel level.

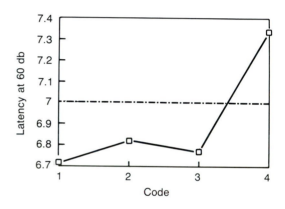

Figure 3 Ear code plotted against latency of a detectable V wave at 60 db.

sistent with the predominantly low frequency conductive loss known to be characteristic of middle ear effusions.

We analyzed the data in order to separate immittance and otoscopy findings and studied the results when analyzed separately (Table 2). The numbers for immittance and ear codes are smaller because ear codes 2 and 3 are excluded, as are all type C tympanograms and all subtype A tympanograms. All three modalities discriminate between the presence and absence of hearing loss at a statistically significant level. There is no marked difference between immittance and otoscopy, and combining data into "ear codes" does not seem to increase one's ability to detect children "at risk" for hearing loss.

TABLE 2   Dallas Cooperative Project

	N	Mean V Latency at 60 db	Mean ABR Threshold	
Otoscopy				
Effusion present	86	7.24 msec	29.5 db	p < 0.0001
Effusion absent	326	6.95 msec	21.8 db	
Immittance				
Type B	85	7.25 msec	30.1 db	p < 0.0001
Type A	82	6.61 msec	21.1 db	
Ear code				
Code 4 (MEE)	82	7.30 msec	31.19 db	p < 0.0001
Code 1 (normal)	156	6.67 msec	20.6 db	

CONCLUSIONS

By combining immittance and otoscopy, we can reliably identify infants at significant risk for hearing loss secondary to middle ear effusion. We are currently working with our statistician to develop a precise measurement of the correlation between immittance, otoscopy, and ear codes and hearing loss. Even though the ear code system is already somewhat weighted toward immittance, we are searching for alternative ways to weight the raw data we acquire so as to improve our ability to select children at risk for hearing loss.

This research was supported by NIH grant 5 RO1 NS 10675–03 and The American Hearing Research Foundation.

The authors wish to thank J. Patrick Hieber, Ellen Formby, and Lisa Howell for their contributions.

REFERENCE

1. Casselbrant ML, Brostoff LM, Cantekin EI, Doyle W, Fria T. Otitis media with effusion in preschool children. Laryngoscope 1985; 95:428–436.

EUSTACHIAN TUBE FUNCTION

PROSPECTIVE STUDY OF EUSTACHIAN TUBE FUNCTION AND OTITIS MEDIA

ERDEM I. CANTEKIN, Ph.D., MARGARETHA L. CASSELBRANT, M.D., Ph.D., WILLIAM J. DOYLE, Ph.D., and LEON M. BROSTOFF, M.D.

Abnormal eustachian tube function is assumed to play a major role in the pathogenesis of otitis media, and in animal models a causal relationship between tubal dysfunction and otitis media has been established.[1] However, there are no prospective studies evaluating this relationship in human subjects, and previous reports concerning the role of eustachian tube function in the pathogenesis of otitis media were limited to populations in which middle ear disease was present before eustachian tube function testing. Therefore, it was never established whether the tubal dysfunction was an a priori condition or the consequence of middle ear disease.

In an attempt to resolve this issue, we conducted several prospective longitudinal studies of eustachian tube function in children and investigated the interrelationships between eustachian tube function and middle ear status. Here we report the findings of the first of these studies, which was conducted in preschool children attending a day care center. The epidemiology of otitis media for this cohort of children was reported previously.[2] That study revealed a 61 percent cumulative incidence of otitis media with effusion, seasonal variations in point prevalence (22 to 33 percent during winter months and less than 10 percent during the summer), and a strong association with the presence of upper respiratory tract infections.

METHODS

The study was conducted between September 1982 and August 1983 at a day care center in a suburb of Pittsburgh, Pennsylvania, as a part of a continuing study of the epidemiology of otitis media in young children.[2] In 57 of these preschool children (2 to 5 years old) with intact tympanic membranes, we evaluated eustachian tube function by the nine step tympanometric inflation-deflation test[3] on different occasions between October and June. Each child was tested at least two times and some children were tested as many as six times; the median number of eustachian tube function tests per child was four. Test results were classified by two different observers into one of five groups according to a schema described previously, with group 1 representing the best function and group 5 representing the poorest function.[4] Then for each ear an average eustachian tube function score was determined by summing up all test results (coded as integers 1 to 5) and by dividing by the number of tests.

According to the protocol of the epidemiology study, these children were examined for the presence or absence of otitis media with effusion and upper respiratory tract infection every month. As described before,[2] at each visit an ear score was assigned based on an arbitrary value system (normal = 0, high negative pressure = 1, and otitis media with effusion = 2) using otoscopic and tympanometric findings. In order to summarize the middle ear status over a 1 year period, visit scores were summed and adjusted with respect to the number of examinations to calculate the yearly score. Also a yearly summary of the upper respiratory tract infections was determined by simply cumulating the number of episodes for the study period.

Eustachian tube function scores were compared with middle ear status scores as well as upper respiratory tract infection scores using univariate and multivariate analysis. Finally, categorical data analyses were performed using functional groupings of eustachian tube function, middle ear status, and upper respiratory tract infection data.

RESULTS

Analysis of the scattergrams and linear regression fits between average eustachian tube function scores and yearly middle ear status scores showed a poor correlation. However, it was evident that average eustachian tube function scores between 1 and 3 were associated mostly with low middle ear status scores. However, the converse was not true: ears with eustachian tube function scores of 5 had a scatter of middle ear status scores ranging from 0 to 16. In other words, children who could never equilibrate applied positive or negative middle ear pressure at every testing session had the same likelihood of having high or low middle ear scores.

In order to simplify the data analysis and to include the known strong association of the middle ear status score with upper respiratory tract infection, we divided the data into two groups—ears with low middle ear scores (0–5) and ears with high middle ear scores (6–16). The low score group corresponded approximately to less than 3 months of otitis media with effusion, and the high score group represented the ears of children who probably would be referred for treatment. Similarly, tubal function and upper respiratory tract experiences were classified dichotomously—good or poor eustachian tube function (defined as an average eustachian tube function score = 5), and children with infrequent episodes of upper respiratory tract infection or those with frequent upper respiratory tract infections (more than two episodes).

With these definitions, the study findings were summarized as shown in Table 1. The analysis was most revealing when eustachian tube function and

upper respiratory tract infection groupings were combined into four groups. Groups A and B represented children with infrequent episodes of upper respiratory tract infection with either good or poor eustachian tube function, and groups C and D included children with frequent episodes of upper respiratory tract infection with good or poor tubal function. Significantly, among children with frequent upper respiratory tract infections and poor eustachian tube function (group D), 50 percent had high middle ear scores in contrast to the other three groups ($p < 0.01$). In group A, for example, only 13 percent of the children had high middle ear scores. For children with infrequent upper respiratory tract infections (groups A and B), eustachian tube function test findings had no demonstrable relation to the pathogenesis. For children with frequent episodes of upper respiratory tract infections, however, the knowledge of tubal function was useful to distinguish those who would have high middle ear scores (i.e., more time with otitis media with effusion) from those with low middle ear scores. These findings imply that the role of tubal function in the development of otitis media with effusion is more pronounced during episodes of inflammation; children with compromised eustachian tube function and frequent episodes of upper respiratory tract infection have an increased likelihood of having otitis media with effusion. Further, upper respiratory tract

TABLE 1   Relationship Between Eustachian Tube Function, Upper Respiratory Tract Infections, and Otitis Media in 57 Preschool Children

	Middle Ear Score			
	Low (0–5)	High (6–16)	Total Ears	
Eustachian tube function class*				
Good	53	11 (17%)	64	$X^2 = 1.75$, dF $= 1$
Poor	31	12 (28%)	43	$p > 0.10$
Upper respiratory tract infections				
≤ 2	64	11 (15%)	75	$X^2 = 6.93$, dF $= 1$
>2	20	12 (38%)	32	$p < 0.01$
Eustachian tube function and upper respiratory tract infection groups+				
A	40	6 (13%)	46	
B	24	5 (17%)	28	$X^2 = 7.75$, dF $= 1$
C	13	5 (28%)	18	$p < 0.01$
D	7	7 (50%)	14	
Total	84	23	107	

* Eustachian tube function class based on child's average tubal function score; good = score 1–4.9 and poor = score 5.
+ Groups defined as A—good eustachian tube function; upper respiratory tract infections ≤ 2; B—poor eustachian tube function, upper respiratory tract infection ≤ 2; C—good eustachian tube function, upper respiratory tract infections >2; D—poor eustachian tube function, upper respiratory tract infections >2.

infection can be one of the factors that compromises tubal function.

DISCUSSION

Evaluation of eustachian tube function in this cohort of preschool children using the nine step tympanometric inflation-deflation test was not difficult. However, the interpretation of changes in tympanometric peak pressure due to small changes in middle ear pressure during the nine step test required careful assessment to ascertain the correctness of eustachian tube function groupings. Although this method of testing in subjects with intact tympanic membranes is simple, it has several limitations, including the inability to test subjects who have flat or high negative pressure type tympanograms. Also the passive eustachian tube function parameters, such as opening and closing pressures, cannot be determined by the nine step tympanometric test. Currently the most reliable method of tubal function assessment in subjects with intact tympanic membranes is digital sonometry. Unfortunately during the conduct of this study that technology was not available.

Given the limitations of eustachian tube function evaluation in a clinical setting, the findings of the present study are encouraging. These results suggest that tubal function in young children is related to their experience with middle ear disease.

Moreover, children with good eustachian tube function had few middle ear problems as reflected by their low middle ear scores. As mentioned earlier, a child's upper respiratory tract infection experience was strongly associated with middle ear problems, but children who had frequent episodes of upper respiratory tract infection and poor eustachian tube function constituted the most otitis prone group, suggesting that tubal function has an important role in the pathogenesis of otitis media with effusion and can be considered a primary risk factor.

Study supported in part by BRSG grant SO7 RR20 awarded by the Biomedical Research Support Grant Program, Division of Research Resources, National Institutes of Health.

REFERENCES

1. Giebink GS, Meyerhoff WL, Cantekin EI. Animal models of otitis media. In: Zak O, Sande MA, eds. Experimental models in antimicrobial chemotherapy. Vol. 1. London: Academic Press, 1986:213–236.
2. Casselbrant ML, Brostoff LM, Cantekin EI, Flaherty MR, Doyle WJ, Bluestone CD, Fria TJ. Otitis media with effusion in preschool children. Laryngoscope 1985; 95:428–436.
3. Bluestone CD, Cantekin EI. Current clinical methods, indications and interpretation of Eustachian tube function tests. Ann Otol Rhinol Laryngol 1981; 90:552–562.
4. Cantekin EI. Physiology and pathophysiology of the eustachian tube in humans with otitis media and related conditions. Ann Otol Rhinol Laryngol 1983; 92:15–16.

ENDOSCOPIC OBSERVATIONS OF EUSTACHIAN TUBE ABNORMALITIES IN CHILDREN WITH PALATAL CLEFTS

SEZELLE A. GEREAU, M.D., DAVID STEVENS, D.D.S., MAHA BASSILA, M.D., AARON E. SHER, M.D., EUGENE J. SIDOTI Jr., M.D., MAXINE MORGAN, M.D., SEISHI OKA, D.D.S., Ph.D., and ROBERT J. SHPRINTZEN, Ph.D.

Recurrent middle ear disease in children with clefts of the palate is a well established observation. The incidence of serous otitis media in cleft patients has been reported to be essentially universal.[1] In his landmark 1971 study, Bluestone radiographically demonstrated obstruction of retrograde flow of contrast material at the nasopharyngeal lumen of the eustachian tube.[2] It has been hypothesized that the

eustachian tube dysfunction is caused by abnormal attachment of the tensor veli palatini with resultant inadequate dilation of the tubal orifice.[3] Other more recent studies have questioned the role of the tensor, citing malformation of the lumen itself as a factor.[4-6]

The purpose of this report is to discuss endoscopic observations of the nasopharyngeal lumen of the eustachian tube in 300 children with palatal clefts. This report represents a preliminary presentation of data from a larger longitudinal study.

MATERIALS AND METHODS

Over 300 subjects from the Center for Craniofacial Disorders of Montefiore Medical Center and from the Lancaster Cleft Palate Clinic were studied with flexible fiberoptic nasopharyngoscopy. Experimental subjects were divided into three subgroups:

Group 1: subjects with cleft palate in the absence of associated anomalies.

Group 2: subjects with cleft lip and cleft palate in the absence of associated anomalies.

Group 3: subjects with common multiple anomaly syndromes of clefting, including velocardiofacial syndrome, Stickler syndrome, Van der Woude syndrome, and fetal alcohol syndrome.

Over 100 noncleft subjects served as normal controls. The age range was 3 years to 60 years, all age groups being well represented.

Direct observations of the eustachian tube orifice were made at rest, during speech, and during swallowing. All studies were videotaped and reviewed in a blind manner by two experienced judges. The position of the orifice, shape and size of the torus tubarius, and patency of the orifice were noted for each study in a blind manner with all studies presented in random order and interspersed with the studies of the 100 controls.

An otologic history was gathered for each subject and an otoscopic examination performed. Chronic serous otitis media was defined as meeting any of the following criteria:

1. Three or more episodes of serous otitis media per year for at least 3 consecutive years.

2. Myringotomy and tube surgery at least twice, excluding the time of initial palate repair.

3. Three or more audiograms over a 3 year period documenting conductive hearing loss.

4. Tympanic membrane changes indicative of chronic serous otitis media.

5. A history of cholesteatoma, permanent perforation, or other signs of chronic serous otitis media.

Data from all studies were stored in a dBase II computer program for eventual analysis.

RESULTS

Preliminary data analysis indicated that only 76 percent of the subjects in groups 1 and 2 combined met the criteria for chronic serous otitis media (Table 1). This figure was even lower (66.7 percent) for the subjects with syndromic clefts (group 3). More female subjects were found to have chronic serous otitis media than male subjects in groups 1 and 2, but not in group 3 in which the numbers were equal (Table 2).

The endoscopic findings in cleft subjects consistently differed from those of normals. The nasopharyngeal orifice of the eustachian tube was found to be posteroinferiorly displaced. The torus tubarius was often hypoplastic, sometimes nearly nonexistent to sight. The orifice was often slitlike in appearance and decidedly smaller than normal (Fig. 1).

The most striking deviation from normal occurred during palatal motion when the interaction of the velum and tubal orifice could be observed. In normal subjects the orifice of the tube was patent at rest. During phonation and swallowing the tube remained patent, or the patency increased as the tube became more rounded (Fig. 2). The sling

TABLE 1 Incidence of Chronic Serous Otitis Media in Groups 1, 2, and 3

	Positive for Chronic Serous Otitis Media (%)	Negative for Chronic Serous Otitis Media (%)
Group 1	75.8	24.2
Group 2	73.5	26.5
Group 3	66.7	33.3

TABLE 2 Incidence of Chronic Serous Otitis Media by Sex in Groups 1, 2, and 3

	Males with Chronic Serous Otitis Media (%)	Females with Chronic Serous Otitis Media (%)
Group 1	58.8	72.4
Group 2	60.4	79.3
Group 3	66.7	66.7

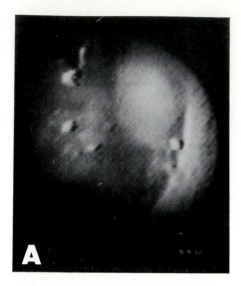

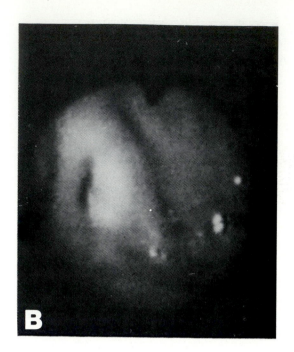

Figure 1 Appearance of the eustachian tube orifice at rest in a normal subject *(A)* and in a subject with cleft palate *(B)*.

of the levator was typically seen to lift the tail of the torus tubarius posterior to the orifice, thus resulting in the rounding effect. In cleft subjects the tube was often nonpatent at rest. This was dependent, in part, on the degree of abnormality of the torus tubarius. During swallowing and speech the orifice of the tube was actually seen to close in the majority of cases (see Fig. 2). The levator sling was seen to fill the orifice, anterior to the position seen in normal subjects. As the levator contracted, it occluded the orifice partially or totally.

DISCUSSION

The universality of middle ear disease in the cleft population has been assumed for the past decade or more. This assumption has led to accepted treatment regimens in many centers involving early and aggressive treatment of serous otitis media. At some major medical centers, cleft patients undergo myringotomy and tube surgery at the time of palate repair, even if the patient has had minimal or no indications of middle ear disease.[2]

In the current study, criteria for inclusion in the chronic serous otitis media group were deliberately liberal. In spite of this, only 76 percent of these subjects could be included in the chronic serous otitis media group. The aggressive use of myringotomy and tube surgery therefore may not be indicated in one quarter of the patients with palatal clefts.

Abnormal anatomy of the nasopharyngeal orifice of the eustachian tube orifice in cleft subjects has been proposed by several authors.[4-6] Therefore, recurrent serous otitis media in patients with clefts may be secondary to malformation of the tubal orifice instead of, or in addition to, the functional obstruction hypothesized by Bluestone.[2]

The mechanism of the functional abnormalities of the eustachian tube in the patient with cleft palate has not yet been conclusively demonstrated. During forced response testing in children with clefts, Doyle et al[7] demonstrated an increased resistance in the eustachian tube during swallowing in 73 percent of their subjects. They postulated that constriction of the tube was secondary to dysfunction of the tensor veli palatini. The findings in the current study indicate that the levator veli palatini sling may be

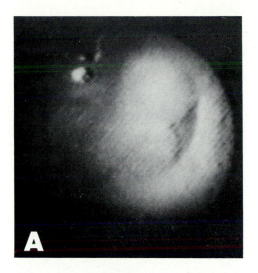

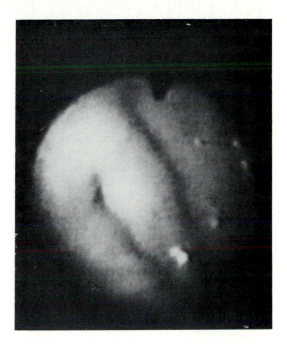

Figure 2 Appearance of the eustachian tube orifice during swallowing in the normal subject shown in *(A)* and the cleft subject shown in *(B)*.

responsible for this observation. In cleft subjects the torus tubarius appears to be in a posteroinferior position relative to that in normal subjects. The abnormal position of the orifice brings it into closer proximity to the velum, more specifically to the levator sling as it enters the lateral pharyngeal wall. As a result, the levator occludes the orifice upon phonation or swallowing. In normal subjects this does not occur because the orifice is positioned well above the palate and anterior to the levator sling. Levator action during swallowing in normal subjects moves the torus upward, which increases the patency of the orifice and tends to make it rounder. Therefore, the posteroinferior positioning of the orifice in the cleft subject places the levator sling directly in the orifice, which would also account for immobility of the torus and closure of the tube.

REFERENCES

1. Paradise JL, Bluestone CD, Felder H. The universality of otitis media in 50 infants with cleft palate. Pediatrics 1969; 44:35–42.
2. Bluestone CD. Eustachian tube obstruction in the infant with cleft palate. Ann Otol (St. Louis) 1971; 80 (Suppl 2):1–30.
3. Honjo I, Okazaki N, Kumazawa T. Experimental study of the eustachian tube function with regard to its related muscles. Acta Otolaryngol 1976; 82:159–163.
4. Maue-Dickson W, Dickson DR, Rood SR. Anatomy of the eustachian tube and related structures in age-matched human fetuses with and without cleft palate. Trans Am Acad Ophthalmol Otolaryngol 1976; 82:159–163.
5. Dickson DR. Anatomy of the normal and cleft palate eustachian tube. Ann Otol (St. Louis) 1976; 85 (Suppl 25):25–29.
6. Shprintzen RJ, Croft CB. Abnormalities of the eustachian tube orifice in individuals with cleft palate. Int J Pediatr Otorhinolaryngol 1981; 3:15–23.
7. Doyle WJ, Cantekin EI, Bluestone CD. Eustachian tube function in cleft palate children. Ann Otol Rhinol Laryngol 1980; 89(Suppl 68):34–40.

EUSTACHIAN TUBE FUNCTION IN CASES OF NASOPHARYNGEAL CARCINOMA

HIROAKI SATO, M.D., KYOSUKE KURATA, M.D., YI-HSIEN YEN, M.D., IWAO HONJO, M.D., YI-HO YOUNG, M.D., and TI HSIEH, M.D.

Nasopharyngeal carcinoma is often associated with otitis media with effusion.[1] The pathogenesis of otitis media with effusion has been considered to involve either tubal blockage[2,3] or functional obstruction of the tube.[4,5] However, the relationship between the tubal function and middle ear disease in patients with nasopharyngeal carcinoma has not been sufficiently elucidated.

We examined the characteristics of tubal dysfunction in patients with nasopharyngeal carcinoma and attempted to define the relationships among tumor extension, otitis media with effusion, and tubal dysfunction.

MATERIALS AND METHODS

One hundred thirteen ears were studied in 60 untreated patients with nasopharyngeal carcinoma. There were 42 men and 18 women ranging in age from 8 to 77 years (mean, 49.3 years). According to histologic classification, the tumors included undifferentiated carcinoma (25 cases), nonkeratinizing carcinoma (21 cases), and squamous cell carcinoma (14 cases). All the examinations were performed before irradiation therapy.

Study 1

Eustachian tube function was examined in 60 cases (113 ears). The ears of patients with nasopharyngeal carcinoma were classified into three groups according to endoscopic findings: those on the tumor side with (group A, 35 ears) and without otitis media with effusion (group B, 55 ears) and those on the unaffected side without otitis media with effusion (group C, 23 ears). On the basis of data from 33 normal ears with traumatic perforation of the drum, tubal function was evaluated as follows:

Ventilatory Function Test (Inflation-Deflation Test[6])

Passive opening of the tube was judged to be

high when the opening pressure was more than 546 mm H_2O. Active opening of the tube with positive pressure was judged to be normal when the applied positive pressure (+200 mm H_2O) dropped below 100 mm H_2O after swallowing several times, while that with negative pressure (−200 mm H_2O) was judged to be normal when any pressure equalization was noted. Other responses were judged to be poor.

Clearance Function Test (Dye Method)

Clearance function was judged to be delayed when the interval between instillation of 0.4 percent indigo carmine solution (0.02 ml) into the middle ear and its initial discharge from the pharyngeal orifice of the tube (which was observed endoscopically) was more than 15 minutes.

Study 2

Tumor extension was evaluated in 37 cases (66 ears) on the basis of computed tomographic findings (GE/CT 8600, 8800, or Pfizer 450) to determine the relationship between tumor extension and tubal dysfunction or otitis media with effusion. Stages were classified as follows: stage I, tumor not occupying the fossa of Rosenmüller (lateral pharyngeal recess); stage II, tumor occupying the fossa; stage III, tumor extending from the fossa to the parapharyngeal space; and stage IV, tumor occupying the parapharyngeal space.

Study 3

To determine the differences in tubal dysfunction between patients with otitis media with effusion with and without nasopharyngeal carcinoma, tubal function of patients in group A was compared with the values obtained in 127 patients with otitis media with effusion but without nasopharyngeal carcinoma (191 ears; 10 to 76 years of age; mean, 48.6 years). The percentage of cases of serous effusion was 85.7 percent in patients with nasopharyngeal carcinoma and 74.0 percent in those without nasopharyngeal carcinoma.

RESULTS

Study 1

Figure 1 shows tubal function in patients with nasopharyngeal carcinoma. Passive opening of the tube was generally less impaired than other tubal functions. The percentage of ears with a high opening pressure was highest in group A, but the differences among the three groups were not significant. The greatest impairment was observed in active opening of the tube, especially negative pressure equalization. Significant differences were found among the three groups for both positive and negative pressure equalization (X^2 test, $p < 0.05$). Clearance function of the tube was impaired only in group A.

Study 2

The incidence of otitis media with effusion and tubal dysfunction according to tumor staging is shown in Figure 2. Active tubal opening with negative pressure was the impairment most frequently seen, followed by active tubal opening with positive pressure, clearance function, and passive opening of the tube, in that order. In stage II, active tubal opening was impaired despite the low incidence of otitis media with effusion. In stage III, otitis media with effusion increased and active tubal opening was markedly impaired, but passive opening of the tube was not impaired.

Study 3

Figure 3 compares tubal function in patients with otitis media with effusion who had nasopharyngeal carcinoma with that in those who did not. All four tubal functions were more impaired in patients with nasopharyngeal carcinoma than in those without. However, no significant differences were observed between the two groups in any of the four tubal function tests.

DISCUSSION

The nearly normal passive opening of the tube, which indicates tubal patency, showed that organic obstruction of the tube was less common in the ears of patients with nasopharyngeal carcinoma. However, active tubal opening was impaired even

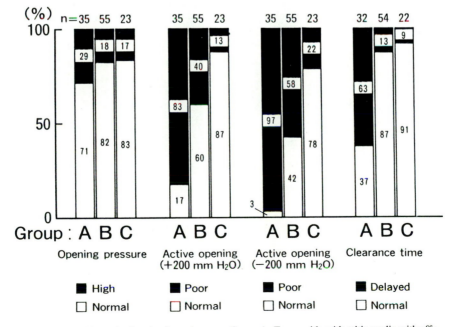

Figure 1 Eustachian tube function in each group. Group A: Tumor side with otitis media with effusion. Group B: Tumor side without otitis media with effusion. Group C: Unaffected side without otitis media with effusion.

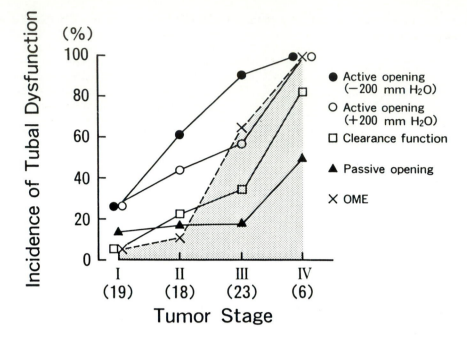

Figure 2 Relationship between tumor stage and otitis media with effusion or tubal dysfunction.

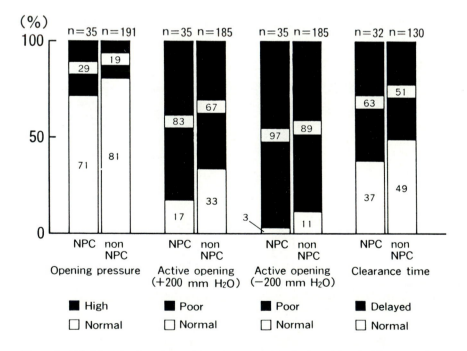

Figure 3 Tubal function in patients with otitis media with effusion with and without nasopharyngeal carcinoma.

in the ears on the tumor side without otitis media with effusion and markedly impaired in those with otitis media with effusion. Therefore, tubal dysfunction in nasopharyngeal carcinoma does not involve organic obstruction but functional impairment, possibly as a result of compression of the tube itself, tumor invasion to the tubal muscles, or inflammation around the tube.

On the other hand, clearance of the tube, which represents mucociliary transport, was poor only in the ears with otitis media with effusion, suggesting that poor clearance is a result of otitis media with effusion rather than its cause. In addition, otitis media with effusion and impairment of active tubal function increased when the tumor extended to the parapharyngeal space. These results indicate that tumor extension to the parapharyngeal space and resultant poor active tubal opening are important etiologic factors in the development of otitis media with effusion in nasopharyngeal carcinoma.

Furthermore, the tubal dysfunction found in patients with otitis media with effusion was similar to that in patients with otitis media with effusion but without nasopharyngeal carcinoma, which suggests

that the pathogenesis of otitis media with effusion both in nasopharyngeal carcinoma and in those without is similar.

REFERENCES

1. Godtfredsen E, Lederman M. Diagnostic and prognostic roles of ophthalmoneurologic signs and symptoms in malignant nasopharyngeal tumors. Am J Ophthalmol 1965; 59: 1063–1069.
2. Wang CC, Little JB, Schulz MD. Cancer of the nasopharynx. Its clinical and radiotherapeutic considerations. Cancer 1962; 15:921–926.
3. Choa G. Nasopharyngeal carcinoma. J Laryngol Otol 1974; 88:145–158.
4. Myers EN, Beery QC, Bluestone CD, Rood SR, Sigler BA. Effect of certain head and neck tumors and their management on the ventilatory function of the eustachian tube. Ann Otol Rhinol Laryngol 1984; 93(Suppl 114):1–16.
5. Takahara T, Sando I, Bluestone CD, Myers EN. Lymphoma invading the anterior eustachian tube. Temporal bone histopathology of functional tubal obstruction. Ann Otol Rhinol Laryngol 1986; 95:101–105.
6. Bluestone CD, Paradise JL, Beery QC. Symposium on prophylaxis and treatment of middle ear effusions. IV. Physiology of the eustachian tube in the pathogenesis and management of middle ear effusions. Laryngoscope 1972; 82: 1654–1670.

INTRANASAL CHALLENGE WITH HISTAMINE AND SALINE: EFFECTS ON TUBAL AND NASAL FUNCTION

DAVID P. SKONER, M.D., WILLIAM J. DOYLE, Ph.D., and PHILIP FIREMAN, M.D.

Recent investigations in both patients with allergic rhinitis and passively sensitized rhesus monkeys have shown that transient eustachian tube obstruction (ETO) is detectable after intranasal allergen challenge.[1-3] Intranasal challenge of nonsensitized rhesus monkeys with histamine, a primary mediator of the immediate allergic reaction, produced similar results, demonstrating that histamine could mediate the development of eustachian tube obstruction.[4] Walker et al[5] reported that following a single intranasal histamine challenge, human atopic subjects developed eustachian tube obstruction more frequently than nonatopic subjects. On the basis of these data, they suggested that the eustachian tube of atopic subjects is hyperresponsive to histamine. The purpose in our study was to

determine the dose-response characteristics of this phenomenon using a double blind crossover design.

Healthy nonsmoking adult subjects (age range, 20 to 31 years) without a history of ear disease or asthma were studied. Subjects with allergic rhinitis had a history of seasonal or perennial nasal symptoms, an elevated total serum IgE level (ranges, 343 to 528 IU per milliliter) by the FAST method,[6] positive skin tests (a wheal larger than 5 mm), and specific serum IgE antibodies (RAST[7]) to ragweed (1.4 to 24.2 percent bound/total radioactivity [BT]), grass (1.5 to 26.2 percent B/T), or house dust mite (0.5 to 30.9 percent B/T). Normal subjects did not have a history of seasonal or perennial nasal symptoms or allergies.

Five subjects with allergic rhinitis and five

nonallergic normal subjects were identified and randomly assigned to a double blinded intranasal challenge study with either increasing doses of histamine or repeated doses of a saline control. Subjects were then challenged with the other solution approximately 1 week later. Nasal and eustachian tube functions were assessed at baseline using anterior rhinomanometric[1] and nine-step tympanometric techniques[8] described previously and again 3 to 5 minutes after each challenge. If at least one eustachian tube maintained normal function, the challenges were repeated 20 minutes later using the next higher dose of histamine. Histamine doses (milligrams of histamine base) were increased as follows: 0.01, 0.1, 0.5, 1.0, 5.0, and 10.0 mg per nostril. Saline concentrations were uniform for each of the six potential challenges. These challenges were repeated until bilateral eustachian tube obstruction was detected or the final challenge dose was administered. Following completion of these challenges, each subject was skin tested intradermally with increasing doses of histamine 0.001, 0.005, 0.01, 0.05, and 0.1 mg of histamine base per milliliter).

The mean areas of skin responses of the allergic rhinitis and nonallergic groups to histamine and saline were compared. A steady increase was observed in the mean areas of wheal and flare with increasing concentration of histamine. However, significant differences were not observed in either wheal or flare for allergic rhinitis and nonallergic subjects.

Before challenge, the nasal airway resistances for both allergic rhinitis and nonallergic subjects were similar to those generated by normal individuals using this instrument. Baseline eustachian tube obstruction was observed unilaterally in one subject with allergic rhinitis. All other subjects had normal eustachian tube function. For the postchallenge nasal resistance data, the logarithm of the histamine dose was plotted against the corresponding logarithm of the nasal resistance for each subject. The median values of the slopes (0.16 and 0.17) and intercepts (0.91 and 0.94) of the fitted regression lines were similar for the allergic rhinitis and nonallergic groups, indicating a similar response in the two groups.

The frequencies with which eustachian tube obstruction was detected following histamine and saline nasal provocations are shown as a cumulative percentage in Figure 1. For the nine ears of subjects with allergic rhinitis, eustachian tube obstruction developed in five (56 percent) at 0.1 mg per nostril and in four (100 percent) at 0.5 mg histamine per nostril. In seven of these nine ears (78 percent), normal function was observed at follow-up examination

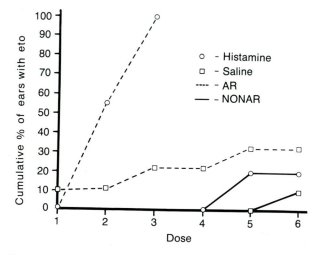

Figure 1   Cumulative percentage of ears with eustachian tube obstruction in patients with allergic rhinitis (broken lines) and in nonallergic patients (solid lines) following provocative intranasal challenge with histamine (open circles) or saline (open squares). The numbers on the horizontal axis indicate the position of each dose in the sequence of challenges (saline doses were uniform for all challenges; histamine dose 1 = 0.01, 2 = 0.1, 3 = 0.5, 4 = 1.0, 5 = 5.0, and 6 = 10.0 mg per nostril). AR = allergic rhinitis; NON-AR = nonallergic. (From Skoner DP, Doyle WJ, Fireman P. Eustachian tube obstruction (ETO) after histamine nasal provocation—a double-blind dose-response study. J Allergy Clin Immunol 1987; 79 (1):27–31.)

1 to 2 hours later. For the 10 ears of nonallergic subjects, eustachian tube obstruction developed in two ears (20 percent) at a dose of 5.0 mg per nostril (same individual) and did not develop in the remaining eight ears at doses up to 10 mg of histamine per nostril. Following the saline challenges, eustachian tube obstruction developed in three ears (33 percent) of two subjects with allergic rhinitis and in one ear (10 percent) of nonallergic subjects.

The results of the dose-response study show that following provocative intranasal histamine challenge, all ears of subjects with allergic rhinitis developed eustachian tube obstruction at relatively low histamine doses (≤ 0.5 mg per nostril). In contrast, even at maximal histamine concentrations (10 mg per nostril), only one nonallergic subject developed eustachian tube obstruction. Thus, subjects with and without allergic rhinitis are easily distinguished by the histamine dose at which eustachian tube obstruction developed. With the methods of the present study, a similar hyperresponsiveness of the nasal mucosa or the dermal skin layer to histamine challenge could not be demonstrated in subjects with allergic rhinitis.

The factors responsible for the observed tubal hyperresponsiveness to histamine are not known. A study to investigate the potential histamine receptor(s) involved has been initiated using specific H_1 and H_2 receptor antagonists.

This chapter is part of an article originally published in The Journal of Allergy and Clinical Immunology. Skoner DP, Doyle WJ, Fireman P. Eustachian tube obstruction (ETO) after histamine nasal provcation—a double-blind dose-response study. J Allergy Clin Immunol 1987; 79(1):27–31. Reprinted with permission from CV Mosby Company.

Study supported in part by grants A1-19262 and MO-1-RR-00084-23S1 from the National Institutes of Health.

REFERENCES

1. Friedman RA, Doyle WJ, Casselbrant ML, Bluestone CD, Fireman P. Immunologic-mediated eustachian tube obstruction: a double-blind crossover study. J Allergy Clin Immunol 1983; 71:442–447.
2. Ackerman MN, Friedman RA, Doyle WJ, Bluestone CD, Fireman P. Antigen-induced eustachian tube obstruction: an intranasal provocative challenge test. J Allergy Clin Immunol 1984; 73:604–609.
3. Doyle WJ, Friedman RA, Fireman P, Bluestone CD. Eustachian tube obstruction after provocative nasal antigen challenge. Arch Otolaryngol 1984; 110:508–511.
4. Doyle WJ, Ingraham A, Fireman P. The effects of intranasal histamine challenge on eustachian tube function. J Allergy Clin Immunol 1985; 76:551–556.
5. Walker SB, Shapiro GG, Bierman CW, Morgan MS, Marshall SG, Furukawa CT, Pierson WE. Induction of eustachian tube dysfunction with histamine nasal provocation. J Allergy Clin Immunol 1985; 76:158–162.
6. Tsay YG, Halpern GM. Fluorescent enzyme immunoassay for serum IgE (total IgE FAST). In: Book of abstracts. Fourth International Symposium on Rapid Methods and Automation in Microbiology and Immunology, Berlin, 1984:w20.
7. Gleich GJ, Yuninger JW. Standardization of allergens. In: Rose NR, Freidman H, eds. Manual of clinical immunology. Washington, DC: American Society for Microbiology, 1976:575.
8. Bluestone CD. Assessment of eustachian tube function. In: Jerger J, ed. Handbook of clinical impedance audiometry. Dobbs Ferry, NY: American Electronics Corp., 1975:127.

EFFECT OF NASAL ALLERGY ON EUSTACHIAN TUBE FUNCTION

YUJI TOYAMA, M.D., CHIYONORI INO, M.D., KEIJI HONDA, M.D., and TADAMI KUMAZAWA, M.D.

The role of allergies in the pathogenesis of middle ear and eustachian tube problems is still a subject of considerable controversy. In clinical and laboratory studies many investigators have reported a high incidence of otitis media with effusion in allergic patients, while an allergic etiology has been denied by others. To clinically observe the effect of nasal allergy on eustachian tube function, we studied 22 adults with a history of nasal allergy but no history of otitis media with effusion.

The patients were confirmed as having hypersensitivity to house dust by a positive skin test reaction to intradermal injection and intranasal challenge. Otologic tests included pneumatic otoscopy and evaluations of hearing and tubal function by the acoustic impedance method and tubotympanoaerodynamic testing. For allergen administration we used two methods.

MATERIAL AND METHODS

We first administered to the anterior part of the inferior turbinate a disk containing a house dust extract as provocation. The second test was direct administration to the pharyngeal opening of the tube through the unblocked side of the nasal cavity by use of an applicator containing the same extract.

A block diagram and a normal pattern for the tubotympanoaerodynamic test are shown in Figure 1. Simultaneous recording of pressures in the external ear canal and nasopharyngeal cavity was carried out during Valsalva inflation and exhalation during swallowing. Thus, inflow and outflow of air through the tube were registered together with the nasopharyngeal pressure change. These consistent pressure changes were recorded as waves. The aerodynamic patterns enable one to evaluate eustachian tube function (Fig. 1).

RESULTS

First Method

No remarkable change was recorded in the inflated segment with the first administration method. In the outflow segment a poor exhalation pattern was observed in three ears of 18 patients, about 17 percent. (Four ears were excluded from the study because of inadequate information or recording error.)

Second Method

With the second administration method, in which the tubal opening was stimulated directly, poor exhalation was observed in three ears. In four ears poor inflation and exhalation were observed. In two ears there was no change. In one ear there was no response.

Of eight ears that showed good inflation and exhalation before administration, one ear showed a normal pattern. In two ears poor exhalation was observed. Poor inflation and exhalation were observed in one ear.

In four ears that showed poor exhalation prior to administration, poor inflation and exhalation were observed in three after administration.

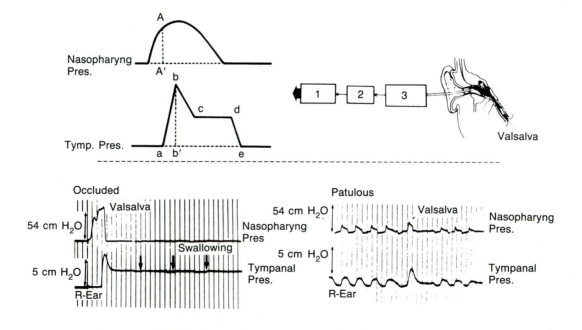

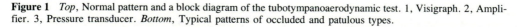

Figure 1 *Top,* Normal pattern and a block diagram of the tubotympanoaerodynamic test. 1, Visigraph. 2, Amplifier. 3, Pressure transducer. *Bottom,* Typical patterns of occluded and patulous types.

Pattern Change with the Passage of Time

The pattern change with the passage of time in the left ear of a 36 year old man is recorded in Figure 1. Before administration the aerodynamic pattern showed good inflation and exhalation. Five minutes later this pattern changed to show poor inflation and exhalation. Seven minutes later the difficulties with inflow and outflow of air through the tube decreased. This tendency continued until recovery was observed, 10 minutes after adminstration.

DISCUSSION

Endoscopic observation of the tubal mouth was successfully conducted in the present study. Mucosal swelling and hypersecretion after provocation were seen with the second method.

Skoner and others have reported the results of studies of eustachian tube function after provocation of the nasal cavity with several extracts, and Skoner (1986) reported changes after inhalation using house dust mites.

In the present study 17 percent of the subjects had poor exhalation after use of the first method. By contrast almost all subjects showed poor inflation and poor exhalation after the use of the second method. It thus can be inferred that the tubal opening can act as a barrier to the eustachian tube to inhaled antigen.

REFERENCES

1. Kumazawa T. Eustachian tube function, physiology and role in otitis media. Workshop report. Ann Otol Rhinol Laryngol 1985; 94:5(Suppl 120):24–26.
2. Skoner DP. Eustachian tube obstruction after intranasal challenge with house dust mite. Arch Otol Head Neck Surg 1984; 110:508–511.
3. McGovern JP. Allergy and secretory otitis media. An analysis of 512 cases. JAMA 1967; 200:134–138.
4. Doyle WJ. Eustachian tube obstruction after provocative nasal antigen challenge. Arch Otolaryngol 1984; 110:508–511.
5. Connell JT. Quantitative intranasal pollen challenges: the priming effect in allergic rhinitis. J Allergy 1969; 43:33–38.
6. Friedman RA. Immunologic mediated eustachian tube obstruction: a double blind crossover study. J Allergy Clin Immunol 1983; 71:442–447.

TYPE I ALLERGIC REACTION IN THE MIDDLE EAR AND EUSTACHIAN TUBE MUCOSA—AN EXPERIMENTAL STUDY

KAZUHIRO TOMONAGA, M.D., YUICHI KURONO, M.D., and GORO MOGI, M.D.

Although allergy has long received attention as a causative factor in secretory otitis media, its exact role in the etiology and pathogenesis of this disease remains unclear. Many clinical studies have supported the allergic etiology because of a high incidence of secretory otitis media in allergic patients.[1-4] However, these observations were made before IgE, a reaginic antibody, was discovered.[5] Since the discovery of IgE in 1966, the mechanisms of atopic allergic reactions (type I immunologic reaction) have been elucidated, resulting in the establishment of accurate diagnostic tests for IgE mediated disorders, such as allergic rhinitis and bronchial asthma. In a previous study we reported that 50 percent of the pediatric patients with secretory otitis media suffered from nasal allergy, that 21 percent of the pediatric patients with nasal allergy suffered from secretory otitis media, and that 17 and 6 percent respectively, of a normal control group suffered from nasal allergy and secretory otitis media.[6] It was also found that the incidence of tubal dysfunction in patients with secretory otitis media associated with nasal allergy was significantly higher than that in patients with secretory otitis media and that the incidence of tubal dysfunction in patients with nasal allergy was significantly higher than that in normal control subjects. This finding is consistent with the results of a study by Skoner et al.[7]

In the present investigation we prepared an animal model of type I allergy and, after provocation, observed changes in the mucosa covering the nasopharynx, eustachian tube, and tympanic cavity. Eustachian tube function was also evaluated before and after the provocation.

MATERIALS AND METHODS

Animals

Healthy male Hartley guinea pigs, weighing 300 to 400 g, were used.

Preparation of Antiserum for Passive Sensitization

Five micrograms of 2, 4-dinitrophenylated Ascaris (DNP Ascaris) was mixed with 5 mg of aluminum hydroxide gel as adjuvant. One milliliter of the mixture was injected into the foot pads of the guinea pigs. The same dose of antigen was administered intracutaneously into the back region twice—2 and 4 weeks—after the initial injection. Serum was obtained 1 week after the final immunization and proven to have an IgE antibody titer greater than 1,024 against DNP Ascaris by passive cutaneous anaphylaxis testing.

Passive Sensitization

The antiserum was injected intravenously into guinea pigs for passive sensitization.

Local Challenge with Antigen in the Nasal and Tympanic Cavities

One week after the passive sensitization, 0.5 ml of DNP ovualbumin (DNP OVA) at a concentration of 5 mg per milliliter was dropped into the nasal cavity, and 0.1 ml of the same antigen solution was injected into the tympanic cavity through the tympanic bulla. Before each challenge the animal was anesthetized with pentobarbital sodium solution.

Evaluation of Eustachian Tube Function

In a total of 40 guinea pigs, tubal function was evaluated by inflation and deflation tests[8] using tympanometry (Amplaid 702, Dana Japan Ltd., Tokyo) after the eardrum was perforated. Inflation and deflation tests were conducted in the passively sensitized animals before the local antigen challenge and 0.5, 1, 2, 3, 4, 5, and 6 hours after the antigen

challenge into the nose to serve as a control, saline solution was administered to five passively sensitized guinea pigs.

Histologic Examination

A total of 35 guinea pigs were used in this examination. Immediately after sacrificing the animals, specimens of the middle ear (both eustachian tube and tympanic cavity), nasopharynx, and nose were fixed with Mota's solution,[9] decalcified by EDTA, and dehydrated with ethanol. Serial tissue sections were stained with hematoxylin-eosin and toluidine blue. Control specimens were obtained from the same sites in guinea pigs at which saline solution was administered. The eustachian tube was usually observed at three points: near the pharyngeal orifice, at the midportion, and near the tympanic orifice (see Fig.3).

RESULTS

Tubal Function Tests

Following all challenges with DNP OVA into the nose, the animals exhibited moderate to severe sneezing, hypersecretion, and open mouth breathing. Sneezing disappeared within 40 minutes, but the hypersecretion and open mouth breathing lasted for 3 hours. As can be seen in Figure 1 an increase in the opening pressure was observed in all animals tested 30 minutes and 1 hour after the antigen challenge into the nose. The mean values of the opening pressure were 478 ± 34.0 mm H_2O (N = 5) at 30 minutes and 463 ± 39.6 mm H_2O (N = 5) at 1 hour. These values were significantly higher ($p < 0.01$) than the value before the antigen challenge and the value in control animals. The mean value of each opening pressure 3 hours after the nasal provocation was almost the same as the value before the provocation as shown in Figure 2.

Histologic Changes

The most remarkable changes seen in mucous membranes were eosinophilic and basophilic infiltrations and edema. Figure 3 summarizes the histologic changes 30 minutes after the local antigen challenge. At that time the histologic changes were usually intense. These changes were seen in the mucous membranes of the nose, nasopharynx, and pharyn-

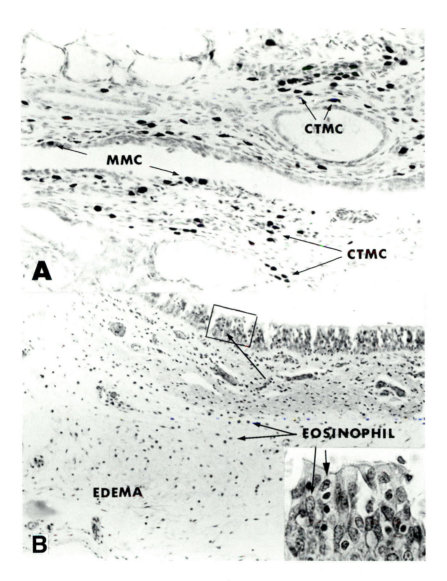

Figure 1 *A*, Mucosal mast cells (MMC) and connective tissue mast cells (CTMC) in the mucous membrane of the eustachian tube near the pharyngeal orifice 30 minutes following administration of antigen to the nasal cavity. (Toluidine blue stain. × 200.) *B*, Eosinophil infiltration and edema in the mucous membrane of the eustachian tube near the pharyngeal orifice 30 minutes following administration of antigen to the nasal cavity. *Inset*, High magnification of the square area. (Toluidine blue stains. × 100, × 400.)

geal orifice and near the pharyngeal orifice of the eustachian tube (but not in the rest of the eustachian tube) upon nasal antigen challenge. When the antigen was administered into the tympanic cavity, histologic changes were limited to the tympanic cavity and eustachian tube (other than near the pharyngeal orifice). Noticeable infiltrations of eosinophils and

basophils were not seen in the mucous membranes of animals sacrificed at 2, 3, 4, 5, and 6 hours after the antigen challenge. Edema lasted 3 hours after the antigen challenge.

Middle ear effusion was not seen, by gross inspection in the tympanic cavity of any animal challenged with the antigen delivered into both the

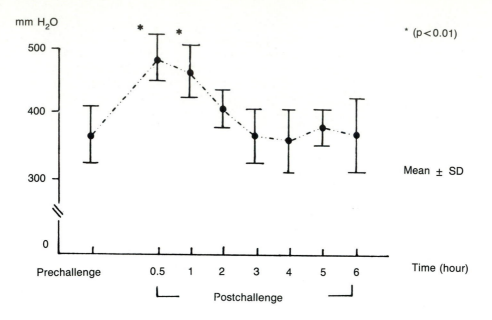

Figure 2 Opening pressures before and after the antigen challenge to the nasal cavity.

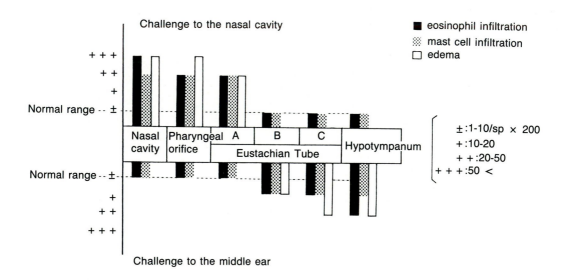

Figure 3 Histologic changes in the mucous membrane 30 minutes following the antigen challenge to the nasal cavity and tympanic cavity.

nasal cavity and the tympanic cavity. However, histologic evidence of effusion was noted in the tympanic cavity and the lumen of eustachian tube in occasional cases.

DISCUSSION

The present investigation showed that the eustachian tube is involved, both functionally and histologically in type I allergic reactions of the nose, even if the histologic changes occurred only up to the area near the pharyngeal orifice. It was also noted that IgE mediated reactions can be induced in the tympanic mucosa upon direct antigenic challenge. This finding supports the supposition, proposed by Miglets,[10] that the tympanic cavity can act as an allergic "shock organ." However, the antigen challenge to the nasal cavity did not induce any allergic change in the tympanic cavity. The histologic change and the dysfunction of the eustachian tube evoked by allergen challenge were transient (a few hours) and did not result in the formation of a middle ear effusion.

Miglets[10] and Doyle et al[11] induced type I allergic reactions in the eustachian tube and tympanic mucosa in rhesus monkeys by allergen challenge (ragweed pollen) to the nose or the eustachian tube following passive sensitization of the animal with allergic (to the ragweed pollen) human serum samples. However, there is a discrepancy between the results of these studies. Miglets observed middle ear effusion, whereas no effusion was detected in the study by Doyle et al even though the pollens reached the tympanic cavity.

Many studies of IgE in human subjects have refuted the hypothesis that middle ear effusion is produced by allergy.[12-14] The results of the present investigation agree with this evidence. Although the middle ear is a "shock organ," it is difficult to believe that inhalant allergens travel up to the tympanic cavity, beyond the barrier (the eustachian tube) that limits the access of many substances to the ear. This function maintains the sterility of the middle ear. Another reason for the lack of generation of middle ear effusion by allergic reactions is that IgE mediated reactions are too transient to cause middle ear effusions. Therefore, we conclude that type I allergy is an otitis prone, or recurrent, factor rather than an etiologic factor in secretory otitis media.

REFERENCES

1. Lewis ER. Otitis media and allergy. Ann Otol Rhinol Laryngol 1929; 38:185–188.
2. Proetz AW. Allergy in the middle and internal ear. Ann Otol Rhinol Laryngol 1931; 40:67–76.
3. Jordan R. Chronic secretory otitis media. Laryngoscope 1949; 59:1002–1015.
4. Derlacki EL. Aural manifestations of allergy. Ann Otol Rhinol Laryngol 1952; 61:179–183.
5. Ishizaka K, Ishizaka T, Hornbrook MM. Physicochemical properties of human reaginic antibodies. IV. Presence of a unique immunoglobulin as a carrier of reaginic activity. J Immunol 1966; 97:75–85.
6. Tomonaga K, et al. Role of nasal allergy in otitis media with effusion. A clinical study. In: Abstracts. Fourth International Symposium on Recent Advances in Otitis Media, Bal Harbour, Florida. 1987:161.
7. Skoner DP, Doyle WJ, Fireman P. Eustachian tube obstruction (ETO) after histamine nasal provocation—double-blind dose-response study. J Allergy Clin Immunol 1987; 79:27–31.
8. Miller GF. Eustachian tubal function in normal and diseased ears. Arch Otolaryngol 1965; 81:41–48.
9. Enerhach L. Mast cells in rat gastrointestinal mucosa. I. Effects of fixation. Acta Path Microbiol Scand 1960; 86:289–294.
10. Miglets A. The experimental production of allergic middle ear effusions. Laryngoscope 1973; 83:1355–1384.
11. Doyle WJ, Takahara T, Fireman P. The role of allergy in the pathogenesis of otitis media with effusion. Arch Otolaryngol 1985; 3:502–506.
12. Mogi G, et al. Radioimmunoassay of IgE in middle ear effusions. Acta Otolaryngol 1976; 82:26–32.
13. Lewis DM, Schram JL, Lim DJ. Immunoglobulin E in chronic middle ear effusions. Comparison of RIST, PRIST and RIA techniques. Ann Otol Rhinol Laryngol 1978; 87:197–201.
14. Bernstein JM, et al. The role of IgE mediated hypersensitivity in recurrent otitis media with effusion. Am J Otol 1983; 5:66–99.

MEASUREMENTS OF BLOOD FLOW VOLUME IN THE EUSTACHIAN TUBE

TOYOHIKO MINAMI, M.D., NOBUO KUBO, M.D., YOSHIRO HORI, HIROYUKI TSUJI, M.D., TOSHIO YAMASHITA, M.D., and TADAMI KUMAZAWA, M.D.

Clinical and physiologic studies have suggested that the volume of blood flow in the eustachian tube mucosa plays an important role in mediating tubal patency. In this study we first examined the regional distribution of blood flow and directly measured the blood flow volume in the eustachian tube. Then we studied autonomic nerve stimulation by histamine and prostaglandin stimulation in order to verify the pathogenetic role of middle ear effusion as a mediator in otitis media with effusion.

MATERIALS AND METHODS

The blood flow volume was measured by two methods.

Microsphere Method

We investigated the regional distribution of the blood flow in the eustachian tube by the microsphere method. Nonradiolabeled microspheres (8 to 15 μm in diameter) were injected directly into the hearts of guinea pigs. Fifteen minutes after the injection a temporal bone specimen including the eustachian tube was dissected out. Then we counted the number of microspheres trapped in the tubal mucosa of each section under light microscopy. Regional distributions of trapped microspheres were calculated.

Hydrogen Gas Clearance Method

The hydrogen gas clearance method is widely used to measure the blood flow volume. In our studies a platinum coated electrode was inserted into the pharyngeal orifice of the eustachian tube of a dog by the palatal approach. Then hydrogen gas was administered for inhalation for a few minutes. A clearance recorder was used to detect the current curve, and the blood flow per unit of tissue was calculated according to Fick's principle. Blood flow volume in the tympanic orifice was measured in the same way through the extra-auditory canal after myringectomy.

Sympathetic stimulation and blocking and parasympathetic stimulation were studied by the topical application of three drugs (norepinephrine 10^{-6} mg per ml; prazosin, 10^{-6} mg per ml; and acetylcholine) on the pharyngeal orifice. The pharmacologic effects were studied after the transtympanic injection of 2–methylhistamine, 10^{-5} mg per ml; 4–methylhistamine, 10^{-5} mg per ml; PGE$_2$, 10^{-4} mg per ml; and PGF$_2$; 10^{-4} mg per ml.

The inflation-deflation test was carried out to determine the effects on patency in the eustachian tube.[2]

RESULTS

The number of trapped microspheres was greatest in the pharyngeal orifice (72 percent). By the hydrogen gas clearance method the blood flow volume in the pharyngeal orifice was found to be 89.6 $\pm$ 2.2 ml per min per 100 g, and it was 42.5 $\pm$ 2.9 ml per min per 100 g in the tympanic orifice. Sympathetic stimulation with norepinephrine and parasympathetic blocking by pterygopalatine ganglion block decreased the blood flow volume. Sympathetic blocking with prazosin and parasympathetic stimulation with acetylcholine increased the blood flow volume.

The blood flow changes in the pharyngeal orifice following transtympanic stimulation with histamines and prostaglandins are shown in Tables 1 and 2. These substances have been reported to be present in middle ear effusion.[3,4] 2–Methylhistamine increased the blood flow volume (133.8 $\pm$ 4.7 ml per min per 100 g). With 4–methylhistamine there was no change (94.7 $\pm$ 7.8 ml per min per 100

TABLE 1 Autonomic and Pharmacologic Effects on Blood Flow Volume in the Pharyngeal Orifice

		Blood Flow Volume (ml/min/100 g)		Patency of Eustachian Tube
		Before	After	
Sympathetic	Stimulation (norepinephrine)	59.8 ± 2	34.3 ± 7	Increased
	Block (prazosin)	91.9	101.2	—
Parasympathetic	Stimulation (acetylcholine)	88.9	97.8	—
	Block (pterygopalatine ganglion)	89.6	71.8	—
Histamine		59.8 ± 2	62.0 ± 9.6	No change

g). PGE_2 increased (108.0 ± 7.7 ml per min per 100 g) but PGF_2 decreased (74.9 ± 6.3 ml per min per 100 g) the blood flow volume in the pharyngeal orifice.

DISCUSSION

With the microsphere method the blood flow volume was found to be highest in the pharyngeal orifice. These results support the argument in several previous reports that vessels are abundant in the pharyngeal orifice of the eustachian tube.[5] In regard to the onset of otitis media with effusion, it is well known that functional obstruction of the eustachian tube plays a significant role. Our study suggests that histamine and PGE_2, whose presence has been demonstrated in middle ear effusions, may increase the blood flow volume and disturb the microcirculation in the eustachian tube by increasing the permeability of the blood vessels in the eustachian tubal mucosa. Middle ear effusion produced by allergy and infections flows out into the pharyngeal orifice by a pumping action and by mucociliary transport, acting on the normal mucosa in the tube. The physiologic effects of histamine and prostaglandins in middle ear effusions may possibly be related to these two possible mechanisms of onset of otitis media with effusion, causing a vicious cycle (Fig. 1).

TABLE 2 Blood Flow Change in Pharyngeal Orifice Following Transtympanic Stimulation with Histamines and Prostaglandins

		Blood Flow Volume (ml/min/100 g)	
		Before	After
Histamine	2-Methylhistamine (H_1 agonist)	86.6	133.8
	4-Methylhistamine (H_2 agonist)	94.7	96.1
Prostaglandin	PGE_2	94.2	108.9
	$PGE_{2\alpha}$	91.9	74.9
Epinephrine		155.0	95.3

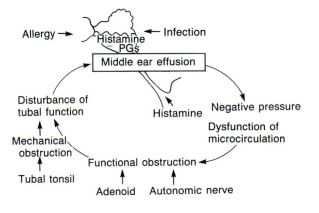

Figure 1 The vicious cycle of otitis media with effusion.

REFERENCES

1. Aukland K. Measurement of local blood flow with hydrogen gas. Circ Res 1964; 14:164–187.
2. Bluestone CD, et al. Panel on experiences with testing eustachian tube function. Ann Otolaryngol 1981; 90:552–562.
3. Jung TK. Identification of prostaglandins and other arachidonic acid metabolites in experimental otitis media. Prostaglandins Leukotrienes Med 1982; 8:249–261.
4. Berger G. Histamine levels in middle ear effusions. Acta Otolaryngol (Stockh) 1984; 98:385–390.
5. Proctor B, et al. Embryology and anatomy of the eustachian tube. Arch Otolaryngol 1967; 86:2–8.

TYMPANOMETRIC FINDINGS IN INFANTS FOLLOWING FEEDING IN UPRIGHT AND SUPINE POSITIONS

MAUREEN COLLISON, M.D., F.R.C.P., COLIN D. MARCHANT, M.D., DAVID SHIPP, M.A., and EUNICE BAND, R.N.

The position of feeding is thought to play a role in the pathogenesis of otitis media.[1-3] Beauregard[1] found that of 183 infants less than 18 months of age with acute otitis media, 85 percent had a history of supine bottle feeding. In contrast, in a control group of 50 infants less than 18 months of age with no history of otitis media, only 8 percent had been bottle fed in this manner. In a study of Canadian Eskimo children Schaefer[2] found a strong association between bottle versus breast feeding in children with chronic otitis media. In a prospective study of 2,565 children by Teele et al,[3] persistent middle ear effusion following acute otitis media was significantly associated with only one factor, and that was giving a child a bottle in bed. The position of feeding is a factor that may explain these findings.

Recently postprandial tympanometric abnormalities were observed in 59.6 percent of the children less than 2 years of age fed in the supine position.[4] Since many of these children may have had previous episodes of otitis media, we studied infants 2 to 7 months of age with no history of ear infection and normal baseline tympanometric findings. Tympanograms were then obtained before and after feeding to determine the incidence of negative peak tympanometric pressure and middle ear effusion after feeding, and whether abnormalities were related to the position of feeding (upright versus supine) or the method of feeding (breast versus bottle).

MATERIALS AND METHODS

The subjects were 21 healthy infants 2 to 7 months of age. Apparently normal infants were recruited either at birth or from private pediatric practices. Subjects were excluded if there was a history of otitis media or concurrent upper respiratory tract infection. Exclusion criteria included head and neck abnormalities (e.g., cleft palate) and significant systemic disease.

Tympanometry was performed using a Grason-Stadler 1723 version II otoadmittance meter. Susceptance tympanograms with a probe tone frequency of 660 Hz were recorded across a pressure range from +300 mm H_2O to −400 mm H_2O at a rate of pressure change of 50 mm per second. Tympanograms were analyzed by drawing a baseline from +300 mm H_2O to −400 mm H_2O and measuring the peak susceptance above the baseline. The peak susceptance was measured at right angles to the abscissa of the X—Y plot.

The following definitions were used:

1. Normal tympanogram: peak susceptance > 0 mmho[5] and peak pressure > −50 mm H_2O.
2. Negative middle ear pressure: susceptance ≤ 0 mmho and peak pressure ≤ 0 −50 mm H_2O.
3. Middle ear effusion peak susceptance ≤ 0 (i.e., a flat tympanogram).
4. An appreciable change was defined as a change in pressure of 50 mm H_2O or more.

Children with flat baseline tympanograms were excluded. Those who demonstrated a peak pressure less than −100 mm H_2O by tympanometry were treated as a separate group.

Children were randomized to feeding in either

the supine or upright position. Infants were either breast or bottle fed for approximately 3 minutes. A postprandial tympanogram was recorded, and if it was normal, the child was fed in the second position. If either negative pressure or a flat tympanogram was observed, the examiner waited for 20 minutes and then repeated the tympanography. If the second tympanogram was normal, the child went on the feeding in the other position. If abnormalities persisted, the patient was scheduled to return within 1 week for feeding in the other position.

RESULTS

We studied 13 breast fed infants and eight bottle fed infants. Tympanograms following feeding are presented in Table 1. In 61 ear examinations only one ear with a normal baseline pressure developed negative pressures of 150 mm H_2O after upright breast feeding. No flat tympanograms were observed.

Several infants had negative peak tympanogram pressures before feeding. We also performed tympanometry in this group after feeding. In the breast fed group, three of seven ears with negative pressures showed no change after feeding. In two ears (supine feeding) the pressure normalized, in one ear (upright) the pressure decreased, and in one ear a flat tympanogram was recorded after upright feeding. In a bottle fed infant one ear had a negative baseline pressure and a flat tympanogram was recorded after feeding.

DISCUSSION

Infection and eustachian tube dysfunction are thought to be important in the pathogenesis of acute otitis media and otitis media with effusion. Whether eustachian tube dysfunction is congenital, secondary to infection, or related to feeding practices such as the position of feeding is unclear. Following feeding a tympanometric finding of negative middle ear pressure suggesting eustachian tube obstruction or a flat tympanogram indicative of middle ear effusion would be highly suggestive of an important role of feeding and position of feeding in the development of otitis media. However, we found these changes to be uncommon in normal infants.

Previous studies have shown a difference in chil-

TABLE 1 Tympanograms After Feeding in Infants With Normal Baseline Tympanograms

Feeding Method	Feeding Position	Tympanograms After Feeding (Ears)		
		Normal	Negative Pressure	Middle Ear Effusion
Breast	Upright	16	1	0
Breast	Supine	20	0	0
Bottle	Upright	12	0	0
Bottle	Supine	12	0	0
Total		60	1	0

dren fed in a supine position, but these children may have had a history of otitis media.[1] Inflammation of the eustachian tube could have predisposed such children to middle ear effusion or negative pressure. Therefore we selected normal infants with no history of otitis media and normal baseline tympanograms prior to feeding. We conclude that:

1. In normal infants without a history of otitis media the position and method of feeding do not affect middle ear pressure as measured by tympanometry.
2. In infants with negative middle ear pressures, flat tympanograms may be recorded after feeding, but further studies in infants with negative middle ear pressures and those with prior otitis media are needed to determine whether changes in middle ear pressure occur after feeding. If these are abnormalities after supine feeding, our finding suggests that they are uncommon in normal infants and therefore must be related to upper respiratory tract infection or prior otitis media.

REFERENCES

1. Beauregard WG. Positional otitis media. J Pediatr 1971; 79:294–296.
2. Schaefer O. Otitis media and bottle feeding. An epidemiological study of infant feeding habits and incidence of recurrent and chronic middle ear disease in Canadian Eskimos. Can J Public Health 1971; 62:478–489.
3. Teele DW, Klein JO, Rosner BA. Epidemiology of otitis media in children. Ann Otol Rhinol Laryngol 1980; 89(Suppl 68):5–6.
4. Tully SB, Bar–Haim Y, Bradley RL. Abnormal tympanography following supine bottle feeding (abstracts). Am J Dis Child 1986; 140:303.

OTITIS MEDIA AND THE BLOCKED NOSE

FINN JÖRGENSEN, M.D. and JÖRGEN HOLMQUIST, M.D., Ph.D.

In several investigations a correlation has been found between the bacterial flora in the nasopharynx and that in the middle ear in acute otitis media as well as in secretory otitis media.[1] This correlation indicates that bacteria found in the middle ear in these diseases may have reached the middle ear by way of the eustachian tube.

The mucociliary system as well as the closed eustachian tube acts to protect the middle ear by preventing bacteria from reaching the middle ear from the nasopharynx. The eustachian tube, however, usually opens during swallowing or yawning. As a result of pressure changes in the nasopharynx during tubal opening, air or secretions may be forced into the middle ear through the eustachian tube. Pressure changes may be created, for example, by blowing the nose as well as by the Toynbee maneuver (swallowing against occluded nostrils).[2]

Pressure changes in the nasopharynx resulting from the Toynbee maneuver may be biphasic or monophasic and positive or negative (Fig. 1). Depending on the time of opening and closing of the tube in relation to nasopharyngeal pressure, the middle ear pressure may be positive, negative, or zero in relation to ambient air pressure.[3]

In the present investigation we measured the final middle ear pressure in normal individuals and in patients with infectious middle ear disease.

MATERIAL AND METHODS

The normal individuals were recruited from medical students or staff without middle ear disease, with normal otomicroscopic findings, and with middle ear pressures within ± 50 mm H_2O. Forty-seven ears in 27 individuals were included in the study.

The pathologic ears were classified into two groups. One group of 25 ears (23 patients) had chronic otitis media and dry perforations of the tympanic membrane. The second group had intact tympanic membranes but a history of recurrent episodes of acute otitis media; the latter group consisted of 49 ears in 32 patients.

In ears with intact tympanic membranes the middle ear impedance changes during the Toynbee maneuver were recorded with an impedance audiometer. Just after the Toynbee maneuver the middle ear pressure was registered by tympanometry.

In ears with tympanic membrane perforations the middle ear pressure was registered with a manometer connected in an air-tight manner to the ear canal.

All individuals were tested in the sitting position, performing the Toynbee maneuver by swallowing against occluded nostrils. The impedance or middle ear pressure was recorded continuously, and when no change was monitored after five repeated maneuvers, the test result was noted as negative.

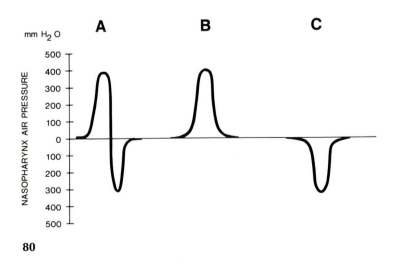

Figure 1 Air pressure changes in nasopharynx during Toynbee's maneuver. A: indicates biphasic; B, monophasic positive; C, monophasic negative.

When changes were noted, the test was halted and the middle ear pressure was monitored by tympanometry or manometry, depending on the condition of the tympanic membrane.

RESULTS

Eighty-three percent of the normal ears and 52 percent of the otitis media ears yielded positive results on the Toynbee test, as illustrated in Figure 2. A positive middle ear pressure after a successfully performed Toynbee maneuver was registered in 2 percent of the normal ears and in 51 percent of the otitis media ears, as seen in Figure 3.

DISCUSSION

Several authors have noted dysfunction of the eustachian tube as the most important factor in the development and maintenance of middle ear disease.[4,5]

The Toynbee phenomenon may be important,

since nasal obstruction is so common in connection with upper respiratory infections; acute and secretory otitis media show the same seasonal variation as upper respiratory infections.[6,7] It is also a common clinical observation that dry chronic otitis media starts draining during upper respiratory infections.

In our study a positive middle ear pressure after the Toynbee maneuver was registered in 51 percent of the otitis media ears but in only 2 percent of the normal ears.

When the eustachian tube opens at a positive nasopharyngeal pressure, air and bacteria containing secretions may be forced into the middle ear. On the other hand, when the middle ear pressure is positive in relation to the air pressure in the nasopharynx, evacuation of the middle ear is facilitated, as seen in Figure 4.

By x-ray examination in 78 children with secretory otitis media it has been shown that radiopaque material passes from the nasopharynx into the middle ear in 56 percent of the cases when the Toynbee maneuver is performed.[8] These findings support the data presented in our study.

We suggest that positive air pressure created at

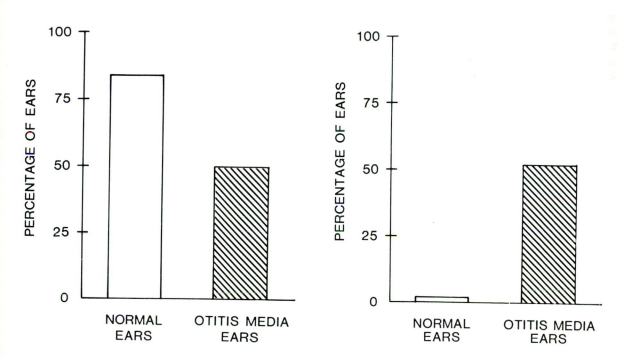

Figure 2 Successfully performed Toynbee test.

Figure 3 Positive middle ear air pressure after Toynbee's maneuver.

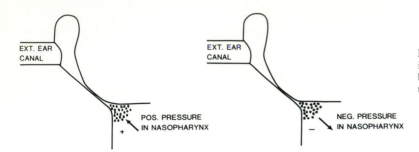

Figure 4 Schematic illustration showing two mechanisms for the transport of bacterial secretion by the eustachian tube.

the time of a Toynbee maneuver plays a role in the initiation and maintenance of middle ear disease. More attention should be paid in keeping the nose unobstructed in order to prevent infectious material from reaching the middle ear during swallowing.

REFERENCES

1. Schwartz RH. Bacteriology of otitis media: a review. Otolaryngol Head Neck Surg 1981; 89:444–450.
2. Thomsen KA. Investigation on Toynbee's experiment in normal individuals. Acta Otolaryngol 1957; Suppl 140:263–268.
3. Ingelstedt S, Örtengren U. Qualitative testing of the eustachian tube function. Acta Otolaryngol 1963; Suppl 182:7–23.
4. Holmquist J, Renvall U. Middle ear ventilation in secretory otitis media. Ann Otol 1976; Suppl 25:178–181.
5. Silverstein H, Miller G, Lindeman R. Eustachian tube dysfunction as a cause for chronic secretory otitis media in children. Laryngoscope 1966; 76:259–273.
6. Meistrup-Larsen KI, Strøyer Andersen M, Helweg J, et al. Variations in tympanograms in children attending group-care during one year period. ORL 1981; 43:153–163.
7. Pukander J, Loutonen J, Sipilä M, et al. Incidence of acute otitis media. Acta Otolaryngol 1982; 93:447–453.
8. Bluestone CD, Paradise JL, Berry QC. Physiology of the eustachian tube in the pathogenesis and management of middle ear effusions. Laryngoscope 1972: 82(9):1654–1670.

EUSTACHIAN TUBE PHYSIOLOGY

MIDDLE EAR PRESSURE AND GAS DIFFUSION

HIDEICHI SHINKAWA, M.D., YUTAKA SASAKI, M.D., NAOKI INAMURA, M.D., TAKUJI OKITSU, M.D., and TOMONORI TAKASAKA, M.D.

The gas in the middle ear is one of the essential factors in middle ear function. However, limited data are available relating to the gas composition in the middle ear because of technologic difficulties.[1-3] Moreover, the gas composition may change depending on the physiologic condition. We determined the middle ear gas content in chinchillas respired spontaneously with air.

Recently a few studies have demonstrated a positive intratympanic pressure after awakening in the morning and before swallowing in the majority of healthy ears.[4,5] During normal sleep the $PaCO_2$ value increases 3 or 4 mm Hg.[6] Therefore the positive pressure is probably caused in part by the diffusion of carbon dioxide into the middle ear.[4] We previously showed that the increase in the $PaCO_2$ level resulting from hypoventilation causes the elevation of pressure in the human middle ear.[5] The results, however, indirectly suggested that the diffusion of carbon dioxide into the middle ear cavity from the surrounding tissue was the cause of the pressure increase in the middle ear. The purpose of the present investigation was to obtain direct evidence of carbon dioxide diffusion into the middle ear during hypoventilation.

MATERIALS AND METHODS

In this experiment tympanometry was always done by measuring the external canal pressure in two ways: from positive to negative and vice versa. The pressure in the external ear canal corresponding to the middle of the two peaks of the tympanogram was taken as the middle ear pressure.[7]

Eleven healthy chinchillas were used, ranging in weight from 390 to 740 g. The animals were anesthetized with diethyl ether and sodium pentobarbital (Nembutal, 32.8 mg per kilogram given by the intraperitoneal route), tracheotomized, and allowed to breathe air spontaneously. The bony bulla was exposed and plastered with a rubber plate with tissue adhesive to avoid admixture of middle ear gas and environmental air. After the middle ear pressures were measured by a tympanometer (Teledyne TA-2C), $20\mu l$ of middle ear gas immediately taken with a gas-tight syringe (Hamilton model 1705-N) in 11 animals. Then the animals were artificially respired with suxamethonium chloride (Relaxin, 15 to 30 mg per kilogram intramuscularly. The rubber plate was taken off the bulla wall and a trepanation hole approximately 1 mm in diameter was made in the bulla wall. The gas composition in the middle ear cavity was confirmed to be equivalent to that of room air.

After determination of the middle ear pressure the tiny hole was closed with a rubber plate and tissue adhesive, and simultaneously 100 percent oxygen (2 L per minute) was administered into an endotracheal tube through the respirator. The respiration rate was kept at 70 to 72 respirations per minute during the procedure. Between 90 and 170 minutes after closure of the hole the animals were hypoventilated for 50 minutes; the tidal volume of the ventilation was reduced by one-third. The middle ear pressure was monitored every 10 minutes by repeated tympanometry in eight chinchillas. In five animals $20 \mu l$ of middle ear gas was obtained before and at the end of hypoventilation. Tympanometry was also performed immediately after the gas sample was taken. The sample was analyzed with a gas chromatograph (Hitachi 063-505U), and the concentrations of carbon dioxide, oxygen and nitrogen were determined.

RESULTS

The middle ear gas composition was determined by gas chromatography in 11 chinchillas that were allowed to breathe air spontaneously. The average concentration and standard deviation (SD) were 6.0

± 0.5 percent for carbon dioxide, 11.9 ± 1.9 percent for oxygen, and 79.8 ± 3.4 percent for nitrogen. Immediately before the evaluation the middle ear pressure was very close to the atmospheric pressure.

Before determinating the changes in middle ear gas composition, we determined whether the middle ear pressure had increased during hypoventilation in three chinchillas. All animals demonstrated elevation of the middle ear pressure from −80, +35, and −150 mm H_2O to +10, +100, and −90 mm H_2O, respectively, after the beginning of hypoventilation.

In five animals we evaluated changes in middle ear pressure and gas composition before and after hypoventilation; one representative case is depicted in Figure 1. Initially the pressure rose rapidly after closure of the hole in the bulla wall and then dropped to a plateau, which varied among the animals. There was a sudden decrease of about 100 mm H_2O in pressure immediately after the gas sample was taken. The intratympanic pressure was elevated in all five animals after the induction of hypoventilation (Figs. 1 and 2). During the experiment there was no equilization of the pressure due to opening of the eustachian tube.

The middle ear gas compositon was identical to that of room air after the bulla was opened—an extremely low content of carbon dioxide and about 21 percent oxygen (Figs. 3 and 4). After closure of the hole in the bulla the carbon dioxide level was elevated, reaching a value of 4 ± 0.8 percent (mean and SD), as shown in Figure 3. At the end of

hypoventilation the carbon dioxide concentration was increased further in all animals. The average concentration and SD were 6.3 ± 1.4 percent (see Fig. 3). In contrast with the change in the level of carbon dioxide, the concentrations of oxygen and nitrogen showed a minimal decline without exception throughout the experiment (see Fig. 4).

DISCUSSION

During sampling of the middle ear gas we were especially careful to prevent the admixture of middle ear gas and environmental air. This was accomplished by covering the bulla wall with a rubber plate and tissue adhesive.

The present study on middle ear gas composition demonstrated an extremely high concentration of carbon dioxide. However, Segal and his colleagues[2] reported a higher concentration of carbon dioxide in guinea pigs respired spontaneously with air, using mass spectrometry. The disagreement may be due to differences in the methods and species. Other reports have shown lower values of carbon dioxide,[1,3] but the results could have been influenced by a state of artificially induced hyperventilation. In regard to the oxygen and nitrogen concentrations, our results are in agreement with those of earlier studies.[1,2]

After closure of the hole in the bulla wall, an initial increase in middle ear pressure was observed, which was followed by a decrease in the pressure to a plateau level. The middle ear gas showed an

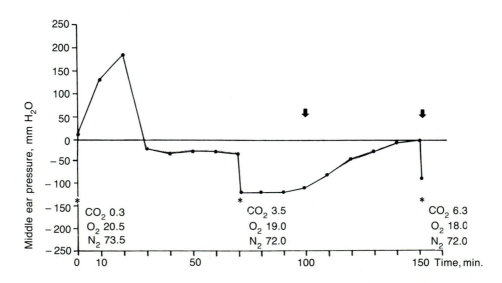

Figure 1 A representative example of changes in pressure and gas composition (%) in the middle ear before and during hypoventilation. The interval between the two arrows indicates a period of hypoventilation. * = 20 μl of gas sample is obtained.

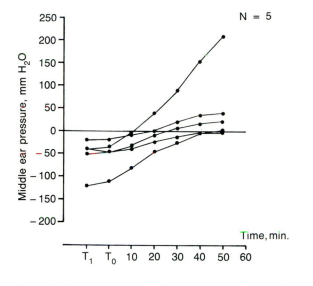

Figure 2 Pressure change in the middle ear during hypoventilation. On the x axis T_1 and T_0 indicate the times before and at the beginning of hypoventilation, respectively.

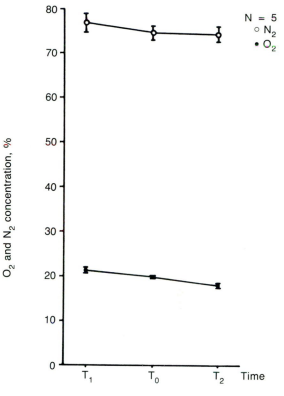

Figure 4 Changes in oxygen and nitrogen concentrations in the middle ear. (Abbreviations are the same as in Figure 3.)

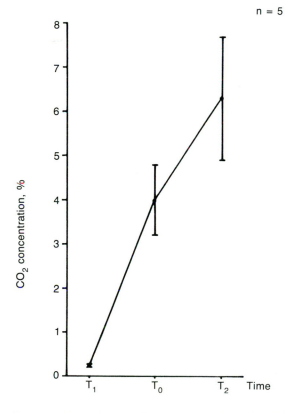

Figure 3 Change in carbon dioxide concentration in the middle ear. T_1, T_0, and T_2 indicate the initial concentration, the concentration before, and that at the end of hypoventilation respectively. The vertical bar represents the standard deviation.

increased concentration of carbon dioxide and slight decreases in oxygen and nitrogen. It is plausible that the initial increase in middle ear pressure is due to the rapid diffusion of carbon dioxide into the middle ear and that the following decrease in the pressure is caused by the slow diffusion of oxygen and nitrogen into the surrounding tissue. This assumption is supported by experiments on subcutaneous gas pockets in rats[8]. Moreover, similar pressure changes in rhesus monkeys were noted by Cantekin et al.[9]

The middle ear pressure was decreased immediately after the sampling of the middle ear gas. Accordingly there is a possibility that the elevation of pressure during hypoventilation is due not only to the diffusion of carbon dioxide but also to the influence of sampling. Further investigation is required to reduce the volume of samples.

In the present study a steady increase in middle ear pressure accompanied the elevation in carbon dioxide concentration in the middle ear cavity by hypoventilation in all animals. The results are in agreement with previous reports[4,5,10] and may suggest that the diffusion of carbon dioxide into the middle ear elevates the middle ear pressure. Furthermore it has been reported that the concentration of carbon dioxide in the middle ear seems to be more sensitive to systemic variations than the oxygen concentration.[11]

REFERENCES

1. Ostfeld E, Blonder J, et al. The middle ear gas composition in air-ventilated dogs. Acta Otolaryngol 1980; 89:105–108.
2. Segal J, Ostfeld E, et al. Mass spectrometric analysis of gas composition in the guinea pig middle ear mastoid system. In: Lim DJ, Bluestone CD, Klein JO, Nelson JD, eds. Recent advances in otitis media with effusion. Proceedings of the Third International Symposium. Toronto: BC Decker, 1984:68.
3. Kusakari J, et al. Gas analysis of the middle ear cavity in normal and pathological conditions. Auris Nasus Larynx (Tokyo) 1985; 12(Suppl 1):114–116.
4. Hergils L, Magnuson B. Morning pressure in the middle ear. Arch Otolaryngol 1985; 111:86–89.
5. Shinkawa H, et al. Positive intratympanic pressure in the morning and its etiology. Acta Otolaryngol 1987; Suppl 435:107–111.
6. West JB. Disorders of regulation of respiration. In: Wintrobe MM, Thorn GW, Adams RD, Bennett IL Jr, Braunwald E, Isselbacher KJ, Petersdorf RG, eds. In: Harrison's principles of internal medicine. 8th ed. Tokyo: McGraw-Hill Kogakusha, 1977:1375.
7. Kobayashi T, Okitsu T, Takasaka T. Forward-backward tracing tympanometry. Acta Otolaryngol 1987; Suppl 435:100–106.
8. Piper J. Physiological equilibria of gas cavities in the body. In: Fenn WO, Rahn H, eds. Handbook of physiology. Section 3, Vol. II. Respiration. Washington: American Physiological Society, 1965:1205.
9. Cantekin EI, et al. Gas absorption in the middle ear. Ann Otol Rhinol Laryngol 1980: 89(Suppl 68):71–75.
10. Buckingham RA, et al. Experimental evidence against middle ear oxygen absorption. Laryngoscope 1985; 95:437–442.
11. Ostfeld E. The limiting effect of blood supply through the microcirculation on gas composition in the canine middle ear. Third International Symposium on Recent Advances in Otitis Media with Effusion, Fort Lauderdale, Florida, 1983:25(A).

DIRECT MEASUREMENT OF MIDDLE EAR GAS COMPOSITION: CLINICAL IMPLICATIONS

JENS U. FELDING, M.D. and TORBEN LILDHOLDT, M.D., Ph.D.

The normal middle ear maintains a neutral or nearly atmospheric pressure by ventilation through the eustachian tube. Decreased ventilation of the middle ear cavity creates negative pressure, which ultimately leads to secretory otitis media. The explanation for these events might be, accordingly, blockage of the eustachian tube, absorption of middle ear air by the middle ear mucosa, and finally formation of transudate. This somewhat teleologic explanation has never been verified.

A recent investigation has revealed that the middle ear gas composition is unique, being in a quasi-equilibrium with the venous blood gases.[1]

In clinical otology, inflation maneuvers (Valsalva, Politzer) are applied to the eustachian tube. They immediately restore the normal middle ear pressure and normal hearing. Nevertheless both experimental and clinical reports have pointed out that this beneficial effect lasts for only a short period.[2,3] The reason is unknown.

Insertion of ventilation tubes is the surgical procedure most often performed in the Western Hemisphere. In Denmark approximately 25,000 such tubes are inserted every year. Although the restoration of normal middle ear pressure and hearing is well documented, the rationale for the procedure is empirical. Likewise, high frequencies of long term sequelae such as tympanic scars have been documented.[4] However, they have never been related to the changes in middle ear physiology introduced by a ventilation tube. Therefore the purpose of this study was to integrate the aforementioned knowledge with common rules in respiration physiology; in this way the physiologic changes in the middle ear caused by insertion of ventilation tubes may be evaluated.

MATERIAL

Results from another part of the study were used to document normal middle ear gas composition.[1] Six men and four women with unilateral ventilation tubes inserted were investigated in order to measure the gas composition of the ventilated ears.

METHOD

The tympanic membrane was punctured through a seal of antibiotic paste and a 300 microliter air sample was aspirated. The tube was sealed with the paste and a Silastic plate (Fig.1). The partial pressures were measured with $pO_2 = CO_2$ electrodes (D–616 5046/36, Radiometer Denmark).

RESULTS

The partial pressure of oxygen in the ventilated middle ear was 138 mm Hg (SD, 5.7 mm Hg; range, 129 to 145 mm). The corresponding figure for carbon dioxide was 15 mm Hg (SD, 6.0 mm Hg; range, 8 to 22 mm Hg).

DISCUSSION

Partial pressures in the middle ear and its relevant surroundings in the normal steady state are outlined in Figure 2. Comparison between the composi-

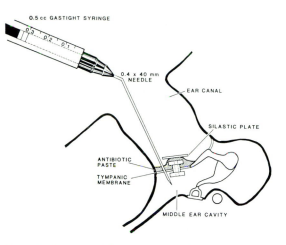

Figure 1 Puncture of the tympanic membrane with an inserted ventilation tube.

tion in the middle ear and in atmospheric air shows that no real ventilation can take place in the normal ear.

Elner[5] showed that normal middle ear gas absorption has a range of 1 to 2 ml per 24 hours; ac-

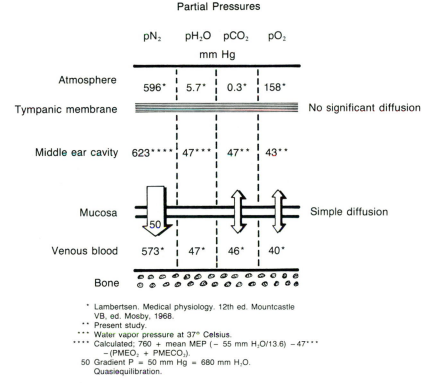

Figure 2 Model of the normal middle ear in a physiologic steady state with net diffusion between middle ear air and blood. The steady state refers to a neutral and constant middle ear pressure, which is due to a balance between diffusion from the cavity to venous blood and microventilation through the eustachian tube.

cordingly the input through the eustachian tube must be of an equal amount (i.e., 1 to 2 μl per minute). This "microventilation" through the eustachian tube may explain normal pressure, but it cannot change the middle ear gas composition significantly, since the ventilated volume is small in comparison with the middle ear volume (1 to 2 per 5,000 microliters). The middle ear is therefore nonventilated but pressure equilibrated.

The gradients in Figure 2 show that only nitrogen has a significant gradient across the mucosa (50 mm Hg). This gas has the lowest diffusion coefficient and is the major factor responsible for the creation of a negative middle ear pressure if "microventilation" is blocked.

Accordingly the absorption or output of middle ear gas is caused by simple diffusion according to Fick's first law. Inflation of atmospheric air would increase the partial pressure of oxygen, which diffuses twice as fast as nitrogen. This may easily explain the rapid recurrence of negative pressure in cases of eustachian tube obstruction, that have been treated with Valsalva or Politzer maneuvers. In such conditions this type of inflation is of short duration and not curative in any sense.

The present study also showed that insertion of a ventilation tube into the tympanic membrane triples the oxygen content in the middle ear cleft.

However, the majority of the cells in the human body, including the cells of the middle ear compartment, are adjusted to a partial pressure of oxygen of about 40 mm Hg. Ingelstedt et al[6] showed that this is also true of the middle ear transudate.

In in vitro cell culture studies similar high oxygen tensions are known to cause changes in RNA-DNA synthesis and cell lysis. In vivo this is known to occur in other organs (lungs, lens, and normal wound healing) to create fibrosis or scar tissue. This process is initiated by the toxic effect of the free radicals of oxygen, especially superoxide oxygen. Depending on susceptibility, duration, and exposure, these radicals can cause damage to the endothelial cells of the vessels in connective tissue; this is followed by transudation, granulation, and an increase in collagen formation and finally fibrosis.[7]

As shown by the high frequency of tympanic membrane sequelae[4] and the experimentally proved thickening of the tympanic membrane,[8] we have some evidence that this sequence of events also could take place in human ears with ventilation tubes. Future studies must show whether oxygen under these circumstances is toxic to the normal ear and/or the ear afflicted by serous otitis media.

CONCLUSIONS

1. The middle ear is an open, pressure equilibrated, and nonventilated gas pocket.
2. Absorption of middle ear gas takes place by simple diffusion.
3. The reason for the short duration of normal pressure after Valsalva or Politzer maneuvers is "superdiffusion" due to an increased oxygen gradient.
4. Insertion of a ventilation tube into the tympanic membrane increases the partial pressure of oxygen three times.

REFERENCES

1. Felding JU, Rasmussen JB, Lildholt T. Gas composition of the normal and the ventilated middle ear cavity. Scand J Clin Lab Invest 1987; 47(Suppl 186):31–41.
2. Cantekin EI, Doyle WJ, Phillips DC, Bluestone CD. Gas absorption in the middle ear. Ann Otol Rhinol Laryngol 1980; 89(Suppl 68):71–75.
3. Gimsing S. Gas absorption in serous otitis, a clinical aspect. Ann Otol Rhinol Laryngol 1983; 92:305–308.
4. Lildholdt T. Ventilation tubes in secretory otitis media. Acta Otolaryngol 1983; Suppl 398.
5. Elner A. Quantitative studies of gas absorption from the normal middle ear. Acta Otolaryngol 1977; 83:25–28.
6. Ingelstedt S, Jonson B, Rundcrantz H. Gas tension and pH in the middle ear effusion. Ann Otol Rhinol Laryngol 1975; 84:198–202.
7. Clark JM, Lambertsen CJ. Pulmonary oxygen toxicity: a review. Pharm Rev 1971; 23:37–133.
8. Søderberg O. Tympanic membrane changes after repeated insertions of ventilation tubes. Acta Otolaryngol 1984; Suppl 414:165–169.

GASEOUS PATHWAYS IN ATELECTATIC EARS

JACOB SADÉ, M.D. and MICHAL LUNTZ, M.D.

According to the classic concept of middle ear aeration, under physiologic conditions oxygen is continuously absorbed from the middle ear into the blood. The gas deficit created is continuously compensated by reentry of air through the eustachian tube.[1] Air is believed to pass through the eustachian tube when swallowing takes place. Several pathologic conditions, of which atelectasis, retraction pockets, and secretory otitis media are the main representatives, are presumed to produce a defect in the return of air into the middle ear, leading to a negative pressure in the middle ear.[2]

This classic dogma, however, was recently questioned by Buckingham et al,[3] Bylander et al,[4] Hergils et al,[5] and Magnuson.[6]

Our study is an attempt to trace the fate of carbon dioxide, oxygen, nitrogen, and air in atelectatic middle ears. It was prompted by the fact that when gas is introduced into an ear with a retracted drum, the drum inflates but tends to revert to its original retracted position.[7] We conceived that the speed or mode of disappearance of the gases introduced into the middle ear may indicate the route a gas takes when it leaves the ear. Should this occur abruptly and with equal speed for different types of gases, it would denote that the gases escaped through the eustachian tube. Conversely, if the gases disappear slowly and with a speed in accordance with the solubility coefficient of the particular gas used, it would indicate that the gases were absorbed into the blood and body tissues.

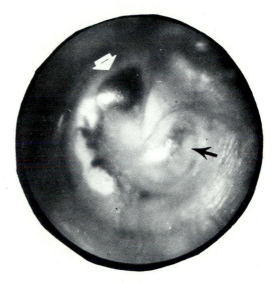

Figure 1 Atelectasis of most of the tympanic membrane. The white arrow points to the anterior region where immediately behind it the drum is atelectatic. The black arrow points to the posterior region where the drum is seen to be collapsed over the incus. The maleus is prominent between the anterior and posterior parts of the drum. Note tympanosclerotic deposits anteroinferiorly.

(Fig. 2). A given middle ear was considered to be filled with the politzerized gas once its tympanic membrane stretched and showed no further retraction (Fig. 3).

MATERIAL AND METHODS

Thirteen patients (average age, 29.7 years; range, 15 to 69 years) with atelectatic ears or retraction served as the experimental model (Fig. 1).

Politzer bags were filled alternately with carbon dioxide, oxygen, air, or nitrogen. The gas concentration was checked periodically using pH–blood gas analyzer ABL3 produced by Radiometer Copenhagen.

Each patient was politzerized with carbon dioxide, oxygen, air, and nitrogen. Altogether 90 such measurements were performed. At the time of politzerization the tympanic membrane was observed under the operating microscope by a second person

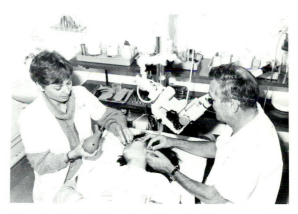

Figure 2 Politzerization performed by a physician; a second physician observes the tympanic membrane at the same time.

After introduction of the gas into the middle ear, we continued to observe the tympanic membrane until it returned to its previous retracted position. The time for the drum to return to its original state was regarded as the time taken by the added gas to leave the ear.

RESULTS

Politzerization with any of the gases in question filled all examined ears, without exception. In some ears this was achieved readily; others required several politzerizations.

Once a given gas was introduced into the middle ear, the tympanic membrane immediately stretched to a nonretracted state. Then the drum usually looked as if it were in its usual place; i.e., it reached its "zero point." Sometimes, however, outward ballooning occurred. This was noted especially in the previously retracted atrophic part of the drum (see Fig. 3).

Eventually all stretched tympanic membranes returned to their exact original retracted position.

The return of the tympanic membrane to its original position took place in all instances very gradually, provided the patients did not sniff, swallow, or perform a Toynbee maneuver.

When the retracted tympanic membrane returned gradually to its original state, it did so at a speed that was different for each gas. The difference in speed was proportional to the diffusion coefficient of the particular gas. The average speeds

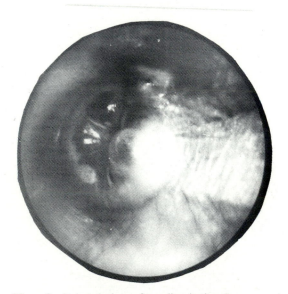

Figure 3 Atelectatic drum after politzerization. Same ear as in Figure 1; note disappearance of atelectasis and ballooning of the posterior "half" of the drum.

for the disappearance of the different gases were as follows: 5.37 minutes (range, 1 to 5 minutes) for carbon dioxide, 33.32 minutes (range, 14 to 90 minutes) for oxygen, 53.37 minutes (range, 15 to 120 minutes) for air, and 104.76 minutes (range, 40 to 335 minutes) for nitrogen.

Once the tympanic membrane was stretched or ballooned after politzerization, some patients could willingly or "on command" cause the membrane to return abruptly to its original retracted level. One patient (7.69 percent) could do this by swallowing, four patients (30.76 percent) by performing the Toynbee maneuver, and four patients (30.76 percent) by sniffing.

Two of our patients informed us that sniffing was a habitual maneuver that they performed to relieve an uncomfortable feeling in the ear. For these patients a situation in which the drum was at zero point and not retracted was uncomfortable. The retracted steady state was for them a comfortable situation.

At least three patients were able to fill atelectatic middle ears with air, one through repeated swallowings and two while yawning.

DISCUSSION

Gases added by politzerization to a middle ear with a retracted drum inflate the retraction immediately—yet for a short time only. Reappearance of the retraction occurs relatively swiftly, and it may be logical to conclude that this happens concomitantly with disappearance of the added gases. Our experiments show that the gases may leave the ear through two alternative paths:

1. When the eustachian tube does not play an active role, the gas disappears gradually. The speed depends regularly on the type of gas used, indicating diffusion into the general circulation. The speed of gas diffusion through semipermeable membranes depends in general on the pressure difference on both sides of the membrane and on the solubility index of the gas.[8] Perfusion conditions may play a significant role as well.[9] Consequently carbon dioxide is expected to pass through a membrane swiftly, nitrogen relatively more slowly, and oxygen and air at a rate between the two. This is indeed how the gases behaved in our study. A previous study demonstrated that gases may similarly pass by diffusion to and from the normal middle ear lining.[3] Our present study establishes, therefore, that in atelectatic ears, oxygen, carbon dioxide, and nitrogen obey the same

laws that govern gas diffusion through biologic semipermeable membranes, as in normal ears.[1,3]

2. We also observed that gas may disappear from the middle ear swiftly, escaping instantly as a single "bolus" of gas pulsed out during sniffing or swallowing. This alternative route was observed in one third of the examined ears and confirms previous communications by Miller[10] and Magnuson.[11] The abruptness with which this happens indicates that the gas could have disappeared only via the eustachian tube.

Our direct observations show that air sometimes can enter the atelectatic middle ear through the eustachian tube during swallowing or yawning. Although we have observed this in three patients, we believe that more persistent tracing of air entry into atelectatic ears through the eustachian tube will show this to happen more often.

Gases thus have two pathways that they may take to enter or leave the normal as well as the atelectatic middle ear. One is through diffusion in or out of the middle ear lining, the other as a bolus of air in or out of the eustachian tube. A balance between the intake and output provides for a physiologic situation. A negative balance may bring about a pathologic situation, as in atelectasis or patients with a retraction pocket. A positive imbalance seldom presents as a clinical problem.

The classic notion that aeration imbalance of the middle ear stems from eustachian tube obstruction now seems to be an oversimplification of a more complex system; indeed recent studies have shown that in secretory otitis media and chronic otitis media, the eustachian tube lumen is not even narrowed.[12-18] It is now known today what brings about a negative aeration balance in these conditions, but information at hand points toward a quantitative difference of aeration in ears with deficient aeration. The lesson learned from this study is that such a quantitative imbalance should take into consideration the entry and exit of gas through the eustachian tube as well as through the circulation.

SUMMARY AND CONCLUSION

1. The eustachian tube in atelectatic ears as a rule is patent to air flow as produced by politzerization.
2. Carbon dioxide, oxygen, air, and nitrogen introduced into atelectatic middle ears are reabsorbed and cause the middle ear to revert to its prepolitzerized state within a relatively short time.
3. The speed of the gas exchange in atelectatic ears

is proportional to the diffusion rate and partial pressure of the particular gases present in the middle ear as in gas pockets or as in normal middle ears.

4. Gas absorption in atelectatic ears provides for subatmospheric pressure as evidenced by the final speedy retraction of tympanic membranes after politzerization.
5. After politzerization, retraction of the tympanic membrane also can occur through sniffing (40 percent), the Toynbee maneuver (35 percent), and swallowing (10 percent). This occurs secondary to loss of a bolus of air through the eustachian tube.
6. We also found that air enters and fills the atelectatic middle ear through the eustachian tube as a result of swallowing or yawning.
7. Gas can pass to and from the atelectatic ear via the same routes as in normal ears, i.e., through the eustachian tube or by diffusion. This does not mean, however, that air passes to and fro in atelectatic ears in the same quantities as it does in normal ears.

REFERENCES

1. Elner A. Indirect determination of gas absorption from the middle ear. Acta Otolaryngol 1972; 74:191–196.
2. Farrior JB, Buckingham RA, Donaldson JA, Rambo JHT, Wright WK, Zöllner F. Management of atelectatic middle ear. Arch Otolaryngol 1969; 89:199–206.
3. Buckingham RA, Stuart DR, Girgis SJ, Geick MR, McGee TJ. Experimental evidence against middle ear oxygen absorption. Laryngoscope 1985; 95:437–442.
4. Bylander A, Tjernström Ö, Ivarsson A, Andreasson L. Eustachian tube function and its relation to middle ear pressure in children. Auris Nasus Larynx (Tokyo) 1985; 12(Suppl 1):43–45.
5. Hergils L, Magnuson B. Morning pressure in the middle ear. Arch Otolaryngol 1985; 111:86–89.
6. Magnuson B. Tubal closing failure in retraction-type cholesteatoma and adhesive middle ear lesions. Acta Otolaryngol 1978; 86:408–417.
7. MacKinnon DM. The sequel to myringotomy for exudative otitis media. J Laryngol Otol 1971; 85:773–793.
8. Van Liew HD. Tissue PO_2 and PCO_2 estimation with rat subcutaneous gas pockets. J Appl Physiol 1962; 17:851–855.
9. Tenney SM, Carpenter FG, Rahn H. Gas transfers in a sulphur hexafluoride pneumoperitoneum. Wright Air Develop Ctr Tech Rept 1953; 55–357:425–432.
10. Miller JB. Patulous eustachian tube. Arch Otolaryngol 1961; 73:310–321.
11. Magnuson B. On the origin of the high negative pressure in the middle ear space. Am J Otolaryngol 1981; 2:1–12.
12. Sadé J, Wolfson S, Sachs Z, Levit I, Abraham S. The infant's eustachian tube lumen: the pharyngeal part. J Laryngol Otol 1986; 100:129–134.
13. Sadé J, Wolfson S, Sachs Z, Abraham S. The eustachian tube midportion in infants. Am J Otolaryngol 1985; 6:205–209.

14. Sadé J, Wolfson S, Sachs Z, Abraham S. Caliber of the lumen of the eustachian tube pre-isthmus in infants and children. Arch Otolaryngol (Stockh) 1985; 242:247–255.
15. Sadé J, Wolfson S, Sachs Z, Levit I, Abraham S. The human eustachian tube lumen in children. I. The isthmus. Acta Otolaryngol (Stockh) 1985; 99:305–309.
16. Sadé J, Luntz M, Berger G. The infant's "post-isthmus" region of the eustachian tube in health and disease. Am J Otol 1986; 7:350–353.
17. Sadé J, Luntz M, Wolfson S, Berger G. The infant's pretympanic region of the eustachian tube in health and disease. Int J Pediatr Otorhinolaryngol 1985; 10:237–243.
18. Sadé J, Luntz M, Yaniv E, Yurovitzki E, Berger G, Galrenter I. The eustachian tube lumen in chronic otitis media. Am J Otol 1986; 7:439–442.

NEW FINDINGS ON MIDDLE EAR VENTILATION USING XENON GAS

TOSHIO YAMASHITA, M.D., NORIO MAEDA, M.D., KEIJI HONDA, M.D., and TADAMI KUMAZAWA, M.D.

The ventilation mechanism of the middle ear is important in regard to the pathogenesis and therapy of middle ear disease, especially otitis media with effusion. Almost all the studies of gas transport in the middle ear in the past have been done by indirect methods—for example, observing pressure changes in the middle ear by the insufflation of various gases.[1,2] One reason for the weakness in this research field might be that gases cannot be observed directly. However, radioisotope techniques have made it possible to observe their images. More than 10 years ago Kirchner[3,4] tried to use radioisotopes in this research field, but unfortunately his reports were preliminary ones and more detailed studies were not performed. In the present study, the ventilation mechanisms of the middle ear were illustrated in clear pictures and numerical values were obtained using radioactive xenon gas.

METHODS AND SUBJECTS

A thin polyethylene tube was placed in the pharyngeal orifice of the eustachian tube through an inserted insufflation catheter. Then 1 ml of 133 xenon gas was insufflated into the middle ear through a syringe connected to the polyethylene tube, and excess gas in the nose, throat, and lung was carefully removed over a 5 minute period. Five minutes after inflation, xenon gas in the middle ear of the subject was represented as an image by a scintiscanner and its numerical value was counted with the passage of time at rest. The insufflation procedure was repeated once or more often in several of the subjects after 2 hours.

In this study there were 12 normal subjects, 7 with occluded eustachian tubes, 4 with patent eustachian tubes, and 1 in whom a tube had been inserted. The tubal function and the degree of development of the mastoid air cells were checked by audiometry, tympanometry, tubotympanoaerodynamic graphy, and simple x-ray examination of the ear.

RESULTS

The real image and the count value of the gas in the middle ear can be visualized with the passage of time (Fig. 1); we found the shape of the radioisotope image to coincide with the configuration of the mastoid air cell represented by the x-ray image in all cases.

Regarding the dynamic movement of gas in normal subjects, initial counts of 1 ml of radioactive xenon gas ("source") were compared with those 5 minutes after insufflation. For example, in case 1, 97 of 1111 K counts inflated into the middle ear resulted in a 9 percentage value; the average in 12 cases was 11 percent (Table 1). This means that 11 percent of the initial amount of the gas entered the middle ear.

Regarding changes with the passage of time, for example, in case 1, 97 counts at 5 minutes diminished to 95, 93, 90, and 83 in the following

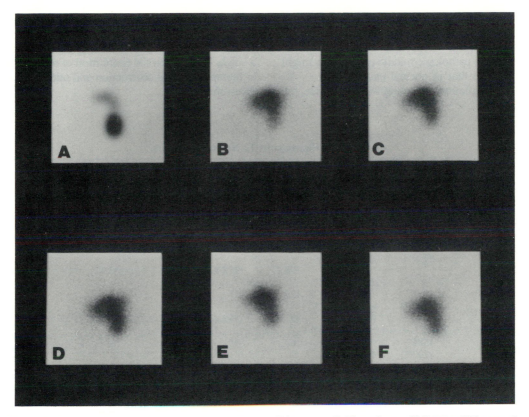

Figure 1 Images and count values versus time. *A*, Source; 606 K count. *B*, Five minutes; 55 K count (100 percent). *C*, Fifteen minutes; 54 K count (98 percent). *D*, Thirty minutes; 54 K count (98 percent). *E*, Sixty minutes; 52 K count (94 percent). *F*, One hundred twenty minutes; 50 K count (90 percent).

2 hours and after insufflation to 57 counts. The diminishing rates during the following 2 hours after inflation were 97, 95, 92, and 88 percent. These data suggest that approximately 8 percent of the gas disappeared in 1 hour in the resting state. After 2 hours, if insufflation was done once, as is shown in cases 8 and 9, the value diminished slightly, but if it was done several times, as is shown in cases 1 and 12, it diminished dramatically.

Regarding the subjects with occluded tubes, for example, in case 1, 37 of 703 initial value counts (source) entered into the middle ear, that is, 5 percent. The average in seven cases was 6 percent. The averages with the passage of time were 91, 84, 72, and 59 percent (Table 2), and approximately 28 percent of the gas disappeared in 1 hour.

On the other hand, in subjects with patent tubes an average of 13 percent of the gas entered into the middle ear. The averages with the passage of time were 90, 72, 63, and 55 percent (Table 2) and approximately 37 percent of the gas disappeared in 1

hour. In the subject with a tube inserted, the rate of decrease in the gas was rapid (Table 2).

DISCUSSION AND CONCLUSIONS

It was clear that air could easily and quickly enter into even the periphery of the mastoid air cell by insufflation via a tube, even though the middle ear and mastoid air cells constitute a closed cavity and are under normal pressure conditions.

The inflation volumes of the initial gas in the middle ear in normal, occluded, and patent tubes were 11, 6, and 13 percent respectively. These data suggest that in occluded tubes the gas had difficulty entering into the middle ear via the tube.

Approximately 8, 28, and 37 percent of the gas volume disappeared in 1 hour in normal, occluded, and patent tubes, respectively. Each diminishing curve is linear in the resting state. Therefore the gas

REFERENCES

1. Cantekin EI, et al. Gas absorption in the middle ear. Ann Otol Rhinol Laryngol 1980; Suppl 68:71–75.
2. Jones GM. Pressure changes in the middle ear after altering the composition of contained gas. Acta Otolaryngol 1961; 53:1–11.
3. Kirchner FR. Radioscanning studies of ear and sinuses. Laryngoscope 1974; 84:1894–1904.
4. Kirchner FR, Robinson R, Smith RF. Study of the ventilation of middle ear using radioactive xenon. Ann Otol 1976; Suppl 25:165–168.

PATTERNS OF RESPONSE OF THE NOSE AND EUSTACHIAN TUBE TO PROVOCATIVE ALLERGEN CHALLENGE

DAVID P. SKONER, M.D., WILLIAM J. DOYLE, Ph.D., SHARON BOEHM, B.S., and PHILIP FIREMAN, M.D.

Provocative challenge of sensitive individuals with allergens causes IgE mediated pathophysiologic responses in the lung, nose, and eustachian tube.[1-3] The "immediate" or "early" responses, which usually occur within 20 minutes after challenge and are of relatively short duration, have been studied most extensively. More recently clinically similar but histopathologically distinct responses of skin, nose, and lung were observed to occur 4 to 9 hours after allergen challenge in approximately 50 percent of allergic individuals.[1,4,5] A number of investigators have suggested that the late phase response is responsible for the perceptible components of human allergic disease, which are manifested as the onset and persistence of symptoms well after allergen exposure. Recently proposed hypotheses of the pathogenesis of the late response provide for a self-perpetuating inflammatory process, with extended pathophysiologic consequences after a single allergen exposure.[6]

Even though early allergen induced eustachian tube obstructive responses characteristically develop in sensitive individuals after intranasal allergen challenge, late phase responses have not been reported for the eustachian tube. The goals in our study were to define the extent and incidence of late responses to nasal allergen challenge in the nose and its extensions in the lung and eustachian tube.

METHOD

Ten young adults (five males, five females) with confirmed ragweed allergic rhinitis, but not asthma or middle ear disease, were enrolled. None of the subjects were smokers, and all were free of infectious and allergic symptoms at the time of study. Studies were conducted at the Children's Hospital Outpatient Clinical Research Center in Pittsburgh. The indoor environmental temperature and humidity remained constant, and subjects refrained from strenuous activities throughout the study period. All studies were performed during months not characterized by seasonal ragweed exposure.

On the day of testing, baseline tests for nasal, pulmonary, and eustachian tube function were performed. A 2.5 mg aliquot of dry ragweed was then placed on a glass slide, and while the contralateral nostril was manually occluded the antigen was inhaled into the nasal cavity via a tube. The procedure was repeated for the contralateral nostril. The function tests were repeated 15 and 30 minutes after the challenge and then hourly for the next 12 hours.

Eustachian tube function was assessed by sonotubometry as previously described.[7] An early response was defined as obstruction of the eustachian tube within 1 hour after the challenge, and a persistent response as continuous eustachian tube obstruction for 6 hours or more after the challenge. A late phase eustachian tube response was defined as the presence of normal function during the 2 to 11 hour observation period, with the subsequent detection of obstruction. In regard to the eustachian tube, subjects could have both a persistent and a late phase response and could have a late phase response without an early or persistent response.

Total nasal conductance was assessed by posterior rhinomanometry using a computer assisted rhinomanometer developed and standardized in our laboratories.[8] Early responders were defined by a greater than 30 percent decrease from baseline conductance within 1 hour after challenge and a persistent response by failure to return to at least 50 percent of baseline conductance within 6 hours after challenge. A late phase response was defined by a return to 50 percent or more of the baseline conductance within 6 hours after challenge and a subsequent decrease of more than 30 percent from the new baseline. Persistent and late phase responses were thus mutually exclusive of each other.

Pulmonary function was measured by the forced expiratory volume (FEV) in 1 second with a flow based, computer assisted spirometer. An early response was defined as a greater than 15 percent decrease in the FEV_1 value from baseline and a persistent response as a failure to return to a greater than 95 percent baseline value within 2 hours. A late phase bronchial response was defined as an increase in the FEV_1 value to more than 95 percent of baseline within 2 hours, followed by a greater than 10 percent decrease from baseline. Alternatively, in a subject without an early response, the late phase response was defined as an isolated decrease in the FEV_1 value of more than 10 percent from baseline during the 4 to 12 hour period.

RESULTS

The baseline nasal conductance in the subjects ranged from 0.147 to 0.425 liter per second per centimeter of water, with a mean ($\pm$S.E.M.) of 0.293 ± 0.029.[9] Early nasal responses were detected in nine of the 10 subjects (Table 1). The nasal conductance in these subjects decreased by an average of 86 ± 5 percent during the early response. The decrease in nasal conductance was persistent in two subjects. Late nasal responses were observed in seven subjects, one of whom did not have an early response. The average nasal conductance during the late response was 0.086 ± 0.031, with an average decrease from the new baseline of 67 ± 5 percent.

Dual late nasal responses were observed in five subjects. The average time of onset of these subjects' first late responses was 6.6 ± 0.8 hours.

All ears of the 10 subjects evidenced normal eustachian tube function prior to challenge. The frequencies of early, persistent, and late responses to allergen challenge are shown in Table 1. Four patterns of eustachian tube response were observed: isolated early, persistent, biphasic early and late, and isolated late (Fig. 1). Early responses were detected in 12 ears of seven subjects, two of whom had persistent bilateral eustachian tube obstruction. Late phase responses were observed in 10 ears (50 percent of all ears) in six patients. Two sequential late eustachian tube responses were observed in three subjects.

Baseline values for FEV_1 ranged from 82 to 107 percent predicted, with a mean value of 95 ± 3. Early bronchial responses were observed in two subjects, neither of whom had persistent responses (Table 1). Late phase bronchial responses were detected in three subjects, one of whom did not have an early response. The FEV_1 value decreased an average of 32 ± 16 and 24 ± 13 percent from baseline for the early and late responses, respectively. The nasal response was persistent in one of the three late bronchial reponders and late in the other two.

Late nasal responses were detected in 70 percent of the subjects. If the persistent responders are added, 90 percent of the subjects responded during the 4 to 10 hour postchallenge period. These figures are much higher than the 3 to 50 percent incidences reported by others, most of whom relied on less objective clinical symptomatology to identify the onset of late responses and evaluated subjects less frequently.[5,10,11] The use of nasal conductance to identify late responses, the objectivity and great sensitivity of the rhinomanometry system, and the ease of frequent monitoring facilitated by the computer are likely explanations for these discrepant percentages.

The results of this study also documented a late

TABLE 1   Early and Late Phase Allergic Reactions Following Intranasal Allergen Challenge

Obstruction	Response		
	Early	Persistent	Late
Eustachian tube patients	7/10	2/10	6/10
Ears	12/20	4/20	10/20
Nasal	9/10	2/10	7/10
Bronchial	2/10	0/10	3/10

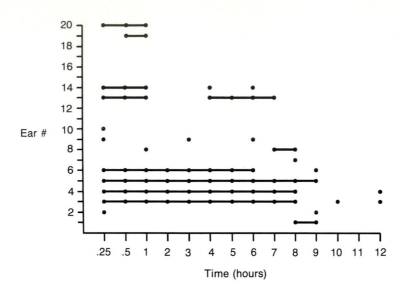

Figure 1 Eustachian tube function for each ear of the 10 study subjects after nasal allergen challenge (15 minutes to 12 hours). Tube obstruction is indicated by closed circles and normal eustachian tube function by an absence of circles. The points are connected by a line when eustachian tube obstruction was detected on two consecutive tests. The ears are pair matched, such that consecutive odd and even numbered ears are from the same patient, e.g., ears 1 and 2, 3 and 4.

phase reaction for the eustachian tube. These responses were observed in 60 percent of the subjects studied and were recurrent in three subjects. The self-perpetuating and self-amplifying nature of the tubal late response, and its occurrence even in the absence of early eustachian tube responses, could provide an important contribution to our understanding of the relationship between allergy and middle ear disease. Specifically, daily allergen exposure, via persistent and late responses, could result in obstruction of sufficient duration to precipitate the development of middle ear disease. Experimental validation of this hypothesis would have important implications for the treatment of allergy mediated nasal and middle ear disease.

Study supported in part by NIH grants AI-19262 and MO-I-RR-00084-23S1.

REFERENCES

1. Durham SR, et al. Immunologic studies in allergen-induced late-phase asthmatic reactions. J Allergy Clin Immunol 1984; 74:49–60.

2. Skoner DP, Doyle WJ, Chamovitz AH, Fireman P. Eustachian tube obstruction after intranasal challenge with house dust mite. Arch Otolaryngol Head Neck Surg 1986; 112:840–842.

3. Friedman RA, et al. Immunologic-mediated eustachian tube obstruction: a double-blind crossover study. J Allergy Clin Immunol 1983; 71:442–447.

4. Solley GO, Gleich GJ, Jordon RE, Schroeter AL. The late phase of the immediate wheal and flare skin reaction. J Clin Invest 1976; 58:408.

5. Pelikan Z. Late and delayed responses of the nasal mucosa to allergen challenge. Ann Allergy 1978; 41:37–47.

6. Kaliner M. Hypotheses on the contribution of late-phase allergic responses to the understanding and treatment of allergic diseases. J Allergy Clin Immunol 1984; 73:311–315.

7. Murti KG, et al. Sonometric evaluation of eustachian tube function using broad-band stimuli. Ann Otol Rhinol Laryngol 1980; 89(Suppl 68):178–184.

8. Stillwagon PK, Doyle WJ, Fireman P. Effect of an antihistamine/decongestant on nasal and eustachian tube function following intranasal pollen challenge. Ann Allergy 1987; 58:442–446.

9. Nolte D, Luder-Luhr I. Comparing measurements of nasal resistance by body plethysmography and by rhinomanometry. Respiration 1973; 30:31–38.

10. Dvoracek JE, Yunginger JW, Kern EB, Hyatt RE, Gleich GJ. Induction of nasal late-phase reactions by insufflation of ragweed-pollen extract. J Allergy Clin Immunol 1984; 73:363–368.

11. Naclerio RM, Proud D, Togias AG, Adkinson NF Jr, Meyers DA, Kagey-Sobotka A, Norman PS, Lichtenstein LM. Inflammatory mediators in late antigen-induced rhinitis. N Engl J Med 1985; 313:65–70.

EFFECT OF PROSTAGLANDIN E₂ AND BACTERIAL ENDOTOXIN ON THE RATE OF DYE TRANSPORT IN THE CHINCHILLA EUSTACHIAN TUBE

LAUREN O. BAKALETZ, Ph.D., STEPHEN R. GRIFFITH, M.D., and
DAVID J. LIM, M.D.

The middle ear is protected by the eustachian tube, including the action of the tubal muscles and the mucociliary apparatus, which are needed for such protective function. The tubal muscles are thought to be involved in pressure equilibration and aeration, and the mucociliary activity of the mucosal surface provides protection against invading organisms from the nasopharynx. Once the middle ear effusion is formed, clearance of fluid and debris from the middle ear space is mediated by both muscular action[1] and mucociliary transport. It has been suggested that disruption of the mucociliary system leads to the development of otitis media, and continued dysfunction of the mucociliary apparatus in the middle ear and eustachian tube may be responsible, in part, for the chronicity of otitis media with effusion.

To assess the effect of various biologically active agents on the mucociliary transport system, it is necessary to establish the normal rate of fluid transport from the middle ear to the nasopharyngeal orifice of the eustachian tube. This study was undertaken to determine baseline transport rates using an in situ system in the chinchilla in which the bulla remains intact. In addition, this animal model was used to assess the effect on transport rates of two biologically active agents commonly found in middle ear effusions, prostaglandin E₂ (PGE₂) and bacterial endotoxin, to test the hypothesis that inflammatory mediators or bacterial products may affect the mucociliary transport mechanism, leading to chronicity of the effusion.

MATERIALS AND METHODS

Healthy adult chinchillas, free of middle ear infection, were used. A total of 84 ears (from 46 animals) were tested. The chinchilla was chosen because of the demonstrated patency of the eustachian tube,[2] which ensures that the transport rates measured are due primarily to mucociliary activity. The animals were anesthetized prior to surgical incision to split the soft palate. Anesthetized animals were placed in a prone position with the jaws clamped open to allow visualization of the orifice with the operating microscope. At the appropriate time, 0.15 ml of either sterile saline, bupivacaine hydrochloride, isoproterenol hydrochloride, *Salmonella typhimurium* lipopolysaccharide (LPS), or prostaglandin E₂ (PGE₂) was injected. Bupivacaine and isoproterenol were used in this system because of their known capacities to decelerate or accelerate ciliary beating, respectively.[3, 4] All were diluted in sterile saline to the desired concentration. Once 0.15 ml was injected into the superior bulla via a tuberculin syringe, with a 25 gauge needle as a vent, the injection of all solutions except lipopolysaccharide was followed exactly 10 minutes later by an injection of 0.15 ml of 5.0 percent Coomassie brilliant blue in 0.01 M phosphate buffered saline. Lipopolysaccharide solutions were allowed to remain in the middle ear for 1 hour before dye injection.

A stopwatch was used to determine the transport time. The watch was started at the moment of dye injection and stopped at the first appearance of dye at the eustachian tube orifice in the nasopharynx. The transport rate was calculated by dividing the average transport time in seconds by 9.5 mm, which is the approximate length of the ciliated portion of the chinchilla middle ear mucosa.[5] Student's t test was used to determine the differences between means. We selected a $p < 0.05$ level of significance for all analyses.

RESULTS

Before initiating transport studies we assessed the effect of volume on transport. Volumes of dye greater than 0.20 ml resulted in the immediate appearance of dye at the eustachian tube orifice, whereas those of 0.10 ml or less failed to appear within the 15 minute limit arbitrarily set for dye transport. A volume of 0.15 ml gave reproducible results and was therefore used throughout these experiments.

The normal transport rate of dye (0.15 ml) from the middle ear cavity to the nasopharyngeal orifice of the eustachian tube (with or without an injection of saline 10 minutes prior to dye) was 130 ±10 seconds (Table 1). To assure ourselves that we were measuring the transport of dye by ciliary activity, we attempted to manipulate the transport rates by accelerating or decelerating the ciliary beating with chemical agents. The beta-adrenergic stimulator isoproterenol caused a significant increase in the rate of dye transport, from an average of 130 seconds to 79 ±7 seconds ($p \leq 0.01$), at a concentration of 0.005 percent (v/v). The local anesthetic bupivacaine had no effect on transport rates at a concentration of 0.0005 percent; however, at concentrations of 0.001, 0.005, and 0.5 percent, dye transport times were prolonged, the majority of times in each category exceeding the 15 minute cutoff. *S. typhimurium* endotoxin did not affect transport rates at concentrations of either 10 or 100 μg per milliliter. At 1,000 μg per milliliter, however, the average dye transport time was 476 ±47 seconds, which was significantly slower than that in controls or with the two lower concentrations of lipopolysaccharide ($p \leq 0.005$). Prostaglandin$_2$ had no effect on transport rates at any concentration tested (10^{-6}, 10^{-8}, 10^{-10} M).

To determine whether the delayed transport of dye noted after brief exposure to high concentrations of lipopolysaccharide or bupivacaine was due to either damage to or swelling of the eustachian tubal epithelium rather than diminished mucociliary transport, we examined cross sections of this tissue by both light and transmission electron microscopy. Both light and transmission electron microscopic findings demonstrated that the lipopolysaccharide or bupivacaine instillation did not alter the morphologic integrity of the ciliated cells in the eustachian tube (Fig. 1), suggesting that the delayed dye transport by these agents was caused by the reduced ciliary activity.

DISCUSSION

The mucociliary apparatus represents a critical defense system of the respiratory tract, including the middle ear, in both animals and man. Through the action of the cilia, debris and fluid are moved from the middle ear space through the eustachian tubes into the nasopharynx for elimination via the upper respiratory or digestive tracts.

Normal transport rates for a mucociliary system vary depending on the origin of the tissue, the particle being carried, and the method used to quantitate the movement as well as the environmental conditions under which the assessment is made (i.e., pH, humidity, temperature). Transport rates for frog palate epithelium vary from 2.1 to 3.2 mm per minute for mucus depleted tissue to 7.2 mm per minute for undepleted tissue.[6] Rat trachea has been reported to have a similar transport rate of 10 to 15 mm per minute.[7] In a study of the movement of tagged particles in the human nasal mucosa, average mucociliary flow rates of 7.5 mm per minute were recorded.[8] Eustachian tube rates have been less thoroughly studied.

TABLE 1   Effect of Biologically Active Agents on the Rate of Dye Transport from the Middle Ear to the Nasopharynx of the Chinchilla

Agent	Concentration	Transport Time (Sec ± SEM; $n \geq 5$ replicates)
Control	—	130±10
Isoproterenol	0.005%	79±7*
Bupivacaine	0.0005%	163±45
Bupivacaine	0.001%	a[†]
Bupivacaine	0.005%	a
Bupivacaine	0.5%	a
S. typhimurium LPS	10 μg/ml	178±44
S. typhimurium LPS	100 μg/ml	110±21
S. typhimurium LPS	1000 μg/ml	476±47*
PGE$_2$	10^{-10} M	115±7
PGE$_2$	10^{-8} M	109±13
PGE$_2$	10^{-6} M	141±29

* Significant difference from controls ($p \leq 0.01$).
† Majority of values exceeded 15 minute limit.

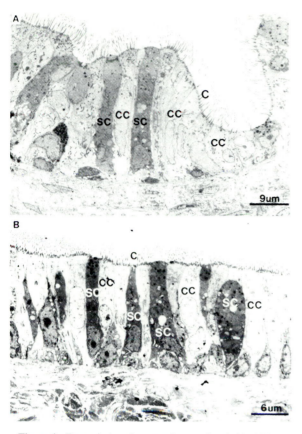

Figure 1 Transmission electron micrographs of chinchilla eustachian tube epithelium following exposure to *A*, 1000 μg lipopolysaccharide per milliliter for 1 hour and *B*, 0.5 percent bupivacaine for 10 minutes. C = cilia; CC = ciliated cell; and SC = secretory cell.

Baseline transport rates obtained in the animal model presented here indicate a calculated transport rate of approximately 4.3 mm per minute, considering that the ciliated portion of the chinchilla middle ear mucosa (from the bony ridge to the nasopharyngeal orifice of the eustachian tube) is approximately 9.5 mm in length.[5] This value includes, by necessity, the time it takes the dye to diffuse from the injection site in the superior bulla to the inferior bulla, where it can pool and be picked up and moved by the ciliated epithelium; therefore the calculated transport rate is likely to be slightly less than the actual rate. This transport rate is well within the range of values reported for other mucociliary systems. Use of the local anesthetic bupivacaine hydrochloride resulted in a delay in the transport of dye, which was not due to ultrastructural damage to the eustachian tube. Although we recorded no effect on transport at 0.0005 percent, there was significant inhibition at 0.001, 0.005, and 0.5 percent. Using a known beta-adrenergic stimulator of rabbit oviduct cilia (isoproterenol),[4] we increased transport rates significantly.

Although we cannot state with absolute certainty that the transport rates reflect ciliary activity exclusively, our ability to readily manipulate the rates with known ciliary accelerators and inhibitors was reassuring. Since the animals were deeply anesthetized throughout the surgical and experimental procedures and therefore did not swallow, thus eliminating any pumping function of the eustachian tube, we believe that the tubal transport rates recorded were predominantly the result of mucociliary activity and not muscular activity. This is particularly true in light of the fact that the chinchilla eustachian tube has been shown to be continually patent.[2]

Middle ear fluids contain a variety of substances, including several biologic mediators of inflammation and lipopolysaccharide, which are also known to have an effect on ciliary activity.[9,10] Lipopolysaccharide or endotoxin is believed to contribute to the pathogenesis of otitis media with effusion. Indeed endotoxin alone can lead to the presence of effusion in the middle ear of the chinchilla and causes capillary engorgement, edema, bleeding, and mononuclear cell infiltration.[11] Endotoxin from *Klebsiella pneumoniae* has been shown by Ohashi et al to result in a dose dependent cessation of ciliary activity in all portions of the middle ear of the guinea pig (see chapter *Ciliary Activity and Lipopolysaccharide*). In addition, endotoxin from type b *H. influenzae* was found to result in a variety of pathologic changes in the middle ear of guinea pigs that the authors attributed to transudation and injury to the mucosa, which disturbed mucociliary transport activity.[12] Our data supported these findings by demonstrating that high concentrations of *S. typhimurium* lipopolysaccharide, which is similar in many respects to that of *H. influenzae*, leads to increased transport rates.

Prostaglandins are also frequently found in middle ear effusions and in relatively high concentrations.[13-15] Prostaglandins E_1 and E_2 have been shown to cause marked increases in permeability and vasodilation edema in dog middle ear and eustachian tube mucosa,[16] which indicates that they may be one cause of middle ear effusions and that their continued presence may contribute to the chronicity of these effusions. The capacity of prostaglandin$_2$ to elevate levels of lactate dehydrogenase, acid and alkaline phosphatase, calcium, and protein in the middle ear demonstrates a potential role for prostaglandins in the inflammation seen in otitis media.[17]

Since prostaglandin$_2$ is also known to stimulate ciliary activity in rabbit oviduct and isolated sheep tracheal epithelial cell cultures,[4, 18] we investigated its effect on the transport rate in the chinchilla eustachian tube. No effect was found over the range of concentrations tested, which may simply reflect the reduced hormonal sensitivity of this non-reproductive tissue or the fact that only minor changes, beneath the sensitivity threshold of this assay, were induced.

CONCLUSIONS

We have established a highly flexible and reproducible system for gross assessment of the rate of transport from the middle ear to the nasopharyngeal orifice of the eustachian tube in the chinchilla. This method offers several advantages over standard in vitro culture techniques, including the maintenance of an intact bulla and mucosa, which allows for better approximation of the in vivo situation. This method can be used to determine the effect of biologically active agents or bacterial products on transport rates. The fact that bacterial endotoxin has been shown to result in significantly delayed transport supports the hypothesis that nonviable bacteria or bacterial components that may be trapped in the tympanic cavity sustain the inflammation and contribute to the chronicity of the middle ear effusion.

This study was supported, in part, by grant NS08854 from the NINCDS/NIH.

REFERENCES

1. Honjo I, Okazaki N, Nozoe T, Ushiro K, Kumazawa T. Experimental study of the pumping function of the eustachian tube. Acta Otolaryngol 1981; 91:85–89.
2. Doyle WJ. Eustachian tube function in the chinchilla. Arch Otolaryngol 1985; 111:305–308.
3. Manawadu BR, Mostow SR, La Force FM. Local anesthetics and tracheal ring ciliary activity. Anesth Analg 1978; 57:448–452.
4. Verdugo P, Rumery RE, Tam PY. Hormonal control of oviductal ciliary activity: effect of prostaglandins. Fertil Steril 1980; 33:193–196.
5. Hanamure Y, Lim DJ. The middle ear and eustachian tube in the chinchilla: a light microscopic study. Am J Otolaryngol 1986; 4:410–425.
6. Spungin B, Silberberg A. Stimulation of mucus secretion, ciliary activity, and transport in frog palate epithelium. Am J Physiol 1984; 247:C299–308.
7. Dalhamn T. Mucous flow and ciliary activity in the trachea of healthy rats and rats exposed to respiratory irritant gases. Acta Physiol Scand 1956; 36 (Suppl 123):1–161.
8. Sakakura Y, Sasaki Y, Harnick RB, Togo Y, Schwartz AR, Wagner HN Jr, Proctor DF. Mucociliary function during experimentally induced rhinovirus infection in man. Ann Otol Rhinol Laryngol 1973; 82:203–211.
9. Bernstein JM, Praino MD, Neter E. Detection of endotoxin in ear specimens from patients with chronic otitis media by means of the limulus amebocyte lysate test. Can J Microbiol 1980; 26:546–548.
10. DeMaria TF, Prior RB, Briggs BR, Lim DJ, Birck HG. Endotoxin in middle ear effusions from patients with chronic otitis media with effusion. J Clin Microbiol 1984; 20:15–17.
11. DeMaria TF, Lim DJ. Inflammatory changes in the middle ear and eustachian tube induced by viable or nonviable *Hemophilus influenzae* or its endotoxin. Ann Otol Rhinol Laryngol 1985; 94 (Suppl 120):14–16.
12. Nonomura N, Nakano Y, Satoh Y, Fujioka O, Niijima H, Fujita M. Otitis media with effusion following inoculation of *Haemophilus influenzae* type b endotoxin. Arch Otorhinolaryngol 1986; 243:31–35.
13. Jackson RT, Waitzman MB, Pickford L, Nathanson SE. Prostaglandins in human middle ear effusions. Prostaglandins 1975; 10:365–371.
14. Bernstein JM. Biological mediators of inflammation in middle ear effusions. Ann Otol Rhinol Laryngol 1976; 85 (Suppl 25):90–96.
15. Smith DM, Jung TTK, Juhn SK, Berlinger NT, Gerrard JM. Prostaglandins in experimental otitis media. Arch Otorhinolaryngol 1979; 225:207–209.
16. Dennis RG, Whitmire RN, Jackson RT. Action of inflammatory mediators on middle ear mucosa. Arch Otolaryngol 1976; 102:420–424.
17. Jung TTK, Smith DM, Juhn SK, Gerrard JH. Effect of prostaglandin on the composition of chinchilla middle ear effusion. Ann Otol Rhinol Laryngol 1980; 89:153–160.
18. Wanner A, Maurer D, Abraham WM, Szepfalusi Z, Sielczak M. Effects of chemical mediators of anaphylaxis on ciliary function. J Allergy Clin Immunol 1983; 72:663–667.

REVERSIBLE FUNCTIONAL OBSTRUCTION OF THE EUSTACHIAN TUBE

MARGARETHA L. CASSELBRANT, M.D., Ph.D., ERDEM I. CANTEKIN, Ph.D.,
DENNIS C. DIRKMAAT, B.A., WILLIAM J. DOYLE, Ph.D.,
and CHARLES D. BLUESTONE, M.D.

Many theories have been proposed in an effort to explain the development of otitis media with effusion. In the early 1970s "functional obstruction of the eustachian tube" was suggested as a pathogenic mechanism.[1,2] The tensor veli palatini muscle has been shown in several mammals, including cats, dogs, and Rhesus monkeys, to be the only muscle that can actively dilate the lumen of the eustachian tube. The integrity of this muscle is essential for normal functioning of the tube.[3-7]

In an attempt to create an animal model of otitis media with effusion congruent with this functional obstruction concept, we performed various surgical manipulations of the tensor veli palatini muscle in Rhesus monkeys. We reported that these surgical procedures created various degrees and durations of functional and mechanical obstruction of the eustachian tube (e.g., negative middle ear pressure) and effusion developed within several days after surgery.[6] One of the interesting but unexplained observations, in Rhesus monkeys with excised tensor muscles, was constriction of the tubal lumen upon swallowing; this observation has also been reported in children and adults with persistent middle ear problems.[8]

The present study was conducted in order to develop a nontraumatic animal model of reversible pure functional obstruction of the eustachian tube and also to investigate the mechanism responsible for constriction of the tube upon swallowing. To eliminate mechanical trauma caused by the surgical procedure, botulinum toxin was injected into the tensor veli palatini to create functional obstruction. Botulinum toxin interferes with acetylcholine release at the nerve terminal at the neuromuscular junction, causing localized muscle paralysis that lasts for weeks to months.

METHODS

Experiments were conducted using botulinum induced tensor veli palatini paralysis to investigate its effect on eustachian tube function and to document changes in the middle ear status. Adult Rhesus monkeys (*Macaca mulatta*) were used in all experiments. During the first experiment with two animals the forced response test was employed to evaluate eustachian tube function.[8] After insertion of bilateral tympanostomy tubes, the tensor veli palatini muscle was injected unilaterally every 6 weeks with increasing doses of botulinum A toxin (5, 8, 10, and 20 ng); the contralateral side served as a control. Following injection the animals were tested weekly for 5 to 6 weeks to assess the effect of the toxin on tubal function. Repeat injections were carried out by alternating the injection side from right to left after the return of tubal function to preinjection levels. In the second experiment with six other animals we documented the effects of tensor veli palatini muscle paralysis on the middle ear status. Initially the left tensor veli palatini muscles were injected with 40 ng of botulinum A toxin; 10 weeks later the right muscles were injected with 40 ng of toxin. Contralateral tensor veli palatini muscles were always injected with normal saline to serve as effective controls. Following injections, daily tympanograms were recorded for both ears. Tympanocentesis was carried out in most ears with tympanograms indicative of an effusion.

RESULTS

Postinjection eustachian tube function was characterized by the absence of active tubal dilations during swallowing, an unchanged opening pressure, and a decreased closing pressure. The average postinjection weekly data for these repeated injections are shown in Figure 1 in regard to tubal dilation efficiency (the ratio of active resistance to passive resistance) as well as two measures of passive function. When compared with the control side, the experimental side showed a significant decrease in dilation efficiency. During the first 3 weeks the injected side had an average dilation efficiency of about 1—equal values for active and passive resistance—indicating complete paralysis of the tensor veli palatini muscle. As shown by the linear regression fit (r=0.72), dilation efficiency gradually returned to preinjection values. Interestingly, forced response test recordings during the paralysis period showed neither dilations nor constrictions secondary to swallowing activity. As shown in Figure 1

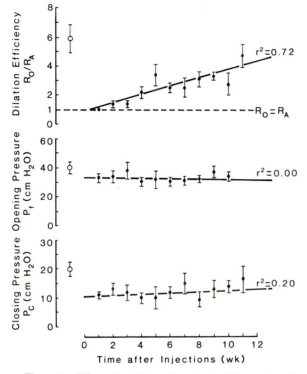

Figure 1 Effect of experimental paralysis of the tensor veli palatini muscle on eustachian tube function. Changes in the dilation efficiency (top) and the response of the passive function parameters—opening pressure (middle) and closing pressure (bottom)—are shown for a forcing flow rate of 24 cc per minute. Data represented by open circles indicate group mean values before injections, and the error bars indicate the standard error of the mean. Also shown are linear regression fits with r^2 values.

illustrating passive function parameters, the opening (P_o) and closing (P_c) pressures were reduced following muscle paralysis. Average closing pressure values were significantly decreased, but these values returned within a standard deviation of the baseline values after 11 weeks. Reductions in the average pressure values were not significant.

The middle ear findings for all 12 ears of the six animals following botulinum toxin injections are summarized in Table 1. Injection of normal saline did not affect the middle ear status. Five of the 12 ears had negative pressures exceeding -100 mm H_2O the day after injections, and within 3 days after injection 10 of the 12 ears had pressures less than -100 mm H_2O. However, the average negative middle pressures never exceeded -300 mm H_2O during the follow-up period. Ten of the 12 ears developed flat tympanogram patterns associated with otitis media with effusion within 8 to 30 days (average, 16 days) after tensor veli palatini paralysis. Tympanocentesis was performed in seven ears with flat tympanograms and serous effusions were recovered from all. In order to avoid the confounding effect of tympanocentesis, the remaining three ears were not tapped. The time for recovery to occur, as measured by tympanometric records for those cases, ranged from 13 to 32 days.

DISCUSSION

We demonstrated that the injection of botulinum toxin A into the tensor veli palatini muscle in Rhesus monkeys creates nontraumatic reversible functional obstruction of the eustachian tube. The duration of paralysis was several weeks, during which time the tensor veli palatini muscle showed no discernible activity that could be recorded by the forced response test. Also of interest was the lack

TABLE 1 Summary of Tympanometric Findings for all Ears and Days to Negative Pressure (-100, -200, -250) and to Middle Ear Effusion

Animal No.													
	336		454		484		506		576		2675		
Side	R	L	R	L	R	L	R	L	R	L	R	L	Group Averages
Middle ear status													
Negative pressure*													
-100 mm H_2O	1	1	2	1	5	1	2	3	1	3	3	12	2.9
-200 mm H_2O	6	7	5	3	NL‡	–	5	7	7	–	10	NL	6.3
-250 mm H_2O	8	7	5	6	NL	–	–	9	14	–	10	NL	8.4
Effusion†	27	30	13	14	NL	8	12	16	17	8	13	NL	15.8

Number of Days for a Given Middle Ear Status to Occur

* Negative pressure determined by the pressure value corresponding to tympanometric peak.
† Effusion—either flat tympanogram, direct observation (tympanocentesis), indirect observation (otomicroscopy), observation of significant change in curve morphology, or relative compliance ratio of tympanometric peak.
‡ NL, returned to normal middle ear status.

of tubal constriction during the paralysis period, suggesting that most dilations as well as constrictions of the eustachian tube lumen recorded during the forced response test are due to activity of the tensor veli palatini muscle. The effect of reversible functional eustachian tube obstruction on the middle ear was the development of negative middle ear pressure, which was a precursor of otitis media with effusion. Middle ear effusions resolved spontaneously, within the same time frame of recovery from functional eustachian tube obstruction. These experiments demonstrated that the middle ear status depends on the integrity of the tensor veli palatini muscle, and pure functional eustachian tube obstruction is one of the possible pathogenic mechanisms in otitis media with effusion.

Study supported in part by NIH–NINCDS grant NS-16337.

REFERENCES

1. Holborow C. Eustachian tube function: changes in anatomy and function with age and the relationship of these changes to aural pathology. Arch Otol 1970; 92:624–626.
2. Bluestone CD. Eustachian tube obstruction in the infant with cleft palate. Ann Otol Rhinol Laryngol 1971; 80:1–30.
3. Rich AR. A physiological study of the eustachian tube and its related muscles. Bull Johns Hopkins Hosp 1920; 31:206–214.
4. Honjo I, Okazaki N, Kumazawa T. Experimental study of the eustachian tube function with respect to its related muscles. Acta Otolaryngol (Stockh) 1979; 87:84–89.
5. Cantekin EI, Doyle WJ, Reichert TJ, Phillips CD. Dilation of the eustachian tube by electrical stimulation of the mandibular nerve. Ann Otol Rhinol Laryngol 1979; 88:40–51.
6. Cantekin EI, Phillips DC, Doyle WJ, Bluestone CD, Kimes KK. Effect of surgical alterations of the tensor veli palatini muscle on eustachian tube function. Ann Otol Rhinol Laryngol 1980; 89 (Suppl 68):47–53.
7. Cantekin EI, Doyle WJ, Bluestone CD. Effect of levator veli palatini muscle excision on eustachian tube function. Arch Otolaryngol 1983; 109:281–284.
8. Cantekin EI, Saez CA, Bluestone CD, Bern SA. Airflow through the eustachian tube. Ann Otol Rhinol Laryngol 1979; 88:603–612.

SELECTED TOPICS ON MIDDLE EAR AND EUSTACHIAN TUBE PHYSIOLOGY OF THE DOMESTIC CAT

KENNY H. CHAN, M.D., J. DOUGLAS SWARTS, B.S., and WILLIAM J. DOYLE, Ph.D.

Mucoid effusion is of great interest to clinicians because it is frequently recovered from ears of children with otitis media with effusion. The more commonly used animal models, such as the rhesus monkey, gerbil, and chinchilla, have failed to produce this type of effusion. The domestic cat may be unique in that obstruction of the eustachian tube by various methods has been reported to consistently produce mucoid effusion.[1-3]

The reason for this species specificity is not known but may lie with corresponding differences in the physiology of the eustachian tube—middle ear system. Although this system has been fairly well characterized in man, the rhesus monkey, and the chinchilla[4,5] no comparable data are available for the domestic cat.

In this article we describe a study designed to define eustachian tube function, middle ear gas absorption characteristics, and the effect of tubal dysfunction on the middle ear in the domestic cat. Through comparison with data from studies in humans and monkeys the pathogenesis of mucoid otitis media with effusion in the domestic cat is explored.

METHODS AND MATERIALS

Six female domestic cats with an average weight of 2.8 kg were acquired from local breeders. The vertical portion of the external ear canal in each cat was ablated to aid in examination and testing. Initially the ears were screened using otomicroscopy and tympanography to insure a disease free status. Three sets of experiments were performed: eustachian tube function testing, middle ear gas absorption, and experiments involving paralysis of the tensor veli palatini muscle.

Eustachian Tube Function Testing

In this set of experiments, the function of the eustachian tube was studied in three animals. Testing was conducted via tympanostomy tubes in two cats and a wide myringotomy in the third. Tubal function was assessed using the forced response test, as described previously.[6] Following the collection of baseline data, tubal function was altered by injecting botulinum toxin into the tensor veli palatini muscles in two cats and transecting the muscles in one cat. Tubal function tests were repeated following these procedures.

Middle Ear Gas Absorption Testing

In the second set of experiments, the longitudinal middle ear gas absorption pattern as reflected by the peaked middle ear pressure of the tympanogram was studied in three cats. The animals were anesthetized with barbiturate and paralyzed with curare. They were then intubated and artificially ventilated with a respirator. Serial tympanograms were recorded every 5 to 15 minutes for a 6 to 8 hour period. In two of the animals the middle ears were then inflated using the technique of politzerization; serial tympanograms were obtained throughout the experiment.

Paralysis of the Tensor Veli Palatini Muscle

In the third set of experiments, the tensor veli palatini muscle in 11 ears of 6 cats was injected with 50 to 100 units of botulinum toxin. The middle ear pressure and status were monitored weekly by repeat tympanometry and otomicroscopy to detect the development of negative pressure and middle ear effusion for up to 7 weeks.

RESULTS

Tubal function was examined before and after a debilitating procedure on the tensor veli palatini muscle by either botulinum toxin injection or transection. Measures of static function, such as opening (P_f), steady state (P_o), and closing pressures (P_c) as well as the passive resistance (R_o), were unchanged before and after the procedures. However, the two measures of active function—active resistance (R_a) and dilation efficiency (R_o/R_a)—were changed. With the resistance ratio as a measure of dilation efficiency, the data give evidence of a significant

decrease in dilation efficiency following muscular injuries.

When interspecies comparisons of eustachian tube function are made, variations among the cat, monkey, and human are evident. Although the opening pressure was substantially greater in the cat, the tubal closing pressures were similar in the three species. Other differences were noted for passive and active resistances (Fig. 1). Both parameters were greater in the cat than those in either the monkey or man. However, Cantekin et al[6] have shown that the ratio of these resistances effectively normalizes the data by controlling for inherent differences in tubal length and diameter. A similarity in the mean values of these ratios for the three species has been noted, suggesting that the cat and monkey are scaled models of the human system with approximately equal tubal dilation efficiencies.

Examples of middle ear gas absorption experiments are depicted by the line tracings shown in Figure 2. Under normal physiologic conditions paralysis of the tensor veli palatini muscle by curare in the cat resulted in the rapid development of a slight underpressure in the middle ear of only −100 mm H_2O. Following politzerization with room air, the induced positive pressures quickly dissipated and a steady state underpressure of −25 to −50 mm H_2O soon developed. This steady state finding was similar to the results reported for the monkey experiments, as noted in the cross hatched area in Figure 2, yet the post inflation value was markedly different from that in the monkey. In that species middle ear gases were quickly absorbed to result in the development of moderate underpressures in the range of −300 to −400 mm H_2O, as depicted by the shaded area in Figure 2. The development of underpressures following politzerization was also observed in the human by Gimsing.[7] These species' differences suggest the existence of a difference in the gas transport properties of the middle ear mucosa in these three species.

The reversible functional obstruction otitis media model in the monkey as described by Casselbrant et al[8] was repeated for the cat. Of the 11 ears injected with botulinum toxin, 9 ears were totally unaffected, 2 developed a negative pressure, and 1 developed an effusion. There was no evidence of the development of severe middle ear underpressures or disease by otoscopy following muscle paralysis. This was distinctly different from results obtained in the monkey model.

DISCUSSION

The domestic cat has long been used in otitis media research, yet the physiologic properties of the

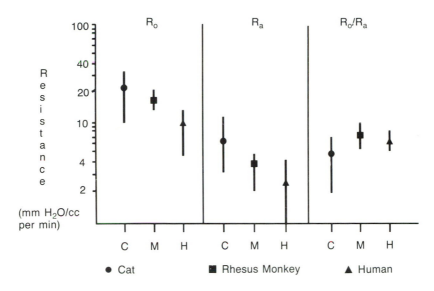

Figure 1   A comparison of the tubal passive resistance (R_o), active resistance (R_a), and dilation efficiency (R_o/R_a) in the cat, monkey, and human.

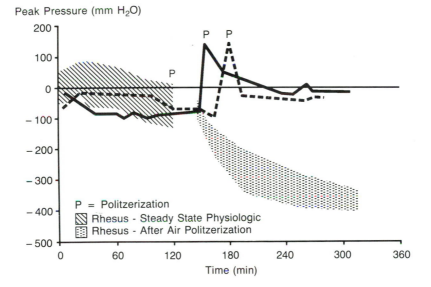

Figure 2   Middle ear gas absorption patterns for the cat and monkey. The line tracings represent two individual ears of two cats. The positive peaks along the line tracings divide the events before and after the politzerization of room air. The cross hatched area represents the range of peak middle ear pressure in the monkey at baseline. The shaded area represents the pressure range following politzerization.

eustachian tube—middle ear system have not been well studied. Selected aspects of the physiology of this system have been presented in this article. It can be concluded that the middle ear physiology in the cat is unique for two reasons. First, in our study no significant underpressures developed following the

insufflation of air into the middle ear. Second, the frequency of effusion formation following tensor veli palatini muscle paralysis was extremely low. Yet eustachian tube function in the cat shared many similarities with that in monkeys and humans. Therefore, it can be postulated that the pathogenesis of mucoid effusion may relate to species specific physiologic and histoanatomic properties of the middle ear. A comparative study of gaseous exchange and histopathology of the middle ear may be necessary to further our understanding of the pathogenesis of mucoid effusion.

Study funded by NIH grants RR550724, NS 07270, and NS 16337.

REFERENCES

1. Proud GO, Odoi H. Effects of eustachian tube ligation. Ann Otol Rhinol Laryngol 1970; 79:1–32.
2. Juhn SK, Paparella MM, Kim CS, Goycoolea MV, Giebink S. Pathogenesis of otitis media. Ann Otol Rhinol Laryngol 1977; 86:481–492.
3. Tos M, Wiederhold M, Larsen P. Experimental long-term tubal occlusion in cats: a quantitative histopathological study. Acta Otolaryngol (Stockh) 1984; 97:580–592.
4. Cantekin EI, Doyle WJ, Bluestone CD. Comparison of normal eustachian tube function in the rhesus monkey and man. Ann Otol Rhinol Laryngol 1982; 91:79–184.
5. Doyle WJ. Eustachian tube function in the chinchilla. Arch Otolaryngol 1985; 111:305–308.
6. Cantekin EI, Saez CA, Bluestone CD, Bern SA. Airflow through the eustachian tube. Ann Otol Rhinol Laryngol 1979; 88:603–612.
7. Gimsing S. Gas absorption in serous otitis: a clinical aspect. Ann Otol Rhinol Laryngol 1983; 92:305–308.
8. Casselbrant ML, Dirkmaat D, Doyle WJ, Cantekin EI, Bluestone CD. Reversible functional obstruction of the eustachian tube. Acta Otolaryngol (In press).

ANATOMY AND MORPHOLOGY

MAGNETIC RESONANCE IMAGING OF THE EUSTACHIAN TUBE

YASUSHI NAITO, M.D., IWAO HONJO, M.D., KAZUMASA HOSHINO, M.D., and KAZUMASA NISHIMURA, M.D.

Diseases in the nasopharynx often cause problems in the middle ear, but the mechanisms involved have not been elucidated clearly. The eustachian tube is thought to play and important role here because it ventilates the middle ears connecting with the nasopharynx. Magnetic resonance imaging is a valuable method for morphologic study of the area around the eustachian tube because it provides extremely high soft tissue contrast resolution.[1] In the present study magnetic resonance images of areas around the eustachian tube were compared with cadaver sections for precise evaluation of the surrounding anatomic areas. Several cases of cleft palate and nasopharyngeal carcinoma are presented here to demonstrate morbid topographic changes around the eustachian tube.

MATERIALS AND METHOD

Magnetic resonance imaging was performed with a superconducting magnet operating at 1.5 Tesla (Signa, GE, Milwaukee). The pulse sequence applied was spin echo. The repetition time was 2000 msec and the echo times were 40 and 80 msec. The scan thickness was 3 mm, and a gap of 1.5 mm separated adjoining scans. Subjects were laid in the supine position with their head extended to obtain an anteriorly tilted transaxial plane parallel to the line including the upper ends of the external auditory canals and the tips of the first upper incisor teeth. Along this tilted plane we could observe the entire picture of the eustachian tube consistently. A cadaver specimen fixed, dehydrated, and embedded in polyester resin was cut serially, parallel to the baseline determined in the same way as with magnetic resonance imaging. Magnetic resonance images of the eustachian tube of a normal volunteer were compared with the corresponding cadaver sections.

NORMAL ANATOMY

The upper part of the eustachian tube is shown in Figure 1. The eustachian tube cartilage is depicted as a low intensity line by magnetic resonance imaging. The mucous lining of the tube is shown as two high intensity lines situated lateral to the tubal cartilage. The mucous membrane of the lateral pharyngeal recess can be seen medial to the tubal cartilage. The tensor veli palatini muscle and the medial pterygoid muscle also can be identified in this section.

Figure 2 shows the lower part of the eustachian tube. The tubal cartilage appears to be slightly curved in this section. The mucous linings of the tube appear thicker than those in the previous section. The venous plexus lateral to the tensor muscle has a high intensity probably because of the long T2 representing the stagnant blood in the plexus.

Cases of cleft palate and nasopharyngeal carcinoma are presented to demonstrate the abnormal anatomic changes around the eustachian tube.

CLEFT PALATE

Three consecutive images in the proximity of the eustachian tube of a 12 year old boy with a submucous cleft palate are shown in Figure 3. The tubal cartilages are cup shaped in their lower part, and the mucous lining of the tube appears much thicker than normal. The levator veli palatini muscles are situated more lateral than normal and do not meet in the midline. This patient had chronic otitis media on the right side and persistent otitis media with effusion on the left side.

The second case is a 50 year old man with an untreated cleft palate. As in the previous case, abnormal curvatures of the lower parts of the tubal

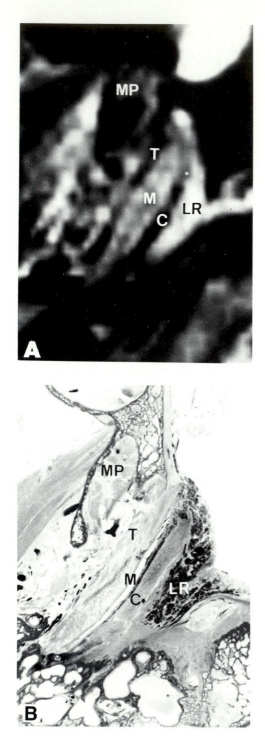

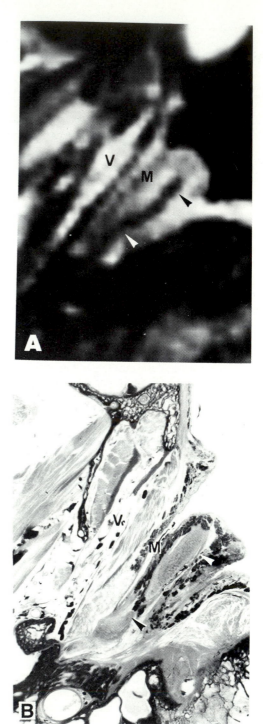

Figure 1 Magnetic resonance image. Left, uppermost part of nasopharyngeal cavity (TR=2000 ms; TE=80 ms); right, corresponding cadaver specimen section. LR indicates lateral pharyngeal recess; C, eustachian tube cartilage; M, mucous lining of eustachian tube; T, tensor veli palatini muscle; MP, medial pterygoid muscle.

Figure 2 Magnetic resonance image (left) 4.5 mm below Figure 1, left (TR=2000 ms, TE=80 ms) and corresponding specimen section (right). V indicates venous plexus. Lower part of eustachian tube cartilage (arrowheads) is slightly curved. Mucous lining of eustachian tube (M) is thicker than in slice shown in Figure 1.

cartilages can be observed. An abnormal lateral position of the levator muscles is also seen in this case. This patient had persistent otitis media with effusion on the right side and chronic otitis media on the left side.

Nine patients with cleft palate were examined, and deformities of the tubal cartilages were found in all cases. By contrast, in 19 normal subjects the curves of the tubal cartilages were not as prominent as in the cleft palate cases.

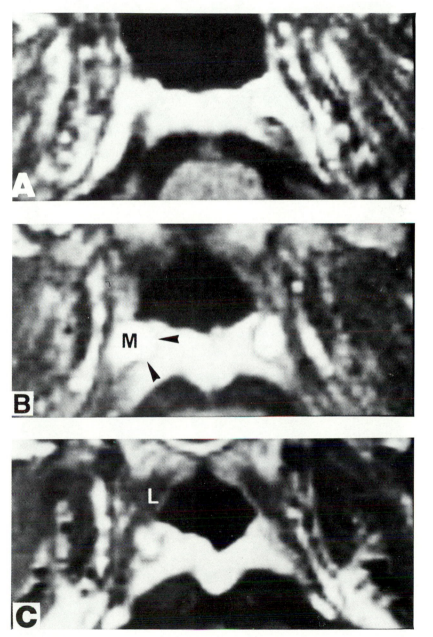

Figure 3 Magnetic resonance images of submucous cleft palate. *A*, Upper part of eustachian tube. *B*, Eustachian tube cartilage (arrowheads) are cup-shaped and mucous lining of tube (M) appears much thicker than normal. *C*, Lower part of eustachian tube. Lavator veli palatini muscle (L) is situated more lateral than normal and does not meet in the midline.

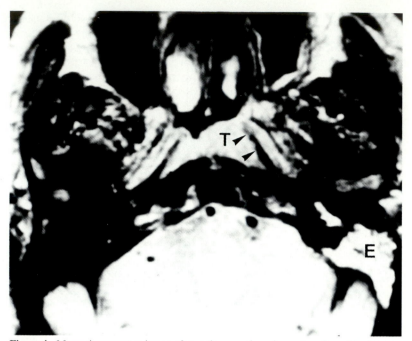

Figure 4 Magnetic resonance image of nasopharyngeal carcinoma together with otitis media with effusion. E indicates middle ear effusion; T, tumor pushed eustachian tube cartilage outward (arrowheads).

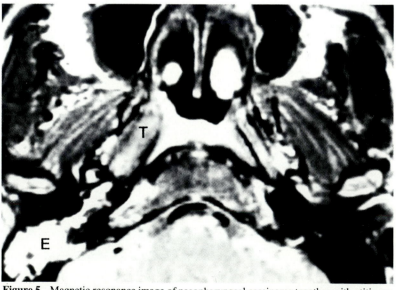

Figure 5 Magnetic resonance image of nasopharyngeal carcinoma together with otitis media with effusion. E indicates middle ear effusion; T, tumor invading eustachian tube.

NASOPHARYNGEAL CARCINOMA

In the first case the tumor was situated in the posterior wall of the nasopharynx. The tubal cartilages remained in the normal position, and there were no abnormal findings in the eustachian tube. This patient had no disease of the middle ear.

In the second case the eustachian tube cartilage on the left side is pushed outward by the tumor in the lateral pharyngeal recess (Fig. 4). The eustachian tube appears to be bent by the lateral shift of the cartilage. The middle ear of this side is filled with effusion, which is shown at high intensity in T2 weighted images.

The third patient has a carcinoma occupying the right lateral wall of the nasopharynx (Fig. 5). The high intensity mass can be seen between the tubal cartilage and the tensor muscle. This sort of direct invasion of the carcinoma into the eustachian tube can also cause otitis media with effusion on the affected side.

Among the 10 patients with nasopharyngeal carcinoma examined by magnetic resonance imaging, eight had otitis media with effusion on the affected side. Either lateral dislocation of the tubal cartilage or direct tumor invasion into the eustachian tube was found in every case with otitis media with effusion.

DISCUSSION

There has been no method developed that provides a clear image of the eustachian tube. Computed tomography, for example, can provide only images of the tensor and levator veli palatini muscles and does not depict the eustachian tube or tubal cartilage. Magnetic resonance imaging, on the other hand, is suitable for the morphologic study of this area because it provides very high soft tissue con-

trast resolution. Routine magnetic resonance imaging at the axial or coronal plane does not yield distinct pictures of the tube. The anteriorly tilted transaxial plane selected in the present study proved to be parallel to the longitudinal axes of the eustachian tubes by anatomic correlation with a cadaver.

Patients with cleft palate have middle ear disease more frequently than those without this anomaly. Morphologic approaches are necessary to determine the etiology of the frequent middle ear disorders. In patients with cleft palate the configuration of the eustachian tube cartilage was different from that in normal subjects, and the levator veli palatini muscles were situated more laterally than normal. This anomaly is suggested as predisposing to eustachian tube dysfunction and middle ear disease in patients with cleft palate.

About one third of the patients with nasopharyngeal carcinoma suffer from middle ear disease, but little is known about how these diseases are caused by the tumor. In our studies of 10 patients with nasopharyngeal carcinoma, lateral dislocation of the eustachian tube cartilage, and direct tumor invasion to the tube have been found to cause otitis media with effusion.

Magnetic resonance imaging along this tilted axial plane provides clear images of the eustachian tube in both normal subjects and patients with disease. This method is expected to become a valuable tool for the study of diseases not only in the nasopharynx but also in the middle ear.

REFERENCES

1. Naito Y, Honjo I, Nishimura K, et al. Magnetic resonance imaging around the eustachian tube. Am J Otolaryngol 1986; 7:402–406.

EUSTACHIAN TUBE CARTILAGE SHAPE AS A FACTOR IN THE EPIDEMIOLOGY OF OTITIS MEDIA

MICHAEL I. SIEGEL, Ph.D., DEBORAH SADLER-KIMES, Ph.D., and
JOHN S. TODHUNTER, Ph.D.

Clinical studies in the last several years have suggested that the incidence of chronic otitis media with effusion is age related, decreasing at or about age 7. It has been further suggested that this may be the result of anatomic variability of the eustachian tube cartilage and its associated musculature (such as improper insertion of the levator veli palatini), resulting in tubal blockage.[1,2] The present study used digital representation of histologically prepared specimens for three dimensional computer reconstruction of the eustachian tube and its associated structures. The resulting data were used to document the normal ontogenetic development and associations of the eustachian tube–middle ear system and to test the hypothesis that epidemiologic findings are related to anatomic variability of cartilage shape. Data from at risk specimens were also examined for similarity of pattern.

METHODS

Twenty-four extended temporal bone specimens were examined and placed into three different groups: normal specimens aged 7 and older, normal specimens aged 6 and younger, and at risk specimens aged 6 and younger. At risk specimens exhibited various structural anomalies of the midface and cranial base regions (e.g., Down syndrome, cleft palate), anomalies associated with a greater than normal prevalence of otitis media with effusion.[3]

Each specimen was histologically prepared and computer reconstructed. Histologic preparation consisted of decalcifying, sagittal sectioning, eosin-hematoxylin staining of every tenth section, and mounting on glass slides. With Kodak Pan X film and a light microscope with a camera attachment, negatives were obtained from the slides, beginning with the one containing the first appearance of tubal cartilage and ending with the last slide in which it was present. Computer reconstruction consisted of digitizing the negatives, extracting the structures to be analyzed, and quantifying selected aspects of the reconstructed structure.

The negatives were placed on a rotating drum scanner, which converted transmitted gray level light intensity to a digitized image, which was stored on the disk of a PDP 11/55 computer. As the images were projected on a Ramtec display screen, they were aligned to correct for displacement errors, and the boundaries of the levator veli palatini, tensor veli palatini, eustachian tube cartilage, and lumen were traced. Computer generated data were obtained for each of the four specimens and analyzed to determine the centers of gravity, cross sectional areas, x and y coordinates of the centers of gravity, second level moments, and longest and shortest points from the center of gravity to the edge of the structure.[4,5] It was then possible to reconstruct the structures and calculate structural volumes.

The x and y coordinates of the second moment were used to analyze the shape of structures in the system. Second moment coordinates represent the energy required to produce rotation around the center of gravity and are physically related to the maximal and minimal axes through the center of gravity (object length and width). The ratio of these coordinates (length/width) has been called the aspect ratio. This ratio, as well as total structural volume, cross sectional area, cartilage length, and distances between centers of gravity, was utilized to compare the four structures among the defined groups.

RESULTS

Eustachian tube cartilage length proved to be an important discriminator among age groups. Cartilage length exhibited a rapid growth rate prior to age 7, but this rate drastically decreased after age 7. By age 7, then, the eustachian tube cartilage had attained adult length. Regression equations for the growth curves reflected this observation. Both the normal less than 6 year and the at risk less than 6 year groups displayed rapid growth rates as evidenced by the steep slopes of the growth curves (y = 1,880x + 10,999; y = 2,396x + 10,145). The slope of the normal more than 7 year group approached zero, indicating a reduced growth rate (y = 53x + 16,588).

Gross measures of eustachian tube cartilage size showed an age related difference between the less than 6 year groups and the more than 7 year group. The mean total volume and cross sectional area of the normal less than 6 year and the at risk less than 6 year groups were significantly smaller than those in the normal more than 7 year group (p < 0.01).

Eustachian tube cartilage shape, however, did not show this age related pattern in all groups. Although the aspect ratio was significantly smaller, indicative of a less elongated structure, in the normal less than 6 year group as compared to the normal more than 7 year group, the results in the at risk less than 6 year group did not differ significantly from those in the normal more than 7 year group (Table 1).

The patterns of shape change in the specimens were similar to the patterns of eustachian tube cartilage size change. Although the groups showed no significant difference in overall configuration, significant differences were observable in the 40 to 80 percent (of total length) region of the specimens (Table 2). It has been reported previously, on the basis of graphed data, that in this region the normal less than 6 year group showed a reduced aspect ratio reflecting a more circular, less elongated shape.[6] Both the at risk less than 6 year and the normal more than 7 year groups maintained a larger aspect ratio, having an elongated shape throughout the specimens.[6] This visual impression from the graphed data is supported by statistical comparison of the slopes of these curves in the present analysis. In the 40 to 80 percent area the normal less than 6 year

TABLE 2 Means and Standard Deviation ( ) for Cartilage Aspect Ratio Slope

	Normal < 6	At Risk < 6	Normal > 7
0–100%	0.012 (0.67)	0.020 (0.25)	0.023 (0.35)
40–80%	−0.040 (0.42)	0.008 (0.19)	0.007 (0.34)

t Values and Probability levels ( ) for Groups Compared

	Normal < 6 Normal > 7	Normal < 6 At Risk < 6	Normal > 7 At Risk < 6
0–100%	0.32 (NS)	0.94 (NS)	0.24 (NS)
40–80%	3.89 (0.05)	5.03 (0.01)	0.06 (NS)

group significantly differed from the normal more than 7 year group, whereas the at risk less than 6 year group did not (see Table 2).

Similarly, lumen cross sectional area and levator veli palatini volume were significantly different in the normal less than 6 year and normal more than 7 year groups, showing the expected age related change. This difference was not present in the at risk less than 6 year group, in which results did not differ from those in the normal more than 7 year group (Table 3). The levator veli palatini–cartilage distance, however, did follow the expected age correlations. In both the normal less than 6 year and the at risk less than 6 year groups, the cartilage and levator veli palatini values were significantly closer than in the normal more than 7 year group (see Table 3).

DISCUSSION

The rate of growth of the cartilage was used to differentiate among the groups. In the less than 6 year group, the cartilage showed rapid growth, as evidenced by the slope of the line showing cartilage growth over time. This rapid growth disappeared in the more than 7 year group. The resulting difference between age groups mirrors the clinical finding of an age related decrease in the incidence of chronic otitis media with effusion.[7] By utilizing these observations, the current sample was divided into three groups. The immature pattern was expected for the normal and at risk less than 6 year groups, whereas the normal more than 7 year group was expected to exhibit the adult morphology.

TABLE 1 Means and Standard Deviation ( ) for Cartilage Aspect Ratio

	Normal < 6	At Risk < 7	Normal > 7
Aspect ratio	2.81 (0.47)	3.08 (0.77)	3.77 (1.13)

t Values and Probability levels ( ) for Groups Compared

Normal < 6 Normal > 7	Normal < 6 At Risk < 6	Normal > 7 At Risk < 6
2.45 (0.05)	0.72 (NS)	1.65 (NS)

TABLE 3   Means and Standard Deviations ( ) for Lumen Area, Levator Veli Palatini Volume and Levator Veli Palatini—Cartilage Distance

	Normal < 6	At Risk < 6	Normal > 7
Lumen area (sq cm)	0.0075 (0.0047)	0.0143 (0.0101)	0.0255 (0.0147)
Levator veli palatini (cu cm)	0.051 (0.034)	0.085 (0.052)	0.163 (0.134)
Levator veli palatini–cartilage distance (micrometers)	4,285 (1,249)	4,147 (1,465)	6,635 (1,135)

t Values and Probability Levels ( ) for Groups Compared

	Normal < 6 Normal > 7	Normal < 6 At Risk < 6	Normal > 7 At Risk < 6
Lumen area	3.83 (0.05)	1.51 (NS)	1.97 (NS)
Levator veli palatini volume	2.73 (0.05)	1.31 (NS)	1.86 (NS)
Levator veli palatini-cartilage distance	3.22 (0.05)	0.17 (NS)	3.75 (.05)

The normal more than 7 year and normal less than 6 year groups showed a pattern of age related differences, although, somewhat surprisingly, in many instances findings in the at risk less than 6 year group more closely resembled those of the adult rather than the immature morphology.

It has been suggested that in a normal more than 7 year group a mature cartilage is functional because some aspects of the system (e.g., cartilage length) make it stable.[6] For the eustachian tube system to function well, the components of the system must be well integrated; i.e., they must work well together. In the at risk group, however, some structures in the system are of the adult pattern whereas others exhibit the immature morphology. The result is an unintegrated system, which performs less efficiently.

The mature regional configuration appeared to consist of a long thin eustachian tube cartilage throughout the specimen, a lumen with a large cross sectional area, a large levator veli palatini muscle volume, and a relatively large distance separating the muscle and the cartilage. The immature configuration consisted of a relatively less elongated eustachian tube cartilage with a significantly rounder shape in the 40 to 80 percent region of the specimen, a smaller cross sectional area of the lumen, a smaller levator veli palatini muscle volume, and a statistically shorter distance between the eustachian tube cartilage and the levator veli palatini.

The morphology in the at risk less than 6 year group resembled the adult morphology in most components. These specimens had a relatively elongated cartilage throughout the specimen and did not significantly differ from the adult in lumen cross sectional area or levator veli palatini volume. Given its similarity to the adult form, it would be expected that the at risk less than 6 year group would also show a greater distance between the cartilage and the levator veli palatini. This was not the case. In the at risk less than 6 year group, the distance between the cartilage and the levator veli palatini muscle was significantly shorter than in the normal more than 7 year group.

If the greater than normal prevalence of otitis media with effusion in the at risk group is the result of structural abnormalities, it may result from the mature morphology of the eustachian tube cartilage and levator veli palatini muscle without the distance buffer between it and the levator veli palatini that is apparent in the normal more than 7 year group.

Study supported in part by NINCDS-NIH grant NS16337.

REFERENCES

1. Bluestone CD, Beery QC, Andries WS. Mechanics of the eustachian tube as it influences susceptibility to and presence of middle ear effusion in children. Ann Otol Rhinol Laryngol 1974; 83:27–34.
2. Sief S, Dellon AL. Anatomic relationships between the human levator and tensor veli palatini and the eustachian tube. Cleft Palate J 1978; 15:329–336.

3. Bluestone CD. Prevalence and pathogens of ear disease and hearing loss. In: Graham M, ed. Cleft palate ear disease and hearing loss. Springfield, Illinois: CC Thomas, 1978.
4. Siegel MI, Todhunter JS, Sadler-Kimes D. New methodology for computer reconstruction of histological preparations. In: Bluestone CD, Doyle WJ, eds. Eustachian tube function: physiology and role in otitis media. Ann Otol Rhinol Laryngol 1985; 94:11–12.
5. Todhunter JS, Siegel MI, Doyle WJ. Computer generated eustachian tube shape analysis. In: Lim DJ, Bluestone CD, Klein JO, Nelson JD, eds. Recent advances in otitis media with effusion. Proceedings of the Third International Symposium. Toronto: BC Decker, 1984:101.
6. Siegel MI, Cantekin EI, Todhunter JS, Sadler-Kimes D. The aspect ratio as a descriptor of ET cartilage shape. Ann Otol Rhinol Laryngol (in press).
7. Casselbrant ML, Brostoff LB, Cantekin EI, Ashoff VM, Bluestone CD. Otitis media in children in the United States. In: Proceedings of the international conference on acute and secretory otitis media. Amsterdam: Kugler, 1986:247.

ORIGIN OF SENSORY FIBERS TO THE TYMPANIC MEMBRANE AND MIDDLE EAR MUCOSA

ROLF UDDMAN, M.D., TORSTEN GRUNDITZ, M.D., AMY LARSSON, M.D., and FRANK SUNDLER, M.D., Ph.D.

The tympanic membrane and the middle ear mucosa are pain sensitive structures. Nerve fibers of a presumed sympathetic, parasympathetic, and sensory nature have been described in these structures.[1,2] Their origin, however, has not been fully elucidated. In the present study we examined the origin and distribution of sensory fibers in the tympanic membrane and middle ear mucosa by retrograde tracing in combination with immunocytochemistry.

MATERIAL AND METHODS

In five anesthetized rats 0.01 μl of true blue was applied to the flaccid part of the tympanic membrane. In another group of five rats a small burr hole was made in the right tympanic bulla. The middle ear mucosa was carefully retracted to form a small cavity into which a small volume (0.05 to 0.1 μl) of true blue was injected by the use of a Hamilton syringe. The hole was sealed with a tissue glue.

After 3 weeks the tympanic membrane, the middle ear mucosa, the trigeminal ganglion, the jugular-nodose ganglionic complex, and the cervical dorsal root ganglia at levels C_2 to C_5 were dissected out. The tissue specimens were immersed in an ice-cold fixative solution of formaldehyde and picric acid for 24 hours and then rinsed in a Tyrode solution containing 10 percent sucrose at 4° C for 48 hours. The tympanic membrane and middle ear mucosa were spread as whole mounts on chrome alum subbed microscope slides. The ganglia were frozen in dry ice and serially cryostat sectioned at 15 μm. Whole mounts and sections were examined for tracer fluorescence.

Sections harboring true blue labeled nerve cell bodies were further processed for immunocytochemistry using the indirect immunofluorescence method.[3] For that purpose antibodies against substance P, neurokinin A, and calcitonin gene related peptide were used. These three peptides are known to occur in sensory neurons. Details about the antisera are given in Table 1. The site of the antigen-antibody reaction was revealed by fluorescein-isothiocyanate labeled second antibodies.

RESULTS AND COMMENTS

True blue applied to the flaccid part of the tympanic membrane and to the middle ear mucosa appeared as a homogeneous accumulation of bright blue fluorescence. Three weeks after application a blue fluorescence appeared in nerve cell bodies in the ganglia examined. In the trigeminal and jugular ganglia small clusters of labeled nerve cell bodies

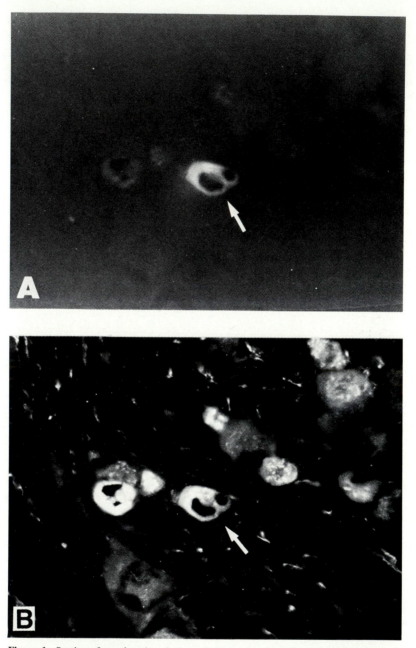

Figure 1 Sections from the trigeminal ganglion, *A*, showing true blue fluorescence and *B*, calcitonin gene related peptide immunofluorescence. The true blue labeled nerve cell body in the ganglion contains immunoreactive calcitonin gene related peptide (arrow). Several additional nerve cell bodies display calcitonin gene related peptide immunofluorescence (300×).

TABLE 1 Details Regarding the Antisera Used for Immunocytochemistry

Antigen	Code	Raised Against	Directed Against	Raised in	Working Dilution	Source
Substance P	SP-8	Protein conjugated substance P	C terminus	Rabbit	1:320	Dr. P.C. Emson M.R.C., Cambridge, U.K.
Neurokinin A	NKA/2	Protein conjugated porcine neurokinin A	C terminus	Rabbit	1:320	Dr. E. Brodin, K.S., Stockholm, Sweden
Calcitonin gene related peptide	8427	Protein conjugated rat calcitonin gene related peptide	—	Rabbit	1:1280	MILAB, Malmö, Sweden

often could be seen. In cervical dorsal root ganglia at levels C_2 to C_4 only single nerve cell bodies were labeled.

In the trigeminal, jugular, and cervical dorsal root ganglia numerous nerve cell bodies contained calcitonin gene related peptide (Fig. 1). A subpopulation of these nerve cell bodies stored, in addition, substance P. All substance P containing nerve cell bodies contained neurokinin A.

In the flaccid part of the tympanic membrane a moderate supply of calcitonin gene related peptide fibers and a rather scarce supply of nerve fibers containing substance P or neurokinin A could be seen. In the tense part only occasional nerve fibers containing these peptides were encountered. In the middle ear mucosa numerous calcitonin gene related peptide and a moderate supply of substance P and neurokinin A-immunoreactive nerve fibers were seen.

True blue is a retrograde tracer, which is taken up by nerve terminals and transported in a centripetal direction to the nerve cell bodies.[4] Only small volumes are needed. No signs of leakage or of transcellular transport have been reported. The principal advantage of using true blue as a retrograde tracer is the possibility to demonstrate the existence of both a retrograde tracer and an antigen in the same nerve cell body. On the other hand, the studies must be interpreted with caution, since it cannot be excluded that the tracer is taken up by fibers of passage.

Another advantage in working with true blue is that time consuming reactions of individual sections with restaining and rephotography can be avoided. Following application of true blue to the tympanic membrane and middle ear mucosa, numerous nerve cell bodies were labeled in the trigeminal and jugular ganglia, suggesting major contributions from these ganglia. The cervical dorsal root ganglia harbored only a few true blue labeled nerve cell bodies, indicating relatively minor contributions from these ganglia. Thus, several sensory ganglia project to the tympanic membrane and the middle ear mucosa, indicating a complex pattern of the sensory innervation. The present and previous studies have shown a comparatively rich supply of nerve fibers storing calcitonin gene related peptide, substance P, and neurokinin A in the middle ear mucosa and a scarce supply in the tympanic membrane.[1,2] Therefore, the reason why the tympanic membrane is highly pain sensitive is still an enigma.

This work was supported by the Swedish Medical Research Council (project number 6859).

REFERENCES

1. Uddman R, Kitajiri M, Sundler F. Autonomic innervation of the tubotympanum. In: Lim DJ, Bluestone CD, Klein JO, Nelson JD, eds. Recent advances in otitis media with effusion. Proceedings of the Third International Symposium Toronto: BC Decker, 1984: 76–78.
2. Widemar L, Hellström S, Schultzberg M, Stenfors L-E. Autonomic innervation of the tympanic membrane. An immunocytochemical and histofluorescence study. Acta Otolaryngol 1985; 100:58–65.
3. Coons AH, Leduc EH, Connolly JM. Studies on antibody production. 1. A method for the histochemical demonstration of specific antibody and its application to a study of the hyperimmune rabbit. J Exp Med 1955; 102:49–60.
4. Sawchenko PE, Swanson LW. A method for tracing biochemically defined pathways in the central nervous system using combined fluorescence retrograde transport and immunohistochemical techniques. Brain Res 1981; 210:31–51.

BRAINSTEM LOCALIZATION OF MOTONEURONS INNERVATING THE TENSORS VELI PALATINI MUSCLE AND THE TENSOR TYMPANI MUSCLE IN THE MONKEY

KENZOU MURANO, M.D., TAKUO NOBORI, M.D., HIROSHI TSURUMARU, M.D.,
ETSUROU OBATA, M.D., RYUZI KIYOTA, M.D., and MASARU OHYAMA, M.D.

The tensor veli palatini, levator veli palatini, and tensor tympani muscles surround the eustachian tube. In order to better understand the regulation of aerodynamics in the tympanic cavity via the eustachian tube, many anatomic and physiologic studies of these muscles have been carried out,[1-9] but their functional morphology has not yet been elucidated in detail. We examined motoneurons innervating the tensor veli palatini and tensor tympani muscles in the monkey using retrograde axonal transport of horseradish peroxidase and wheat germ agglutinin conjugated to horseradish peroxidase.

MATERIAL AND METHOD

Twenty-five normal adult Japanese monkeys were used in this experiment. The tensor veli palatini and tensor tympani muscles were exposed by microsurgical technique and the tensor veli palatini muscle was identified by using an electric stimulator with the animal under general anesthesia with sodium pentobarbital and ketamine (1 mg per kilogram). Fifty percent horseradish peroxidase (Toyobo grade-1-C) or 5 percent wheat germ agglutinin conjugated to horseradish peroxidase (Toyobo) was injected unilaterally into the tensor veli palatini muscle in nine adult Japanese monkeys and into the tensor tympani muscle in 16 adult Japanese monkeys; pressure injection of 1 to 4 μl of the 50 percent horseradish peroxidase or the 5 percent wheat germ agglutinin conjugated to horseradish peroxidase dissolved in 0.9 percent saline was carried out manually through a fine glass pipette connected to a 10 μl Hamilton microsyringe with a short length of polyethylene tubing. After 24 to 48 hours the animals were reanesthetized deeply and perfused transcardially with 5,000 ml of 0.9 percent saline, 1.25 percent glutaraldehyde, and 2 percent paraformaldehyde in 0.1 M phosphate buffer (pH 7.4), followed by 1,500 ml of the same buffer containing 10 percent sucrose. The lower brainstem was immediately removed, saturated with a solution of 30 percent sucrose in the same buffer at 4° C until it sank, and cut serially in the horizontal plane at 50 μm thickness on a freezing microtome. For histochemical demonstration of horseradish peroxidase the sections were treated with diaminobenzidine or tetramethylbenzidine and then mounted on gelatin coated slides and counterstained with cresyl violet for the diaminobenzidine reaction or with 1.0 percent neutral red for the tetramethylbenzidine reaction. The sections were examined microscopically using bright and darkfield illumination.

RESULTS

Injection of horseradish peroxidase or wheat germ agglutinin conjugated to horseradish peroxidase into the tensor veli palatini muscle produced retrograde labeling of cells ipsilaterally. The labeled cells were clustered in the ventromedial division of the trigeminal motor nucleus dorsal to the motoneurons of the lateral pterygoid and mylohyoid muscles (Fig. 1A).[8] The tensor veli palatini motoneurons extended from caudal to rostral in relation to the trigeminal motor nucleus and were not present at the pole of the motor nucleus (Fig. 2A). The cell bodies of the labeled tensor veli palatini motoneurons were medium sized and multipolar (Fig. 3A).

Injection of horseradish peroxidase or wheat germ agglutinin conjugated to horseradish peroxidase into the tensor tympani muscle produced retrograde labeling of cells ipsilaterally as in the tensor veli palatini muscle. The horseradish peroxidase labeled cells were clustered within the small area of the brainstem reticular formation located ventral or ventrolateral to the trigeminal motoneurons (Fig. 1B). Like the tensor veli palatini motoneurons, tensor tympani motoneurons were located at the rostral two thirds of the trigeminal motoneurons (Fig. 2B). The cell bodies of the labeled tensor tympani motoneurons were medium sized and multipolar as were the tensor veli palatini motoneurons (Fig. 3B).

DISCUSSION

The results of our studies in the monkey generally agree with those of various experimental studies in the rat, guinea pig, and cat that describe tensor veli palatini motoneurons localized in the ventromedial division of the trigeminal motor nucleus and tensor tympani motoneurons clustering within the small area of the brainstem reticular formation located ventral or ventrolateral to the trigeminal motoneurons.[2,7,10]

The tensor veli palatini motoneurons in the monkey are located in the regions dorsal to the motoneurons of the lateral pterygoid and mylohyoid muscles.[8] Mizuno et al[10] reported that labeled cells were located in the region medial to the cluster of lateral pterygoid motoneurons in both the guinea pig and the cat.

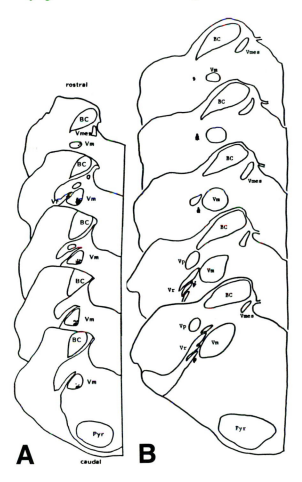

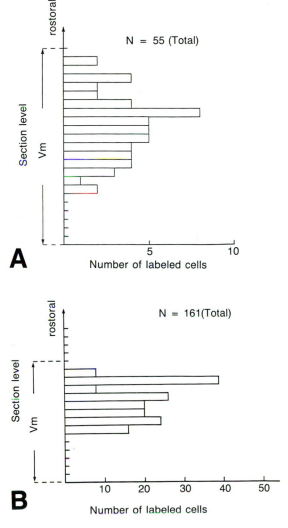

Figure 1 Projection drawings of serial cross sections through the brainstem of a monkey, showing the location of the tensor veli palatini and tensor tympani motoneurons. Horseradish peroxidase labeled cell bodies are represented by dots in a one to one fashion. The drawings are arranged from rostral to caudal. A, tensor veli palatini. B, tensor tympani. BC, brachium conjunctivum. Vm, trigeminal motor nucleus. Vr, motor root of trigeminal nerve. Vmes, trigeminal nucleus. Vp, principal sensory nucleus of trigeminal nerve.

Figure 2 Comparison of levels between horseradish peroxidase labeled cells and trigeminal motor nucleus. A, tensor veli palatini. B, tensor tympani. Vm, trigeminal motor nucleus.

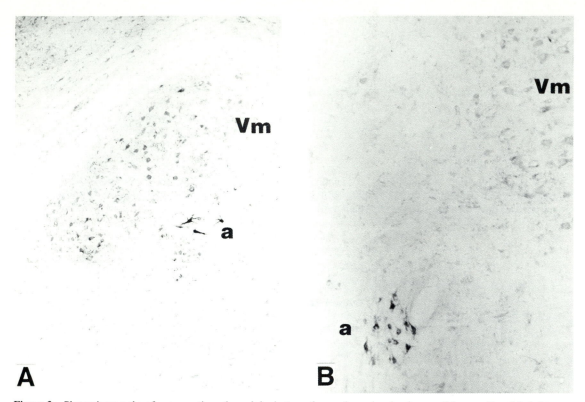

Figure 3   Photomicrographs of cross sections through brainstem of a monkey, showing horseradish peroxidase labeled tensor veli palatini motoneurons and tensor tympanimotoneurons. *A*, tensor veli palatini. *B*, tensor tympani. a, horseradish peroxidase labeled tensor veli palatini motoneurons and tensor tympani motoneurons. Vm, trigeminal motor nucleus.

In the monkey the tensor tympani motoneurons are more closely clustered than in the guinea pig, the cat, and the rabbit and more distinctly separated from the trigeminal motoneuron.

Our experiments show that tensor veli palatini and tensor tympani motoneurons in the monkey are located in two separate areas. We may conclude that there are no interrelations between the two types of motoneurons.

Recently in physiologic studies of the eustachian tube it was reported that the tensor veli palatini muscle plays the most important role in tubal function, whereas the tensor tympani muscle has no effect on eustachian tube function.[4,5] However, there is electromyographic evidence that the tensor tympani muscle functions actively during generalized motor events, including vocalization and swallowing.[3]

From the neuroanatomic viewpoint our study of tensor veli palatini motoneurons confirms physiologic and clinical phenomena in demonstrating that the tensor veli palatini muscle has a function in mastication and swallowing. The results of tensor tympani support the idea that action of the tensor tympani muscle is related to the reticular reflexes of the brainstem.

REFERENCES

1. Kusama T, Mabuchi M. Stereotaxic atlas of the brain of Macaca fuscata. Tokyo: University of Tokyo Press, 1970:1–79.
2. Jeffrey TK, et al. Identification of motoneurons innervating the tensor veli palatini and the tensor tympani muscle in the cat. Brain Res 1983; 270:209–215.
3. Salomon G, Starr A. Electromyography of middle ear muscles in man during motor activity. Acta Neurol Scand 1963;

39:161–168.

4. Honjo I, Okazaki N, et al. Experimental study of the eustachian tube function with regard to its related muscles. Acta Otolaryngol 1979; 87:84–89.
5. Honjo I, Ushiro K, et al. Role of the tensor tympani muscle in eustachian tube function. Acta Otolaryngol 1983; 95:329–332.
6. Szentagothai J. Functional representation in the motor trigeminal nucleus. J Comp Neurol 1949; 90:111–120.
7. Mizuno N, Nomura S, et al. Localization of motoneurons innervating the tensor tympani muscles: a horseradish peroxidase study in the guinea pig and cat. Neurosci Lett 1982; 31:205–208.

8. Mizuno N, Matsuda K, et al. Myotopical arrangement and synaptic morphology of masticatory motoneurons, with special reference to commissural interneurons. In: Kawamura Y, Dubner R, eds. Oral-facial sensory and motor functions. Tokyo: Quintessence, 1981:113–120.
9. Murano K, Nobori T, Ohyama M, et al. Brain stem localization of motoneurons innervating the tensor tympani muscle in the monkey. A horseradish peroxidase study. Ear Res Jpn 1985; 16:155–159.
10. Mizuno N, Nomura S, et al. Identification of motoneurons supplying the tensor veil palatini muscle in the guinea pig and cat: a horseradish peroxidase study. Neurosci Lett 1982; 32:17–21.

ULTRASTRUCTURAL COMPARISON OF MIDDLE EAR MUCOSA FROM DIFFERENT AGE GROUPS OF SECRETORY OTITIS MEDIA PATIENTS

TOMONORI TAKASAKA, M.D., YOSHIHIRO SHIBAHARA, M.D., D.M.S.,
MAMORU SHIBUYA, M.D., MITSUKO SUETAKE, M.D., ATSUSHI KURIHARA, Ph.D.,
and HIDEAKI SUZUKI, M.D.

Study of the age distribution of patients in our clinic with secretory otitis media revealed that the majority belonged to one of two age groups. Sixty-eight of the 145 patients (46.9 percent) were children between 4 and 7 years of age and 37 (25.5 percent) were adult patients over 50 years of age. In Japan it is generally accepted that secretory otitis media has been common in adults in the past 50 years, whereas cases in children have only recently been found and are still increasing in number. It also has been evident in our clinic that serous middle ear effusions are found more frequently in adults, whereas mucoid effusions are common in children (p < 0.001). These facts indicate that there are differences in the pathogenesis between the two age groups. The purpose of this study was to study the ultrastructural histopathologic changes in the middle ear mucosa in patients with secretory otitis media in both age groups and to discover whether there is any significant difference between them.

MATERIALS AND METHODS

Biopsy specimens of middle ear mucosa obtained from 28 ears in children with secretory otitis media and five ears in adult patients were immediately fixed with 2.0 percent glutaraldehyde in 0.1 M phosphate buffer and postosmificated after several washings in the buffer solutions. Dehydration was performed with graded ethanols and propylene oxide. After complete polymerization of the epoxy resin, 1.0 μm sections were cut for light microscopy and ultrathin 80 nm sections for electron microscopy using a Sorvall ultramicrotome MT-5000. The specimens were observed with a Hitachi H-600 or JEOL 100C electron microscope with an accelerating voltage of 80 kv.

Middle ear effusions were classified as serous, low viscous mucoid, and highly viscous mucoid types. Effusions that were easily collected through a suction tube with an average diameter were designated as the serous type, and effusions that could not be collected in this fashion because of their tenacity were classified as highly viscous mucoid type; the remainder were classified as low viscous mucoid type. The age distribution for each type of effusion is shown in Figure 1.

RESULTS

Light microscopic observation of a serous type of mucosa revealed a thin epithelial lining consisting of a single layer of cuboidal cells and associated basal cells. Infiltrating cells in the lamina propria were scanty, but tissue edema was remarkable. Electron micrographs of a serous type of secretory otitis media in a 10 year old boy showed remarkably widened epithelial intercellular spaces filled with a homogeneous fluid-like substance, as well as subepithelial tissue edema with a dispersed cellular infiltrate (Fig. 2A).

Figure 2B, an electron micrograph of a 46 year old male patient with a serous middle ear effusion reveals a single cuboidal ciliated cell among nonciliated cells and an enlarged intercellular space containing a homogeneous transudate. In the epithelial

cell cytoplasm we observe mitochondria and endoplasmic reticulums but no obvious secretory elements.

We examined specimens from eight cases of serous type of otitis media in children and in one adult patient, and it was almost impossible to differentiate characteristic features of the middle ear mucosa in the children from those in adults.

No remarkable ultrastructural difference was found in the middle ear mucosa of mucoid effusions from the two age groups. Figure 3, showing sections from a 4 year old girl and a 57 year old male, reveals large numbers of secretory granules in the apical cytoplasm of goblet cells. The apical surface of these secretory cells bulges into the lumen. The intercellular space is tight, but inflammatory cells, mainly polymorphonuclear leukocytes infiltrate into the space. The secretory activity of the epithelial cells varied from specimen to specimen, but it was generally mild in the low viscous mucoid type of secretory otitis media when compared to the cells in the highly viscous mucoid type.

Marked proliferation of epithelial cells was seen in specimens from highly viscous mucoid otitis in a 5 year old girl (Fig. 4) and a 64 year old male patient. Increased macroapocrine secretions were

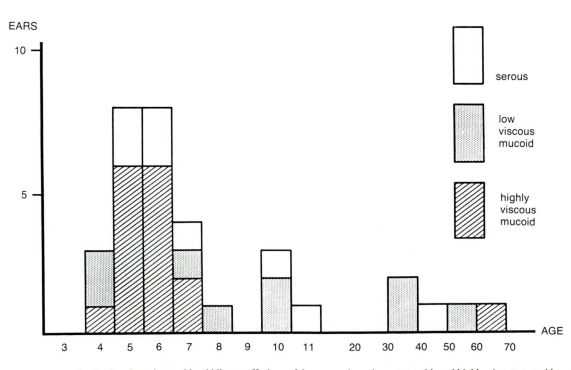

Figure 1   Age distributions in patients with middle ear effusions of the serous, low viscous mucoid, and highly viscous mucoid types.

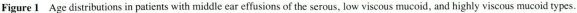

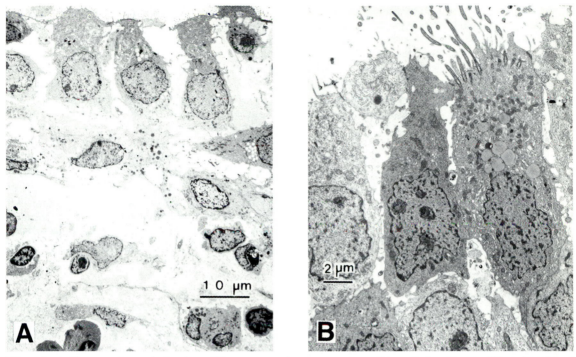

Figure 2 *A*, Electron micrograph showing middle ear mucosa in serous secretory otitis media in a 10 year old boy. An enlarged intercellular space and subepithelial tissue edema are evident. The epithelium is composed of a single layer of cuboidal cells and associated flat basal cells. *B*, Electron micrograph showing the epithelium in serous secretory otitis media in a 46 year old male. There are no marked ultrastructural differences between Figures 2*A* and 2*B*.

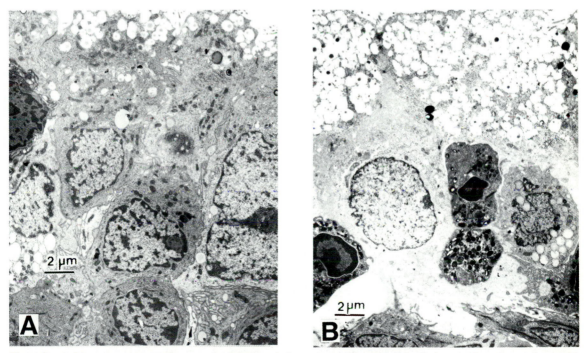

Figure 3 *A*, Many secretory granules are present in the apical cytoplasm of the epithelial cells in a specimen from a 4 year old girl with low viscous mucoid secretory otitis media. The intercellular space is not enlarged and the junctional complexes between the cells are intact. *B*, Secretory cell transformations are evident in this specimen from a 57 year old male. A large number of secretory granules with a central core are present in the apical cytoplasm. Polymorphonuclear leukocyte infiltrations are also seen in the intercellular space.

common on the apical free surface of the cells, which contained massive accumulations of secretory granules with electron dense cores. Abundant cellular debris and infiltrated polymorphonuclear leukocytes were seen in the lumen.

These characteristic features indicate that secretory cell transformations of the epithelial cells were increased in the highly viscous mucoid type of otitis and secretory activity was also enhanced. Balloon-like cytoplasmic protrusions on the ciliated cells also revealed the hypersecretory activity of the cells. A mucociliary coupling disorder was also found in the highly viscous mucoid type of secretory otitis media.

DISCUSSION

As previously described,[1-5] we observed prominent secretory cell transformation of the epithelial cells in most specimens from both age groups. Tall goblet cells containing numerous secretory granules with or without a dense core showed apical bulging into the lumen. Neutrophil infiltrates

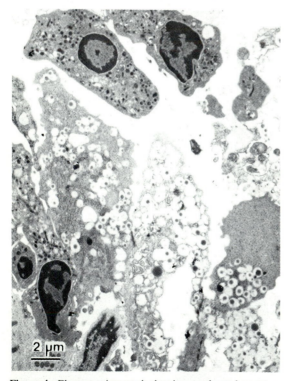

Figure 4 Electron micrograph showing accelerated secretory activity of a highly viscous mucoid type in a 5 year old girl with secretory otitis media. There is marked proliferation of epithelial cells and abundant cell debris associated with polymorphonuclear leukocytes, characteristic features of the highly viscous mucoid type of secretory otitis media.

in the intercellular space were also commonly seen, and some of them had been released from the epithelial surface through open junctions. Ciliated cells were observed occasionally but were fewer in number; the ciliary bundles were surrounded by tenacious mucoid effusions.

So far it has been difficult to demonstrate a significant difference in the middle ear mucosa in the two age groups, although each type of effusion had characteristic features in the epithelial lining, as Lim et al[1] have mentioned. However, we still do not know why the mucoid type of effusion is more frequently observed in children. Our previous study of the endotoxin content of middle ear effusions revealed remarkably high concentration of endotoxin in children.[6] It was also confirmed that effusions from children with secretory otitis contain a higher PGE_2 concentration than those from adults.[7] These biochemical analyses seem to indicate that the etiopathogenesis of secretory otitis in the two age groups is not the same and thus the character of the effusions is different in the two groups. The floppy eustachian tube and hypertrophied adenoids may increase the hypoventilated condition of the tubotympanum in children, and the anaerobic conditions may favor epithelial metaplasia with the development of secretory elements, as suggested by Zechner.[8] Although we could not find ultrastructural differences in the two age groups, we believe that further multifocal investigations in the two age groups will provide a better understanding of the remaining unanswered questions about the etiopathogenesis of secretory otitis media.

REFERENCES

1. Lim DJ, Birck H. Ultrastructural pathology of the middle ear mucosa in serous otitis media. Ann Otol Rhinol Laryngol 1971; 80:838–853.
2. Hentzer E. Ultrastructure of the middle ear mucosa in secretory otitis media. I. Serous effusion. Acta Otolaryngol (Stockh) 1972; 73:394–401.
3. Hentzer E. Ultrastructure of the middle ear mucosa in secretory otitis media. II. Mucous effusion. Acta Otolaryngol (Stockh) 1972; 73:467–475.
4. Tos M, Bak-Pedersen K. Goblet cell population in the normal middle ear and eustachian tube of children and adults. Ann Otol Rhinol Laryngol 1976; 85(Suppl 25):44–50.
5. Albiin N, Hellström S, Stenfors L-E, Cerne A. Middle ear mucosa in rats and humans. Ann Otol Rhinol Laryngol 1986; 95(Suppl 126):1–15.
6. Iino Y, et al. Endotoxin in middle ear effusion in chronic otitis media tested with Limulus assay. Acta Otolaryngol (Stockh) 1985; 100:42–50.
7. Kurihara A. Personal communication.
8. Zechner G. Auditory tube and middle ear mucosa in nonpurulent otitis media. Ann Otol Rhinol Laryngol 1980; 89(Suppl 68):87–90.

MASTOID PNEUMATIZATION AND SECRETORY OTITIS MEDIA

YRJÖ QVARNBERG, M.D., HENRIK MALMBERG, M.D., JORMA RAHNASTO, M.D., and TAUNO PALVA, M.D.

Pneumatization of the mastoid bone depends on adequate aeration of the tympanic cleft and a normally functioning eustachian tube.[1] Prolonged dysfunction arrests the growth of air cells. In addition, secretory otitis media may cause chronic inflammatory changes in existing mastoid cells, especially in the cells around the antrum. Blockage of the aditus causes absorption of air from the mastoid, resulting in capillary leakage and consequent mucosal proliferation.[2-5] The involvement of the mastoid in secretory otitis media may range from a nearly normal condition with air filled cells to an advanced stage with mucoid fluid filled air cells and bone breakdown, depending upon the initial infectious process and the time of the first surgical intervention.[5] In part it is related to the course of the disease, i.e., whether secretory otitis media is the result of an initial episode of acute purulent or recurrent otitis media or has developed insidiously without noticeable inflammatory acute episodes. In the treatment of secretory otitis media one should not neglect the mastoid process because it communicates directly with the middle ear.

MATERIAL AND METHODS

This prospective study of mastoid involvement in secretory otitis media was carried out in 208 children who had had symptoms of secretory otitis media for at least 3 months and were receiving their first ventilation tube treatment in the period from October 1981 to April 1983. The mean age of the children was 2.7 years (SD, 2.6; range, 6 months to 15 years). There were 80 girls (38 percent) and 128 boys (62 percent). In all the children the mobility of the tympanic membrane was decreased and the tympanograms, when obtained, were all flat.

Both ears were subjected to radiographic examination by lateral projection on the day before surgery. The area of pneumatization was measured with a planimeter, and the mastoid was classified as large, medium sized, or small as described by Qvarnberg.[6,7] Air cell appearance was also classified into three categories: normal, partially cloudy, and cloudy. Destruction of bony air cell septa or their thickening was recorded.

Tympanostomy was done under general anesthesia with nitrous oxide, and adenoidectomy was performed under direct and mirror control. The ear canal was sterilized for 90 seconds with 70 percent ethyl alcohol before myringotomy. The middle ear secretion was analyzed for bacteria in a routine manner. If there was a discharge from the tube postoperatively, the patient was given the potassium salt of penicillin V for 7 to 10 days, the dosage being adjusted according to sensitivity test results. If the discharge continued and the mastoid was cloudy, thorough simple mastoidectomy was considered.

The patients were first seen at 1 month and after intervals of 3 to 6 months. If the disease recurred after extrusion of the tube, a new tube was inserted. If the tympanic cavity normalized, the child was seen at a final follow-up examination 3 to 6 months later and, if cooperative, examined by tympanometry and audiometry. All patients were followed for at least 2 years and some of them for over 4 years.

RESULTS

A ventilation tube was inserted in 403 ears—in 13 children only unilaterally. There was mucoid secretion in 227 ears (56 percent). In the remaining 176 ears (44 percent) a secretion was not found on incision of the tympanic membrane, although the mucosa was thickened. Bacterial cultures were positive for 54 specimens (24 percent) and negative for 173 (76 percent). The most common pathogenic strain was *Haemophilus influenzae* (25 ears, 46 percent), followed by pneumococci and Branhamella. The percentage of beta-lactamase producing strains was 19.

The air cell system was large in 2 percent, medium sized in 63 percent, and small in 35 percent of the ears. At the initial examination the mastoid air cells were normal in 13 percent, partially cloudy in 44.5 percent, and cloudy in 42.5 percent. Ears without secretion had a significantly larger air cell system than those with a mucoid secretion. On the other hand, the size of the cellular system did not correlate with the presence of pathogenic bacteria ($p < 0.25$).

Clouding of the mastoid correlated significantly with the presence of secretion in the middle ear as well as with the presence of bacteria. During the follow-up time of 2 years, healing occurred in 136 patients (65 percent); 72 (35 percent) at this writing either have the tube in situ or await the final check-up. Healing did not correlate with the presence or absence of secretion at the first insertion of the tube, and the absence of secretion was probably related to general anesthesia, which forced the fluid out of the middle ear. In the group of 142 nonhealed ears, 73 (51 percent) had at least one episode of discharge from the tube during the follow-up period. In the group of healed ears the corresponding figures were 90 and 34 percent ($p < 0.005$). Discharge during tube treatment did not correlate with the size of the air cell system, but the correlation with cloudiness of the mastoid was statistically significant at the level of $p < 0.05$ (Table 1).

Retympanostomy was necessary in 117 ears (28 percent), i.e., in 24 children (18 percent) in the group with healed secretory otitis media and in 47 children (65 percent) in the nonhealed group. The size of the mastoid air cell system correlated with the number of retympanostomies, these being most frequent in ears with small mastoids (Table 2). Cloudiness of the mastoid showed a highly significant correlation with the need for retympanostomies (Table 3).

Mastoidectomy was done in three patients (1.4 percent)—four ears (1 percent). The mastoid cells were cloudy in all these ears, and the pneumatized area was small in two and medium sized in two. At this writing the child who underwent bilateral mastoidectomy has been followed for 2 years, is free of disease, and has normal hearing. The other two

TABLE 1 Discharge During Follow-up in Relation to Mastoid Cloudiness

Air Cell Appearance	No Discharge No. Ears	Episode(s) No. Ears	Total No. Ears
Clear	40	13	53
Partially cloudy	106	73	179
Totally cloudy	94	77	171
Total no.	240	163	403

$x^2 = 6.6$, df = 2, $p < 0.05$

TABLE 2 Mastoid Pneumatization in Relation to Retympanostomy

Mastoid Size	Ears Requiring Tympanostomy		
	Once Only (No.)	Twice or More (No.)	Total
Large	6	1	7
Medium	191	62	253
Small	89	54	143
Total no.	286	117	403

$x^2 = 7.9$, df = 2, $p < 0.05$

still have tubes in their ears. The number of perforations after tube extrusion was 13 (3.2 percent); all these ears have been included in the group of nonhealed ears.

DISCUSSION

The patients included in this study represent three different geographic areas of Finland. All patients had had middle ear problems of varying duration before a decision was made to insert a ventilation tube. It is worth noting that at insertion only 13 percent of the 403 mastoid x-ray views showed normal aeration and that 42.5 percent showed overall cloudiness. This finding is in agreement with Qvarnberg's earlier data[6,7] from patients with acute purulent otitis media, many of whom showed chronic mastoid changes as a sign of earlier middle ear problems. Mastoid cloudiness is always a sign of mastoid participation in the disease process. Its nature may range from simple air resorption and replacement by serous capillary fluid to bone breakdown, the formation of granulation tissue, and masked mastoiditis.

TABLE 3 Mastoid Cloudiness in Relation to Retympanostomy

Air Cell Appearance	Ears Requiring Tympanostomy		
	Once Only (No.)	Twice or More (No.)	Total
Clear	45	8	53
Partially cloudy	134	45	179
Totally cloudy	107	64	171
Total	286	117	403

$x^2 = 11.4$, df = 2, $p < 0.005$

Involvement of the mastoid bone prolongs the healing process in secretory otitis media. In these ears the need for retympanostomies was greater and the periods of discharge more frequent. The mastoid should be examined radiographically at the latest when tympanostomy tube insertion is considered. If the air cell system is well developed with no noteworthy cloudiness, the condition may resolve with conservative methods. If there are marked signs of mastoid involvement, insertion of a tube should be carried out quickly to achieve resolution of the process in the air cells.

Mastoidectomy was necessary in only 1.5 percent of the children in this study, the figure being similar to that (1.3 percent) reported earlier by Palva et al.[5]

It is probable, however, that we have been too conservative, for the disease persisted in as many as 35 percent of the children after follow-up for 2 years or more. Especially in the younger age groups latent involvement of the mastoid may maintain a nonhealing condition for years, and even lead to frank chronic otitis media in some of the children.

The adverse effect of secretory otitis media on the growth of mastoid air cells was also apparent in this study. The proportion of ears that, in rela-

tion to age, showed a large pneumatic mastoid was only 2 percent in our series, but it was 14 percent in Qvarnberg's acute purulent otitis media series.[6] Arrested pneumatization in connection with cloudiness is a poor prognostic sign and calls for active measures, such as early adenoidectomy and long term ventilation. If longer periods of discharge occur, mastoidectomy should be seriously considered.

REFERENCES

1. Ojala L. Pathogenesis and histopathology of chronic adhesive otitis. Arch Otolaryngol 1953; 57:378–401.
2. Palva T. Mastoiditis in children. Laryngoscope 1962; 72:353–360.
3. Palva T, Karma P, Kärjä J, Palva A. Secretory otitis media in chronic lymphatic leukaemia. J Laryngol Otol 1976; 90:773–783.
4. Palva T, Pulkkinen K. Mastoiditis. J Laryngol Otol 1959; 78:573–588.
5. Palva T, Virtanen H, Mäkinen J. Acute and latent mastoiditis in children. J Laryngol Otol 1985; 99:127–136.
6. Qvarnberg Y. Acute otitis media; a prospective clinical study of myringotomy and antimicrobial treatment. Acta Otolaryngol [Suppl] (Stockh) 1981; 375:1–157.
7. Qvarnberg Y. Acute otitis media and radiographic findings in the mastoid air cell system. Int J Pediatr Otorhinolaryngol 1982; 4:333–342.

ROUND WINDOW PERMEABILITY

MARCOS V. GOYCOOLEA, M.D., M.S., Ph.D., DAVID MUCHOW, ANNA-MARY CARPENTER, M.D., Ph.D., PATRICIA A. SCHACHERN, B.S., and MICHAEL M. PAPARELLA, M.D.

Otitis media is a multifaceted disease that can evolve or resolve in a number of different unpredictable ways. Its study can involve different aspects of its many forms, complications, and sequelae. Stimulated by hypotheses regarding the subtle inner ear complications of otitis media, 11 years ago we initiated a systematic experimental approach to study this aspect of the disease.

One possible mechanism for the subtle inner ear complications of otitis media is the passage of harmful substances from the middle to the inner ear through the round window membrane.[1] Although passage of substances via the round window membrane has been documented in cats and rodents,[2-7]

there have been no studies to date that show that such passage occurs in primates.

The purpose of this study was to determine whether cationic ferritin placed in the middle ear side in normal primates (rhesus monkeys) can be observed to pass through the round window membrane.

METHODS AND MATERIALS

Two healthy adult rhesus monkeys were anesthetized with sodium pentobarbital (30 mg per kilogram). After a tracheostomy had been performed, the middle ear was exposed via a posterior bulla approach. The round window niche was identified. Cationic ferritin (0.1 ml) was placed in the niche using a micropipette and left for 1 hour. The middle ear cavity was injected with 3 percent glutaraldehyde in 0.2 ml of phosphate buffer, pH 7.2. After the animals were decapitated, the temporal bones were trimmed of excess bone and tissue. Two pin sized holes were made in the cochlea, one at the helicotrema and the other in the scala tympani, approximately 2 mm apical from the round window. The cochleas were fixed with glutaraldehyde solution injected through the basal hole. Bones were rinsed and postfixed in 1 percent osmium tetroxide in 0.15 M phosphate buffer at pH 7.2 for 2 hours at 4° C. After several buffer rinses the round window membrane was removed. Round window membranes were dehydrated and embedded separately in epoxy resin (EPON 812). Sections 200 to 400 Å thick were cut with glass knives using an ultramicrotome (LKB ultratome); mounted on Formvar coated, single hole or 50 mesh copper grids; stained with alcoholic uranyl acetate—lead citrate; and examined with an electron microscope (Phillips 201).

RESULTS

After 1 hour of exposure to cationic ferritin, the tracer was found in the round window in the three layers—within outer epithelial cells (Fig. 1) and between outer epithelial cells medial to the level of the tight junctions (Fig. 2). Ferritin was observed within the connective tissue layer, mainly within connective tissue cells. In the inner epithelial cells it was found to be present but in fewer vesicles than in the outer layers (Fig. 3).

DISCUSSION

It has been suggested that the round window membrane, despite being three layered, behaves like a semipermeable membrane. Antibiotics placed in the middle ear side have been reported to cause inner ear changes.[8] Studies of permeability to macromolecules such as albumin and toxins have shown that when these tritiated macromolecules are placed on the middle ear side in normal cats, they can be recovered in the perilymph.[5-7] By immunoelectrophoresis it has been verified that what is recovered is indeed albumin and not the tritium alone.[9]

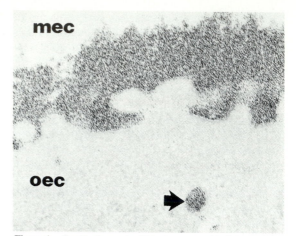

Figure 1 Ferritin (arrows) within the outer epithelial cells (oec). mec, middle ear cavity (82, 500 X).

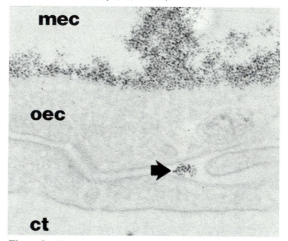

Figure 2 Ferritin (arrow) in the intercellular space of the outer epithelial cells (oec). mec, middle ear cavity. ct, connective tissue layer (15, 2000 ×).

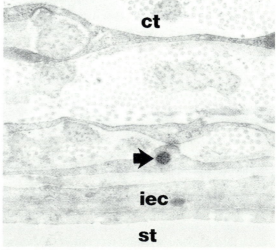

Figure 3 Ferritin (arrow) within the inner epithelial cells (iec). ct, connective tissue layer. st, scala tympani (48, 000 ×).

Cationic ferritin placed in the middle ear side in cats for 2 hours has been observed in the three layers of the round window membrane,[2] as has been shown to be the case with horseradish peroxidase in chinchillas and guinea pigs.[3,4]

Because there are general morphologic similarities among different species, there are also significant differences, which could affect permeability and the significance of experimental results.[2] For these reasons we decided to investigate the passage of cationic ferritin in primates and selected the rhesus monkey.

Our results show that cationic ferritin does traverse the round window membrane in primates, just as in cats and rodents, in spite of a thicker membrane rich with connective tissue in monkeys.

This study was supported in part by grant NS—14538 from the NINCDS and a grant from the 3M Company of Minnesota, and a grant from Audia Chile, Santiago, Chile.

REFERENCES

1. Goycoolea MV, Paparella MM, Juhn SK, Carpenter AM. Oval and round windows in otitis media: potential pathways between middle and inner ear. Laryngoscope 1980; 90:1387–1391.
2. Goycoolea MV, Carpenter AM, Muchow D. Ultrastructural studies of the round window membrane of the cat. Arch Otolaryngol 1987; 113:617–624.
3. Tanaka K, Motomura S. Permeability of labyrinthine windows in guinea pigs. Arch Otolaryngol Head Neck Surg 1981; 233:67–75.
4. Schachern P, Paparella MM, Goycoolea MV, Duvall AJ, Choo YB. The permeability of the round window membrane during otitis media. Arch Otolaryngol Head Neck Surg 1987; 113:625–629.
5. Goycoolea MV, Paparella MM, Goldberg B, Carpenter AM. Permeability of the round window in otitis media. Arch Otolaryngol 1980; 106:430–433.
6. Goycoolea MV, Paparella MV, Goldberg B, Schlievert P, Carpenter AM. Permeability of the round window membrane to staphylococcal pyrogenic exotoxin. Int Pediatr Otolaryngol 1980; 1:301–308.
7. Goycoolea MV. Passage of macromolecules and pyrogenic staphylococcal exotoxin from middle to inner ear. Masters Thesis, University of Minnesota, 1979.
8. Proud GO, Mittlebaum H, Seiden GD. Ototoxicity of topically applied chloramphenicol. Arch Otol 1968; 87:580–587.
9. Goldberg B, Goycoolea MV, Schlievert P, Schachern P, Carpenter AM. Passage of albumin from middle to inner ear in otitis media in the chinchilla. Am J Otol 1981; 2:210–214.

IMMUNOLOGY

SPECIAL LECTURE: ONTOGENY AND FUNCTION OF CELLULAR IMMUNE RESPONSE IN INFANCY

ANTHONY R. HAYWARD, M.D., Ph.D.

Cell mediated immune responses extend beyond the prototypes of delayed type hypersensitivity and foreign graft rejection to include antigen specific help for antibody responses by B cells and the production of lymphokines (IL2 and gamma interferon), which alter the behavior of macrophages and natural killer cells. These responses are mediated by thymus derived (T) lymphocytes, and it is with the development and function of this subset in infancy that this review is primarily concerned. As a necessary background, the fetal development of T cells of diverse specificities is summarized first.

DEVELOPMENT OF LYMPHOID TISSUES AND LYMPHOCYTE POPULATIONS

Lymphocytes are derived from hemopoietic precursors,[1] which are first found in the yolk sac and are present in the liver during fetal life and in the marrow during adult life. Cell transfer experiments indicate that a very small number of precursors suffices to repopulate the lymphoid system in mice and that as cells mature, their potential becomes restricted. The cells that ultimately compose the T cell compartment are therefore derived from specialized precursors, which migrate into the epithelial thymus in fetal life.

The thymic anlage in man is formed between 5 and 6 weeks of gestation by the invagination of the third and fourth pharyngeal pouches into the neck, followed by their growth into the mediastinum. The first lymphocytes appear among these epithelial cells between 9 and 10 weeks of gestation. These cells are stained with a broadly reactive anti-T cell antibody called 3A1, but they lack CD3, CD5, CD4, and CD8. A densely packed lymphoid medulla is visible by 12 weeks and Hassals corpuscles are present by 14 weeks' gestation. By 10 weeks of gestation, cells that are simultaneously positive for CD5, CD4, and CD8 are present, whereas CD3 and CD1

positive cells do not appear until about 12 weeks.[2] The significance of simultaneous CD4 + CD8 expression by thymocytes is not known, although a relationship to the development of the HLA restriction of antigen recognition seems likely. Other studies suggest that the CD2 antigen is expressed on cells soon after they arrive in the thymus, and that these cells have the potential to express an IL2 receptor.

The frequency of T cells of different subsets in the fetal thymus by 18 weeks is generally similar to that in adults.[3] There is little direct information about the early emigration of fetal T cells from the thymus into the periphery. The proliferative response of spleen cell suspensions at 15 weeks' gestation to PHA is positive though weak, which suggests that some T cells have arrived in the spleen by this time. Aggregates of $CD4^+$ and $CD8^+$ lymphocytes appear in gut associated lymphoid tissue from about 14 weeks of gestation.[4] Fetal blood samples obtained between 16 and 20 weeks' gestation have percentages of $CD3^+$, $CD4^+$, and $CD8^+$ cells very similar to those in adults: this allows infants with severe congenital immunodeficiencies to be identified early enough in gestation for termination to be considered.[5] Differences reported between newborn and adult T cells include the expression of the T10 antigen on newborn $CD3^+$ T cells, the occasional presence of increased numbers of $CD1^+$ cells,[6] the presence of PNA receptors on $CD8^+$ cells, and the presence of some $CD4^+$ + $CD8^+$ cells.[7]

The development of lymph nodes accelerates following birth and external antigen stimulus, and the nodes remain small in experimental animals kept under antigen deprived conditions.[8] Interestingly, these animals have normal numbers of lymphocytes in the spleen, suggesting that endogenous stimulus may be sufficient to achieve full development in this organ.

SPECIFICITY AND THE DEVELOPMENT OF THE T CELL REPERTOIRE

The antigen specificity of a T lymphocyte is determined by the shape of the variable regions that make up the binding site of the antigen receptor. This is in turn determined by the variable (V), D, and J region gene segments that were selected during the development of the cell in the thymus. T cell receptor gene rearrangement starts in the thymus, and beta chain V, D, and J genes on chromosome 7 are rearranged with genes for the constant regions of the receptor before the corresponding alpha chain genes (located on chromosome 14).[9] The phenotype of the cells in which these rearrangements are taking place is CD4[+], CD8[+], CD1[+], and CD3[-]. Expression of the antigen receptor on the cell surface is associated with the expression of CD3, and the cell loses CD1 and either CD4 or CD8. In mice, thymus cells with beta chains in their cytoplasm are detectable in the cortex of the thymus by 15 days of gestation, and surface expression of beta chains (presumably together with alpha chains) follows at 16 days.[10] The fetal thymus in addition is rich in cells with receptors encoded by two other T cell receptor genes: gamma and possibly delta chains.[11] Because gamma and delta genes are utilized by only a minor population of T cells in adults, little is known about their specificity or function.

The range of antigens that can be distinguished by the developing population of T cells (the repertoire) depends on the sequence with which different V, D, and J gene segments are rearranged to generate functional receptors. This process appears to be at least partially regulated rather than random, at least as judged by the way in which certain V region families are selected for rearrangement. Immunoglobulin V region genes (about whose development there is more information than T cell receptor V genes) tend to be rearranged starting from the more proximal genes, and this restricts the diversity of specificity during fetal development. If the selection and rearrangement processes are analogous for B and T cells, some ordered expansion of the T cell repertoire during development is to be expected.

A major requirement for a developing immune system is to distinguish self from not-self. In the case of T cell development this might be achieved by the elimination of self-reactive clones within the thymus, perhaps supplemented by selective inactivation of cells in the periphery. Recent evidence supporting the former mechanism comes from the apparent elimination of cells with specificity for a self histocompatibility antigen in the thymus, at the stage of immature thymocyte.[12]

ACCESSORY CELLS

Accessory cells (such as mononuclear phagocytes and dendritic cells) play an essential role in the development of immune responses through the uptake and processing of antigens and by the production of interleukin 1, a necessary second signal for T cell activation. The antigen processing function of mononuclear phagocytes is important, because CD4 T cells recognize small antigenic fragments in association with membrane class II major histocompatibility antigens (HLA-DP, DQ, and DR in humans; IA and IE in mice). Several studies of newborn rats and mice indicate impaired presentation of antigen by neonatal macrophages. This correlates with reduced Ia antigen expression on the neonatal cells. The gestation period in humans is much longer than that in rodents, and experiments designed to test in vitro presentation of antigens such as tetanus toxoid and herpesviruses by neonatal macrophages have shown normal function.[13]

NATURAL KILLER CELLS

Natural killer cells are a subpopulation of blood mononuclear cells that lyse neoplastic and virus infected cells without prior immunization and without any requirement for major histocompatibility complex (MHC) matching. Natural killer cells develop in the human fetal bone marrow from about 13 weeks' gestation, and they subsequently appear and differentiate in the fetal liver, spleen, lymph nodes, thymus, and bone marrow. The lytic activity of these cells was amplified by exposure to either interleukin-2 or gamma-interferon from 20 weeks and 27 weeks, respectively. Despite an increase in natural killer activity of cells from fetal blood during gestation, the level of their cytotoxicity to tumor or virus infected target cells at birth remains low when compared with adult cells. Although the percentage of natural killer cells in the blood of newborns is lower than in adults, reduced binding of newborn natural killer cells to targets[14] and reduced responses to cytokines[15] are also important. Newborn natural killer cell activity is amplified by both interleukin-2 and alpha interferon, but the increase is again less than is seen with lymphokine stimulated adult natural killer cells. The reduced responses to herpesviruses on newborn natural killer cells may contribute to the increased pathogenicity of these viruses for newborns compared with adults. Natural killer cells achieve adult levels of cytotoxicity during childhood.

DEVELOPMENT AND CELL INTERACTIONS

It is rare to detect specific proliferative responses by lymphocytes from newborns to anything other than foreign histocompatibility antigens. This most likely reflects the small number of T cells in the circulation with specificity for the antigen under test. Following encounter with antigen (as infections and immunizations), responder T cells proliferate and their frequency increases. For example, prior to varicella zoster virus (VZV) infection the frequency of VZV specific T cells in the blood is $< 1:10^6$ cells. After infection this frequency increases to about $1:10^4$. Increases follow immunization too, although with the Oka strain of varicella zoster virus vaccine the rise is less than that following natural infection. Immunization with nonreplicating antigens such as tetanus toxoid elicit responder T cell frequencies of about 1:25,000.

A major unanswered question is whether antibodies to T cell receptors (anti-idiotype antibodies) contribute to the proliferation of T cells, and hence to the development of the T cell repertoire during infancy and childhood. Antibodies to immunoglobulin idiotypes are made by B cells in the course of immune responses and may regulate the continued production of antibody. Antibodies with specificity for T cell idiotypes are less well studied. They can suppress the development of parts of the T cell repertoire, and in the presence of costimulators such as interleukin 1 they might trigger T cells to proliferate. Apart from providing a model for the development or control of autoimmune disease, anti-idiotype antibodies have a potential role as antigens for immunization.

EARLY INFECTIONS CAUSING SECONDARY DEFECTS OF DEVELOPMENT

Some pathogens are eliminated much less effectively by newborns compared with adults. For example, infants with congenital rubella continue to excrete the virus in the urine for the first years of life. Cytomegalovirus also is excreted in the urine of babies infected congenitally or neonatally for many years. This suggests that the response to some infections acquired early in life is inefficient. Our own studies have dealt primarily with immune responses to herpes simplex virus and cytomegalovirus following perinatal infection, and they show that these infections are followed by a smaller increase in the numbers of circulating virus specific T cells than in primary herpes simplex virus infections in adults.[16] The reasons for this difference are incompletely understood, but they do not appear to involve any defect of antigen processing by monocytes. The survivors of neonatal herpes simplex virus infections are clearly not immunologically tolerant of the virus, since they make antiherpes simplex virus antibody.[17] Cells with the potential for proliferating in response to the virus are not eliminated either, as shown by the production of low levels of soluble mediators following stimulation of the infants' cells with viral antigen.

An increased incidence of immunodeficiency and autoimmunity is another adverse consequence of congenital rubella infection but apparently not of other congenital infections. The immunodeficiency is most often selective IgA deficiency (occasionally IgG is deficient too), and the best documented autoimmune association is with insulin dependent (type 1) diabetes mellitus. Because selective IgA deficiency sometimes occurs with autoimmune disorders, a single mechanism could account for both associations. The observation that infants with congenital rubella who develop type 1 diabetes mellitus have the same HLA DR 3 and 4 antigens as other type 1 diabetics suggests that the congenital infection increases autoantibody production only in genetically susceptible individuals.

REFERENCES

1. Keller G, Paige C, Gilboa E, Wagner EF. Expression of a foreign gene in myeloid and lymphoid cells derived from multipotent haematopoietic precursors. Nature 1985; 318:149–154.
2. Lobach DF, Hensley LL, Ho W, Haynes BF. Human T cell antigen expression during the early stages of fetal thymic maturation. J Immunol 1985; 135:1752–1759.
3. Rosenthal P, Rimm IJ, Umiel T, et al. Ontogeny of human hemopoietic cells: analysis using monoclonal antibodies. J Immunol 1983; 31:232–237.
4. Spencer J, Macdonald TT, Finn T, Isaacson PG. The development of gut associated lymphoid tissue in the terminal ileum of human fetal intestine. Clin Exp Immunol 1986; 64:536–543.
5. Durandy A, Oury C, Griscelli C, Dumez Y, Oury JF, Henrion R. Prenatal testing for inherited immune deficiencies by fetal blood sampling. Prenat Diag 1982; 2:109–113.
6. Wilson M. Immunology of the fetus and newborn: lymphocyte phenotype and function. Clin Immunol Allergy 1985; 5:271–286.
7. Griffiths-Chu S, Patterson JAK, Berger CL, Edelson RL, Chu AC. Characterization of immature T cell subpopulations in neonatal blood. Blood 1984; 64:296–300.

8. Pereira P, Forni L, Larsson EL, Cooper M, Heusser C, Coutinho A. Autonomous activation of B and T cells in antigen free mice. Eur J Immunol 1986; 16:685–688.

9. Born W, Yogue J, Palmer E, Kappler J, Marrack P. Rearrangements of T cell receptor beta chain genes during T cell development. Proc Natl Acad Sci USA 1985; 82:2925–2930.

10. Owen JJT, Kingston R, Jenkinson EJ. Generation of cells expressing cytoplasmic and/or surface T cell receptor beta chains during the development of mouse fetal thymus. Immunology 1986; 59:23–27.

11. Pardoll DM, Fowlkes BJ, Bluestone JA, Kruisbeek A, Maloy WL, Coligan JE, Schwartz RH. Differential expression of two distinct T-cell receptors during thymocyte development. Nature 1987; 326:79–81.

12. Kappler JW, Roehm N, Marrack P. T cell tolerance by clonal elimination in the thymus. Cell 1987; 49:273–280.

13. Chilmonczyk B, Levin MJ, McDuffie R, Hayward AR. Characterization of the newborn response to herpesvirus antigens. J Immunol 1985; 134:4184–4188.

14. Baley JE, Schacter BZ. Mechanism of diminished natural killer cell activity in pregnant women and neonates. J Immunol 1985; 134:3042–3048.

15. Leibson PJ, Hunter-Laszlo M, Douvas GS, Hayward AR. Impaired neonatal natural killer cell activity to herpes simplex virus: decreased inhibition of viral replication and altered response to lymphokines. J Clin Immunol 1986; 6:216–224.

16. Hayward AR, Herberger M, Groothuis J, Levin MJ. Specific immunity after congenital or neonatal infection with cytomegalovirus or herpes simplex virus. J Immunol 1984; 133:2469–2473.

17. Hayward AR, Leibson P, Arvin A. Development of lymphocyte responses to herpes simplex virus following neonatal infection. In: Burgio GR, ed. Immunology of the neonate. New York: Springer, 1986:112.

SPECIAL LECTURE: IMPORTANCE OF IgG SUBCLASSES AND GENETIC FACTORS IN PREDICTING SUSCEPTIBILITY TO BACTERIAL INFECTIONS

GEORGE R. SIBER, M.D.

Several lines of evidence indicate that the formation of antibodies to bacterial capsular polysaccharides is a key mechanism of protection against many bacteria, including pneumococci, *H. influenzae* b, meningococci, and group B streptococci. Epidemiologic evidence includes the observation that children are at highest risk from invasive infections between the ages of 6 and 18 months when anticapsular antibody levels are lowest. In vitro anticapsular antibodies are bactericidal or opsonic together with complement. Passive immunization with anticapsular antibodies is protective in animal models and in humans.[1,2] Active immunization with purified capsular polysaccharide vaccines is also protective.

The capacity to respond to capsular polysaccharide antigens is remarkably variable. As an example, the postimmunization concentrations of antibody to the *H. influenzae* b capsular polysaccharide in healthy white adults vary over a more than 100-fold range. It seems likely that variation in antibody response results in variation in susceptibility to infection.

For several years my collaborators and I have been interested in the basis for this variation in responsiveness. Before describing some of our findings, I should like to review briefly some of the evidence suggesting that genetic factors may be important in regulating the antibody response to capsular polysaccharides and describe some of the peculiarities of antibodies to capsular polysaccharides.

NATURE OF POLYSACCHARIDE ANTIBODY RESPONSES

Polysaccharides are considered to be "T cell independent" antigens, in contrast to most proteins, which are T cell dependent. This means that, unlike proteins, polysaccharides can elicit an antibody response without the participation of major histocompatibility complex restricted T cell help. It does not mean, however, that T cells cannot play a role in modulating the magnitude of the response to some degree. It is also possible that T cells are necessary in the initial induction of the capsular polysaccharide antibody response responsible for "natural" antibody that is present in most individuals prior to immunization. Perhaps because of the limited role of T cells, there is little class switching during the antibody response; typically IgG, IgM, and IgA antibody levels increase simultaneously after immunization with purified polysaccharide vaccines. There is little maturation in affinity and no booster response to repeated immunization.

Immune response genes that control the capacity to respond to protein antigens typically map to the major histocompatibility complex locus on chromosome 6. In contrast, the capacity to respond to polysaccharides appears to be regulated by genes mapping primarily to the immunoglobulin constant regions.

Another difference of particular interest to pediatricians is that capsular polysaccharide antibody responses tend to mature later than protein antibody responses.

A peculiarity of capsular polysaccharide antibodies is that they typically differ in composition from protein antibody and total immunoglobulin. For example, in the adult response to many capsular polysaccharides there is preferential and frequently predominant use of IgG2 heavy chains.[3] IgG2 composes only 20 percent of total IgG. In contrast, most proteins elicit predominantly IgG1 responses; IgG1 is the major IgG subclass, comprising 70 percent of the total IgG. Because of this heavy chain restriction, we looked for and found a relationship between total IgG2 levels and an allotype marker of the IgG2 heavy chain and the capacity to respond to capsular polysaccharides. I will describe these findings in more detail.

It should be noted that the IgG2 preference or predominance may vary with different capsular polysaccharide antigens in adults and is generally less prominent or even absent in children. For example, children immunized with *H. influenzae* b vaccine, particularly the new protein—capsular polysaccharide conjugate vaccines, make predominantly IgG1 class antibodies.

A second form of restriction relates to the preferential use of one of the two available types of light chains. For example, *H. influenzae* b and meningococcal C antibodies contain mostly kappa chains in most white adults, whereas pneumococcus type 3 antibodies contain mostly lambda light chains.[5] For kappa predominant antibodies, an allotypic marker expressed on the constant region of kappa chains appears to correlate with responses.

Finally, capsular polysaccharide antibodies are also restricted in their diversity. Only a limited number of antibody clones are expressed in any one individual.[6] We therefore were interested in determining whether individuals capable of expressing a more diverse repertoire have greater capsular polysaccharide antibody responses than individuals with a more restricted repertoire.

EVIDENCE THAT GENETIC FACTORS INFLUENCE POLYSACCHARIDE ANTIBODY RESPONSES

Both epidemiologic and immunologic evidence indicates that the immune response to the *H. influenzae* b capsular polysaccharide may be under genetic control. The incidence of *H. influenzae* b infections may be as much as 100 times higher in certain racial groups, such as Alaskan Eskimos and American Indians, than in whites.[7] Clinical expression of the disease also differs; for example, epiglottitis is seen mainly in whites and only rarely in these high risk populations. Finally, we have seen families with several episodes of *H. influenzae* b infection occurring over long periods of time.

Immunologic evidence that genetic factors are important includes the observation that patients who have recovered from *H. influenzae* b meningitis, when studied at a later time, have lower antibody concentrations and poorer responses to immunization than age matched siblings.[8,9] The siblings in turn have lower antibody responses to immunization than matched healthy controls, suggesting that the hyporesponsiveness may be familial.[10]

CORRELATION BETWEEN IgG2 LEVELS AND POLYSACCHARIDE ANTIBODY RESPONSES

I first became interested in polysaccharide antibody responses several years ago when we attempted to immunize splenectomized patients who had completed therapy for Hodgkin's disease. The intensively treated patients had markedly impaired antibody responses to pneumococcal vaccine but normal responses to influenza virus vaccine.[11] Study of the total immunoglobulin levels revealed a normal total IgG level but a selective decrease in the IgG2 subclass, which was probably induced by the therapy.[12] Indeed the concentration of IgG2 was significantly correlated with the mean response to the pneumococcal vaccine (r = +0.71; p < 0.001). A similar correlation was found in healthy control subjects, although subsequent larger studies indicated that the correlations tend to be lower in healthy adults.[13] Intensive treatment for Hodgkin's disease thus induces a selective decrease in the IgG2 subclass and a selective defect in capsular polysaccharide antibody responsiveness. Similar correlations between total IgG2 concentrations and natural pneumococcal antibody levels were found recently in a group of children with recurrent otitis media.* This correlation remained significant after adjustment for age, which also correlates with IgG2 levels.

Recently we also immunized children with recurrent infections and selective IgG subclass deficiencies.[14] The group with low IgG2 levels for age had significantly lower antibody responses to *H. influenzae* b vaccine than healthy controls or IgG3 deficient children. This defect appears to be selective for polysaccharides, since their diphtheria antibody concentrations were normal. Their normal response to protein antigens may have practical significance for successful immunization of these children. Insel and Anderson[15] recently reported that children with selective IgG2 deficiencies are capable of responding to new vaccines in which the *H. influenzae* b capsular polysaccharide is covalently linked to diphtheria toxoid.

Although low total IgG2 levels appear to be a convenient marker for poor antibody responsiveness to capsular polysaccharides, it is important to remember that all individuals with low IgG2 levels are not poor responders. Indeed individuals have been described who have a complete absence of IgG2 because of a deletion of the G2 heavy chain gene and yet appear to have no problems with infections. There clearly are compensatory mechanisms.

IMMUNOGLOBULIN ALLOTYPES AND POLYSACCHARIDE ANTIBODY RESPONSES

Immunoglobulin allotypes are serologically detected markers on immunoglobulins that represent, typically, single amino acid changes in the constant regions of heavy or light chains. Any given marker is found in only a portion of the population and is inherited as a mendelian dominant trait. This system is analogous to but not nearly as polymorphic as the HLA system. The only two markers I will mention further are the G2m(n) marker carried on the IgG2 heavy chain and the Km(1) marker carried on the kappa light chain. The n marker is present in 70 percent of whites and absent or null in the remaining 30 percent. It is only rarely found in blacks, Eskimos, and Native Americans.

It has been known for some time that in whites

the n marker is correlated with higher concentrations of total IgG2 and IgG4. Recently, in studying a large group of Swiss Army recruits, we also noted that the n(+) group had slightly but significantly lower IgG1 levels than the n(−) group.[16] Total IgG levels did not differ. It appeared as if n(+) individuals preferentially switched to IgG2 at the expense of IgG1.

N(+) individuals also have higher concentrations of antibodies to many polysaccharides, including *H. influenzae* b and most pneumococcal serotypes.[13] Shown in Table 1 are total antibody levels measured by radioimmunoassay. The magnitude of the difference is only about two-fold, and thus a large number of individuals must be examined to detect this effect. When class specific levels are examined, in the case of *H. influenzae* b antibodies, it is apparent that only IgG class antibody is correlated with the n marker.

When the subclass of the IgG antibodies is examined, it is apparent that only the IgG2 subclass differs significantly between n(+) and n(−) groups. However, the magnitude of the difference is much more dramatic than for the total antibody level—about six fold.

G2M(N) ALLOTYPE AS A MARKER OF SUSCEPTIBILITY TO INFECTION

In order to determine whether the serologic correlations of the n allotype were also reflected in the susceptibility to infection, we performed a case control study of children with bacteremic *H. influenzae* b infections and healthy controls matched for age, sex, race, and postal code.[13] In white children with infections other than epiglottitis, the frequency of the n marker, as expected, was significantly lower than in controls. The relative risk of infection for n(−) versus n(+) children was 2.4. The difference was greater when the youngest group, aged less than 18 months, was analyzed separately. Here the relative risk was 5.1 in n(−) children.

Recently Granoff et al[17] confirmed the clinical significance of the n marker in children with vaccine failure. The n allotype occurred less commonly than expected in children who developed *H. influenzae* b infections despite immunization with the currently available *H. influenzae* b capsular polysaccharide vaccine.

In summary, the 70 percent of whites who have the n marker have higher total IgG2 levels, have higher antibody levels to many capsular polysaccharide antigens, have only the IgG2 component of the antibody response affected, are at lower risk of de-

---

* Pelton S, Teele D, Siber G. Unpublished observations.

TABLE 1 Relationship of G2m(n) Allotype and Antipolysaccharide Antibody Concentrations After Immunization in 130 Healthy Adults

	Geometric Mean Antibody Concentration		
	G2m(n)$^+$ (n=88)	G2m(n)$^-$ (n=42)	p Value
Total Ab by RIA to:			
Mean pneumococcal (ng protein N/ml)*	1870	1220	0.0005
H. influenzae b (Hib) (µg/ml)	35	21.3	0.024
Class specific Ab to Hib (ELISA units)			
IgG	12950	5740	0.005
IgM	1425	1201	NS
IgA	1408	1425	NS
Subclass specific Ab to Hib (ELISA units)			
IgG1	617	401	NS
IgG2	2440	391	<0.0001
G2/G1 ratio	3.96	0.98	<0.0001

* Geometric mean of 11 types measured.

veloping severe *H. influenzae* b infections particularly when very young, and are less likely to be vaccine failures.

The n allotype is rare in certain racial groups that are at high risk of infection by encapsulated bacteria, such as Native Americans and Alaskan Eskimos. However, it is not known whether the absence of the n marker is related to the risk of infection in these racial groups. A recent study in Alaskan Eskimos found no difference in the proportion of n(+) markers in children with *H. influenzae* b infection and in controls.[18] However, the proportion of n(+) individuals is only 5 percent in this population, making the power of the comparison very low.

The mechanism of the n allotype associated effect is currently unknown and is the subject of further investigation in our laboratories. One possibility is that genes closely linked to the G2 heavy chains coding for the n allele function as enhancers or promoters that selectively increase transcription of the G2 heavy chain, as switch regions that preferentially switch to G2 or as regulatory genes that result in earlier maturation of the capacity to switch to G2. Another possibility is that the n marker itself is recognized by regulatory T cells on IgG2 bearing B cells.

KM9(1) ALLOTYPE AND POLYSACCHARIDE ANTIBODY RESPONSES

The published literature relating to correlations between the Km(1) allotype and polysaccharide antibody responses and disease susceptibility appears to be contradictory.[5,19] The most probable explanation for this is that the same serologic determinant appears to be associated with opposite effects in whites and blacks.

We have shown that the Km(1) marker, which is present in only 10 to 15 percent of whites, is a "low responder" marker.[5] Km(1)$^+$ individuals make lower levels of kappa light chain containing Ig and lower levels of antibody to capsular polysaccharides which contain predominantly kappa chains. Only the kappa containing antibody, not the lambda containing antibody is affected. As expected, since all Ig classes utilize kappa light chains, all Ig classes are affected.

In whites the Km(1) marker has not been shown to be a risk factor for infection. However, a large number of cases need to be studied because the proportion of whites that are Km(1)$^+$ is so low.

In contrast, 75 percent of blacks are Km(1)$^+$. Granoff and colleagues[19] have shown that Km(1)$^+$ black children have higher antibody responses to *H.*

influenzae b vaccine and are at lower risk of *H. influenzae* b infection.

ANTIBODY DIVERSITY AND CAPSULAR POLYSACCHARIDE ANTIBODY RESPONSES

The last factor influencing the antibody response to capsular polysaccharide that I will discuss is the diversity of the antibodies produced. Isoelectric focusing analyses suggest that most adults have between two and 10 clones of antibody to the *H. influenzae* b polysaccharide after immunization.[6] We wondered whether individuals with more clones made more antibody. We simply correlated the total number of bands on isoelectric focusing gels and the antibody responses. Individuals expressing more diverse repertoires did have higher antibody levels to *H. influenzae* b capsular polysaccharide than individuals with relatively restricted repertoires.[†] This was true for IgG and IgA class antibodies but not for IgM clan antibodies.

OTHER GROUPS WITH DEFECTIVE ANTIBODY RESPONSES TO POLYSACCHARIDE ANTIGENS

I have already mentioned the selective hyporesponsiveness to *H. influenzae* b capsular polysaccharide immunization in children with recurrent infections and IgG2 deficiency. I should like to conclude by mentioning several other groups that we have recently studied with defects in capsular polysaccharide antibody responses. In collaboration with Donna Ambrosino and Raif Geha, we recently immunized a group of 15 children with recurrent infections and normal IgG subclass levels as well as 15 age matched healthy controls.[20] We found that the frequently infected children had lower *H. influenzae* b capsular polysaccharide antibody responses than their controls. The differences reached significance for IgG class antibodies. Dr. Geha and colleagues have been treating many of these children with immunoglobulin and have seen clinical improvements. A controlled trial is needed to assess the efficacy of immunoglobulin replacement in such patients.

Recently we saw a 30 year old patient with recurrent episodes of pneumococcal pneumonia since childhood, which continued after immunization with pneumococcal vaccine as an adult. An im-

munologic investigation revealed no abnormalities, including normal Ig and subclass levels. However, after immunization this patient made no detectable IgG or IgA class antibodies and only very low levels of IgM antibodies to capsular polysaccharide antigens.[21] His antibody concentrations to protein antigens were similar to those in healthy adults. This individual was also given intravenous globulin therapy and at the time of this writing has had no further infections.

Finally we examined the antibody responses in Apache children to *H. influenzae* b vaccine. These children have much higher incidences of bacteremia and meningitis than whites as well as ear infections due to encapsulated bacteria. When compared to white children, the Apache children had significantly lower antibody concentrations before immunization and an even greater difference after immunization.[22] Thus, deficiency in capsular polysaccharide antibody responsiveness may explain, at least in part, the high infection incidences in this population.

Taken together, these studies suggest that the measurement of specific antibody responses to relatively poor immunogens such as polysaccharide vaccines may be a sensitive method for detecting immunologic defects that predispose children to frequent infections. These studies of the role of IgG subclasses, low responder allotypes, and selective unresponsiveness to polysaccharide vaccines may lead us to a better understanding of human immunity to encapsulated bacteria.

One should be cautious, however, to avoid concluding that defective polysaccharide antibody responses are themselves, necessarily, responsible for the increased susceptibility to infection. Indeed the most common sites of infection are mucosal, and many of the pathogens are nonencapsulated bacteria such as nontypable *H. influenzae* or viruses. It may well be that IgG2 levels or capsular polysaccharide antibody responses, both of which undergo rapid maturation in the first years of life, may merely provide a convenient index of the state of immunologic maturation of the individual. In other words, the maturation of other immunologic functions important in protection from mucosal infections may parallel the maturation of capsular polysaccharide antibody responses.

Should measurements of IgG subclasses, antibody responses to capsular polysaccharide vaccines, or Ig allotypes be part of the clinical investigation of children with recurrent infections? In my view it is currently not clear whether these measurements have practical value for patient management. Although several authors have suggested that in-

---

[†] Siber G, Insel R. Unpublished observations.

dividuals with selective IgG subclass deficiencies or selective antibody deficiencies may be candidates for immunoglobulin replacement therapy, well controlled studies documenting the efficacy of this approach have not yet been reported. For the moment, it is therefore most reasonable to use clinical judgment rather than laboratory measurements to guide decisions about immunoglobulin prophylaxis. This expensive modality might be reserved for patients with particularly severe infections who have failed to benefit from more conventional therapy, such as prophylactic antibiotic therapy.

I should like to recognize the important contributions of my co-workers, Doctors Donna M. Ambrosino, Gerda de Lange, Raif Geha, Richard Insel, Andreas Morell, Steven Pelton, Mathuram Santosham, and Peter Schur.

Study supported by grants AI18125, AI20738, and AI24996 from the National Institutes of Health and a grant from the Thrasher Foundation.

REFERENCES

1. Ambrosino DM, Schreiber JR, Daum RS, Siber GR. Efficacy of human hyperimmune globulin in prevention of *Haemophilus influenzae* type b disease in infant rats. Infect Immun 1983; 39:709–714.
2. Santosham M, Reid R, Ambrosino DM, Priehs C, Aspery KM, Garrett S, Croll L, Foster S, Burge G, Page P, Zacher B, Moxon R, Siber GR. Prevention of *Haemophilus influenzae* type b infections in high risk infants with bacterial polysaccharide immune globulin. N Engl J Med 1987; 317:923–929.
3. Yount WH, Dorner MM, Kunkel HG, Kabat EA. Studies on human antibodies. VI. Selecting variations in subgroup composition and genetic markers. J Exp Med 1968; 127:633–646.
4. Weinbergt GA, Einhorn MS, Lenoir AA, Granoff PD, Granoff DM. Immunization of infants with *Haemophilus influenzae* type b (Hib) polysaccharide-outer membrane protein (PS-OMP) conjugate vaccine primes for IgG1 booster responses to conventional Hib PS vaccine. Pediatr Res 1987; 320A (abstract 879).
5. Ambrosino DM, Barrus VA, deLange GG, Siber GR. Correlation of the Km(1) immunoglobulin allotype with anti-polysaccharide antibodies in caucasian adults. J Clin Invest 1986; 78:361–365.
6. Insel RA, Kittelberger A, Anderson P. Isoelectric focusing of human antibody to the *Haemophilus influenzae* b capsular polysaccharide: restricted and identical spectrotypes in adults. J Immunol 1985; 135:2810–2816.
7. Losonsky GA, Santosham M, Sehgal VM, Zwahlen A, Moxon ER. *Haemophilus influenzae* disease in the White Mountain Apaches: molecular epidemiology of a high risk population. Pediatr Infect Dis 1984; 3:539–547.
8. Whisnant JK, Rogentine GN, Gralnick MA, Schlesselman JJ, Robbins JB. Host factors and antibody response in *Haemophilus influenzae* type b meningitis and epiglottitis. J Infect Dis 1976; 133:448–455.
9. Gorden CW, Michaels RH, Melish M. Effect of previous infection on antibody response of children to vaccination with capsular polysaccharide of *Haemophilus influenzae* type b. J Infect Dis 1975; 132:69-74.
10. Granoff DM, Squires JE, Munson RS, Suarez B. Siblings of patients with *Haemophilus meningitis* have impaired anticapsular antibody responses to *Haemophilus* vaccine. J Pediatr 1983; 103:185–191.
11. Siber GR, Weitzman SA, Aisenberg AC. The humoral immune response to protein and polysaccharide antigens in patient with Hodgkin's disease before and after treatment. Rev Infect Dis 1981; 3:S144–S159.
12. Siber GR, Schur PH, Aisenberg AC, Weitzman SA, Schiffman G. Relationship between serum IgG-2 concentrations and the antibody response to bacterial polysaccharide vaccines. N Engl J Med 1980; 303:178–182.
13. Ambrosino DM, Schiffman G, Gotschlich EC, Schur PH, Rosenberg GA, deLange GG, van Loghem E, Siber GR. Correlation between G2m(n) immunoglobulin allotype and the human antibody response and susceptibility to polysaccharide encapsulated bacteria. J Clin Invest 1985; 75: 1935–1942.
14. Umetsu DT, Ambrosino DM, Quinti I, Siber GR, Geha RS. Recurrent infections in children and selective IgG subclass deficiency. N Engl J Med 1985; 313:1247–1251.
15. Insel RA, Anderson PW. Response to oligosaccharide-protein conjugate vaccine against *Hemophilus influenzae* b in two patients with IgG2 deficiency unresponsive to capsular polysaccharide vaccine. N Engl J Med 1986; 315:449–503.
16. Morell A, Vassalli G, deLange GG, Skvaril F, Ambrosino DM, Siber GR. Class and subclass composition of natural antibodies to group A streptococcal carbohydrate: correlations with serum immunoglobulin concentrations and allotypes. J Clin Invest 1987 (Submitted for publication).
17. Granoff DM, Shackelford PG, Suarez BK, Nahm MH, Cates KL, Murphy TV, Karasic R, Osterholm MT, Pandey JP, Daum RS, the Collaborative Group. *Hemophilus influenzae* type b disease in children vaccinated with type b polysaccharide vaccine. N Engl J Med 1986; 315: 1584–1590.
18. Petersen GM, Silimperi DR, Rotter JI, Terasaki PI, Schanfield MS, Park MS, Ward JI. Genetic factors in *Haemophilus influenzae* type b disease susceptibility and antibody acquisition. J Pediatr 1987; 110:228–233.
19. Granoff DM, Shackelford PG, Pandey JP, Boies EG. Antibody responses to *Haemophilus influenzae* type b polysaccharide vaccine in relation to Km(1) and G2m(23) immunoglobulin allotypes. J Infect Dis 1986; 154:257–263.
20. Ambrosino DM, Umetsu DT, Geha RS, Michaels RS, Noyes J, Goularte TA, Howie, Siber GR. Impaired antibody response to polysaccharide antigen in children with recurrent sinopulmonary infections and normal IgG subclass concentrations. Interscience Conference on Antimicrobial Agents and Chemotherapy. 1986 (abstract 860).
21. Ambrosino DM, Siber GR, Chilmonczyk BA, Jernberg JB, Finberg RW. An immunodeficiency characterized by impaired antibody responses to polysaccharides. N Engl J Med 1987; 316:790–793.
22. Siber GR, Santosham M, Priehs CM, Reid R, Letson W, Madore D, Eby R. Impaired antibody response to H. influenzae b. Capsular polysaccharide in Native American children. Interscience Conference on Antimicrobial Agents and Chemotherapy 1987 (Abstract 326).

HUMORAL IMMUNE FACTORS FOLLOWED FROM BIRTH TO THE AGE OF THREE—COMPARISON BETWEEN OTITIS PRONE AND NONOTITIS PRONE CHILDREN

KARIN PRELLNER, M.D., Ph.D., GÖRAN HARSTEN, M.D., JESPER HELDRUP, M.D., OLOF KALM, M.D., Ph.D., and RAGNHILD KORNFÄLT, M.D.

Because deficiencies of immunoglobulins or complement factors usually become apparent through recurrent severe bacterial infections,[1] it has been proposed that such defects might contribute also to the appearance of recurrent episodes of acute otitis media in some children. Children suffering from recurrent acute otitis media, compared to healthy age matched control subjects, often exhibit lower total serum levels of the IgG_2 subclass,[2] lower concentrations of specific IgG antibodies against certain pneumococcal types,[3,4] and complement aberrations including low C1q levels and high concentrations of C1r-C1s complexes,[3] findings that support the assumption just made. Examination of immune factors in children with recurrent acute otitis media, however, was not performed until the children had already sustained at least one episode of acute otitis media. It is therefore difficult to determine whether the aforementioned aberrations were present prior to the disease period or whether they might have appeared as a consequence of the infections. The purpose of the present study was to further clarify the pathogenetic role of immunologic factors in recurrent acute otitis media.

MATERIAL AND METHODS

Patients, Samples, and Follow-up

The parents of all children born at the University Hospital of Lund, Sweden, during a certain period were asked to participate, but only those who gave written consent were included. The study finally comprised 122 children.

At the beginning of the study, data concerning living conditions, smoking habits, allergic diseases, and susceptibility of family members to otitis media were obtained by questionnaires. All the children were observed up to the age of 3, and the data mentioned were kept up to date for each child and completed with notations regarding feeding habits and type of day care.

The children were subjected to a standard Swedish vaccination program, including vaccination against measles, mumps, and rubella. The children and their parents could easily reach one of two pediatricians and one of two ENT specialists when needed. Special forms detailing the condition, diagnosis, and treatment of the child were filled in at every disease episode.

Acute otitis media was defined as an episode of earache in a child with red bulging eardrum(s) (as judged by pneumatic otomicroscopy) who occasionally was febrile and had signs of upper respiratory tract infection. Tympanocentesis generally was performed in children who are less than 1 year of age. Recurrent acute otitis media was defined as six or more episodes of acute otitis media during a 12 month period.

Blood samples were obtained at regular intervals, starting with the cord blood and followed by samples at the age of 6 weeks and at 3, 6, 12, 18, 24, 30, and 36 months of age. Samples also were obtained during the acute and convalescent phases of infection.

Laboratory Methods

The total serum concentrations of IgG were determined by electroimmunoassay and results were expressed in grams per liter.

Specific IgG, IgM, and IgA antibodies against the pneumococcal capsular polysaccharide types 3, 6A, and 19F were determined by the ELISA method.

Specific antibodies against rubella were determined by a hemolysin-gel test and results were expressed as the diameter (mm) of the area of hemolysis.

Complement components were analyzed by electroimmunoassay, and the results were expressed as percentages of the concentrations in a pool of normal adult serum. C1r-C1s proenzyme complexes were demonstrated by crossed immunoelectrophoresis and, owing to the area under the curve, judged as $-$, $+$, $++$, or $+++$.

RESULTS

Pattern of Episodes of Acute Otitis Media

One hundred thirteen children remained in the study group during the 3 year period. Of these, 13 children turned out to have suffered from recurrent acute otitis media; 29 had very few episodes of upper respiratory tract infection and no episode of acute otitis media (these were designated as "healthy children"). In the present study analysis of immune factors was restricted to these two groups of children.

Six of the 13 children with recurrent acute otitis media had the first episode of acute otitis media before or at the age of 6 months (Fig. 1). The total number of episodes of acute otitis media per child (of the children with recurrent acute otitis media) varied from six to 23. The seven children with an early onset had a mean total number of 15.1 episodes of acute otitis media as compared to 6.8 episodes in the six children with a later onset (see Fig. 1).

Total IgG

The mean total IgG concentration in cord blood was 10.5 g per liter (range, 7.1 to 13.0) in children with recurrent acute otitis media and 10.5 g per liter (range, 7.2 to 15.9) in the healthy children. At 6 months of age the mean concentrations were 5.3 g per liter (range, 3.3 to 8.0) and 4.4 g per liter (range, 2.4 to 7.7), respectively.

Specific Pneumococcal Antibodies

The serum concentrations of specific IgG antibodies against pneumococcus type 6A were lower in the children with recurrent acute otitis media when compared to the healthy children. At the ages of 18 and 24 months, respectively, 9 of 13 and 7 of 11 children with recurrent acute otitis media had concentrations less than 10 ELISA units. In the healthy children, 8 of 28 and 9 of 25, respectively, exhibited concentrations below this limit.

No other difference in the levels of specific antibodies of the different Ig classes for any of the pneumococcal types was observed between the two groups of children when tested at the ages of 18, 24, 30, and 36 months.

Antibodies Against Rubella

None of the prevaccination sera of the children had any demonstrable antibodies. The postvaccination sera of "healthy children" had significantly higher antibody levels than those of the children with recurrent acute otitis media ($p < 0.02$). The median hemolytic zones were 10 and 8.5 mm, respectively.

Complement Component and Complexes

The C1q levels in cord blood were significantly lower in the children with recurrent acute otitis media than in the healthy children ($p < 0.05$). The mean levels were 65 and 75 percent, respectively. The lowest levels (40 and 50 percent) were obtained in the children with recurrent acute otitis media who had the earliest onset of acute otitis media. A large variation in the C1q levels was seen in the children with recurrent acute otitis media during the 3 year follow-up.

C1r-C1s complexes in amounts equal to or greater than ++ were seen only in the children with

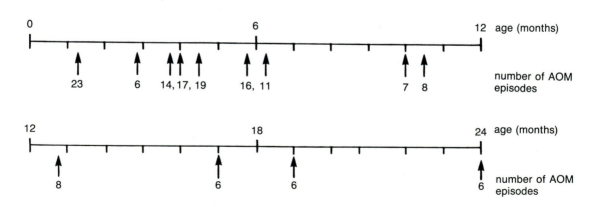

Figure 1 Time of the first episode of acute otitis media (AOM) (↑) in children with recurrent acute otitis media (rAOM) as related to the total number of episodes during the first 3 years of life.

recurrent acute otitis media. The complexes were not present in cord blood and did not appear until the onset of acute otitis media.

DISCUSSION

The present study demonstrates that the common assumption that children below the age of 6 months are usually protected from acute otitis media is not true for those who eventually suffer from recurrent episodes. Thus, in six of 13 children (children with recurrent acute otitis media) onset of acute otitis media occurred before this age.

Despite a rather strict definition of recurrent acute otitis media, it was obvious that children with recurrent acute otitis media constituted a heterogeneous group. The time of onset of the first episode of acute otitis media was a factor having a high predictive value, and the children with an early onset of acute otitis media were thus almost inevitably frequently affected.

It has been suggested that children with recurrent acute otitis media have a delayed capacity to respond with antibody production following stimulation with polysaccharide antigens, such as those of pneumococci.[5] The finding of poorer antibody responses following rubella vaccination in children with recurrent acute otitis media compared with nonotitis prone children indicates a lower degree of responsiveness in children with recurrent acute otitis media to protein antigens also.

Sequential analyses of serum complement components from birth through the first years of life enable us to demonstrate that C1r-C1s complexes are not present prior to the onset of acute otitis media. Thus, the appearance of large amounts of C1r-C1s proenzyme complexes in most children with recurrent acute otitis media seems most probably to be a secondary effect of the infections.

Since by far the lowest C1q levels were found in children with the earliest onset of acute otitis media, it might be possible to use cord blood C1q levels as a tool to predict whether a child is at risk of being frequently afflicted with acute otitis media.

This work was supported by the Swedish Medical Research Council (grant B87–16 ×–06857–004C), the Medical Faculty of the University of Lund, and the Åke Wiberg Trust.

REFERENCES

1. Dwyer JM. Thirty years of supplying the missing link. History of gamma globulin therapy for immunodeficient states. Am J Med 1984; 76:46-52.
2. Freijd A, Oxelius V, Rynnel-Dagöö B. IgG subclass levels in otitis-prone children. In: Lim DJ, Bluestone CD, Klein JO, Nelson JD, eds. Recent advances in otitis media with effusion. Proceedings of the Third International Symposium. Toronto: BC Decker, 1984:153-155.
3. Prellner K, Kalm O, Pedersen FK. Pneumococcal antibodies and complement during and after periods of recurrent otitis. Int J Pediatr Otorhinolaryngol 1984; 7:39-49.
4. Freijd A, Hammarström L, Persson MAA, Smith CIE. Plasma antipneumococcal antibody activity of the IgG class and subclasses in otitis prone children. Clin Exp Immunol 1984; 56:233-238.
5. Kalm O, Prellner K, Pedersen FK. Pneumococcal antibodies in families with recurrent otitis media. Int Arch Allergy Appl Immunol 1984; 75:139-142.

IMMUNOLOGIC CHARACTERISTICS OF CHILDREN WITH FREQUENT RECURRENCES OF OTITIS MEDIA

STEPHEN I. PELTON, M.D., DAVID W. TEELE, M.D., CHARLES B. REIMER, M.D., GERDA G. DE LANGE, Ph.D., GEORGE R. SIBER, M.D., and the Greater Boston Otitis Media Study Group: LLOYD TARLIN, M.D., PETER STRINGHAM, M.D., SIDNEY STAROBIN, M.D., LILLIAN McMAHON, M.D., MIRJANA KOSTICH, M.D., GILBERT FISCH, M.D., LORNA BRATTON, M.B., Ch.B., and CAROLE ALLEN, M.D.

An immunologic defect has been proposed as one mechanism for enhanced susceptibility in children with frequent recurrences of acute otitis media. A lower mean IgG$_2$ subclass level has been observed in children with recurrent otitis media when compared to otitis free children.[1] Children with recurrent sinopulmonary infections, with and without IgG subclass deficiency, have been found to respond less well to immunization with capsular polysaccharide of *Haemophilus influenzae* type b, suggesting that an impairment of antibody response in this population predisposes to recurrent infection.[2,3] These investigators suggest that a response to *H. influenzae* type b may be a marker of susceptibility to infection even in the absence of IgG subclass deficiency.

In children with recurrent otitis media we evaluated immunologic characteristics associated with susceptibility to infection and responsiveness to polysaccharide vaccines. We observed an association between antibody concentration to selected pneumococcal polysaccharides and frequent recurrences of acute otitis media after controlling for confounding variables.

METHODS

Patient Population

Serum specimens from 114 Caucasian children enrolled in a study of pneumococcal vaccine for the prevention of recurrent otitis media were available for analysis.[4] These children had been followed from birth and immunized after the third episode of acute otitis media with one of two pneumococcal vaccines (Eli Lilly). The children were followed for 24 months after immunization, and each episode of acute otitis media was diagnosed by clinical criteria, as described by Teele.[4] New episodes required the presence of fluid in the middle ear and one of the following symptoms: fever, irritability, lethargy, earache, diarrhea, or vomiting.

Measurement of IgG, IgM, IgA, IgG$_2$, and Pneumococcal Antibody

IgG, IgM, and IgA levels were measured by rate nephelometry. IgG$_2$ subclass levels were measured employing a mouse antihuman IgG$_2$ monoclonal antibody. Monoclonal antibody* was utilized as a capture antibody and goat antimouse IgG as a developing antibody in an ELISA technique.[5] Pneumococcal antibody levels were measured in 1978 using radiolabeled polysaccharide antigens in Dr. Gerald Schiffman's laboratory.

---

* HP 6014 provided by Dr. Charles Reimer.

Ig Allotypes

Immunoglobulin allotypes were determined by hemagglutination inhibition in the laboratory of Dr. Gerda de Lange.

Statistical Analysis

Data analysis and organization were performed by use of the PROPHET system, a national computer system sponsored by the Chemical/Biological Information Handling Program, National Institutes of Health. The mean preimmunization pneumococcal antibody value was defined as the geometric mean of that individual's antibody concentration to 11 vaccine serotypes (1, 3, 4, 6A, 7F, 8, 9, 12, 14, 18C, 23F). We performed multiple linear regression analysis utilizing numerical values directly, or their logarithms in the case of antibody concentration. "Dummy" variables were created for Km allotypes or Gm haplotypes; i.e., the presence of Km(1), Gm(f,n,b), Gm(f,..,b), Gm(za,..,g), or Gm(zax,..,g) was coded as 1 and the absence as 0.

RESULTS

Characteristics of Children with Frequent Recurrences of Otitis Media

Univariate analysis revealed a significant correlation between the age at the third episode (same as age at immunization) and the number of recurrences of otitis media. Twenty-three of 47 children (49 percent) who sustained the third episode of otitis media before 12 months of age had three or more episodes during the 24 month follow-up period, compared with only 11 of 48 children (23 percent) 12 months or older at the time of the third episode. The relative risk of three or more recurrences of acute otitis media was 3.2 in children with three episodes before 12 months of age compared with those with three episodes after 12 months of age.

Univariate analysis also revealed a negative correlation between the mean "natural" (preimmunization) pneumococcal antibody level and the number of recurrences. Significant negative correlations were also found for postimmunization antibody concentrations for each vaccine, but the correlations were lower than for "natural" antibody concentrations; therefore, results are presented only for "natural" antibody concentrations. Twenty-seven of the 49 children (55 percent) in whom the antibody level was less than the 50th percentile for the cohort had three or more episodes, compared with only seven of 46 (15 percent) children in whom the antibody level was greater than the 50th percentile. The relative risk of three or more recurrences of acute otitis media was 6.8 in children with values below the 50th percentile in natural pneumococcal antibody concentration compared to those with values above the 50th percentile.

Total IgG$_2$, IgG, IgM, and IgA levels at the time of immunization did not significantly correlate with the number of episodes observed during follow-up.

Multiple regression analysis revealed that both age at the time of immunization (same as the time of the third episode) and mean preimmunization pneumococcal antibody levels were independently correlated with the frequency of subsequent episodes of acute otitis media. Children who had lower mean preimmunization pneumococcal antibody levels had more episodes of otitis media during the 24 month follow-up period (partial r = −0.46; p = 0.001). Children who had the third episode at a younger age had more episodes during the next 24 months (partial r = −0.37; p = 0.046).

Ig Allotypes in Children with Frequent Recurrences of Otitis Media

Ig allotypes in children with recurrent otitis media were compared with those in two other Caucasian populations—children admitted for surgery to the Children's Hospital, Boston and adults residing in Boston. The Gm(n) allotype was identified in 68 percent of the children with recurrent otitis media. This was similar to the percentage of pediatric surgical admissions and adults with the Gm(n) allotype. The Km(1) allotype was identified in 22 percent of the children with recurrent otitis media. This frequency was greater that in the control populations, but the difference was not statistically significant (p = 0.07).

We compared the distributions of all allotypes in children with three or more episodes of otitis media during follow-up with those with two or fewer episodes. No difference in allotype distribution was identified (χ^2 = 0.26; p = NS).

DISCUSSION

Our studies have identified two factors predictive of frequent recurrences of acute otitis media—the occurrence of several episodes at a young age and the presence of low antibody concentrations of pneumococcal polysaccharides. Both findings are consistent with previous reports.[6,7]

The biologic significance of low pneumococcal antibody levels in the pathogenesis of recurrent otitis media is not defined by our studies. The low levels in children with three or more recurrences might merely have been a reflection of the younger age of this group. However, a multiple linear regression analysis indicated that the children with frequent recurrences of acute otitis media had low pneumococcal antibody levels even after controlling for age. A second possibility is that these children had less natural exposure to polysaccharide antigens and therefore had not developed as much "natural" antibody as the children with fewer recurrences of acute otitis media. This seems improbable, since it is likely that children with recurrent infections have greater exposure to encapsulated organisms. A third possibility is that children with frequent recurrences of acute otitis media have developed partial immunologic tolerance to polysaccharide antigens because of the nature of their exposure to these antigens (early age, route, dose). However, there is only limited evidence of the occurrence of tolerance to pneumococcal antigens in humans.[8] We therefore propose that the most likely explanation for the low antibody concentrations in the children with frequent recurrences of acute otitis media is a genetically determined immunologic hyporesponsiveness. These children may have a maturational delay of immune development that is conveniently identified by immunologic measurements, such as IgG$_2$ levels and polysaccharide antibody levels, that show marked maturational increases during the first years of life. This concept implies that neither low IgG$_2$ levels nor low pneumococcal antibody levels are themselves necessarily responsible for the pathogenesis of recurrent infections but merely provide a "marker" of a more global immunologic immaturity. This hypothesis is also consistent with observations that children with recurrent sinopulmonary infections have a low antibody response to a polysaccharide antigen (Hib vaccine). This hyporesponsiveness is found in the subgroup with low total IgG$_2$ levels[2] as well as in the larger group with normal Ig and IgG subclass levels.[3] Additional support for a maturation delay is provided by Kalm et al, who reported that children with recurrent acute otitis media have fewer mature circulating B cells as judged by surface markers (see chapter *Humoral Immune Factors Followed from Birth to the Age of Three—Comparison Between Otitis Prone and Nonotitis Prone Children*). Our hypothesis is also consistent with the observation that adults with a history of recurrent acute otitis media have IgG class antibody concentrations to six pneumococcal types similar to those in adults without such a history.[9]

In animals and humans, immune responses to polysaccharides are regulated in part by genes mapping to the Ig heavy and light chain coding regions. Ig allotypes provide convenient markers, analogous to HLA markers, for these genes. In Caucasians a marker of the IgG_2 constant region, G2m(n), is correlated with high adult antibody responses to many polysaccharides and an increased risk of infection due to *Haemophilus influenzae* type b in young children.[10] In Caucasians (but not in blacks) a marker of kappa chain constant regions, Km(1), is correlated with low antibody responses to polysaccharides that preferentially utilize kappa chains.[11] We found no differences in the frequency of the G2m(n) marker between children with recurrent acute otitis media and two Boston control populations. However, there was a statistical trend toward a higher frequency of the "low responder" Km(1) marker. The validity of this correlation requires further study in larger Caucasian populations.

Our results suggest that children with frequent recurrences of otitis media differ from children with fewer recurrences of otitis media in their response to pneumococcal polysaccharide antigens. Responses to these antigens, which are relatively poor immunogens in infants, may be sensitive indicators of the maturational status of immune function in children. It would follow that children whose immune system matures more slowly are at greater risk for recurrent episodes of otitis media. It would also follow that immune function is important in protecting against recurrences of otitis media.

REFERENCES

1. Freijd A, Oxelius V, Rynnel-Dagöö B. A prospective study demonstrating an association between plasma IgG_2 concentration and susceptibility to otitis media in children. Scand J Infect Dis 1985; 17:115–120.
2. Umetsu DT, Ambrosino DM, Quinti I, Siber GR, Geha RS. Recurrent sinopulmonary infection and impaired antibody response to bacterial capsular polysaccharide antigen in children with selective IgG-subclass deficiency. N Engl J Med 1985; 313:1247–1251.
3. Ambrosino DM, Umetsu DT, Siber GR, et al. Selective defect in the antibody response to *Haemophilus influenzae* type b in children with recurrent infections and normal serum IgG subclass levels. Accepted for Publication, Journal of Allergy and Clinical Immunology. J Allergy Clin Immunol (In press).
4. Teele DW, Klein JO, et al. Use of pneumococcal vaccine for prevention of acute otitis media in infants in Boston. Rev Infect Dis 1981; 3:S113–S118.
5. Jefferis R, Reimer CB, Skvaril F, et al. Evaluation of monoclonal antibodies having specificity for human IgG subclasses: results of an IUIS/WHO collaborative study. Immunol Lett 1985; 10:223–252.
6. Marchant CD, Shurin PA, Turczyk VA, et al. Course and outcome of otitis media in early infancy: a prospective study. J Pediatr 1984; 104:826–831.
7. Freijd A, Hammarström L, Persson MAA, Smith CIE. Plasma anti-pneumococcal antibody activity of the IgG class and subclasses in otitis prone children. Clin Exp Immunol 1984; 56:233–238.
8. Pichichero ME. Immunological paralysis to pneumococcal polysaccharide in man. Lancet 1985; 2:468–471.
9. Kalm O, Prellner K, Pedersen FK. Pneumococcal antibodies in families with recurrent otitis media. Int Arch Allergy Appl Immunol 1984; 75:139–142.
10. Ambrosino DM, Schiffman G, Goschlich EC, et al. Correlation between G2m(n) immunoglobulin allotype and human antibody response and susceptibility to polysaccharide encapsulated bacteria. J Clin Invest 1985; 75:1935–1942.
11. Ambrosino DM, Barrus VA, DeLange GG, Siber GR. Correlation of the Km(1) immunoglobulin allotype with anti-polysaccharide antibodies in Caucasian adults. J Clin Invest 1986; 78:361–365.

LYMPHOCYTE SUBPOPULATIONS IN OTITIS PRONE AND NONOTITIS PRONE CHILDREN

JESPER HELDRUP, M.D., OLOF KALM, M.D., Ph.D., and KARIN PRELLNER, M.D., Ph.D.

Among other effects on the defense system of the human body, acute infections generate an increased immunoglobulin production by plasma cells, which, together with their precursors, are called B lineage cells. The degree of differentiation and maturation of lymphoid cells can be studied using fluorochrome labeled monoclonal antibodies against structures (antigens) on the cell surfaces, analyzed by flow cytometry.[1] At various defined stages of their "maturation," cells have on their surfaces different sugar and protein structures called CD (cluster of differentiation) structures according to a nomenclature proposed by the WHO Study Group on Differentiation Antigens on Human Leukocytes.[2,3]

It has been proposed that during the maturation of B lineage cells, there occurs a sequential expression of the different surface antigens from precursor cells to immunoglobulin producing plasma cells.[4] HLA-DR, CD 19, CD 24, CD 20, and CD 22 thus appear sequentially on the surface of B lineage precursor cells in the bone marrow where they are produced.[3,5] When leaving the bone marrow, they express surface immunoglobulin M and are then by definition B cells, although they do not express CD 21. These immunoglobulin bearing B lineage cells in the circulation and in lymph nodes mature further to a CD 21- bearing B cell as yet not able to produce immunoglobulins. When meeting their specific antigen they transform into plasma cells through a CD 23-positive lymphoblastic stage.

In children with recurrent acute otitis media, lower total levels of the IgG_2 subclass have been observed[6] as well as lower concentrations of specific IgG antibodies against certain pneumococcal types.[7] A delayed switchover from IgM to IgG antibody production has been proposed in these children.[7]

The low levels of IgG_2 and specific antibodies in children with recurrent acute otitis media theoretically could be due to humoral or cellular factors. The humoral factor was studied in a trial of intravenous immunoglobulin treatment in which, however, no reduction in the frequency of acute otitis media was attained.[8]

The cellular factor investigated in the present study concerned possible differences in blood B cell and T cell subpopulations between children with recurrent acute otitis media and nonotitis prone children. Flow cytometry was used, and the possible influence of immunoglobulin therapy on these subpopulations was studied.

MATERIAL AND METHODS

Patients and Samples

Nine children with recurrent acute otitis media (defined as six or more episodes of acute otitis media during the previous 12 months) were investigated for surface antigens on blood lymphocytes immediately before a 5-month trial of treatment with serial infusions of human immunoglobulin[8] and at follow-up 6 months later. Since one child did not take part in the first sampling and another one not in the second sampling, eight children were analyzed on each occasion. The first sampling was performed at a mean age of 1.8 years (range, 1.1 to 2.9 years) and the second sampling at a mean age of 2.8 years (range, 1.7 to 5.2 years).

For comparison, blood samples were also obtained from two age matched nonotitis prone child groups—one of five children with a mean age of 1.8 years (range, 1.7 to 1.9 years) and the other of five children with a mean age of 2.7 years (range, 2.0 to 3.3 years). According to the medical records at the University Hospital of Lund, where the blood samples were analyzed, all these children were free from infection at the time of sampling and had no history of episodes of acute otitis media.

For flow cytometry analysis, venous whole blood samples were obtained from the children and immediately delivered to the laboratory. In the children with recurrent acute otitis media the white blood cell counts and differential counts were analyzed both at the time of the first sampling and repeatedly during the interval between samplings.

Immunoglobulin Administration

In the children with recurrent acute otitis media, immunoglobulin (0.2 g per kilogram of body weight) was infused intravenously five times (with a mean interval of 25 days) over a period of 5 months, as described earlier.[8]

Laboratory Methods

Peripheral blood cells were separated on a Ficoll-Hypaque gradient, and the isolated mononuclear cells were resuspended in modified McCoy solution containing fetal calf serum. A standard panel of monoclonal antibodies was used to detect membrane antigens by a microplate and indirect immunofluorescence technique.[1,9] The B lineage antibodies used were defined at the third Workshop on Leukocyte Differentiation Antigens (Oxford, 1986).[2] The T lineage and HLA-DR antibodies were purchased from Becton-Dickinson, Stockholm, Sweden. After labeling with primary and secondary antibodies (Nordic goat antimouse GAM-m-Ig-FITC), 10,000 cells were analyzed by flow cytometry (Ortho 50 H). The following B lineage surface structures were studied: HLA-DR, CD 19, CD 24, CD 20, CD 22, IgM, CD 21, and CD 23; of the T cell lineage, antigens CD 7, CD 2, CD 4, CD 8, and CD 3.

Statistical Methods

The Mann-Whitney U test was used when comparing results in children with recurrent acute otitis media with those in healthy children, and the Sign test was used for comparing values before and after immunoglobulin treatment in the children with disease.

RESULTS

Before immunoglobulin therapy, blood specimens in the children with recurrent acute otitis media exhibited significantly higher concentrations of the early B lineage antigens CD 19, CD 24, CD 20, and CD 22 and of HLA-DR (p = 0.001 to 0.009) than did those in age matched controls (Fig. 1). No differences were found between children with recurrent acute otitis media and controls for the B cell surface antigens IgM, CD 21, and CD 23. At follow-up 6 months later, no differences were seen between children with recurrent acute otitis media and age matched controls in any of the eight B lineage surface antigens analyzed. As for the T lineage antigens, the children with recurrent acute otitis media exhibited lower frequencies of CD 2 (p = 0.009) before immunoglobulin treatment than did the controls. No other difference was found among the T cells.

In comparing the two groups of healthy children, it was found that the older group had slightly higher concentrations of CD 20 (p = 0.048) and slightly lower concentrations of CD 21 (p = 0.048) than those in the younger ones. No other differences were found between the healthy children groups.

In six of the nine children with recurrent acute otitis media, values for all 13 surface antigens were analyzed both before treatment and at follow-up. The concentrations of CD 19, CD 24, CD 20, and CD 22 (but not HLA-DR) were lower in all six children at follow-up than before treatment (p = 0.0156; Fig. 2).

The mean white cell count in the nine children with acute recurrent otitis media at the time of the first sampling was 7.8×10^9 per liter (normal range, 5.2 to 10.5×10^9 per liter). In the differential count the mean number of lymphocytes was 4.6×10^9 per liter (normal range, 4.0 to 9.0×10^9 per liter).

DISCUSSION

With the leukocyte and differential counts essentially within normal ranges, our findings indicate that children with recurrent acute otitis media have nearly twice the normal concentrations of blood B lineage cells. The B lineage cells found in our children with recurrent acute otitis media had an unusual immature phenotype without IgM and CD 21 on the cell surface, and not the more mature B cell phenotype, expressing both surface IgM and CD 21, seen in the nonotitis prone controls. The content of blood T lineage cells in the children with recurrent acute otitis media was normal and essentially without abnormalities. The results can be interpreted

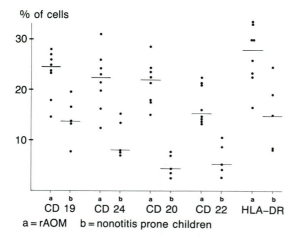

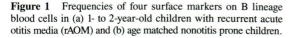

Figure 1 Frequencies of four surface markers on B lineage blood cells in (a) 1- to 2-year-old children with recurrent acute otitis media (rAOM) and (b) age matched nonotitis prone children.

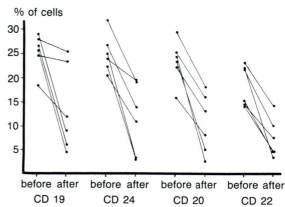

Figure 2 Frequencies of four surface markers on B lineage blood cells in 6 rAOM children before and after intravenous immunoglobulin treatment. The interval between samplings was 6 months.

as reflecting either an enduring stimulative effect on the bone marrow of frequent infections with "leakage" of immature cells into peripheral blood, or an age dependent delay in the sequential differentiation of early B lineage cells into more mature B lymphocytes. After immunoglobulin treatment the B lineage cells normalized. Recent in vitro studies, however, have demonstrated an inhibitory effect of immunoglobulin on the differentiation of B cells.[10] The normalization of the B lineage cells seen in the present study thus might only be a result of the increasing age of the children with recurrent acute otitis media rather than a beneficial effect of the immunoglobulin treatment.

Children with recurrent acute otitis media have a higher frequency of immature blood B lineage cells than age matched nonotitis prone children. Whether any relationship exists between this finding and the poor ability to produce certain specific antibodies is yet not known.

This work was supported by the Swedish Medical Research Council (B87–16X–06857–04C), the Medical Faculty of the University of Lund, and the Åke Wiberg Trust.

REFERENCES

1. Alpert NL. Flow cytometers are coming. Clin Instr Systems 1984; 5:1–14.
2. Shaw S. Characterization of human leukocyte differentiation antigens. Immunology Today 1987; 8:1–3.
3. Reinherz EL, Haynes BF, Nadler LM, Bernstein ID. Human B lymphocytes. New York: Springer Verlag, 1986.
4. Foon KA, Schroff RW, Gale RP. Surface markers on leukemia and lymphoma cells: recent advances. Blood 1982; 60:1–19.
5. Campana D, Janossy G, Bofill M, Trejdosiewicz LK, Ma D, Hoffbrand AV, Mason DY, Lebacq A-M, Forster HK. Human B cell development. I. Phenotypic differences of B lymphocytes in the bone marrow and peripheral lymphoid tissue. J Immunol 1985; 134:1524–1530.
6. Freijd A, Oxelius V-A, Rynnel-Dagöö B. A prospective study demonstrating an association between plasma IgG$_2$ concentrations and susceptibility to otitis media in children. Scand J Infect Dis 1985; 17:115–120.
7. Kalm O, Prellner K, Pedersen FK. Pneumococcal antibodies in families with recurrent otitis media. Int Arch Allergy Appl Immunol 1984; 75:139–142.
8. Kalm O, Prellner K, Christensen P. The effect of intravenous immunoglobulin treatment in recurrent acute otitis media. Int J Pediatr Otorhinolaryngol 1986; 11:237–246.
9. Janossy G, Campana D, Coustan-Smith E. Immunofluorescence. In: Cawley JC, ed. Leukocyte methods. Edinburgh: Churchill Livingstone, 1986.
10. Stohl W. Cellular mechanisms in the in vitro inhibition of pokeweed mitogen-induced B cell differentiation by immunoglobulin for intravenous use. J Immunol 1986; 136:4407–4413.

DECREASED LEVELS OF NASOPHARYNGEAL SECRETORY IGM AND INCREASED LEVELS OF PLASMA IGG1, IN OTITIS PRONE CHILDREN

CHRISTINA H. SØRENSEN, M.D. and LARS K. NIELSEN, M.D.

Various dysfunctions have been demonstrated in both the humoral and the cellular immune apparatus in children with recurrent acute otitis media as well as in those with secretory otitis media.[1] The susceptibility to otitis has been associated with low levels of plasma IgG2[2] and plasma antipneumococcal antibodies and complement factors,[3] which to some extent could explain recurrent infections of the upper respiratory tract. In contrast to acute otitis media, secretory otitis media usually appears without clinical signs of acute inflammation, although increased nasopharyngeal colonization of microorganisms and dysfunction of the eustachian tube are important factors in the pathogenesis of both.[4,5] Therefore, in theory, a decreased nasopharyngeal capacity for immune exclusion is to be expected in children with recurrent acute otitis media as compared with that in those with secretory otitis media and healthy controls. In the present study we describe quantitatively the secretory immunoglobulins, SIgA and SIgM, in nasopharyngeal secretions and plasma samples and the levels of plasma IgG and IgG subclasses in children with different degrees of susceptibility to otitis.

SUBJECTS AND METHODS

Plasma samples (EDTA) were obtained from 196 children, classified into the following three groups according to the medical history and records supplemented by otoscopy and tympanometry:

1A.   100 children (median age, 52 months; interquartile range, 37 to 64) with recurrent acute otitis media, hospitalized for insertion of grommets or adenoidectomy. All the children had had secretory otitis media during the preceding 3 to 6 months. Of the 100 children, 52 had had one to five episodes of acute otitis media during the preceding 1 to 2 years; and 48 were termed "otitis prone," having had more than six episodes of acute otitis media.[6]

2A.   53 children (median age, 54 months; interquartile range 41 to 70) who had had secretory otitis media for at least 3 to 6 months but without previous episodes of acute otitis media.

3A.   43 healthy children (median age, 63 months; interquartile range 47 to 109) hospitalized for noninfectious disorders (e.g., operations for hernia, phimosis). None of these children had had episodes of acute otitis media or known periods of secretory otitis media, and normal otoscopic findings were verified in all cases.

Quantitation of plasma IgA, IgM, and IgG levels was done by means of turbidimetry and ELISA.[6-8] Levels of plasma IgG subclasses were determined by means of the Manzini technique, using antisera from the Central Laboratory of the Netherlands Red Cross Transfusion Service.[8] Because of the scarcity of plasma samples, IgG subclass measurements were performed in only 156 children classified as follows:

1B.   81 children with recurrent acute otitis media. Of these, 35 were otitis prone according to the previously mentioned criteria; and the remaining 46 had had one to five episodes of acute otitis media.

2B.   41 children who had had secretory otitis media at least 3 to 6 months but without previous episodes of acute otitis media.

3B.   34 healthy children.

Nasopharyngeal secretions were aspirated directly under visual guidance[7] from 100 children who were classified as follows:

1C.   54 children with recurrent acute otitis media (median age, 55 months; interquartile range 41 to 66). Of these, 34 were considered otitis prone.

2C.   34 children with secretory otitis media (median age, 58 months; interquartile range 44 to 69).

3C.   7 healthy children (median age, 63 months; interquartile range 17 to 109) with symptoms of snoring and moderate hyperplasia of the adenoids but without previous episodes of acute and secretory otitis media.

Quantitation of SIgA and SIgM levels in both nasopharyngeal secretions and plasma samples was carried out using ELISA, as previously reported.[7,8] The albumin content in nasopharyngeal secretions and in paired plasma samples was measured by routine rocket immunoelectrophoresis.[6] The concentration ratio of nasopharyngeal secretion albumin to plasma albumin was regarded as the index of transudation of plasma proteins through the nasopharyngeal mucosal barrier.

Nonparametric statistical analyses were employed because of nongaussian distributions of groups of data.

RESULTS

Plasma IgA and IgM levels in 196 children are shown in Table 1. A steady increase in IgA with age was observed, but no differences could be calculated between children with and without recurrent acute otitis media ($p > 0.15$; see Table 1). By contrast, an uneven distribution of plasma IgM was observed, and although the median age of the healthy group of children was somewhat higher than that of the two other groups, significantly higher levels of IgM were found in plasma from children with recurrent acute and secretory otitis media than in the healthy group ($p < 0.01$; see Table 1).

Levels of secretory IgA and IgM in 100 nasopharyngeal secretion specimens are shown in Table 2. No statistically significant differences in the levels of secretory IgA were found in three

TABLE 1   Plasma IgA and IgM Levels in 196 Children with Recurrent Acute Otitis Media and Secretory Otitis Media and in Healthy Children*

	Recurrent Acute Otitis (n = 100)	Secretory Otitis Media (n = 53)	Healthy Children (n = 43)	Significance[+]
IgA (g/l)	0.97 (0.72–1.34)	1.10 (0.71–1.35)	0.81 (0.64–1.28)	p>0.15
IgM (g/l)	1.08 (0.90–1.39)	1.05 (0.86–1.62)	0.82 (0.72–1.12)	p<0.01

* Median levels and interquartile ranges (in parentheses) are given.
+ Kruskal-Wallis one way analysis of variance.

TABLE 2   Secretory IgA and Secretory IgM in 100 Nasopharyngeal Secretions and Secretory IgA in Plasma Samples from Children with Recurrent Acute Otitis Media and Secretory Otitis Media and from Healthy Controls*

N = 100	Recurrent Acute Otitis (n = 59)	Secretory Otitis Media (n = 34)	Healthy Children (n = 7)	Significance[+]
Secretory IgA (g/l)	1.18 (0.57–1.94)	1.21 (0.80–2.33)	1.42 (0.46–3.85)	$p > 0.4$
Secretory IgM (U/l)	66.6 (33.3–120.1)	82.5 (51.7–152.6)	116.5 (50.1–264.8)	$p < 0.01$
Plasma Secretory IgA (mg/l)	3.8 (2.7–4.5)	3.8 (3.3–5.2)	2.4 (1.6–4.3)	$p < 0.005$
Albumin (nasopharyngeal secretion/plasma, %)	10 (6–18)	12 (6–22)	9 (6–21)	$p > 0.8$

* The transudation index of albumin from plasma to nasopharyngeal secretions is also listed. Median levels and interquartile ranges (in parentheses) are given.
+ Kruskal-Wallis one way analysis of variance.

groups of children ($p > 0.4$). In contrast to the levels of plasma IgM, children with recurrent otitis media had significantly lower nasopharyngeal secretion SIgM levels than those in the secretory otitis media and healthy groups of children ($p < 0.06$ and $p < 0.02$, respectively; see Table 2). For both SIgA and SIgM there was no correlation with age (Spearman rho = 0.03 and 0.05, respectively). Also there was no correlation between plasma IgA and nasopharyngeal secretion SIgA or between plasma IgM and nasopharyngeal SIgM (Spearman rho = 0.07 and -0.17, respectively). By contrast, a close correlation was found between the two secretory Ig levels in the nasopharyngeal secretions (Spearman rho = 0.85; $p < 0.001$). An even distribution of the transudation index of albumin was found in the three groups of children, as shown in Table 2. A significant but negative correlation was observed between the transudation index of albumin and the ratio of SIgA to total IgA (Fig. 1). As the regression line indicates, a transudation index of 8 percent corresponds to a 100 percent ratio of SIgA to total IgA.

Levels of SIgA in the plasma samples are shown in Table 2. Significantly higher levels of SIgA were found in plasma samples from children with recurrent acute and secretory otitis media than in the healthy group ($p < 0.05$). In all plasma samples SIgM was undetectable.

Although the healthy children were somewhat older than the other groups of children investigated, significantly higher levels of plasma IgG and, in particular, of IgG1 were measured in samples from chil-

dren with recurrent acute and secretory otitis media than in those from the healthy group (Table 3). Moreover, as shown in Table 3, there seems to be a correlation between low levels of plasma IgG2 and susceptibility to otitis, but the difference between the groups of children disappeared when age matched groups were tested ($p > 0.25$).

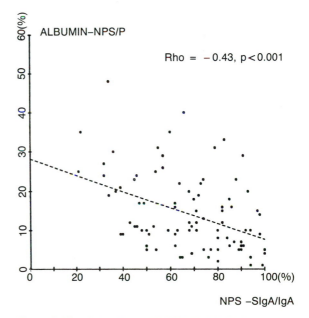

Figure 1   Correlation (Spearman rho) between ratios of secretory IgA to total IgA in nasopharyngeal secretions (NPS-SIgA/IgA) and the corresponding transudation index of albumin from plasma to NPS (albumin-NPS/P). Regression is illustrated by the dotted line.

TABLE 3   Plasma IgG and IgG Subclasses in Otitis Prone Children, in Children with Recurrent Acute Otitis Media and Secretory Otitis Media, and in Healthy Children*

	Otitis Prone Children (n = 35)	Recurrent Acute Otitis Media (n = 46)	Secretory Otitis Media (n = 41)	Healthy Children (n = 34)	Significance+
IgG (g/l)	10.2 (7.7–11.8)	10.4 (9.6–12.1)	9.9 (8.5–11.3)	8.5 (7.4–11.2)	$p < 0.02$
IgG1 (g/l)	6.5 (5.3–8.1)	6.8 (5.9–8.1)	6.5 (5.6–7.4)	5.6 (4.3–6.8)	$p < 0.002$
IgG2 (g/l)	1.0 (0.7–1.4)	1.3 (0.9–1.6)	1.4 (0.9–1.6)	1.5 (1.2–1.8)	$p < 0.03$
≤months IgG2 (g/l)	(n = 28) 0.9 (0.7–1.3)	(n = 27) 1.2 (0.9–1.6)	(n = 19) 0.9 (0.7–1.2)	(n = 13) 1.4 (0.7–1.7)	$p > 0.25$

*   Median levels and interquartile ranges (in parentheses) are given.
+   Kruskal-Wallis one way analysis of variance.

DISCUSSION

The ease of transmission of acute and secretory otitis media during early childhood has often been attributed to immaturity of the immune apparatus. However, the precise pathogenic roles of the various dysfunctions previously reported in such children have also been difficult to establish.[1] In general, the susceptibility to otitis does not seem to be associated with deficiencies in plasma Ig levels. On the contrary, as shown in Table 1, we found normal plasma Ig levels and even increased plasma levels of IgM and IgG in otitis prone children, indicating a systemic immune response to recurrent upper respiratory tract infections. In this regard it is of interest that children suffering only from "simple" secretory otitis media has Ig levels ranging between those of otitis prone children and healthy children (see Table 1).

The mucosal lining of the nasopharynx is provided with a secretory immune system, in principle like that of other mucosal surfaces in humans.[7] Sustained integrity of the nasopharyngeal epithelial barrier seems important in order to minimize the mucosal leakage of plasma proteins and inflammatory cells. In children with both recurrent acute and secretory otitis media high plasma levels of SIgA could be explained in part by an increased reabsorption of nasopharyngeal secretion SIgA as a result of recurrent leakage of the mucous membrane. As shown in Table 2, equally high levels of SIgA were found in nasopharyngeal secretions from the three groups of children investigated, and the median concentrations were even higher than the corresponding levels of plasma IgA (see Tables 1

and 2). Because of the calculations of the transudation index of plasma proteins to the nasopharynx and the lack of correlation between nasopharyngeal secretion SIgA and plasma IgA levels, it seems obvious that the majority of the IgA antibodies found in nasopharyngeal secretions are secreted locally. These matters have fundamental importance in efforts to design new approaches in vaccine prophylaxis.

In contrast to the increase in the plasma IgM level in children with recurrent acute and secretory otitis media, a significant decrease in SIgM was calculated in nasopharyngeal secretions, especially in otitis prone children (see Table 2). This decrease could be ascribed only partly to increased consumption of Ig, because none of the children suffered from acute upper respiratory tract infections at the time of the investigation, an observation in agreement with the even distribution of the albumin transudation index (see Table 2). More likely the nasopharyngeal overload of microbial antigens, which appears from time to time in children with recurrent acute and secretory otitis media, may contribute to insufficient induction of specific immunity, rendering the child more susceptible to new infections.

Little is known about the function of SIgM during the initial phase of a viral infection, but low levels of SIgM may contribute in some way to decreased integrity of the nasopharyngeal epithelial barrier, which, as shown in Figure 1, may yield decreased concentrations of secretory immunoglobulins. Consequently increased nasopharyngeal colonization of pathogens may occur. It is interesting that the colonization of pathogens in cases of acute and secretory otitis media seems to differ quantitatively but not qualitatively.[4,5] Such results are in line with the difference in levels of secretory immunoglobulins between children with recurrent acute and secretory otitis media, as indicated in Table 2.

Freijd et al[2] demonstrated low levels of plasma IgG2 in 20 otitis prone children, investigated at both 12 and 36 months of age. Such an association could not be demonstrated in the present study (see Table 3). On the contrary, we found significantly higher levels of plasma IgG1 in otitis prone children than in healthy children.

The results of the present study indicate a secretory hyporesponsiveness in regard to low nasopharyngeal secretion SIgM in otitis prone children, whereas these children seem to be well furnished with locally produced SIgA antibodies at the nasopharyngeal level. In children suffering from secretory otitis media the hyporesponsiveness seems to be less pronounced than that in otitis prone children.

REFERENCES

1. Bernstein JM, Prellner K, Rynnell-Dagoo B, Sipila P, Palva T. Otitis media: the immunological factor. In: Sade J, ed. Acute and secretory otitis media. Amsterdam: Kugler, 1986:203–210.
2. Freijd A, Oxelius V, Rynnel-Dagoo B. A prospective study demonstrating an association between plasma IgG2 concentrations and susceptibility to otitis media in children. Scand J Infect Dis 1985; 17:115–120.
3. Prellner K, Kalm O, Pedersen FK. Pneumococcal antibodies and complement during and after periods of recurrent otitis. Int J Pediatr Otorhinolaryngol 1984; 7:39–49.
4. Long SS, Henretig FM, Teter MJ, McGowan KL. Nasopharyngeal flora and acute otitis media. Infect Immun 1983; 41:987–991.
5. Sørensen CH, Andersen LP, Tos M, Thomsen J, Holm-Jensen S. Nasopharyngeal bacteriology and secretory otitis media in young children. Acta Otolaryngol 1988; 105:126–131.
6. Sørensen CH, Nielsen LK. Nasopharyngeal secretory immunoglobulins in children with recurrent acute otitis media and secretory otitis media. Acta Pathol Microbiol Immunol Scand (in press).
7. Sørensen CH. Secretory IgA enzyme immunoassay. Application of a model for computation of the standard curve. Scand J Clin Lab Invest 1982; 42:577–583.
8. Sørensen CH, Nielsen LK. Plasma IgG, IgG subclasses and acute-phase proteins in children with recurrent acute otitis media. Acta Pathol Microbiol Immunol Scand (in press).

IMMUNOGENESIS OF OTITIS MEDIA WITH EFFUSION—WITH SPECIAL REFERENCE TO IMMUNOSUPPRESSIVE FACTORS IN THE MIDDLE EAR

HIROMU KAKIUCHI, M.D., YOSHIHIRO DAKE, M.D., and TOSHIHIDE TABATA, M.D.

Close attention has been paid recently to immunologic factors in the mechanism of onset and prevalence of otitis media with effusion. Yamanaka et al[1,2] reported that serous middle ear effusion inhibits both cell mediated immunity and humoral immunity as a result of soluble fractions with a molecular weight of about 50,000. These substances that inhibit immunity include immunosuppressive substance and immunosuppressive acidic protein.

Immunosuppressive substance is a glycoprotein with a molecular weight of 52,000 and an isoelectric point of pH 2.7 to 3.3. It was detected in ascitic fluid from patients with advanced colon cancer by Fujii et al[3] and has various immunosuppressive activities. For example, it suppresses PHA, ConA, PWN stimulated lymphocyte blast formation, NK activity, delayed type hypersensitivity in mice, and SRBC induced antibody production in mice.

Immunosuppressive acidic protein has a molecular weight of 50,000 and an isoelectric point of pH 3.0. It was detected in sera from cancer patients by Tamura et al[4] and has immunosuppressive activities similar to those of immunosuppressive substance. Both substances vary in their effects on the recurrence, and prognosis of cancer.

The present study was designed to measure the levels of immunosuppressive substance and immunosuppressive acidic protein in serous middle ear effusions. In studies using rats, immunosuppressive substance was administered into the middle ear cavity in order to determine whether otitis media with effusion could be produced experimentally. In addition, immunosuppressive substance was instilled into the middle ear cavity in nonviable *H. influenzae* produced otitis media with effusion models in order to determine whether immunosuppressive substance would cause prolongation of otitis media with effusion.

MATERIALS AND METHODS

The levels of immunosuppressive substance and immunosuppressive acidic protein in middle ear effusions and sera were measured by single radial immunodiffusion in 38 patients with serous otitis media with effusion. Serum samples serving as controls were taken from 24 healthy donors.

Sprague and Dowley rats weighing 200 to 300 g were used in the animal experiments. In an effort to determine whether otitis media with effusion could be produced experimentally, the test rats were administered 2,000 μg per milliliter of rat immunosuppressive substance. The animals were decapitated 1, 3, and 7 days after administration to observe changes in the mucosa of the middle ear. The controls were administered physiologic saline. The rat immunosuppressive substance was diluted with physiologic saline.

In the other study a model of otitis media with effusion was prepared according to the report of DeMaria et al.[5] Nontypable *H. influenzae* isolated from middle ear effusion from a patient with otitis media with effusion was treated with 0.3 percent formalin and diluted with phosphate buffered saline to a concentration of 3×10^7 per ml. Then 50 μl of the killed bacterial solution was injected into the right middle ear of the rats. On the first day after the administration of killed *H. influenzae,* immunosuppressive substance was administered to those that were to be decapitated at days 3 and 7 for observation. Immunosuppressive substance was administered in alternate weeks to those that were to be decapitated at 2 weeks and later. The controls were given physiologic saline in a similar fashion; they were decapitated at days 3, 7, 14, 21, 28, and 35 to observe the condition of the middle ear.

RESULTS

The mean levels of immunosuppressive substance and immunosuppressive acidic protein in middle ear effusions in patients with serous otitis media with effusion were 1,115.0 $\pm$ 347.9 μg per milliliter and 774.4 $\pm$ 315.7 μg per milliliter, respectively, levels that were significantly elevated (p < 0.01) compared to those in serum specimens from patients (706.2 $\pm$ 226.0 μg per milliliter and 406.3 $\pm$ 176.5 μg per milliliter, respectively) and healthy donors (509.7 $\pm$ 104.4 μg per milliliter and 381.3 $\pm$ 104.5 μg per milliliter, respectively).

The administration of rat immunosuppressive substance into the middle ear cavity did not cause otitis media with effusion in rats (Fig. 1). Otitis media with effusion was produced, however, by the administration of formalin killed *H. influenzae* into the middle ear cavity, and when rat immunosuppressive substance was administered afterward, there was a prolongation of histologic features of inflammation in comparison to the controls, which were given physiologic saline (Fig. 2). Histologic examination revealed that the 25 μm thick connective tissue disappeared in about 2 to 3 weeks in the controls, whereas it persisted for 4 to 5 weeks in the rats treated with immunosuppressive substance (Fig. 3).

DISCUSSION

The present study showed that the levels of immunosuppressive substances were higher than normal in serous middle ear effusion. However, we do not know whether this was due to concentrated effusion or to the local production of these immunosuppressive substances; both mechanisms are feasible.

Immunosuppressive substance has an isoelectric point of pH 2.7 to 3.3. Its molecular weight varies slightly with the species, being 52,000 for the human variety and 50,000 for the rat variety. However, the biologic properties are essentially the same.

In this study we used rat immunosuppressive substance. Otitis media with effusion was not caused by the administration of immunosuppressive substance into the middle ear alone. When it was administered to rats in which otitis media with effusion had been induced by the injection of formalin killed *H. influenzae*, no effusion was found, but there were indications that histologic changes might persist. This may be explained by the prolongation of the inflammatory responses because of the various immunosuppressive activities of immunosuppressive substance. Another possible cause is delayed clearance of the endotoxin of *H. influenzae*. It has been reported that immunosuppressive substance influences IL_2 and PGE production by macrophages. Thus one may suppose that it may suppress phagocytosis and affect macrophages and neutrophils to delay the clearance of endotoxin. This may account for the widespread histologic changes.

We have not conducted any experiments on immunosuppressive acidic protein, but we assume that it has actions similar to those of immunosuppressive substance. These immunosuppressive substances may be one of the causes of the prolongation of otitis media with effusion.

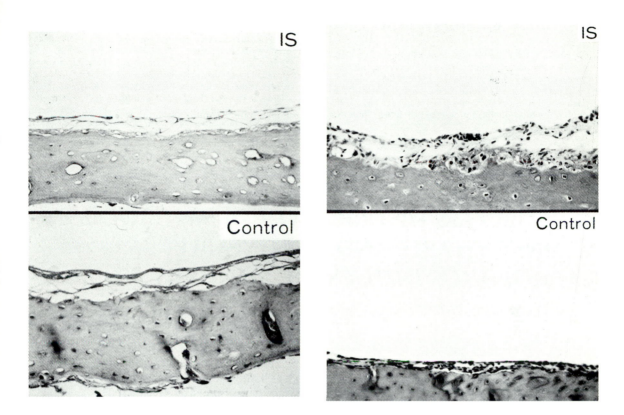

Figure 1 Three days after the administration of immunosuppressive substance. No effusion was found in the middle ear, and there were no significant differences in changes in the mucosa of the middle ear between the rats given immunosuppressive substance (IS) and those given physiologic saline (Control).

Figure 2 Two weeks after injection of formalin killed nontypable *H. influenzae*. Histologic changes stopped and features began to return to normal in the controls (Control), whereas in the rats treated with immunosuppressive substance (IS), edema was still present and the connective tissue was 25 μm or more in thickness in all rats.

1 . Control Group

(14 rats)

Sacrificed day	0	3	7	14	21	28	35
Effusion		2/2	0/2	0/2	0/3	0/3	0/2
Histological change of mucous membrane		2/2	2/2	1/2	1/3	0/3	0/2

2 . IS Group

(18 rats)

Sacrificed day	0	3	7	14	21	28	35
Effusion		2/2	0/2	0/4	0/4	0/4	0/2
Histological change of mucous membrane		2/2	2/2	4/4	3/4	4/4	1/2

Figure 3 Results of immunosuppressive substance (IS) treatment using nonviable *H. influenzae* induced models with otitis media with effusion. When the connective tissue was 25 μm or more in thickness, histologic change was regarded as positive.

REFERENCES

1. Yamanaka T, Bernstein TB, et al. Immunologic aspects of otitis media with effusion: characteristics of lymphocyte and macrophage activity. J Infect Dis 1982; 145:804–810.
2. Yamanaka T, Cumella T, et al. Immunologic aspects of otitis media with effusion. II. Nature of cell-mediated immunosuppressive activity in middle ear fluid. J Infect Dis 1983; 147:794–799.
3. Fujii M, et al. Purification and characterization of immunosuppressive (IS) substance obtained from ascitic fluids of patients with gastrointestinal cancer. Clin Biochem 1987; 20:183–189.
4. Tamura K, Ishida N, et al. Isolation and characterization of an immunosuppressive acidic protein from ascitic fluids of cancer patients. Can Res 1981; 41:3244–3252.
5. DeMaria TF, et al. Experimental otitis media with effusion following middle ear inoculation of nonviable H. influenzae. Ann Otol Rhinol Laryngol 1984; 93:93–100.

IGG SUBCLASS DISTRIBUTION OF ANTIBODIES AGAINST TYPABLE AND NONTYPABLE *HAEMOPHILUS INFLUENZAE* ANTIGENS

BRITTA RYNNEL-DAGÖÖ, M.D., Ph.D. and ANDERS FREIJD, M.D.

H. influenzae is one of the dominating pathogens in early childhood during the period of physiologic hypogammaglobulinemia. Capsulated strains of *H. influenzae* type b give rise to invasive infections, whereas nontypable strains are a common cause of acute otitis media and sinusitis.

Investigations of host resistance to *H. influenzae* type b disease have shown that anticapsular antibodies are important in the protection against such infections.[1] Shurin and co-workers[2] have demonstrated that otitis media due to nontypable *H. influenzae* induced a systemic antibody response and that absence of antibody in serum was associated with susceptibility to infection.

Outer membrane proteins and lipopolysaccharides are the dominant noncapsular antigens on the *H. influenzae* surface and have been prepared from both typable and nontypable strains.[3,4] Preparations of *H. influenzae* type b capsule as well as outer membrane proteins and lipopolysaccharides from typable and nontypable strains were used for the detection of humoral antibodies of the four IgG subclasses in healthy individuals of various age groups and in otitis prone children.

MATERIAL AND METHODS

Patients

Plasma samples were collected from healthy children of various ages and from adults, as well as from children participating in a prospective study of healthy and otitis prone children.[5]

Antigens

Tyraminated *H. influenzae* type b capsular polysaccharide was obtained from Dr. R. A. Insel, Department of Pediatrics, University of Rochester, School of Medicine, New York. Outer membrane proteins and lipopolysaccharides from *H. influenzae* strain Eagan were obtained from Dr. Ian Allan, Oxford. Outer membrane proteins and lipopolysaccharides from nontypable *H. influenzae* were obtained from Dr. Loek van Alphen, Amsterdam.

Enzyme Linked Immunosorbent Assay (ELISA)

The ELISA was performed as described previously, using monoclonal subclass antibodies.[6]

RESULTS

Specific Antibody Activity Against *H. influenzae* Type b Polysaccharide

In children and in adults a substantial amount of the activity was of the IgG_1 subclass, which often dominated IgG$_2$ activity. No clear age dependent differences in activity were seen.

Specific Antibody Activity Against *H. influenzae* Outer Membrane Proteins in Healthy Donors of Different Age Groups and in Healthy and Otitis Prone Children

Antibody activity of the IgG$_1$ subclass resembled the pattern of total IgG. It was high neonatally, declined at 6 to 12 months of age, and increased to adult levels in the age group 3 to 6 years. Antibody activity of the IgG$_2$ subclass was lacking in small children. Some activity was seen in older age groups.

Figure 1 shows the specific antibody activity of IgG subclasses 1 and 3 in otitis prone children and age matched controls at 12 months of age. No significant differences were observed between the age groups.

Specific Antibody Activity Against *H. influenzae* Lipopolysaccharides

Antibody activity was derived mainly from the IgG$_1$ and IgG$_3$ subclasses but also was exhibited

by IgG$_2$. The activity was significantly higher in infants than in adults. No difference between healthy and otitis prone children was seen. Outer membrane protein and lipopolysaccharide preparations from typable and nontypable strains were tested and the patterns were the same.

DISCUSSION

Since the early work of Yount and co-workers[7] in 1968, antibodies against polysaccharides have been claimed to be mainly of the IgG$_2$ subclass. The poor response to bacterial polysaccharide antigens in early childhood both to natural infection and to vaccination has been explained by the slow maturation of the IgG$_2$ subclass compared to the earlier maturation of the IgG$_1$ subclass. Antibodies against the *H. influenzae* capsule were found to be mainly of the IgG$_2$ subclass.[8]

However, our study shows that a substantial amount of the activity against the *H. influenzae* polysaccharide is of the IgG$_1$ subclass, and this finding is in accordance with a report of an extensive investigation recently published by Shackelford and co-workers.[9]

H. influenzae lipopolysaccharide induces mainly IgG$_1$ and IgG$_3$ activity, which is greater in infants than in adults. This subclass restriction has not

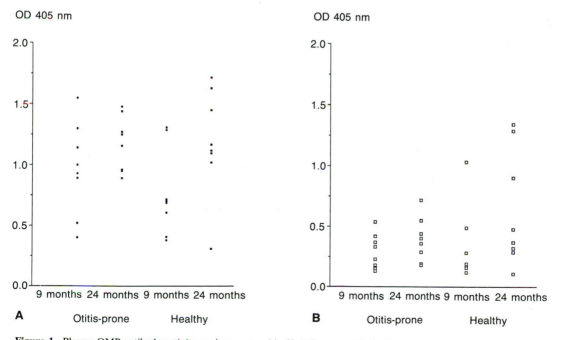

Figure 1 Plasma OMP antibody activity against nontypable *H. influenzae* of IgG subclasses expressed as optical density. *A*, IgG$_1$ and *B*, IgG$_3$ subclass determinations in healthy and otitis prone children 9 and 24 months of age.

been demonstrated before and is the same as for lipopolysaccharides from *Salmonella* whereas *Shigella* lipopolysaccharide antibodies are of the IgG_2 subclass.

Antibody activity against outer membrane proteins from both typable and nontypable strains are mainly of the IgG_1 subclass and show an age dependent pattern, reaching adult levels at 3 to 6 years of age. There is no difference in regard to antibody levels between otitis prone and healthy children. This is in contrast with our earlier findings. Significantly lower levels of specific antibody activity against *S. pneumoniae* type 6A of both the IgG_1 and IgG_2 subclasses were found in the otitis prone children.[10]

The different patterns of outer membrane protein and lipopolysaccharide antibody activity, especially in adults, might reflect differences in the protective role of antibodies against these antigens.

The present study indicates that a good response to *H. influenzae* outer membrane proteins and lipopolysaccharides also occurs in otitis prone children. However, outer membrane proteins from non-capsulated strains are highly heterogeneous in regard to protein composition. Preparations of outer membrane proteins consist of at least six proteins, several of which have been characterized in regard to molecular weight and protective efficiency. Such preparations have to be further studied in order to elucidate the mechanism of regulation of antibody response of the IgG_1 subclass in infection prone individuals.

This study was supported by grants from The Swedish Medical Research Council (B89–17K–06257–01) and Swedish Society for Medical Sciences (134).

REFERENCES

1. Andersson P, Smith DH, Ingram DL, Wilkins J, Wehrle P, Howie VM. Antibody to polyribophosphate of *Haemophilus influenzae* type b in infants and children: effect of immunization with polyribophosphates. J Infect Dis 1977; 136:857–862.
2. Shurin PA, Pelton SI, Tager IB, Kasper DL. Bactericidal antibody and susceptibility to otitis media caused by nontypable strains of *Haemophilus influenzae*. J Pediatr 1980; 97:364–369.
3. Loeb MR, Smith DA. Outer membrane protein composition in disease isolates of *Haemophilus influenzae*: pathogenic and epidemiological implications. Infect Immun 1980; 30:709–717.
4. Flesher AR, Insel RA. Characterization of lipopolysaccharide of *Haemophilus influenzae*. J Infect Dis 1978; 138:719–730.
5. Freijd A, Oxelius V-A, Rynnel-Dagöö B. A prospective study demonstrating an association between plasma IgG_2 concentrations and susceptibility to otitis media in children. Scand J Infect Dis 1985; 17:115–120.
6. Persson MAA, Hammarström L, Smith CIE. Enzyme-linked immunosorbent assay for subclass distribution of human IgG and IgA antigen-specific antibodies. J Immunol Methods 1985; 78:109–121.
7. Yount WJ, Doyner MM, Kunkel HG, Kabat EA. Studies on human antibodies. VI. Selective variations in subgroup composition and genetic markers. J Exp Med 1968; 127:633–646.
8. Johnston RB, Andersson P, Rosen S, Smith DH. Characterization of human antibody to polyribophosphate, the capsular antigen of *Haemophilus influenzae* type b. Clin Immunol Immunopathol 1973; 1:234–240.
9. Shackelford PG, Granoff DM, Nelson SJ, Scott MG, Smith DS, Nahm MH. Subclass distribution of human antibodies to *Haemophilus influenzae* type b polysaccharide. J Immunol 1987; 138:587–592.
10. Freijd A, Hammarström L, Persson M, Smith E. Plasma anti-pneumococcal antibody activity of the IgG class and subclasses in otitis-prone children. Clin Exp Immunol 1984; 56:233–238.

SPECIFIC ANTIBODY LEVELS IN OTITIS PRONE CHILDREN: SUBCLASS RESTRICTION OF PNEUMOCOCCAL POLYSACCHARIDE AND PHOSPHORYLCHOLINE ANTIBODIES

ANDERS FREIJD, M.D. and BRITTA RYNNEL-DAGÖÖ, M.D., Ph.D.

The peak incidence of otitis proneness, coinciding with physiologic hypogammaglobulinemia, raises the hypothesis that an immunologic deficiency is of pathogenic importance in otitis media. In collaboration with Dr. Vivianne Oxelius, Lund,

Sweden,[1] we showed that a group of heavily otitis prone children, prospectively monitored after the first episode of otitis media, had significantly lower levels of the IgG_2 subclass than those in a healthy age matched group of children. Yount and co-workers[2] described an association between the IgG_2 type of antibody and antibodies to certain polysaccharides. Siber and co-workers[3] found a correlation between serum IgG_2 levels and the capacity to respond to a pneumococcal polysaccharide vaccine. These findings thus could form a basis for the concept that otitis proneness could be due to an unresponsiveness to polysaccharide antigens. To further explore this hypothesis, specific antibody levels to a number of pneumococcal polysaccharides as well as the small carbohydrate molecule phosphorylcholine were determined in the sera from children with otitis media.

MATERIAL AND METHODS

Patients

Of 150 children who had had at least one episode of otitis media before 1 year of age and who had been monitored prospectively up to 48 months of age, 15 were selected as being highly otitis prone (eight to 17 episodes) and 15 were considered to be healthy controls (one to two episodes).

Plasma specimens collected at various ages and kept at $-70°$ C were analyzed as well as samples from healthy adults.

Methods

A subclass specific ELISA utilizing monoclonal mouse antihuman subclass sera was used. This method has been described in detail elsewhere.[4]

Antigens

Phosphorylcholine (Sigma) was coupled to human serum albumin to make it adhere to the plastic surface. Pneumococcal polysaccharide antigens were obtained through the kindness of Smith, Kline & French Laboratories and their purity with regard to C polysaccharide was analyzed by nuclear mass resonance (NMR) spectrum analysis.

RESULTS

Antibody activity toward pneumococcal serotypes 3, 6, and 23 was analyzed. Analysis of IgG activity showed the same pattern for the two groups of children as well as for the healthy adults (that is, otitis prone children, healthy children, and adults; Fig. 1A). The IgG_2 analysis disclosed significant differences between the two groups of children only for type 6A. IgG_1 activity was generally higher in

children than in adults (Fig. 1B). Thus for these polysaccharides the majority of antibodies seem to be of the IgG_2 type, since the IgG_2 distribution among the patient groups investigated resembled that of IgG.

Antibody activity against phosphorylcholine of the IgG isotype was at almost the same level in all groups (Fig. 2). However, the distribution of the IgG_1 values resembled that for the pneumococcal polysaccharides, and there was no difference in IgG_2 levels between the two groups of children, the levels in the adults being slightly higher.

The dependence of the subclass pattern on age was further investigated in healthy children of various ages.[5] The IgG_1 antitype 6A levels were high in 12 month old children and then subsequently declined. IgG_2 levels were high in cord blood, reflecting maternal antibodies, declining during childhood and rising in school and preschool children.

In collaboration with Dr. K. Prellner, Lund, Sweden, the subclass pattern after pneumococcal vaccination was investigated in healthy individuals of various ages. The number of patients responding to vaccination increased with age, and in both older children and adults the response consisted mainly of an increase in the IgG_1 levels (data not shown).[6]

DISCUSSION

Analysis of the plasma activity levels (assayed by ELISA) of various pneumococcal polysaccharide antigens commonly found in association with otitis media showed different degrees of correlation with the otitis prone condition. The highest correlation was obtained with serotype 6A, one of the most common pneumococcal isolates in otitis media. The immunogenicity of this antigen is considered to be poor in vitro as well as in vivo.

Antibody activity against the small hapten sized carbohydrate molecule phosphorylcholine has been extensively studied in mouse protection systems, and such antibodies induce protection against pneumococcal infections in mice.[7] It has been proposed that IgG antiphosphorylcholine antibodies belong to the IgG_2 subclass in man,[8] and it has been established that the mice germ line genome contains the genetic code for antibodies phosphorylcholine. These findings indicate that antiphosphorylcholine immunocompetence is a basic requirement for integrity of the organism. Since phosphorylcholine is included in the pneumococcal C polysaccharide cell wall antigen and is common for all serotypes, the purpose of this study was to investigate whether anti-

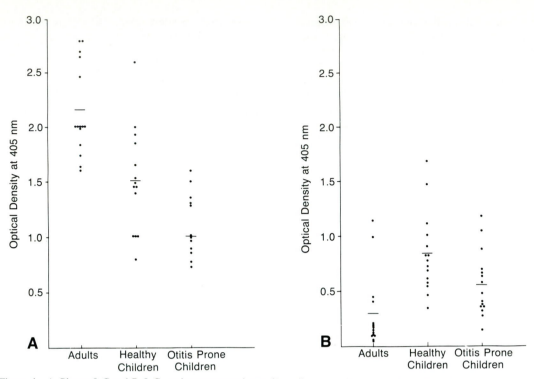

Figure 1 *A*, Plasma IgG and *B*, IgG_1 antipneumococcal type 6A antibody activity expressed as optical density in healthy and otitis prone children at 32 months of age and in adults.

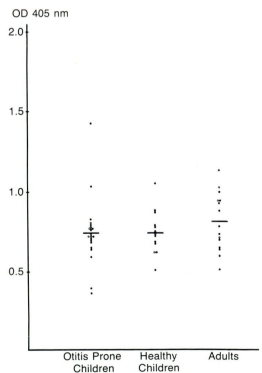

Figure 2 Plasma IgG antiphosphorylcholine antibody activity in healthy and otitis prone children at 23 months of age and in adults, expressed as optical density.

phosphorylcholine deficiency is a common denominator in the infectious prone state. This was not found to be the case. We observed the same IgG antiphosphorylcholine levels in adults and in small children. This finding shows that antiphosphorylcholine antibody activity is not subject to the same age dependence found, for example, with pneumococcal polysaccharide antigens.[9]

The data of this study demonstrate a shift in the age group 7 to 15 years of the IgG subclass pattern from a higher IgG_1 level than IgG_2 level in childhood, to an adult pattern with a higher level of IgG_2 than of IgG_1. This shift occurs too late to be linked to the decrease in the infection prone condition generally seen at 3 to 4 years of age.

Studies are in progress in order to improve the response after pneumococcal polysaccharide vaccination by coupling the polysaccharide molecules to a protein carrier, thus inducing a thymus dependent antibody response and a shift of the IgG_2 response to IgG_1. IgG_2 antibodies are believed to be less efficient than IgG_1 antibodies in activating antibacterial defense mechanisms. Our data, however, show that children as well as adults even without conjugated vaccines respond with IgG_1 antibody formation.

We do not believe that our earlier observation of low IgG_2 levels in otitis prone children gives a simple answer to the question why some children are susceptible to infections. More likely it reflects a wider although still undefined immunologic immaturity. To further complicate the picture, different polysaccharides induce different IgG subclass patterns, and since the age of the individual seems to be of importance, different immunization principles could be essential.

These studies were supported by grants from the Swedish Medical Research Council (B89=17K=06257=01) and the Swedish Society for Medical Sciences (134).

REFERENCES

1. Freijd A, Oxelius V-A, Rynnel-Dagöö B. A prospective study demonstrating an association between plasma IgG_2 concentration and susceptibility to otitis media in children. Scand J Infect Dis 1985; 17:115–120.
2. Yount W, Dorner M, Kunkel H, Kabat E. Studies on human antibodies. VI. Selective variations in subgroup composition and genetic markers. J Exp Med 1968; 127:633–646.
3. Siber G, Schur P, Aisenberg A, Weitzman S, Schiffman G. Correlation between serum IgG_2 concentration and the antibody response to bacterial polysaccharide antigens. N Engl J Med 1980; 303:178–182.
4. Persson MAA, Hammarström L, Smith CIE. Enzyme-linked immunosorbant assay for subclass distribution of human IgG and IgA antigen-specific antibodies. J Immunol Methods 1985; 78:109–121.
5. Rynnel-Dagöö B, Freijd A, Hammarström L, Oxelius V-A, Persson M, Smith C. Pneumococcal antibodies of different immunoglobulin subclasses in normal and immunodeficient individuals of various ages. Acta Otolaryngol 1986; 101: 146–151.
6. Rynnel-Dagöö B, Freijd A, Prellner K. Antibody activity of IgG subclasses against pneumococcal polysaccharide after vaccination. Am J Otolaryngol 1985; 6:275–279.
7. Briles D, et al. Antiphosphorylcholine antibodies found in normal mouse serum are protective against intravenous infection with type 3 *Streptococcus pneumoniae*. J Exp Med 1981; 153:694–705.
8. Brown B, Schiffman G, Rittenberg M. Subpopulations of antibodies to phosphorylcholine in human serum. J Immunol 1984; 132:1323–1328.
9. Freijd A, Hammarström L, Persson M, Smith C. Plasma antipneumococcal antibody levels of the IgG class and subclasses in otitis prone children. Clin Exp Immunol 1984; 56:233–238.

NEUTROPHIL FUNCTION IN OTITIS MEDIA WITH EFFUSION: A 1987 UPDATE

JOEL M. BERNSTEIN, M.D., Ph.D., ELINOR SCHOENFELD, Ph.D., LINDA MOORE, Ph.D., JAMES R. HUMBERT, M.D., ROBERT C. WELLIVER, M.D., LEONARD J. LASCOLEA, M.D., DIANE M. DRYJA, B.S., and PEARAY L. OGRA, M.D.

It is imperative to understand the functional characteristics of polymorphonuclear leukocytes in middle ear infections because the resolution of acute otitis media caused by both gram positive and gram negative organisms requires specific antibody, complement, and normal phagocytic cells. Furthermore, mechanisms that may be employed by the organism to counter host defenses must be considered. The purpose of this presentation is to review work from our laboratory concerning neutrophil function in both acute otitis media and otitis media with effusion.

MATERIALS AND METHODS

Oxygen Consumption of Middle Ear and Peripheral Blood Neutrophils in Suppurative Otitis Media

The population studied consisted of 15 children with symptomatic acute otitis media who had had the disease for 24 to 72 hours. None of the children was taking antibiotics at the time of tympanocentesis. The neutrophil counts in the peripheral blood samples were adjusted as closely as possible to the neutrophil counts in the ear fluid samples, a problem that was not addressed in our previous communication.[1] Oxygen consumption was measured by means of a Clark oxygen electrode as described by Nakamura et al[2] by using a standard 2 ml water jacketed cell with the reagent volumes adjusted proportionately. Phagocyte connected oxygen consumption was induced by the addition of opsonized zymosan particles. The resting state oxygen consumption and the stimulated oxygen consumption values were expressed as nmols of oxygen per minute per 10^6 neutrophils. In all experiments results were calculated at $37°$ and $40°$ C. Results were analyzed statistically by the Student's t test.

Phagocytosis and Killing of *Candida Albicans* and *Staphylococcus Aureus* by Middle Ear and Peripheral Blood Neutrophils in Otitis Media with Effusion

Forty-eight children whose ages ranged from 10 months to 15 years were studied. Specimens of middle ear effusions were obtained by tympanocentesis. Nasopharyngeal swabs were used to collect viral and bacterial specimens. In addition, middle ear supernatants were analyzed for viral antigen using an ELISA technique. In this study viruses were isolated in six of 48 cases, or 12.5 percent of the population studied. The distribution of bacterial isolates from the middle ear were as follows: *Streptococcus pneumoniae*, 6; nontypable *Haemophilus influenzae*, 11; *Staphylococcus aureus*, 5; coagulase negative *Staphylococcus*, 12; and *Branhamella catarrhalis*, 3. The nasopharyngeal flora included *S. pneumoniae*, 13; nontypable *Haemophilus influenzae*, 26; beta hemolytic Streptococcus, 4; *S. aureus*, 17; and coagulase negative Staphylococcus, 2.

The correlation between nasopharyngeal and middle ear bacteria and viruses and blood neutrophil and middle ear function was assessed. Phagocytosis was assessed using the acridine orange supravital stain technique of Pantazis and Kniker.[3] Blood and ear samples were collected at the time of the tympanostomy procedure, and the phagocytic cells were deposited on glass cover-slips of monolayer preparations. The technique of adding acridine orange and enumerating the bacteria under fluorescence microscopy has been described previously.[4]

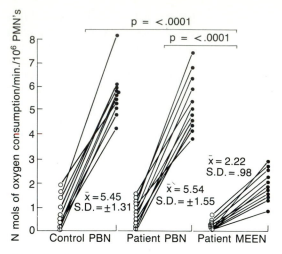

Figure 1 Oxygen consumption in peripheral blood neutrophils PBN and middle ear effusion neutrophils (MEEN) in acute suppurative otitis media. There is a significant depression of oxygen consumption by middle ear neutrophils. ○ = baseline oxygen consumption at 37° C. ● = oxygen consumption 60 minutes after activation with zymosan.

RESULTS

Figure 1 summarizes the findings from the oxygen consumption assay. The oxygen consumption of middle ear neutrophils was significantly less (p < 0.001) in both the corresponding peripheral blood neutrophils and the controlled peripheral blood neutrophils. Middle ear neutrophil oxygen consumption for opsonized zymosan was found to be less than 50 percent of the oxygen consumption of peripheral blood neutrophils from the same patient. Furthermore, as seen in Figure 2, oxygen consumption when assessed at 40° C always disclosed an increase in oxygen consumption by the peripheral blood neutrophils. However, middle ear neutrophils never consumed more oxygen at 40° C. In general, middle ear fluid neutrophils consumed less oxygen at 40° C, a temperature that has been found to accelerate oxygen consumption.[5]

These results suggest that the middle ear neutrophils are metabolically active, but when placed in an in vitro assay are not capable of utilizing oxygen as well as the resting neutrophil characterized by polymorphonuclear leukocytes in the peripheral blood. Therefore, even though oxygen consumption by middle ear neutrophils is significantly less than that in the corresponding peripheral blood neutro-

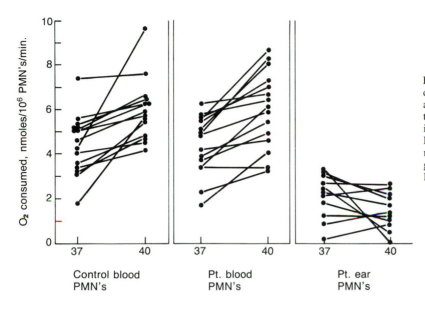

Figure 2 This figure demonstrates the difference between oxygen consumption at 37° and 40° C. In general, there is a trend for increased oxygen consumption in peripheral blood neutrophils at 40° C. However, middle ear fluid neutrophils rarely perform better at 40° C and, in general, perform poorly. Pt.=Patient; PMN=Polymorphonuclear leukocyte.

phils, the question arises whether this decrease could have an effect on the capacity of the middle ear neutrophils to phagocytose and kill a target organism.

To address this question we studied the phagocytosis and killing properties of middle ear and peripheral blood neutrophils in different middle ear effusions as they relate to both bacterial and viral flora in the nasopharynx and the middle ear effusion. Despite the decreased oxygen consumption seen in middle ear fluid neutrophils in acute suppurative otitis media, phagocytosis and killing by middle ear fluid neutrophils in otitis media with effusion are as good as that by the corresponding peripheral blood neutrophils when using *C. albicans* or *S. aureus* 502A as the target organism. The relationship between the bacteria flora in the nasopharynx and phagocytosis and killing of opsonized *C. albicans* is reviewed in Tables 1 and 2. Table 1 summarizes the relationship between phago-

cytosis and killing by peripheral blood neutrophils as related to nasopharyngeal bacteria. In general, there is no significant difference in peripheral blood neutrophil function as related to nasopharyngeal bacterial flora. Table 2 summarizes the relationship of middle ear effusion neutrophil function to nasopharyngeal flora. In general, there is no significant relationship of neutrophil function to nasopharyngeal flora.

Phagocytosis is an oxygen independent mechanism, and it is interesting that there is little difference in phagocytosis and killing in between middle ear neutrophils and peripheral blood neutrophils. There is also no relationship between neutrophil function and the nasopharyngeal bacterial flora. However, the relationship of the middle ear fluid bacterial flora to neutrophil middle ear function suggests a depression of phagocytosis and killing when nontypable *H. influenzae* and *B. catarrhalis* are present. There is a statistically significant depression of neutrophil

TABLE 1 Relationship of Phagocytosis and Killing by Peripheral Blood Neutrophils and Nasopharyngeal Bacteria

	S. Pneumoniae (n=13)	H. Influenzae (n=26)	Beta Hemolytic Streptococcus (n=4)	S. aureus (n=17)	Coag. Neg. Staph. (n=2)
Neutrophil phagocytosis	237±104	239±103	192±34	223±87	335±176
Neutrophil killing	113±60	113±78	86±44	112±65	182±88

TABLE 2 Relationship of Middle Ear Effusion Neutrophil Function to Nasopharyngeal Flora

	S. Pneumoniae (n=13)	H. Influenzae (n=26)	Beta Hemolytic Streptococcus (n=4)	S. aureus (n=17)	Coag. Neg. Staph. (n=2)
Neutrophil phagocytosis	216±73	203±96	180±63	226±95	270±127
Neutrophil killing	110±53	100±54	81±30	112±51	98±40

phagocytosis and killing from middle ear neutrophils when these gram negative bacilla are isolated from the middle ear fluid. Table 3 demonstrates the relationship of middle ear effusion neutrophil function to middle ear bacteria. In general, there is a significant difference between the capacity of middle ear neutrophils to phagocytose and kill when *H. influenzae* and *B. catarrhalis* are present, suggesting the possible release of local mediators that depress neutrophil function in the middle ear when these gram negative bacteria are present. Table 4 tabulates the results of neutrophil function in the peripheral blood and middle ear when virus is present in either the nasopharynx or the middle ear. There does not appear to be any significant difference between blood and ear neutrophil function regardless of whether virus is present or absent.

DISCUSSION

Previous investigations of the role of neutrophil function in otitis media have consistently suggested that neutrophil function is defective in this disease. However, less than 25 percent of children have this problem.[6] Furthermore, all these studies have been performed with in vitro techniques. Therefore, it is difficult to determine whether there is truly a defect intrinsic to the phagocyte or whether the phagocyte has been metabolically fatigued when tested in an in vitro assay.

As a result of our studies of neutrophil function, we suggest that although oxygen consumption by middle ear effusion neutrophils in acute suppurative otitis media is depressed, the middle ear neutrophil as well as the peripheral blood neutrophil still

TABLE 3 Relationship of Middle Ear Effusion Neutrophil Function to Middle Ear Bacteria

	S. Pneumoniae (n=6)	H. Influenzae (n=11)	S. aureus (n=5)	Coag. Neg. Staph. (n=12)	B. Catarrhalis (n=3)
Neutrophil phagocytosis	313±109	172±70	246±100	245±92	162±39
	⌐——p<0.001——⌐				
Neutrophil killing	148±45	84±36	134±69	118±71	81±30
	⌐——p<0.001——⌐				

TABLE 4 Neutrophil Function in Blood and Middle Ear Effusion

	Blood	Ear (n=48)	Virus Present Blood	Ear (n=6)
Neutrophil phagocytosis*	219±95	201±92	209±31	189±87
Neutrophil killing	108±65	97±49	93±20	88±43

* Number of *Candida albicans* organisms per 100 neutrophils.

has significant reserve capacity to phagocytose and kill when *S. aureus* 502A or *C. albicans* is used as the target organism. Whether the middle ear effusion neutrophil can function as well against *S. pneumoniae* or nontypable *H. influenzae* is not known at this time.

Whereas the oxygen consumption of the peripheral blood neutrophil always increases at 40° C, the middle ear neutrophil does not appear to perform better at this temperature. This finding also suggests that the middle ear neutrophil is not defective, but more likely is metabolically exhausted.

REFERENCES

1. Bernstein JM, Humbert JR, Hliwa MM. Oxygen consumption of middle ear and peripheral blood neutrophils in acute suppurative otitis media. Am J Otolaryngol 1985; 6:169–172.
2. Nakamura M, Nakamura MA, Wanai M. Polorographic micromethods for the rapid assay of phagocytosis-connected oxygen consumption by leukocytes in diluted peripheral blood. J Lab Clin Med 1981; 97:31–38.
3. Pantazis CG, Kniker WT. Assessment of blood leukocyte microbial killing using a new fluorochrome microassay. J Reticuloendothel Soc 1979; 23:155.
4. Bernstein JM, Moore LL, Ogra PL. Defective phagocytic and antibacterial activity of middle ear neutrophils. In: Lim DJ, Bluestone CD, Klein JO, Nelson JD, eds. Recent advances in otitis media with effusion. Proceedings of the Third International Symposium. Toronto: BC Decker, 1984:129–131.
5. Van Oss CJ, Absolom DR, Moore LL, et al. Effects of temperature on the chemotaxis, phagocytic engulfment, digestion and oxygen consumption of human polymorphonuclear leukocytes. J Reticuloendothel Soc 1980; 27:561–565.
6. Giebink GS, Payne EE, Mills EL, et al. Experimental otitis media due to *Streptococcus pneumoniae*: immunopathogenic response in the chinchilla. J Infect Dis 1976; 134:595–604.

PRESENCE OF SPECIFIC ANTIBODIES AGAINST OUTER MEMBRANE PROTEINS OF NONTYPABLE *HAEMOPHILUS INFLUENZAE* IN MIDDLE EAR EFFUSIONS: FUNCTIONAL AND ISOTYPIC CHARACTERISTICS

JOEL M. BERNSTEIN, M.D., Ph.D., MARK E. WILSON, Ph.D., TIMOTHY F. MURPHY, M.D., DIANE M. DRYJA, B.S., and PEARAY L. OGRA, M.D.

The recognition of nontypable *Haemophilus influenzae* as one of the predominant human pathogens in otitis media in children of all ages has stimulated interest in studying the pathogenesis and the immune response to this infection in both sera and middle ear effusions. There is increasing evidence that outer membrane proteins of nontypable *H. influenzae* may be targets for bactericidal antibodies.[1,2] Although there is great heterogeneity of outer membrane protein profiles among nontypable *H. influenzae,* there is some conservation of these proteins in all strains.[3] Therefore, antibody directed against outer membrane proteins that are conserved not only might be important in eradication of the existing middle ear infection with one species of nontypable *H. influenzae*, but also may be protective in a subsequent infection by another strain.

The purpose of this communication is to report a study of the presence of specific antibodies directed against outer membrane proteins of nontypable *H. influenzae* isolates from middle ear effusions and to describe their functional and isotypic characteristics.

MATERIALS AND METHODS

Bacteria

Isolates of nontypable *H. influenzae* were recovered from eight middle ear fluid specimens obtained by tympanocentesis in children with acute suppurative otitis media.

Outer Membrane Complex

The preparation of the outer membrane complex and separation of outer membrane proteins by the use of sodium dodecyl sulfate polyacrylamide gel electrophoresis and the use of Western blot assay for identification of specific antibody directed against these outer membrane proteins have been described previously.[2–4]

Dot Assay

The semiquantitative dot assay using nitrocellulose has also been previously described.[2]

Bactericidal Assay

Cultures of Nontypable *H. influenzae* were prepared in Mueller-Hinton broth and incubated overnight in 37° C incubators and supplemented with 5 percent carbon dioxide. Aliquots were diluted 1:100 in Gey's balanced salt solution, and 0.1 ml aliquots of adjusted bacterial suspension were transferred to sterile culture tubes containing variable amounts of 10 percent normal human serum, middle ear IgG, Gey's buffer alone, or normal human serum heat inactivated at 56° C for 30 minutes. Colony forming units were enumerated and expressed as the number of units per milliliter of reaction mixture.

RESULTS

Analyses of the serum sensitivity of nontypable *H. influenzae* clinical isolates from the eight middle ear strains and seven corresponding nasopharyngeal strains demonstrated that more than 90 percent killing occurred in 1 hour in five strains. Conversely, nine isolates were totally resistant to 10 percent pooled normal human sera. The pooled normal human sera consisted of six adult serum specimens, and all these sera demonstrated, by Western blot analysis, antibody against all outer membrane proteins. Thus, the pooled sera contained antibody to all outer membrane proteins, which apparently conveyed bactericidal antibody to serum sensitive strains but was not necessarily bactericidal for all strains of nontypable *H. influenzae*. This finding suggests the significant heterogeneity of different isolates of nontypable *H. influenzae* in human middle ear disease. When IgG from the patient's middle ear was added to the bactericidal assay, there was no evidence of blocking of the bactericidal killing of the serum sensitive strain, nor was there enhancement of killing with a serum resistant strain. Thus, in six middle ear fluid specimens tested in which the IgG fraction was isolated, this IgG fraction of middle ear fluid possessed neither blocking antibody nor specific bactericidal antibody.

Figure 1 summarizes the results of study of the serum sensitive strain 9274. Ten percent pooled normal human serum completely destroyed the organism within 10 minutes, whereas heated pooled serum allowed bacterial growth to flourish. This experiment suggests that antibody in addition to complement is necessary for bactericidal killing of nontypable *H. influenzae* in this assay system. Similarly, in Western blot analysis with the serum sensitive organism 9274, antibody of all isotypes was present in both the patient's serum and the patient's middle ear fluid, as seen in Figure 2. Nevertheless the organism was viable at the time of isolation. Furthermore, antibody as measured by the immunodot assay demonstrated that at the time of the first and second clinical infections with nontypable *H. influenzae*, specific IgG as well as specific IgA and IgM was present in the serum of the child. IgG was present in very high titers. Thus, even though there is specific antibody in high titers directed against all the outer membrane proteins, the patient develops acute suppurative otitis media. The Western blot analysis confirms the findings of the bactericidal assay in suggesting that the presence of specific antibody in serum or middle ear fluid directed against all outer membrane proteins does not necessarily convey functional antibacterial activity.

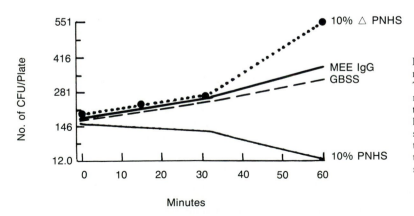

Figure 1 The serum sensitivity for nontypable *H. influenzae* 9274 is shown. Ten percent pooled normal human serum is capable of destroying this bacterial isolate within 60 minutes, whereas heat inactivated pooled normal human serum is unable to do this. Most important, middle ear fluid IgG cannot block the serum bactericidal activity against strain 9274.

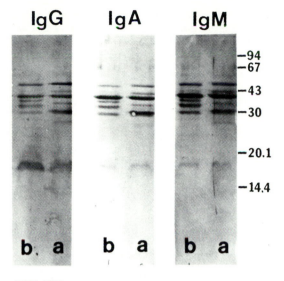

MEF 1/86

Figure 2   This figure represents a Western blot assay. Lane b represents an isolate of nontypable *H. influenzae* from a patient in May 1986. Lane a represents the outer membrane profile of the isolate in January 1986. There is antibody present against all outer membrane proteins for all immunoglobulin isotypes. The major outer membrane proteins consist of protein 1 at approximately 50,000 daltons, protein 2 at approximately 40,000 daltons, protein 4 at 30,000 daltons, and protein 6 at 16,600 daltons. At the time of the first infection, specific antibody directed against outer membrane proteins of the isolate that occurred 6 months later was already present in the sera. These findings strongly suggest that although antibody against outer membrane proteins may be present prior to an infection with an isolate of nontypable *H. influenzae*, these antibodies apparently may not be protective and cannot lead to resolution of the disease.

DISCUSSION

Previous studies in our laboratory have demonstrated that nontypable *H. influenzae* isolates from middle ear specimens in different patients have different outer membrane profiles, and that nontypable *H. influenzae* middle ear isolates from the same child but during different episodes of otitis media with nontypable *H. influenzae* have different outer membrane profiles.[5] We demonstrated this in five patients who had multiple recurrent episodes caused by nontypable *H. influenzae*. Furthermore, restriction endonuclease analysis of DNA of the bacterial genome was carried out in the same isolates, and as with outer membrane protein analysis, there was marked heterogeneity of the DNA in different isolates of nontypable *H. influenzae* from patient to patient and also from the same patient during different episodes.

The results of the present study suggest that a child may produce an adequate antibody response against all outer membrane proteins with the major immunoglobulin isotypes and yet the organism may survive. Therefore, despite adequate specific antibody levels directed against effective antigens, these antibodies are not capable of resolving the infection.

There are a number of theoretical reasons for this inadequate in vivo destruction of the bacteria. First, the antibody may be cytophilic for the organism and surround the bacteria and actually prevent bactericidal antibody from attaching to receptors of effective antigen. This mechanism is thought to play a role in other gram negative diseases, including infection by *Neisseria gonorrhoeae*, *Brucella abortus*, and chronic bronchitis from nontypable *H. influenzae*.[6-9] The results from our laboratory, however, cannot confirm that blocking IgG antibody exists in the middle ear. IgA would be a more logical candidate as a blocking antibody because it is antiopsonic and does not fix complement. Both mechanisms appear to be necessary for the effective killing of nontypable *H. influenzae*. Other possible reasons for the inability of outer membrane protein antibody to destroy the organism may be suggested. Antibody can be directed against the outer membrane protein but not against the effective epitope of that protein. Antibody may be directed against the correct epitope but may not present in amounts adequate to destroy the organism. Antibody may be directed against the effective epitope and be quantitatively sufficient, but the epitope may be hidden in the membrane of the bacterium. Neutrophil function may be defective and may be important in the resolution of the nontypable *H. influenzae* infection. Thus, specific antibody and complement as well as adequate neutrophil function may be necessary for the effective eradication of nontypable *H. influenzae* in otitis media. Unlike the situation in the experimental animal, in which passive immunization may protect an animal with the homologous organism,[10] the situation in human otitis media is far more complex because of the tremendous heterogeneity of different isolates of nontypable *H. influenzae* from patient to patient and in different episodes of otitis media in the same patient.

Study supported in part by NICHD grant HD19679.

REFERENCES

1.   Murphy TF, Bartos LC, Rice PA, et al. Identification of a 16,000-dalton outer membrane protein on nontypable *Hae-*

mophilus influenzae as a target for human serum bactericidal antibody. J Clin Invest 1986; 78:1020–1027.

2. Murphy TF, Bartos LC, Campagnari AA, et al. Antigenic characterization of the P6 protein of nontypable *Haemophilus influenzae*. Infect Immun 1986; 54:774–779.

3. Murphy TF, Nelson MB, Dudas KC, et al. Identification of a specific epitope of *Haemophilus influenzae* in a 16,600-dalton outer-membrane protein. J Infect Dis 1985; 152:1300–1307.

4. Murphy TF, Dudas KC, Mylotte JM, et al. A subtyping system for nontypable *Haemophilus influenzae* based on outer-membrane proteins. J Infect Dis 1983; 147:838–846.

5. Murphy TF, Bernstein JM, Dryja DM, et al. Outer membrane protein and lipooligosaccharide analysis of paired nasopharyngeal and middle ear isolates in otitis media due to nontypable *Haemophilus influenzae*. J Infect Dis 1987; 156:723–731.

6. Rice PA, Kasper DL. Characterization of serum resistance of *Neisseria gonorrhoeae* that disseminate. J Clin Invest 1982; 70:157–167.

7. McCutchan JA, Katzenstein D, Norquist D, et al. Role of blocking antibody in disseminated gonococcal infection. J Immunol 1978; 121:1884–1888.

8. Hall WH, Manion RE, Zinneman HH. Blocking serum lysis of *Brucella abortus* by hyperimmune rabbit immunoglobulin A. J Immunol 1971; 107:41–46.

9. Musher DM, Goree A, Baughn RE, Birdsdall HF. Immunoglobulin A from bronchopulmonary secretions blocks bactericidal and opsonizing effects of antibody to nontypable *Haemophilus influenzae*. Infect Immun 1984; 45:36–40.

10. Barenkamp SJ, Munson RS, Jr, Granoff DM. Outer membrane protein and biotype analysis of pathogenetic nontypable *Haemophilus influenzae*. Infect Immun 1985; 36:535–540.

PATHOGEN SPECIFIC ANTIBODIES IN THE MIDDLE EAR EFFUSION DURING THE EARLY PHASE OF ACUTE OTITIS MEDIA

PEKKA SIPILÄ, M.D., HEINO KARJALAINEN, M.D., MARKKU KOSKELA, M.D., and JUKKA LUOTONEN, M.D.

The main causative pathogenic bacteria in acute otitis media are *Streptococcus pneumoniae*, *Haemophilus influenzae* and *Branhamella catarrhalis*.[1] As a sign of the immune response, it has been reported that middle ear effusion usually contains immunoglobulins specific to these pathogens.[2–4] The nature of the immune response during acute otitis media, however, continues to be obscure, and the specificity of the humoral immune response against the pathogenic bacteria is poorly documented. The aim of this study was to characterize the immunoglobulin response specific to the pathogenic bacteria during the first 12 hours of disease.

MATERIAL AND METHODS

Eighty-two children with acute otitis media (37 males, 45 females) aged 2 months to 15 years (mean, 4 years 2 months) were included in this series. All the children had symptoms of acute otitis media, and the duration of the symptoms involving the ear at the time of the first visit did not exceed 12 hours. Patients with otitis media and those who had received antimicrobial therapy within the previous 3 months were excluded.

Serum and middle ear effusion antibodies specific to *S. pneumoniae*, *H. influenzae*, and *B. catarrhalis* were measured by enzyme linked immunosorbent assay (ELISA) as described earlier.[3–5] IgG, IgM, and IgA class antibody levels (except IgM for *B. catarrhalis*) were measured. Pneumococcal antibodies were determined against the capsular polysaccharide of the homologous serotype isolated from the corresponding middle ear effusion sample. If the bacterial culture yielded no pneumococci, the pneumococcal antibodies were measured against the type 3 capsular polysaccharide. Antibodies against *H. influenzae* and *B. catarrhalis* were measured against the whole bacterial cell antigen, as described earlier.[3] The specific antibodies were measured against all three pathogens from each sample, if the volume of the sample was sufficient.

RESULTS

We analyzed 102 middle ear effusion samples and 46 serum samples. In the bacterial cultures

S. pneumoniae was the main pathogen in 34 middle ear effusion samples, *H. influenzae* in 12, and *B. catarrhalis* in 8 samples. In 48 samples none of the aforementioned three pathogens could be detected.

Antibodies against at least one of the three pathogens were found in 57 (55.9 percent) of the 102 middle ear effusion samples and in 60.5 percent of the patients. Effusion antibodies against all the three bacteria were found in 17.3 percent of the patients, against two bacteria in 27.1 percent, and against one bacterium in 16.1 percent of the patients (Table 1). Antibodies were also detected in 20 (51.1 percent) of the 39 patients without any pathogens in bacterial cultures.

Table 2 shows the incidence of appearance of the specific antibodies against the three pathogens in the different effusion culture groups. Antibodies against *H. influenzae* and *B. catarrhalis* were found more frequently than those against *S. pneumoniae*. This difference may be due to the difference in the antigens used in the ELISA assay. All in all, antibodies specific to the different pathogens were detected with almost equal frequencies irrespective of the bacterial culture result. Even the effusions in which none of the pathogens could be cultured contained specific antibodies in about the same percentages as the culture positive effusions.

Both IgG and IgM class antibodies against *S. pneumoniae* were found in two effusions, only IgG in five effusions, and only IgM in 12 effusions. IgA class antibody to *S. pneumoniae* was found in one effusion. Antibodies against *H. influenzae* were of both IgG and IgA types in 33 effusions, only IgG in seven effusions, and IgA in 10 effusions. No IgM class antibodies could be found. Antibodies against *B. catarrhalis* were of the IgG and IgA types in 23 effusions, only IgG in two effusions, and only IgA in 19 effusions. IgM class antibodies were not determined, because they could not be found in the earlier study.[3]

There was a correlation between the serum titers and the effusion levels of the specific antibodies. Figure 1 shows the serum antibody titers and the effusion levels of the specific antibodies against *H. influenzae*. The antibody level in the effusion sample was considered negative at an absorbance value lower than 0.3, positive at an absorbance value of 0.3 to 0.5, and strongly positive at an absorbance value higher than 0.5. The patients whose sera revealed strongly positive absor-

TABLE 1 Incidence of Appearance of Specific Antibodies Against Three Pathogens in Middle Ear Effusion Compared with Culture Result

Pathogen in Middle Ear Effusion Culture	Patients with Antibodies Against			Patient with No Antibodies
	One Pathogen	Two Pathogens	Three Pathogens	
S. pneumoniae	5	8	6	8
H. influenzae	2	2	1	5
B. catarrhalis	1	2	2	0
No pathogens	5	10	5	19
Total	13 (16.1%)	22 (27.1%)	14 (17.3%)	32 (39.5%)

TABLE 2 Incidence of Appearance of Specific Antibodies Against Three Pathogens in Middle Ear Effusion Culture Groups

Pathogen in Middle Ear Effusion Culture	Number of Effusions (Percentages) with Antibodies Against			Number of Effusions with No Antibodies
	S. pneumoniae	*H. influenzae*	*B. catarrhalis*	
S. pneumoniae	10/34 (29.4%)*	14/31 (45.2%)	14/22 (63.3%)	15/34 (44.1%)
H. influenzae	1/7 (14.3%)+	5/12 (41.7%)	5/12 (41.7%)	5/12 (41.7%)
B. catarrhalis	4/4 (100%)+	4/7 (57.1%)	5/8 (62.5%)	1/8 (12.5%)
No pathogens	8/39 (20.5%)+	23/48 (47.9%)	16/48 (33.3%)	24/48 (50.0%)
Total	23/84 (27.4%)	46/98 (46.9%)	40/90 (44.4%)	45/102 (44.1%)

*Antibodies to capsular polysaccharide of homologous serotype found in the bacterial culture.
+Antibodies against type 3 capsular polysaccharide.

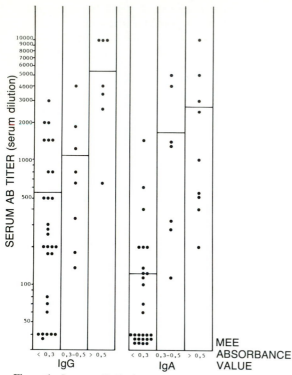

Figure 1 Serum antibody titers and middle ear effusion absorbance values of the antibodies against *Haemophilus influenzae.*

bance values against *H. influenzae* in the effusion had statistically significantly higher serum titers of both IgG and IgA class antibodies than the patients who did not have antibodies against *H. influenzae* in the middle ear effusion (p < 0.01 and p < 0.02, respectively). All the patients who had antibodies in the middle ear effusion had antibodies in the serum too. The same pattern was seen for the specific antibodies against *S. pneumoniae* and *B. catarrhalis.*

The appearance of the middle ear effusion antibodies was not related to the number of preceding attacks of acute otitis media nor was the appearance of the IgG class antibodies related to age. However, the IgA class antibodies against *H. influenzae* and *B. catarrhalis* in middle ear effusions appeared more frequently in older patients than in those who were 1 year old or younger.

DISCUSSION

In this series none of the patients had acute otitis media during a period of at least 3 months prior to the study. Therefore it can be postulated that the middle ear mucosa of the patients had no or only minimal pathologic changes. Normal middle ear mucosa is probably not an immunocompetent organ, because it contains only a few immunocompetent cells.[6] All the samples were taken within 12 hours after the beginning of the symptoms of acute otitis media. Accordingly the results of this study characterize the very early humoral immune response in acute otitis media.

The findings of the present study indicate that the humoral immune response in the very early phase of acute otitis media seems to occur quite extensively even against bacteria other than the causative pathogen, and antibodies specific to the pathogens can be found even in the effusions without any culturable pathogen. The antibodies in middle ear effusions in the early phase of acute otitis media are probably mainly transudates from the serum, because the middle ear effusion and serum levels of the specific antibodies correlated and the same antibody was found in the serum and the middle ear effusion at same time. It thus seems that the initial humoral immune response in acute otitis media is mediated by systemic immune mechanisms. The pathologic changes in the middle ear mucosa also support this idea. In purulent otitis media the main pathologic features are vasodilatation, extravasation, and edema in the subepithelial space.[6]

The antibody response in the effusions against *S. pneumoniae* was mediated mainly by IgG and IgM or both. IgA class antibodies were found in only one effusion. There were also no or very few IgA class antibodies against *S. pneumoniae* in the serum. In our earlier analysis, however, we found both serum type and secretory type IgA class antibodies in the middle ear effusion in the later phase of otitis media.[4] It therefore seems that the IgA response against *S. pneumoniae* develops more slowly during otitis media than the IgG and IgM responses and is mediated, at least partly, by local immune mechanisms. In this material the specific antibodies against *H. influenzae* and *B. catarrhalis* were IgG and IgA class antibodies, but in the earlier analysis we found IgM class antibodies in the later phase of otitis media.[7]

It has also been shown that lymphocytes, plasma cells, and macrophages appear in the subepithelial space in secretory otitis media.[6] According to these findings, it seems that systemically mediated humoral immune responses predominate in the early phase of otitis media and the middle ear mucosa matures immunologically during otitis media along with the development of the local immune mechanisms.

It should be noted that this material is part of a more extensive study, in which our purpose is to describe the natural immune response during otitis media. The findings in this series indicate that at the very early phase of acute otitis media, the initial humoral immune response seems to occur fairly extensively even against bacteria other than the causative pathogen. The humoral immune response is mediated mainly by systemic immune mechanisms.

REFERENCES

1. Luotonen J, Herva E, Karma P, Timonen M, Leinonen M, Mäkelä PH. The bacteriology of acute otitis media in children with special reference to *Streptococcus pneumoniae* as studied by bacteriological and antigen detection methods. Scand J Infect Dis 1981; 13:177–183.
2. Sloyer JL, Howie VM, Ploussard JH, Amman AJ, Austrian R, Johnston RB Jr. Immune response to acute otitis media in children. I. Serotypes isolated and serum and middle ear fluid antibody in pneumococcal otitis media. Infect Immun 1974; 9:1028–1032.
3. Leinonen M, Luotonen J, Herva E, Valkonen K, Mäkelä PH. Preliminary serologic evidence for a pathogenic role of *Branhamella catarrhalis*. J Infect Dis 1981; 144:570–574.
4. Luotonen JP, Koskela MJ, Karjalainen HK, Sipilä PT. Secretory IgA and pathogen specific secretory antibodies in the middle ear effusion in acute otitis media. In: Acute and secretory otitis media. Amsterdam: Kugler, 1986:217.
5. Koskela M, Luotonen J. Recurrent pneumococcal otitis media: presence of pneumococcal antigen and antibody in middle ear effusion compared with antibody levels in serum. In: Lim DJ, Bluestone CD, Klein JO, Nelson JD, eds. Recent Advances in otitis media with effusion. Proceedings of the Third International Symposium. Toronto: BC Decker, 1984:251.
6. Paparella MM, Sipilä PT, Juhn SK, Jung TTK. Subepithelial space in otitis media. Laryngoscope 1985; 95:414–420.
7. Sipilä P, Koskela M, Karjalainen H, Luotonen J. Secretory IgA, secretory component and pathogen specific antibodies in the middle ear effusion during an attack of acute and secretory otitis media. Auris Nasus Larynx 1985; 12 (Suppl 1):180–182.

ANTIBODY ACTIVITY AGAINST PNEUMOCOCCAL ANTIGENS AND THE LEVEL OF SERUM IgG SUBCLASS OF OTITIS MEDIA WITH EFFUSION

YOSHIHIRO DAKE, M.D., HIROMU KAKIUCHI, M.D., and TOSHIHIDE TABATA, M.D.

Bacterial infections play an important role in the etiology of otitis media with effusion, and *S. pneumoniae* has been identified as one of the major pathogens. Therefore examination of host defense mechanisms against this pathogen may help to understand the pathogenesis of this disorder as well as the mechanism involving its progression to the chronic stage. To study humoral immunity we measured *S. pneumoniae* specific antibodies and IgG subclass antibodies in the blood.

MATERIALS AND METHODS

The 46 patients selected for this study had chronic otitis media with effusion. There were 26 males and 20 females ranging in age from 1 to 12 years (mean, 6.5 years).

Pneumococcal antibody levels were measured by the ELISA technique. Pneumococcal capsular antigens were prepared as a solid layer in the microplate and then reacted with serum diluted 32-fold. After reaction with alkaline phosphatase-labeled goat antihuman IgG, IgM, and IgA antibodies (Miles Corporation), the preparations were stained with p-nitrophenyl phosphate. The reaction times were 20, 30, and 60 minutes for IgG, IgM, and IgA antibodies, respectively. The absorbance of these antibodies was measured at 405 nm. Eight types of pneumococcal capsular antigens, including the 23-valant vaccine Pneumovax and type 3, 6A, 6B, 9V, 19A, 19F, and 23F antigens were provided by the Merck Corporation. The IgG subclass in the blood was measured by radial immunodiffusion technique, using an immunoglobulin kit (Miles Corporation).

RESULTS

The IgG antibody reaction to pneumococcus was expressed as the absorbance at 405 nm, and a

tated the same proteins as the unabsorbed convalescent sample, reassuring us that the proteins were not being coprecipitated with LPS by anti-LPS antibodies, as has been reported previously for certain proteins closely associated with LPS in the bacterial membrane.

Shown in lanes 5–7 are the results of an assay of samples from a second patient. The acute serum sample (lane 6) does precipitate a few proteins. The convalescent sample (lane 7) again shows substantial increases in activity directed primarily against two high molecular weight proteins. The results demonstrated by these two patients are representative of those observed with the other six patients. Acute phase serum samples generally precipitated few proteins, whereas the convalescent samples demonstrated substantial increases in activity, most often directed against one or more proteins with apparent molecular weights of 100kDa or greater.

DISCUSSION

Our investigation has focused on antibodies present in the serum of patients with nontypable Haemophilus otitis media. In young children the absence of serum bactericidal activity has been associated with susceptibility to Haemophilus otitis.[4] Whether serum antibodies have a direct role in protection of the host against nontypable Haemophilus otitis is unclear. Organisms present in mucosal surface infections such as otitis media may not be accessible to antibodies present in the serum. However, pathogen specific antibodies of the IgG, IgM, and IgA classes have been demonstrated in middle ear fluid collected during the course of Haemophilus otitis media.[1] This suggests that some local transudation of serum antibodies occurs in the course of the disease. Furthermore, in an animal model of infection, passive immunization with immune serum was capable of preventing experimentally induced nontypable Haemophilus otitis.[9] Thus it is conceivable that serum antibodies have a direct role in protecting the host against Haemophilus otitis media.

Antibodies likely to be important in a protective host immune response will probably be directed against antigens that are exposed on the bacterial surface. We focused our investigation on two major classes of surface exposed antigens of nontypable *Haemophilus influenzae*—lipopolysaccharide and outer membrane proteins. Previous work suggested that nontypable Haemophilus outer membrane proteins are the principal targets of naturally occurring bactericidal antibodies.[10] In our investigation removal of anti-LPS antibodies from convalescent

sera led to a decrease in bactericidal activity in three of our eight patients, and purified anti-LPS antibodies were bactericidal in two instances. However, substantial bactericidal activity remained in all samples. Thus our results are consistent with the earlier observations and suggest that non-LPS determinants, possibly outer membrane proteins, may be the principal targets of bactericidal antibody in serum samples of children convalescing from nontypable Haemophilus otitis media.

Identification of specific outer membrane proteins that are immunogenic in the course of infection and that are accessible to antibody may allow one to predict which proteins are targets of bactericidal antibody. To identify such proteins, we made use of the whole cell radioimmunoprecipitation assay. One or several minor outer membrane proteins with molecular weights of 100kDa or greater appeared to be the principal proteins against which substantial increases in antibody were noted in convalescent sera. These findings are similar to those previously reported on children recovering from invasive type b Haemophilus disease in whom high molecular weight minor outer membrane proteins were found to be major targets of antibody in convalescent sera.[11] Although we did not demonstrate directly that antibodies directed against these high molecular weight proteins were bactericidal, further studies of these proteins would seem to be warranted on the basis of these results.

This study was supported in part by grant RO1 AI21707 from the National Institute of Allergy and Infectious Diseases and by grant 2796–4 from the Thrasher Research Fund.

REFERENCES

1. Sloyer JL Jr, Cate CC, Howie VM, Ploussard JH, Johnston RB Jr. The immune response to acute otitis media in children. II. Serum and middle ear fluid antibody in otitis media due to *Haemophilus influenzae*. J Infect Dis 1975; 132:685–688.
2. Bjuggren G, Tunevall G. Otitis in childhood: a clinical and serobacteriological study with special reference to the significance of *Haemophilus influenzae* in relapses. Acta Otolaryngol 1952; 42:311–328.
3. Branefors-Helander P, Nylen O, Jeppson PH. Acute otitis media: assay of complement-fixing antibody against *Haemophilus influenzae* as a diagnostic tool in acute otitis media. Acta Pathol Microbiol Scand (Sect B) 1973; 81:508–518.
4. Shurin PA, Pelton SI, Tager IB, Kasper DL. Bactericidal antibody and susceptibility to otitis media caused by nontypable strains of *Haemophilus influenzae*. J Pediatr 1980; 97:364–369.
5. Sloyer JL Jr, Howie VM, Ploussard JH, Schiffman G, Johnston RB Jr. Immune response to acute otitis media: association between middle ear fluid antibody and the clearing of clinical infection. J Clin Microbiol 1976; 4:306–308.

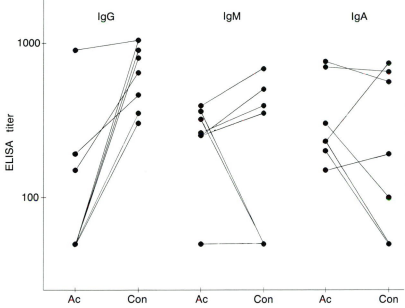

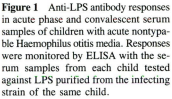

Figure 1 Anti-LPS antibody responses in acute phase and convalescent serum samples of children with acute nontypable Haemophilus otitis media. Responses were monitored by ELISA with the serum samples from each child tested against LPS purified from the infecting strain of the same child.

ies were recovered from the affinity columns and were also monitored for activity in the bactericidal assay. The LPS-absorbed convalescent samples had the same bactericidal titers as the original samples in most instances (see Table 1). In three cases two- to fourfold decreases in activity were noted. The affinity purified anti-LPS antibodies had no bactericidal activity against the majority of strains. Two anti-LPS preparations, derived from convalescent samples that demonstrated decreases in bactericidal activity following LPS absorption, did have demonstrable activity.

Antibody Against Surface Exposed Outer Membrane Proteins

The presence of persisting bactericidal antibody in the LPS-absorbed samples suggested that other bacterial antigens such as outer membrane proteins were also targets of bactericidal antibody. To identify those surface exposed outer membrane proteins against which antibody was developing in convalescent serum samples, use was made of the whole cell radioimmunoprecipitation assay. Figure 2 demonstrates the results of such an assay when acute phase and convalescent serum samples from two of our patients were tested against the respective infecting strains. The acute phase serum sample of the first patient (lane 2) had no significant activity. In contrast, the convalescent sample (lane 3) precipitated several proteins in the 100kDa and greater weight range. The LPS-absorbed sample (lane 4) precipi-

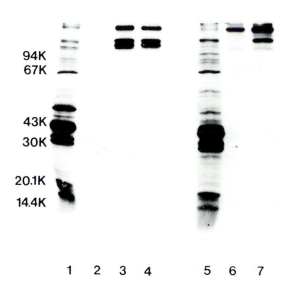

Figure 2 Whole cell radioimmunoprecipitation assay with serum samples from two children with acute nontypable Haemophilus otitis media. Each serum sample was tested against the nontypable Haemophilus strain isolated from the middle ear fluid specimen of the same child. Lane 1 demonstrates the radiolabeled proteins present in the labeled cells of strain 1. Proteins immunoprecipitated by the serum samples from patient 1 are shown as follows: lane 2, acute phase serum; lane 3, convalescent serum; lane 4, LPS absorbed convalescent serum. Lane 5 demonstrates the radiolabeled proteins present in the labeled cells of strain 2. Proteins immunoprecipitated by the serum samples of patient 2 are shown as follows: lane 6, acute phase serum; lane 7, convalescent serum.

SERUM ANTIBODY RESPONSES TO BACTERIAL SURFACE ANTIGENS OF NONTYPABLE *HAEMOPHILUS INFLUENZAE* FOLLOWING ACUTE OTITIS MEDIA IN YOUNG CHILDREN

STEPHEN J. BARENKAMP, M.D. and FRANK F. BODOR, M.D.

Host immunity appears to play an important role in protection of the human host against Haemophilus otitis media. Serum and middle ear fluid antibodies directed against the infecting organism develop during the course of Haemophilus otitis,[1-4] and the presence of these antibodies is associated with a more rapid resolution of infection.[3,5] During the course of the disease, serum bactericidal antibodies develop, and susceptibility to Haemophilus otitis appears to correlate with the absence of bactericidal antibody in acute phase serum samples.[4] Identification of bacterial surface antigens against which bactericidal antibodies are directed is important for our understanding of host immunity. Two major classes of Haemophilus antigens—lipopolysaccharide and outer membrane proteins—are accessible on the bacterial surface and are potential targets of bactericidal antibodies. In this investigation we monitored serum samples from children with acute Haemophilus otitis for the development of bactericidal antibodies and attempted to correlate their development with the appearance of antibodies directed against lipopolysaccharide and outer membrane proteins of the infecting strain.

METHODS

Bacterial Strains and Serum Samples

Nontypable *Haemophilus influenzae* was isolated in pure culture from middle ear fluid specimens of each of the eight children described in this report. Identification of bacteria was performed using standard methods.[6] Organisms were classified as nontypable on the basis of their failure to agglutinate with a panel of typing antisera (a to f) for encapsulated *Haemophilus influenzae*. Acute phase serum samples were collected from the children at the time of presentation with acute otitis media, and convalescent samples were collected 4 to 6 weeks later.

Bactericidal Assay

Serum bactericidal activity was monitored using a previously described assay.[7] Frozen serum collected from an individual with untreated agammaglobulinemia served as the source of complement.[7] Reaction mixtures consisted of 20 μl of complement, 25 μl of a test serum or serum fraction dilution, 12.5 μl of the bacterial suspension, and 67.5 μl of veronal buffered saline with 0.5 percent bovine serum albumin. Calcium chloride and magnesium chloride were added to final concentrations of 0.15 mM and 0.5 mM, respectively. Bacterial test organisms were freshly grown to mid-log phase in brain-heart infusion broth supplemented with nicotinamide-adenine dinucleotide and hemin, each at a level of 4 μg per milliliter. After the bacteria were washed with veronal buffered saline, they were diluted to a concentration of 10^4 cfu per milliliter in the final reaction mixture. The reaction mixtures were incubated at 37° C in a water bath, and viable colony counts were performed at 0 and 60 minutes by plating 12.5 μl samples of the mixtures onto chocolate agar. The bactericidal titer was defined as the dilution of serum that resulted in 90 percent killing of the test strain. Active complement controls and serum controls with heat inactivated complement were included in all assays.

Preparation of LPS Absorbed Serum Fractions

Lipopolysaccharide (LPS) was purified from bacterial strains using the technique of Galanos and co-workers.[8] Solid phase affinity columns were prepared with each of the purified LPS preparations using previously described techniques.[9] Absorption of anti-LPS antibodies from convalescent sera and recovery of affinity purified antibodies were performed as described previously.[9] Efficiency of absorption and recovery were monitored by ELISA using commercially prepared alkaline phosphatase labeled conjugates to human IgG, IgM, and IgA to detect bound antibody.

Measurement of Anti-LPS Antibodies by ELISA

Serum binding activity against LPS antigens was determined by ELISA using techniques modified slightly from those previously described.[9] Serum samples from each child were assayed using LPS purified from the nontypable Haemophilus strain isolated from middle ear fluid of the same child as antigen. All serum samples were assayed simultaneously against their respective LPS preparations. One convalescent serum sample with substantial levels of IgG, IgM, and IgA anti-LPS antibody was selected as the reference standard. Test reactions were read when a 1:300 dilution of this sample reached an optical density of 0.3. Serum titers were defined as the limiting dilution that gave an optical density of 0.3 at the same time as the reference standard. Reaction times required for the reference standard to reach this optical density were approximately 45 minutes, 150 minutes, and 10 hours for the IgG, IgM, and IgA conjugates, respectively. Negative controls were included as previously described.[9]

Detection of Antibodies Against Surface Exposed Outer Membrane Proteins

The whole cell radioimmunoprecipitation assay was performed as previously described.[9] Serum samples from each child were assayed using the bacterial strain isolated from the same child as the test strain.

RESULTS

Acute stage and convalescent serum samples from eight children with acute nontypable *Haemophilus influenzae* otitis media were assayed. Acute phase samples were collected at the time of presentation with acute otitis, and convalescent samples were collected 4 to 6 weeks later. The children ranged in age from 7 to 58 months.

Serum Bactericidal Activity

Paired serum samples from each of the eight children were monitored for serum bactericidal activity (Table 1). In each instance the acute phase serum sample lacked bactericidal activity. In contrast, the convalescent samples demonstrated bactericidal activity against the respective infecting strains with titers ranging from 1:8 to 1:32.

Anti-LPS Antibody Responses

Possible targets of bactericidal antibody include LPS determinants, outer membrane proteins, and pilus proteins. To explore the possible contribution of anti-LPS antibodies to the observed bactericidal activity, paired serum samples from each child were monitored for the presence of and change in levels of anti-LPS antibodies (Fig. 1). Five of the eight children had low or no IgG anti-LPS activity in the acute phase samples. Each of these children demonstrated a fivefold or greater increase in titer in the respective convalescent samples. Three of the children had higher preexisting levels and their corresponding convalescent samples demonstrated smaller increases. In contrast to the IgG responses, the IgM and IgA responses were quite variable. A few patients demonstrated small increases in titer, and several patients with preexisting antibody in acute phase samples demonstrated apparent falls in titer in the convalescent samples. The IgG, IgM, and IgA responses are shown on the same scale in Figure 1, but no attempt was made to quantitate the relative amounts of antibody.

Bactericidal Activity of LPS Absorbed Convalescent Samples and Affinity Purified Anti-LPS Antibody

To more directly assess the contribution of anti-LPS antibodies to the bactericidal activity in convalescent samples, anti-LPS antibodies were removed from the samples by affinity chromatography, and the LPS-absorbed samples were monitored for persisting bactericidal activity. Anti-LPS antibod-

TABLE 1   Bactericidal Activity in Serum Samples from Children with Acute Nontypable Haemophilus Otitis Media

Patient No.	Acute Phase	Convalescent	LPS Absorbed Convalescent	Affinity Pure Anti-LPS
1	<1	1:16	1:16	<1
2	<1	1:16	1:16	<1
3	<1	1:16	1:16	<1
4	<1	1:8	1:4	<1
5	<1	1:16	1:8	1:1
6	<1	1:16	1:16	<1
7	<1	1:16	1:4	1:2
8	<1	1:32	1:32	<1

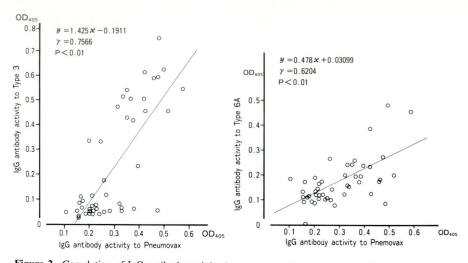

Figure 2 Correlation of IgG antibody activity in response to Pneumovax and other capsular antigens.

either low levels or a deficiency of IgG_2 among IgG subclasses.[1] Also children with recurrent otitis media are said to have low pneumococcal antibody titers and low levels or a deficiency of IgG_2 antibody to pneumococcal capsular polysaccharide.[2-4] Therefore, in regard to the immune response to bacterial infection in otitis media with effusion to which children were predisposed, it was postulated that defense mechanisms might be premature or deficient in these children. However, our study demonstrated no abnormal IgG subclass values in such children. Also no correlation was observed between IgG_2 and pneumococcal antibodies. Furthermore, pneumococcal antibody levels, as assessed according to antigen types, revealed no specific trend except for types 3 and 6A. These results could be attributable to different bacterial pathogens in individual patients or varying potencies of antigen types. However, when Pneumovax containing 23 types of capsular antigens was used as an antigen, pneumococcal anti IgG antibody levels were low in infants and rose with increasing age. This suggests that an antibody production system against bacterial invasion may not be fully developed in infants.

In view of the fact that children of older age groups who are considered to have high pneumococcal antibody also develop this disease, it is necessary to examine not only humoral immunity but also nonspecific defense mechanisms and cellular immunity. Although in this study we assessed the systemic immune response, we believe that the role of local immunity in the middle ear itself should be studied in the future.

REFERENCES

1. Shackelford PG, Polmar SH, Mayus JL, Johnson WL, Corry JM, Nahm MH. Spectrum of IgG_2 subclass deficiency in children with recurrent infections: prospective study. J Pediatr 1986; 108:647–653.
2. Freijd A, Hammarström L, Persson MAA, Smith CIE. Plasma anti-pneumococcal antibody activity of the IgG class and subclasses in otitis prone children. Clin Exp Immunol 1984; 56:233–238.
3. Kalm O, Prellner K, Pedersen HK. Pneumococcal antibodies in families with recurrent otitis media. Int Arch Allergy Appl Immunol 1984; 75:139–142.
4. Kalm O, Prellner K, Freijd A. Antibody activity before and after pneumococcal vaccination of otitis-prone and non-otitis-prone children. Acta Otolaryngol (Stockh) 1986; 101:467–474.

TABLE 1 IgG Antibody Activity Against Pneumococcal Capsular Antigens

		Type						
Age	Pneumovax	3	6A	6B	9V	19A	19F	23F
1 (1)	0.104*	0.054	0.188	0.050	0.042	ND	0.064	0.030
2 (1)	0.204	0.045	0.131	0.006	0.007	0.185	0.217	0.000
3 (3)	0.248	0.181	0.176	0.194	0.087	0.189	0.116	0.103
4 (7)	0.239	0.168	0.109	0.040	0.058	0.153	0.152	0.078
5 (7)	0.236	0.181	0.134	0.102	0.188	0.196	0.178	0.035
6 (9)	0.268	0.153	0.164	0.115	0.157	0.193	0.144	0.105
7 (3)	0.297	0.338	0.239	0.071	0.087	0.239	0.127	0.139
8 (3)	0.455	0.600	0.251	0.248	0.272	0.144	0.248	0.100
9 (3)	0.337	0.354	0.130	0.080	0.136	0.266	0.206	0.046
10 (4)	0.443	0.377	0.278	0.250	0.302	0.272	0.164	0.059
11 (3)	0.368	0.121	0.194	0.135	0.114	0.247	0.097	0.152
12 (2)	0.426	0.334	0.302	0.166	0.087	0.238	0.111	0.227

* mean absorbance value at 405 nm
ND = not done
( ) = number of cases

mean value was obtained for each age group (Table 1). Mean antibody levels in response to reactions to the various antigens were as follows: 0.300 when induced by Pneumovax, 0.236 by type 3, 0.174 by type 6A, 0.121 by type 6B, 0.154 by type 9V, 0.205 by type 19A, 0.155 by type 19F, and 0.088 by type 23F. Thus, type 23F provoked a low antibody reaction compared with the other capsular antigens.

An assessment of a correlation between age and pneumococcal antibody indicated that antibody levels were low in infants when Pneumovax was used as an antigen and rose with increasing age with a statistical significance of 1 percent (Fig.1). Antibody to type 3 was also correlated with age at a significance level of 5 percent. Antibody to type 6A also demonstrated an age related increase with a significance of 1 percent. However, no such correlation was observed in the other capsular antigen types 6B, 9V, 19A, 19F, and 23F.

When a correlation of IgG antibody levels between Pneumovax and the other antigens was assessed, types 3 and 6A showed a correlation with significance of 1 percent but not the other antigens (Fig.2). When IgM and IgA antibodies to pneumococcus were measured using Pneumovax as the antigen, specific IgM antibody levels were low at all ages. The levels of pneumococcal IgA antibody were also either low or undetectable at all ages. In all cases IgG subclass levels were within a normal range established for each age group, and none had a low value or showed a deficiency.

The mean IgG subclass values were 10,426 mg per liter for IgG_1, 2,667 mg per liter for IgG_2, 421 mg per liter for IgG_3, and 299 mg per liter for IgG_4.

When a correlation between age and IgG subclass values was assessed, IgG_1 showed a correlation with age with a statistical significance of 2 percent, but not the other subclasses. Antipneumococcal antibody levels revealed no relation to IgG subclasses 1, 2, 3, and 4.

DISCUSSION

Children who experience relapses of upper respiratory infections have been reported to have

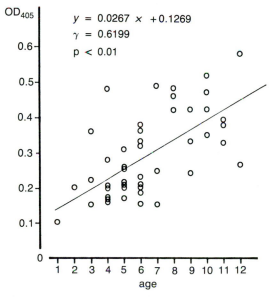

Figure 1 Correlation between age and IgG antibody activity in response to Pneumovax.

6. Kilian M. *Haemophilus*. In: Lennette EH, Balows A, Hausler WJ Jr, Shadomy HJ, eds. Manual of clinical microbiology. 4th ed. Washington, DC: American Society for Microbiology, 1985:387–393.
7. Steele NP, Munson RS Jr, Granoff DM, Cummins JE, Levine RP. Antibody-dependent alternative pathway killing of *Haemophilus influenzae* type b. Infect Immun 1984; 44:452–458.
8. Galanos C, Luderitz O, Westphal O. A new method for the extraction of R lipopolysaccharides. Eur J Biochem 1969; 9:245–249.
9. Barenkamp SJ. Protection by serum antibodies in experimental nontypable *Haemophilus influenzae* otitis media. Infect Immun 1986; 52:572–578.
10. Gnehm HE, Pelton SI, Gulati S, Rice PA. Characterization of antigens from nontypable *Haemophilus influenzae* recognized by human bactericidal antibodies: role of *Haemophilus* outer membrane proteins. J Clin Invest 1985; 75:1645–1658.
11. Gulig PA, McCracken GH Jr, Frisch CF, Johnston KH, Hansen EJ. Antibody response of infants to cell surface-exposed outer membrane proteins of *Haemophilus influenzae* type b after systemic *Haemophilus* disease. Infect Immun 1982; 37:82–88.

STUDY OF B AND T LYMPHOCYTES AND SUBPOPULATIONS IN MIDDLE EAR EFFUSIONS

PAUL van CAUWENBERGE, M.D., JEAN PLUM, M.D., Ph.D., and MAGDA DE SMEDT

It has been suggested that defective immunoregulation is associated with otitis media with effusion in children,[1] that the disorder could be due to a type IV (cellular) hypersensitivity reaction,[2] but also that children with well documented T and B cell immunodeficiencies still can develop otitis media with effusion.[3]

Some of the research concerning cellular immunology in cases of otitis media deals with findings in the peripheral blood and suggests that children with otitis media have subtle immunologic defects, such as depressed helper-suppressor ratios, defective interleukin 2 production, and a decreased mitogenic effect of T lymphocytes and B lymphocytes on nonspecific mitogens.[1]

Earlier cytologic studies of the cellular pattern in serous and mucoid effusions showed that two cells dominate: lymphocytes and neutrophils.[4,5] Palva et al[6] and van Cauwenberge et al[7] reported that in the majority of serous and mucoid effusions granulocytes were the dominant cells. In both types, however, there was a nonneglectable percentage of cases that were very poor in cells.

The relative numbers of T lymphocytes in another study by Palva et al[8] were similar (60 percent of all lymphocytes) in serous and mucoid effusions, regardless of whether granulocytes or mononuclear lymphocytes were the dominant cells. Study of mucosal biopsy specimens, however, showed that the lamina propria is infiltrated mainly by mononuclear cells and that granulocytes only pass through the propria to accumulate in the effusions. This suggests that (bacterial) infection takes place only in the effusion—as can be deduced from the presence of granulocytes—whereas in the mucosa itself a chronic inflammation takes place involving an active cellular immunologic response with mononuclear cells. Study of subpopulations of T lymphocytes showed 70 to 80 percent OKT3 positive cells (mature T lymphocytes) and a predominance of T helper over T suppressor cells, with a ratio of about 2:1.[8]

It was the aim in our study to determine the population of T and B lymphocytes and the subsets of T lymphocytes in a well defined patient group—young children with chronic otitis media—in order to discover whether specific abnormalities could be detected in these children.

MATERIAL AND METHODS

Effusions (total 64) from 48 children, aged 2 to 7 years, were obtained by myringotomy prior to the insertion of tympanostomy tubes. All the children had suffered from otitis media with effusion for at least 2 months, and at the time of collection of the sample there were no signs of acute otitis media.

The ear canal was not sterilized. The effusions were collected in disposable sterile collectors (Juhn Tym Tap) and brought to the immunology laboratory with a maximal delay of 20 minutes. All specimens were processed within 2 hours after collection.

The middle ear effusions were liquefied with acetylcysteine as much as necessary. The cells were centrifuged at 200 g for 10 minutes and the cell pellets were resuspended in phosphate buffered saline containing 1 percent bovine serum albumin and 0.1 percent sodium azide.

The number and distribution of B and T lymphocytes and T lymphocyte subsets were determined as described previously.[9,10] Briefly, monoclonal antibodies (Ortho-Mune, OKT3, OKT4, OKT8, OKT11, and OKB7), fluorescein conjugated goat antimouse IgG, and a flow microcytometer were used. Cells were monitored by measuring forward scatter versus right angle scatter and the green fluorescence simultaneously. The lymphocytes represented a distinct spot within a cytogram of forward versus right angle. The percentage of lymphocytes in each specimen was determined by gating the scatter signal of the lymphocytes with a cytofluorimeter.

RESULTS

Of the 64 samples collected, 34 yielded an insufficient number of lymphocytes to be examined with the computerized method. In most instances neutrophils or bacteria dominated the picture, and in fewer cases there were nearly no cells present. Of the 30 samples yielding enough lymphocytes to be examined, eight were not examined fully because of lack of a sufficient number of lymphocytes. The majority of the samples were mucoid (23); there were only three serous and four (muco-) purulent effusions.

The results of study of the 30 samples that could be examined are listed in Table 1 and the mean values with standard deviations of the mucoid effusions are shown in Figure 1. If we focus on the mucoid effusions, it is obvious that there is no uniform pattern of lymphocytes present in the effusions despite the similar clinical picture of middle ear disease in the children.

Lymphocytes accounted for not more than 17.4 (± 10.8) percent of the cellular components if we consider the mean value of all 23 specimens of mucoid effusions; the range was 4 to 49 percent. In only two samples lymphocytes accounted for more than 30 percent of the cells in the effusions. Neutrophils were the predominant cells. T lymphocytes were the predominant component among the lymphocytes with the OKT11 monoclonal antibody technique, with which the mean value was 55.8 (± 20.6) percent, as well as with the OKT3 technique, with which the mean value was 55.3 (± 20.5) percent. This demonstrates that nearly all T lymphocytes (T11) are mature lymphocytes (T3). The range here was 16 to 88 percent for T11 and 12 to 89 percent for T3. In only two samples (from the same child) the percentage of OKB7 (total of B lymphocytes) exceeded the percentage of OKT11 and OKT3. The mean value for OKB7 positivity was 14.7 (± 12) percent, with a wide range from 0 to 39 percent. T helper-inducer lymphocytes (OKT4) in most samples (17 of 19) were more numerous than T suppressor-cytotoxic lymphocytes (OKT8). The mean value for OKT4 was 32.3 (± 16.7) percent and for OKT8, 19.8 (± 12.1) percent. Only in two samples (of 19) was the percentage of OKT8 positive cells more than 40, and in these two cases the T4:T8 ratio was less than 1.

Although the number of serous and (muco-) purulent effusions examined is small, it seems that the lymphocyte population is different from that of the mucoid effusions. Two of the three serous effusions had a T4:T8 ratio of less than 1 (in contrast to only two of 19 mucoid effusions), whereas three of four (muco-) purulent effusions had a very high T4:T8 ratio.

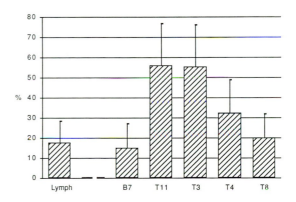

Figure 1 Lymphocytes in 23 mucoid effusions. Incidence of detection of lymphocytes (percentage of total number of cells in the effusions) and their subpopulations (percentage of total number of lymphocytes), with standard deviations. B7 = B lymphocytes; T11 = E rosette receptor, pan T; T3 = mature T lymphocytes; T4 = T helper-inducer; T8 = T cytotoxic-suppressor.

TABLE 1   **Populations and Subpopulations of T and B Lymphocytes in 30 Middle Ear Effusions***

Sample	% LY	B 7	T 11	T 3	T 4	T 8	4/8 Ratio
Mucoid							
1	14	3	88	89	48	22	2.18
2	23	39	46	63	14	43	0.33
3	7	ND	64	ND	ND	ND	NA
4	18	ND	40	33	19	16	1.17
5	18	11	48	39	30	15	2.00
6	14	ND	44	ND	ND	ND	NA
7	35	33	77	ND	ND	ND	NA
8	8	3	76	76	54	8	7.11
13	10	10	76	74	58	10	5.69
14	25	3	49	63	27	22	1.27
15	30	0	80	75	10	43	0.25
16	25	7	55	35	38	2	23.81
17	18	10	54	48	24	23	1.06
18	49	ND	25	ND	16	8	2.03
19	27	8	27	42	20	ND	NA
20	15	12	54	69	27	18	1.49
21	15	17	54	49	29	17	1.73
24	4	0	65	66	43	22	1.91
25	5	17	59	69	58	32	1.81
26	13	27	81	59	43	26	1.64
27	9	33	81	68	51	35	1.44
29	12	23	16	21	7	0	°°
30	7	25	24	12	19	14	1.36
Serous							
9	15	5	80	75	55	5	11.00
22	31	ND	73	ND	30	45	0.67
28	19	27	90	76	38	39	0.97
(Muco-) purulent							
10	20	21	40	38	32	1	39.62
11	9	43	45	38	35	6	5.65
12	19	58	55	56	37	6	6.15
23	36	6	ND	63	36	20	1.86

* LY = lymphocytes; ND, = not done; NA, = not applicable; °° = indefinitely high; numbers grouped together with } indicate both samples are from one child.

DISCUSSION

Our results correlate well with those of Palva et al[7] and confirm that the lymphocyte population in middle ear effusions is not a uniform picture and that there is a wide range in the distribution patterns in the different patients. Probably acute exacerbations of infection in the chronically infected middle ear cavity influence the cellular pattern considerably. Lymphocytes are not the major cellular component in mucoid and mucopurulent middle ear effusions in children with otitis media with effusion. In the presence of abundant granulocytes or bacteria, for example, lymphocytes are absent or present only in very small numbers. This is in contrast to earlier reports.[1,5]

T helper-inducer lymphocytes in most cases (17 of 19) outnumber the T cytotoxic-suppressor lymphocytes in the effusions. There is consequently no deficiency of T helper cells in most of the children.

As in the study by Palva et al,[7] it was obvious that there was no lack of essential defense mechanisms and that the cellular picture in mucoid otitis media with effusion may vary depending upon the stage of the disease and probably also the treatment of the ear disorder. We believe that, on the basis of our results and those of Palva et al, there is no reason to assume in the majority of children with mucoid otitis media that the cellular immunologic processes in the middle ear differ from those of chronic infections in other closed cavities of the body. Further research on serous and (muco-) purulent effusions is needed.

REFERENCES

1. Bernstein JM, Yamanaka T, Cumella J, Ogra PL, Park B. Some observations on lymphocyte and macrophage function in middle ear effusions. In: Veldman JE, McCabe BF, Huizing EH, Mygind N, eds. Immunobiology, autoimmunity, transplantation in otorhinolaryngology. Amsterdam: Kugler Publications, 1985:51.
2. Bernstein JM. Immunological reactivity in otitis media with effusion. In: Oehling A, ed. Advances in allergology and clinical immunology. Oxford: Pergamon Press, 1980:139.
3. Veldman JE, Roord JJ, Kuis W, Stoop JW, Huizing EH. In vivo immunology: serous otitis media in children with immunodeficiency disorders. In: Lim DJ, Bluestone CD, Klein JO, Nelson JD, eds. Recent advances in otitis media with effusion. Proceedings of the Third International Symposium. Toronto: BC Decker, 1984:178.
4. Palva T, Holopainen E, Karma P. Protein cellular pattern of glue ear secretions. Ann Otol Rhinol Laryngol 1976; 85 (Suppl 25):103–109.
5. Bryan MP, Bryan WTK. Cytologic and immunologic response revealed in middle ear effusions. Ann Otol Rhinol Laryngol 1976; 85 (Suppl 25):238–244.
6. Palva T, Häyry P, Ylikoski J. Lymphocyte morphology in middle ear effusions. Ann Otol Rhinol Laryngol 1980; 89 (Suppl 68):143–146.
7. van Cauwenberge P, Rysselaere M, Waelkens B. Bacteriological and cytological findings according to the macroscopic characteristics of the middle ear effusions. Auris Nasus Larynx 1985; 12 (Suppl 1):73–76.
8. Palva T, Taskinen E, Häyry P. T lymphocytes in secretory otitis media. In: Veldman JE, McCabe BF, Huizing EH, Mygind N, eds. Immunobiology, autoimmunity, transplantation in otorhinolaryngology. Amsterdam: Kugler Publications, 1985:45.
9. Plum J, van Cauwenberge P, de Smedt M. Phenotyping of mononuclear cells from tonsils and corresponding biopsies using a cytofluorimeter. Acta Otolaryngol (Stockh) 1986; 101:129–134.
10. Plum J, van Cauwenberge P, de Smedt M. Human tonsillar T lymphocytes: an immature or activated T-lymphocyte population. Clin Immun Immunopathol 1986; 39:14–23.

MORPHOLOGIC STUDY ON MACROPHAGES AND LYMPHOCYTES IN MIDDLE EAR EFFUSION

MAMORU SHIBUYA, M.D., KOJI HOZAWA, M.D., MASAKO ISHIDOYA, M.D., HIDEICHI SHINKAWA, M.D., and TOMONORI TAKASAKA, M.D.

The first pathologic studies of the infiltrated cells in middle ear effusions were recorded by Bryan[1] in 1953. Later Lim et al,[2] Bernstein et al,[3] Sipilä and Karma,[4] Palva et al,[5] and McGhee et al[6] reported cytologic and ultrastructural investigations of middle ear effusions. However, the immunopathologic details of otitis media with effusion remained uncertain. To clarify the cell mediated immunologic aspects of middle ear effusions, the distributions of infiltrated cells and the biologic activities of macrophages were studied by monoclonal antibody staining and a peroxidase staining method.

MATERIAL AND METHODS

Analysis of Cellular Components in Middle Ear Effusions

Therapeutic myringotomy and aspiration of middle ear effusions were performed in 53 pediatric patients with otitis media with effusion. The subjects ranged in age from 3 to 10 years (Fig. 1). The effusions were classified into three groups, based on the following criteria.

In collecting the middle ear effusions we always

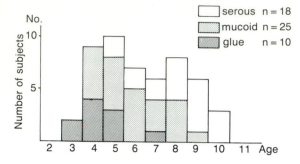

Figure 1 Relationship between the types of effusions and the distribution of patients' ages (analysis of cellular components in middle ear effusion).

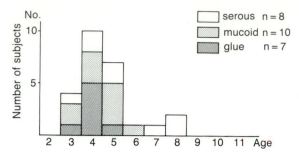

Figure 2 Relationship between the types of effusions and the distribution of patients' ages (investigation of biologic activities of macrophages in middle ear effusion).

used the same size aspiration tube. An effusion that was easily aspirated was classified as a "serous effusion." A "mucoid effusion" was defined as one that required a long time for aspiration by the same suction tube. When it was too tenacious to be aspirated by the same size suction tube and a larger tube was used for the collection, the effusion was classified as a "glue effusion." According to our rheologic classification, 18 effusions were classified as serous, 25 as mucoid, and 10 as glue type. The collected effusions were immediately diluted with 2 ml of physiologic sodium chloride solution and were centrifuged by Cytospin II* for 7 minutes at 500 rpm into six slide glasses. The five centrifuged samples were incubated with normal horse serum and one was incubated with normal goat serum.

We used Leu 4, 14, 2a, 3a, HLA-DR, and Ml as primary antibodies. Biotinylated antimouse IgG and IgM were also employed with normal human serum.[†]

Investigation of Biologic Activities of Macrophages in Middle Ear Effusions

Middle ear effusions were collected from 25 patients ranging in age from 3 to 11 years who had undergone myringotomy (Fig. 2). The effusions (eight serous, ten mucoid, and seven glue) were immediately prefixed in 2.5 percent phosphate buffered glutaraldehyde for 60 minutes. Only serous samples were centrifuged at 400 rpm for 10 minutes during prefixation. Karnovsky's method using the 3-3′-diaminobenzidine reaction was performed with the sediments of serous, mucoid, and glue middle ear effusions for 5 minutes. Then they were postfixed

* Shandon Southern Instruments Inc., 515 Broad Street, Sewickley, PA 15143
† Antibodies were supplied by Becton Dickinson Immunocytometry Systems, Mountain View, CA 94039

with 1 percent osurium tetroxide, dehydrated with graded alcohols, and embedded in Epon 812. Three serial sections 500 nm thick were made for light microscopic observation with and without toluidine blue staining and electron microscopic study with a high voltage electron microscope (1,000 kv of accelerating voltage). Several thin (75 nm) sections were prepared for ultrastructural observation.

RESULTS

Analysis of Cellular Components in Middle Ear Effusions

With the Miller ocular disc the number of Leu positive cells and the total cells in the same field were counted under a magnification of 200 X. The percentage of Leu positive cells in the total number of cells was calculated. The counts and calculations were repeated for 10 fields of the same specimen. The mean percentage of the 10 fields was regarded as the reaction positive frequency in the specimen.

By these procedures the Leu 4 positive frequencies were determined in 17 serous and 24 mucoid effusions (16.2 and 14.6 percent, respectively) and showed no significant differences (Table 1).[5] There were small numbers of Leu 14 positive cells in both types of effusion, and the Leu 14 positive frequencies also showed no significant differences. Although the Leu 2a positive frequency in serous effusions approximated that in mucoid effusions the Leu 3a positive frequency in mucoid effusions was significantly greater than that of the serous group. The Leu Ml positive frequency in mucoid effusions was higher than that of the serous effusion. Ten glue effusions were examined by the same techniques, but the infiltrated cells showed no diaminobenzidine positive reaction. It seemed that the surface markers of lymphocytes and the other cells were covered with

TABLE 1   Distributions of Leu Positive Cells in Different Middle Ear Effusions

	Serous		Mucoid	
	M±SD (%)	n	M±SD (%)	n
Leu 4[+]	16.2±9.3	17	14.6±8.5	24
Leu 14[+]	2.4±2.0	16	1.4±1.1	23
Leu 2a[+]	6.4±4.3	17	5.8±4.2	24
Leu 3a[+]	7.0±2.8	18	19.7±13.0	25
Leu HLA-DR[+]	26.0±11.0	17	18.6±16.2	25
Leu M1[+]	18.1±11.9	17	23.8±13.8	24

M = mean reaction positive frequency (number of Leu positive cells per total number of cells in same field, 100x).

tenacious materials and that the primary antigen antibody reaction was disturbed physically.

The relationship between the helper-suppressor T ratio and the macrophage occurrence frequency was investigated in 14 serous and 19 mucoid effusions (Fig. 3). Most serous effusions showed a small percentage of macrophages and a low helper-suppressor ratio, but many mucoid effusions showed a greater percentage and a higher ratio. The higher helper-suppressor ratio tended to correlate with a greater percentage of macrophages. Accumulation of helper T lymphocytes and macrophages in the mucoid effusion indicated the presence of active cellular interaction and cellular immunity.[5]

Investigation of Biologic Activities of Macrophages in Middle Ear Effusions

The numbers of macrophages were light microscopically counted under a magnification of 200 X following toluidine blue staining. Then the diaminobenzidine reaction positive macrophages were counted in serial sections without staining. To count the macrophages more accurately, a third serial thick section was examined under the electron

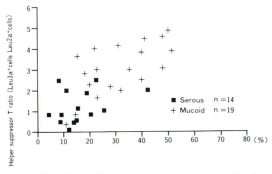

Figure 3   Relationship between helper-suppressor T ratio and M1 reaction positive frequency. M1 reaction positive frequency: number of Leu M1 positive cells per total number of cells in same field (100 X).

microscope. Ultrastructural study showed that most macrophages in serous effusions had numerous diaminobenzidine reaction positive granules in the intracytoplasm and phagosomes (Fig. 4). Some were phagocytosing actively (Fig. 4B). Many macrophages of mucoid effusions had a small number of peroxidase reaction positive precipitates (Fig. 5). Macrophages of glue effusions frequently showed many vacuoles but no diaminobenzidine reaction positive material (Fig. 6A). Most glue sections contained many degenerating cells and much cellular debris (Fig. 6B). The electron density of the ground substance was higher than in the other groups, and some of the glue specimens also showed cholesterin crystals.

With these procedures the number of macrophages and the number of diaminobenzidine reaction positive macrophages were counted in eight serous, ten mucoid, and seven glue effusions (Table 2). The greatest number of macrophages was found in mucoid effusions and the smallest number in serous effusions. The mean number of diaminobenzidine reaction positive macrophages was also greatest in mucoid effusions and smallest in serous effusions, but the diaminobenzidine positive frequency was highest in serous effusions and lowest in glue effusions.

DISCUSSION

It is widely accepted that many diaminobenzidine reaction positive granules are found in the cytoplasm of activated macrophages. One activator, lymphokine, is released from effector or helper T lymphocyte. By examining the histochemical characteristics of macrophages, we noted that the frequency of occurrence of biologically activated macrophages was highest in serous effusions. Although the greatest number of macrophages was counted in mucoid effusions, nearly 40 percent of them showed depressed activity that seemed to interfere with their

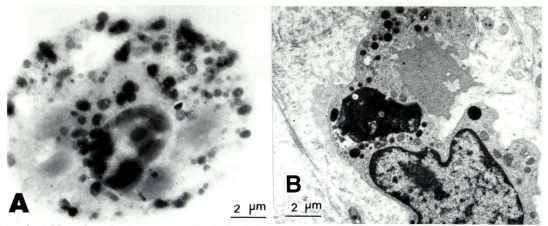

Figure 4 *A*, Macrophage showing numerous diaminobenzidine reaction positive granules in a serous effusion (500 nm thick section without staining under high voltage electron microscopy). *B*, A macrophage in a serous effusion containing diaminobenzidine positive material and a phagosome, phagocytosing actively (75 nm thin section with double staining).

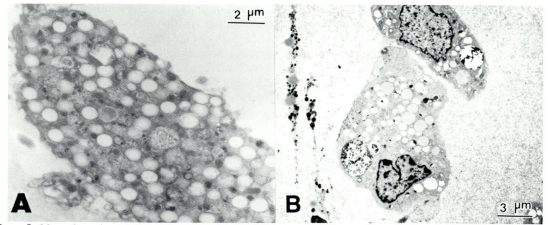

Figure 5 Macrophages in mucoid effusions had a small number of peroxidase reaction positive granules and showed lower electron densities than those of serous effusions. *A*, 500 nm thick section without double staining. *B*, 75 nm thin section with double staining.

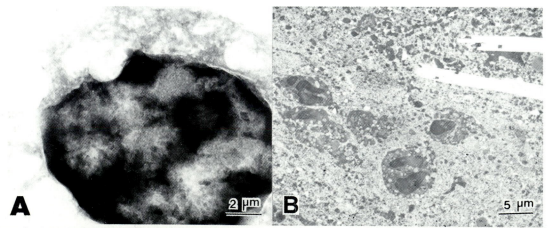

Figure 6 *A*, Macrophage in a 500 nm thick section of a glue effusion showed many vacuoles but no diaminobenzidine reaction positive material without staining. *B*, A 75 nm thin section of a glue effusion contained many degenerating cells and much cellular debris. Cholesterin crystals were also found in this specimen with double staining.

TABLE 2 **Relationship Between Type of Middle Ear Effusion and Diaminobenzidine Reaction of Macrophages**

	$M\phi/F \pm SD$	$DAB(+)M\phi/F \pm SD$	$DAB(+)Rate(\%) \pm SD$	$n \times (Fs)$
Serous	1.08 ± 0.44	0.92 ± 0.39	82.6 ± 18.3	8(10)
Mucoid	9.51 ± 8.58	5.52 ± 4.88	60.8 ± 16.1	10(10)
Glue	7.00 ± 5.13	2.54 ± 1.52	34.3 ± 20.8	7(10)

$M\phi/F$ = mean number of macrophages in one field; $DAB(+)M\phi/F$ = mean number of diaminobenzidine reaction positive macrophages in one field; $DAB(+)$Rate = mean diaminobenzidine reaction positive frequency $(M = \frac{1}{\eta} \sum_{i=1}^{\eta} DAB(+)M\phi_i / M\phi_i)$; n = number of specimens; Fs = number of observation fields.

function. In glue effusions 65 percent of the macrophages showed evidence of biologic dysfunction, characterized by vacuoles and cellular collapse. Because intracytoplasmic granules and organelles maintained the activities of lysosomal enzyme, collapse of the infiltrated cells added to the tenacity as well as cytotoxicity of the effusions.[2,7]

Accumulation of helper T lymphocytes and macrophages indicated intensive cellular immunity of mucoid effusion.[5] However, some of the infiltrated cells exhausted their own intracellular energy and gradually lost their biologic activity.

REFERENCES

1. Bryan WTK. The identification and clinical significance of large phagocytes in the exudates of acute otitis media and mastoiditis. Laryngoscope 1953; 63:559–580.
2. Lim DJ, Lewis DM, Schram SL, et al. Otitis media with effusion: cytological and microbiological correlates. Arch Otolaryngol 1979; 105:404–412.
3. Bernstein JM, Szymanski B, Albini B, et al. Lymphocyte subpopulations in otitis media with effusion. Pediatr Res 1978; 12:786–788.
4. Sipilä P, Karma P. Inflammatory cells in mucoid effusion of secretory otitis media. Acta Otolaryngol 1982; 94:467–472.
5. Palva T, Häyry P, Ylikoski J. Lymphocyte morphology in mucoid ear effusion. Ann Otol Rhinol Laryngol 1978; 87:421–425.
6. McGhee RB Jr, Demaria TF, Okazaki N, Lim DJ. Selective induction of macrophages in the middle ear. Ann Otol Rhinol Laryngol 1983; 92:510–517.
7. Juhn SK, Paparella MM, Kim LS, et al. Pathogenesis of otitis media. Ann Otol Rhinol Laryngol 1977; 86:481–492.

IMMUNOGLOBULINS IN MIDDLE EAR EFFUSIONS: A STUDY IN EXPERIMENTALLY INDUCED SEROUS AND PURULENT OTITIS MEDIA

ULF JOHANSSON, M.D., STEN O.M. HELLSTRÖM, M.D., Ph.D., and TORGNY STIGBRAND, M.D.

Otitis media is defined as an inflammation of the middle ear cleft with an accumulation of fluid—middle ear effusion. The effusion can be serous, mucoid, or purulent. The fluid composition may be indicative of different inflammatory conditions with varying etiologic and pathogenetic factors. Much information on this subject is available from clinical studies. However, in clinical work various factors are difficult to control. Most patients present with middle ear effusion in which the time course is unknown, and the effusion material may include both serous and mucoid components. In the present study two well defined types of otitis media, serous and purulent, were induced in rats, and the effusion material was sequentially analyzed with respect to the pattern of immunoglobulins and some other serum proteins, e.g., albumin and transferrin.

MATERIALS AND METHODS

Serous and purulent forms of otitis media were induced in rats by obstruction of the eustachian tube and clefting of the soft palate, respectively.[1,2] The inflammatory response was observed over a 6 week period, and samples of middle ear effusion and serum were analyzed electrophoretically and immunochemically at 1, 2, 3, 4, and 6 weeks after the

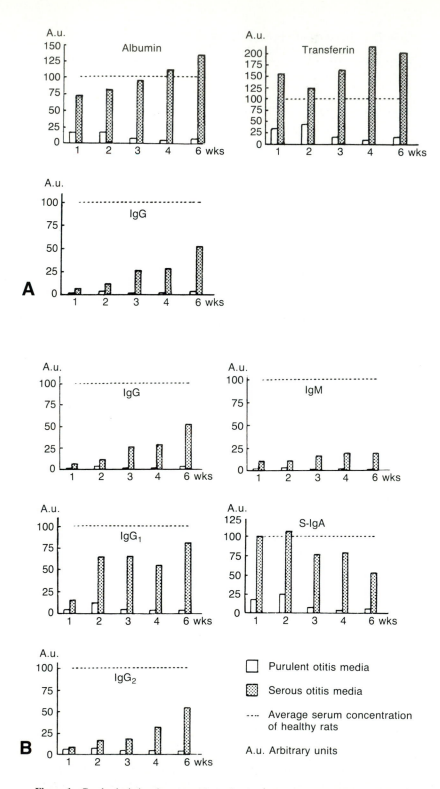

Figure 1   Graphs depicting the mean values of various serum proteins determined by rocket immunoelectrophoresis in serous and purulent middle ear effusions. The dotted lines represent the average serum concentrations in healthy Sprague-Dawley rats. *A*, Albumin, transferrin, and IgG. *B*, IgG, IgG$_1$, IgG$_2$, IgM, and s-IgA.

initiation of otitis media. The content of albumin, transferrin, total IgG, IgG_1, IgG_2, IgM, and s-IgA was determined. The microbiologic pattern for these two conditions was characterized at the same time intervals.

RESULTS

Significantly higher levels of all investigated proteins were found in middle ear effusion in the serous otitis media group amounting to three- to 15-fold the concentration found in the purulent otitis media group (Fig. 1). With time higher ratios tended to occur. Some of the proteins of the effusion—transferrin, albumin, and IgG—were seen to increase during the course of serous otitis media, whereas levels in the purulent otitis groups showed the opposite change. The serous effusion was culture negative (Fig. 2). As expected, the otomicroscopically puslike effusion material was culture positive, initially gram positive but turning gram negative over the time period observed. The changed microbiologic flora did not seem to result in a changed immunoglobulin pattern of the middle ear effusion.

DISCUSSION

The content of the middle ear effusion in serous and purulent otitis media changed throughout the observation period. These changes differed between the two types of otitis media, indicating different mechanisms for the generation of the middle ear effusion content in these inflammatory conditions. The study puts emphasis on the dynamics observed

Nasopharynx (day 0):	α-Streptococcus, S. aureus, S. epidermidis, P. mirabilis, S. faecalis
Middle ear effusions:	SOM: culture negative POM: gram + ⟶ gram −

None of the samples showed any growth of anaerobic bacteria.

Figure 2 The bacteriologic pattern in serous and purulent middle ear effusion. The figure also depicts the normal nasopharyngeal flora of the rat.

during the course of otitis media, with characteristic changes seen in both experimental groups. The possibility of identifying and utilizing selected parameters to describe specific inflammatory reactions may make possible the proper evaluation of the types of otitis media, staging of the inflammation, therapy assessments, and prediction of prognosis.

Study supported by grants from the Swedish Medical Research Council (17X-6578) and the Ragnar and Torsten Söderbergs Foundation.

REFERENCES

1. Hellström S, Salén B, Stenfors L-E, Söderberg O. Appearance of effusion material in the attic space correlated to an impaired eustachian tube function. Int J Pediatr Otorhinolaryngol 1983; 6:127–134.
2. Hellström S, Salén B, Stenfors L-E. The site of initial production and transport of effusion materials in otitis media serosa. Acta Otolaryngol 1982; 93:435–440.

INDUCTION OF ANTIGEN SPECIFIC IgA FORMING CELLS IN THE EUSTACHIAN TUBE AND MIDDLE EAR MUCOSAE

GORO MOGI, M.D., NORITAKE WATANABE, M.D., HIROYUKI YOSHIMURA, M.D., and HIROFUMI KATO, M.D.

Many studies have suggested that mucosal immunity is present in the middle ear during otitis media.[1,2] Since mucosal immunity is one of the important defense mechanisms, enhancement of its activity may prevent otitis media. However, the exact source of IgA forming cells and their route to the eustachian tube and middle ear are not known. In order to clarify these questions we attempted to induce IgA forming cells in the eustachian tube and middle ear mucosa and to discover whether mucosal immunization suppresses immune mediated otitis media.

MATERIALS AND METHODS

Animals

Healthy male Hartley quinea pigs (250 to 300 g) were used.

Immunization Schedule

Figure 1 indicates the schedule for immunization. The animals were divided into three groups; the number in each group are noted in Figure 1. The footpads of all the animals in each group were injected with 200 μg of dinitrophenylated ovalbumin (DNP-OVA) mixed with Freund's adjuvant. One week late 200 μg of DNP-OVA coupled to polyacrylamide gel beads (DNP-OVA-Pa) was injected into the duodenal lumen during laparotomy (group A) and into the tracheal lumen (group B). Group C animals, serving as controls, received no intraduodenal or intratracheal immunization. Two weeks after the initial immunization the right tympanic cavity of all animals in each group was injected with 200 μg of DNP-OVA-Pa in 100 μl of 0.8 percent hydroxypropyl cellulose solution was injected into the left ear. One week after immunization of the tympanic cavity, animals of the three groups were killed for evaluation.

Collection of Saliva, Middle Ear Effusion, and Serum

Seven days after the intratympanic inoculation of the antigen, salivary secretions, serum samples, and specimens of middle ear effusion collected. To stimulate the secretion of saliva, pilocarpin was injected intraperitoneally (1.0 mg per 100 grams of body weight). Blood samples for serum were obtained by heart puncture. After the collection of sali-

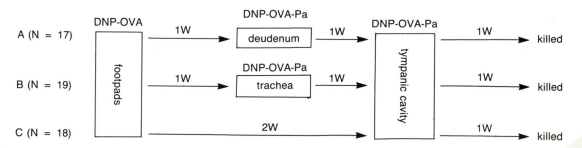

Figure 1 Immunization schedule for the induction of antigen specific IgA forming cells. DNP-OVA-Pa: dinitrophenyl ovalbumin coupled with polyacrylamide gel beads.

va and sera, the animals were killed. Regardless of the absence or presence of a middle ear effusion, the tympanic cavity was irrigated with 100 μl of saline. The saline was aspirated and submitted for biochemical analysis as the middle ear effusion sample.

Determination of Antibody Titers of IgA and IgG in Response to DNP-OVA-Pa

An indirect ELISA technique was employed. Rabbit antiserum against the alpha-chain of guinea pig serum was used as the first antibody, and goat antiserum against rabbit IgG conjugated with horseradish peroxidase was employed as the second antibody.

Identification of Anti-DNP-OVA IgA Forming Cells

Immediately after the animals were killed, tissue specimens obtained from various organs were frozen by a dry ice–ethanol technique to yield frozen sections or were fixed in cold ethanol (95 percent) for paraffin sections. To identify anti-DNP-OVA IgA forming cells, double staining techniques were used according to the method reported by Kawamura.[3] Two serial sections were treated separately. One section was incubated with rabbit antiguinea pig alpha-chain serum, followed by treatment with goat antirabbit IgG labeled with rhodamine. The other section was stained with DNP-OVA conjugated with FITC. Rhodamine stained sections were observed under a 546 nm green exciting beam with a 590 nm barrier filter, and FITC stained sections under a 495 nm blue exciting beam with a 510 nm barrier filter. If a cell was positive for both stains, it was defined as an anti-DNP-OVA IgA forming cell. Blocking tests were performed by supplying appropriate unconjugated antibodies to consecutive tissue sections prior to staining with FITC or rhodamine conjugates.

RESULTS

Antibody titers of IgA and IgG to DNP-OVA in Saliva, Serum, and Middle Ear Effusion

As illustrated in Figure 2, the mean titers of salivary IgA activity in groups A and B were significantly greater than the mean titer in group C. The mean titer of the serum IgG in group C signifi-

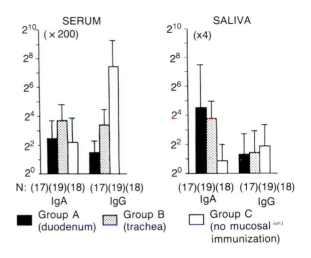

Figure 2 Antibody titers of IgA and IgG to DNP-OVA in saliva and serum.

cantly exceeded the mean titers in groups A and B. Titers of IgA activity in middle ear effusions in groups A and B were greater than the titer in group C, while titers of IgG activity in middle ear effusions of groups B and C exceeded the titer in group A. However, there was no significant difference between these values of the ear effusion samples.

Occurrence of Otitis Media

Otitis media was seen in 3 of 17 (17.6 percent) guinea pigs of group A, in 4 of 17 (21.1 percent) in group B, and in all 18 animals in group C. The left ears of all animals were found to have no evidence of otitis media. Otitis media was defined by the presence of a middle ear effusion and the thickness of the tympanic mucosa.

Histologic Findings in Middle Ear Mucosa

Figure 3 summarizes the histologic findings in the tympanic mucosa in each group. Moderate cell infiltration was seen in the mucosa of some animals in group A, which were determined by gross appearance to have no otitis media.

Antigen Specific IgA Forming Cells

Considerable numbers of anti-DNP-OVA antibody forming IgA immunocytes were detected in the eustachian tube mucosa (through the pharyngeal orifice to the cartilaginous portion) in group A and

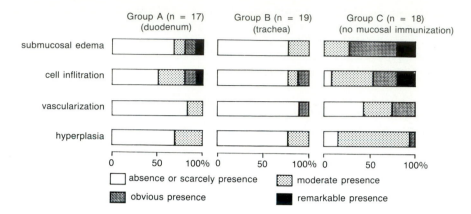

Figure 3 Histologic findings in middle ear mucosa.

B animals. As seen in Figure 4, antigen specific IgA immunocytes were demonstrated in the tympanic mucosa of group A and B animals that developed otitis media. Although IgA forming cells were detected in the tympanic mucosa in group C animals, these cells were not antigen specific. Antigen specific IgA immunocytes were also demonstrated in various secretory sites, such as intestine, trachea, nasopharynx, and nose. However, the liver and spleen were found to have no antigen specific IgA immunocytes.

DISCUSSION

Our study demonstrated the induction of antigen specific IgA forming cells in the mucous membranes of the eustachian tube and tympanic cavity of animals that underwent mucosal immunization of the duodenal or tracheal lumen followed by intratympanic immunization. Precursors of IgA forming cells are abundant in gut associated lymphoid tissue and bronchus associated lymphoid tissue, but other peripheral lymphoid organs contain few IgA bearing lymphocytes.[4,5] After sensitization with antigen in gut or bronchus associated lymphoid tissue, precursors of IgA forming cells enter the circulation through the thoracic duct and eventually settle either in the mucosal tissue of the antigen stimulated organ itself or at a distant secretory site. The presence of antigen specific IgA forming cells in distant mucosal tissues in considered evidence for a common mucosal immune system. Results of the present investigation show that IgA forming cells in the mucous membrane of the eustachian tube and tympanic cavity originate from the gut and bronchus associated lymphoid tissue. However, it is still not known whether other organs, such as the tonsils,

nasopharynx, and nose, are a source of precursors of IgA immunocytes in the middle ear and eustachian tube mucosa. Our study suggests that in otitis media, findings in the middle ear mucosa bear a striking resemblance to the immunologic features observed in peripheral mucosal sites of the common mucosal system.

It has been postulated that mucosal immunity is independent of systemic immunity, since the antigen encountered by the enteric or respiratory route can stimulate an antibody response in the intestinal or respiratory tract in the absence of an apparent systemic immune response. However, recent studies have demonstrated that important regulatory interactions take place between the systemic and mucosal immune systems. Antigen impinging on the immune

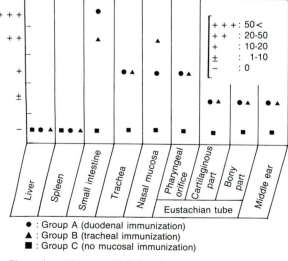

● : Group A (duodenal immunization)
▲ : Group B (tracheal immunization)
■ : Group C (no mucosal immunization)

Figure 4 Antigen specific IgA immunocytes in various organs. Cells are observed and counted by 400 μ magnification.

system via mucosal surfaces generally leads to unresponsiveness after subsequent parenteral challenge with the same antigen. Tomasi[6] called this phenomenon "oral tolerance." These regulatory mechanisms occur because the oral administration of antigen induces the formation of mucosa derived T suppressor cells, which act on the IgG and IgM plasma cell precursors (B lymphocytes) but not on the precursors of IgA forming plasma cells. In contrast, the IgA response is enhanced following mucosal antigen administration because of the induction of antigen specific T helper cells.[7] The present study demonstrated that mucosal antigen administration restrains the induction of immune mediated otitis media. Suzuki et al report in the chapter *Immune Mediated Otitis Media With Effusion* that the transfer of spleen derived suppressor T cells of antigen fed mice suppressed immune mediated otitis media. This evidence indicates that IgG mediated otitis media can be suppressed to some extent by the induction of antigen specific mucosa derived T suppressor cells.

Our study suggests that mucosal immunization of the intestinal and respiratory tracts enhances the mucosal defense of the eustachian tube, the gateway to the tympanic cavity.

REFERENCES

1. Mogi G, et al. Secretory immunoglobulin A (SIgA) in middle ear effusion. A further report. Ann Otol Rhinol Laryngol 1974; 82:92–101.
2. Bernstein JM, Tomasi TB Jr, Ogra PL. The immunochemistry of middle ear effusions. Arch Otolaryngol 1974; 99:320–326.
3. Kawamura A. Fluorescent antibody techniques and their applications. 2nd ed. Tokyo: University of Tokyo Press, 1977.
4. Craig SW, Cebra JJ. Peyer's patches, an enriched source of precursors for IgA producing immunocytes in the rabbit. J Exp Med 1971; 134:188–200.
5. Bienenstock J. Bronchus-associated lymphoid tissue. Int Arch Allergy Appl Immunol 1985; 76(Suppl 1):62–69.
6. Tomasi TB Jr. Oral tolerance. Transplantation 1980; 29:353–356.
7. Richman LK, et al. Simultaneous induction of antigen-specific IgA helper T cells and IgG suppressor T cells in the murine Peyer's patches after protein feeding. J Immunol 1981; 126:2079–2083.

IMMUNE MEDIATED OTITIS MEDIA WITH EFFUSION

MASASHI SUZUKI, M.D., HIDEYUKI KAWAUCHI, M.D., SHIGEHIRO UEYAMA, M.D., TATSUYA FUJIYOSHI, M.D., and GORO MOGI, M.D.

Data accumulating over the past decade have demonstrated that an immune response or immune reactions are involved in inflammatory diseases of the middle ear. In order to clarify the role of immune reactions in otitis media with effusion, the disease was induced in chinchillas. Characteristics of the experimental disease were evaluated biochemically, cytologically, and histologically.

MATERIALS AND METHODS

Animals

We used healthy chinchillas, weighing 400 to 550 g, that were free of middle ear infection.

Antigens

Keyhole limpet hemocyanin, a potent immunogen, was used as the antigen.

Measurement of Antibody Titers

Antibody titers in sera and middle ear effusions were measured by an indirect enzyme linked immunosorbent assay method utilizing rabbit antichinchilla IgG serum and peroxidase conjugated goat antirabbit IgG.

Induction of Immune Mediated Otitis Media with Effusion

Thirteen chinchillas (group A) that had been systemically sensitized with 1 mg of keyhole limpet hemocyanin in complete Freund's adjuvant underwent intratympanic inoculation with 300 μg of keyhole limpet hemocyanin in 200 μl of 0.8 percent hydroxypropylcellulose–phosphate buffered saline (pH 7.2) solution four times at 2 day intervals, 2 weeks after the systemic immunization. Four animals (group B) that were systemically sensitized

8 weeks earlier were injected with keyhole limpet hemocyanin intratympanically 4 times. Four chinchillas (group C) that had been intradermally immunized underwent a booster injection of keyhole limpet hemocyanin 8 weeks after the initial injection and 2 weeks later received four successive injections into the tympanic cavity. Eight chinchillas (group D) that had no systemic immunization were challenged in the middle ear with keyhole limpet hemocyanin four times. All the animals were injected with keyhole limpet hemocyanin in one ear, while 200 μl of the hydroxypropylcellulose solution was introduced into the other ear. These procedures were carried out under sterile conditions. The middle ears of the chinchillas were monitored daily by tympanometry, and microscopic observation of the eardrum was undertaken after the initial injection of keyhole limpet hemocyanin into the tympanic bulla until sacrifice 8 days after the first middle ear injection.

Induction of Immune Mediated Short and Long Term Otitis Media with Effusion

Eight chinchillas that had been systemically sensitized with keyhole limpet hemocyanin underwent intratympanic inoculation only once with 300 μg of keyhole limpet hemocyanin in 200 μl of 0.8 percent hydroxypropylcellulose–phosphate buffered saline solution. These animals were sacrificed 4 days after the intratympanic injection (short term experiment).

Seventeen chinchillas intradermally immunized with keyhole limpet hemocyanin 2 weeks earlier were systemically sensitized again and inoculated with 300 μg of keyhole limpet hemocyanin in 200 μl of the hydroxypropylcellulose solution, and then boosted two times by intradermal and intratympanic injections at intervals of 1 week. All animals were killed 7 days after the final injection (long term experiment).

Preparation of Immune Complexes

Immune complexes were prepared by mixing 5 ml of a high titer chinchilla antiserum against keyhole limpet hemocyanin (incubated at 56° C for 30 minutes to inactivate complement) with 20 mg of keyhole limpet hemocyanin at the optimal ratio. Five hundred milligrams of a well washed pellet of the immune complex was suspended in 10 ml of the hydroxypropylcellulose solution.

Induction of Otitis Media with Effusion by Immune Complexes

Twelve chinchillas were inoculated with 200 μl of the immune complex suspension delivered into the tympanic cavity of one ear through the superior bulla. To serve as a control, the other ear was injected with 300 μg of keyhole limpet hemocyanin in 200 μl of the hydroxypropylcellulose solution. Six of 12 chinchillas were killed at 4 days after the inoculation, and the remaining animals were killed at 7 days for aspiration of the middle ear effusion and morphologic study of the middle ear mucosa.

Collection of Effusion Samples and Histologic Study

Middle ear effusions were aspirated aseptically through the eardrum with a 26 gauge disposable syringe and processed for analysis. The effusions were divided immediately into cellular and liquid components by centrifugation at 150 g for 10 minutes. The cellular components were distilled in phosphate buffered saline and placed in a cytocentrifuge for staining with hematoxylin and eosin; some samples were prepared for immune peroxidase staining.

Immune Peroxidase Method

The cells were fixed in 95 percent alcohol and washed in phosphate buffered saline. The slides were incubated in 0.114 percent periodic acid solution and washed in phosphate buffered saline. Then the rabbit antikeyhole limpet hemocyanin IgG antibody was applied at a 1:200 dilution. The slides were incubated in a humidified chamber at room temperature and subsequently washed in phosphate buffered saline. The goat antirabbit IgG antibody conjugated with peroxidase diluted at 1:50 was applied, and the specimen was incubated in the humidified moisture chamber. The specimens were washed in phosphate buffered saline, and 0.02 percent 3,3′ - diaminobenzidine with 0.005 percent hydrogen peroxide was applied in the moisture chamber. The slides were washed in distilled water, and the cells were stained with methylgreen.

Biochemical Analysis

The liquid components of the middle ear effusion were divided into three aliquots and submitted for measurement of the antikeyhole limpet hemocyanin IgG titer and histamine and prostaglandin E_2 levels. The histamine content in the effusions was determined by high speed liquid chromatography, described by Tsuruta et al.[1] Prostaglandin E_2 measurement was carried out by radioimmunoassay, as described by Inagawa.[2]

Light and Electron Microscopy

The middle ear and eustachian tube mucosa specimens from the chinchillas were examined by light and electron microscopy. For light microscopy the tissues were stained routinely with periodic acid–Schiff stain. For electron microscopy the specimens were fixed with 2.5 percent glutaraldehyde in 0.1 M phosphate buffered saline. The specimens dissected from the bony wall were postfixed with 1 percent osmic acid and embedded in epoxy resin. Ultrathin sections were prepared for transmission and phase electron microscopy.

RESULTS

Immune Mediated Otitis Media

All chinchillas in groups A and C, which had a high serum antibody titer to keyhole limpet hemocyanin, developed otitis media with effusion, whereas no effusion was detected in groups B and D in which the serum antibody titers were low. The effusion specimens were submitted for bacterial culture and were found to be negative. Cells in the effusions included substantial numbers of neutrophils with a few macrophages, lymphocytes, basophils, and eosinophils. Antikeyhole limpet hemocyanin IgG activity was detected in the effusions, but the

levels were lower than those in the sera. The mean histamine level of the three effusion samples was 112 ±3.7 ng per milliliter (SE), which significantly exceeded the mean level in corresponding sera (6.2±1.4 ng per milliliter). The lining membrane of the bullae was edematous and thickened. The epithelial cells (both ciliated and nonciliated) were swollen. Infiltration of neutrophils, basophils, eosinophils, and lymphocytes was seen in the epithelial layer where dilation and rupture of blood capillaries were apparent. These morphologic findings indicated increased vascular permeability of the middle ear mucosa and exudation of the blood elements.

Comparison of Short and Long Term Models of Otitis Media with Effusion

All chinchillas in the short term experiment developed otitis media with effusion (short term model). In the long term experiment middle ear effusions developed in seven of the 17 animals (long term model); in the remaining animals effusions developed but eventually disappeared and the tympanogram returned to type A (failed long term model). Antibody titers in the sera of failed long term models (17.2±3.40) were significantly lower (p < 0.05) than those in long term models (21.4±3.89).

Cells in the effusions of short term models consisted of equal numbers of macrophages and neutrophils and a few lymphocytes, basophils, and eosinophils. In effusions of long term models neutrophils were dominant.

The mean histamine level in all effusions of short term models was 98.7±8.4 ng per milliliter and that in long term models was 86.5±9.1 ng per milliliter. The mean prostaglandin E_2 concentrations in the effusions of short and long term models were 3.75±0.61 and 3.20±0.74 ng per milliliter, respectively (Table 1). All the levels were signifi-

TABLE 1 Histamine and Prostaglandin E_2 Concentrations in Middle Ear Effusions in Immune Mediated Otitis Media with Effusion and Immune Complex Mediated Otitis Media with Effusion

	Histamine (ng/ml)		Prostaglandin E_2 (ng/ml)	
	Middle Ear Effusions	Sera	Middle Ear Effusions	Sera
Immune mediated otitis media				
Short term otitis media (n=8)	98.7±8.4	6.1±1.8	3.75±0.61	2.13±0.62
Long term otitis media (n=7)	86.5±9.1	5.7±1.3	3.20±0.74	1.91±0.57
Immune complex mediated otitis media (n=4)	36.6±2.4	6.2±1.4	3.54±0.50	1.64±0.31

cantly higher than those in corresponding sera.

The light microscopic findings in the middle ear mucosa in long term models included more infiltrative cells with lymphoid follicles, larger mucous glands in the epithelial layer, and more goblet cells than in the short term models (Fig. 1). Capillary dilation in short and long term models was similar in degree. Goblet cells in the eustachian tube increased in both models. Cell infiltrations in the subepithelial layers of the eustachian tube mucosa were seen only in the long term model.

Immune Complex Mediated Otitis Media with Effusion

Middle ear effusions appeared within 4 days after the injection in all ears inoculated with immune complexes and disappeared spontaneously 8 or 9 days after the injection. No effusion was observed in the control ears. Cells in the effusions obtained at the fourth day consisted predominantly of macrophages, neutrophils, and lymphocytes, in that order, and a few eosinophils and basophils. In effusions at 7 days neutrophils dominated. With the immune

peroxidase method, neutrophils phagocytosing immune complexes were seen in the effusions (Fig. 2). The mean histamine and prostaglandin E_2 concentrations of the four effusion samples were significantly higher than those in the corresponding sera. Electron microscopic findings in the middle ear mucosa in chinchillas with otitis induced by immune complexes were similar to those in immune mediated otitis media with effusion (Fig. 3).

DISCUSSION

Studies by Ryan et al[3,4] and the present investigation demonstrated that a secondary immune response in the middle ear produces otitis media with effusion. IgG antibodies and their immune complexes are likely a key factor in the generation of immune mediated otitis. The presence of soluble immune complexes in middle ear fluids has been reported.[5,6] The present investigation also showed the production of effusions in experimental animals by inoculation of immune complexes into the tympanic cavity. Therefore, it is suggested that immune complexes may be responsible for immunopathologic changes in the middle ear.

Immune complexes can activate the complement system via the classic pathway. C3a and C5a are anaphylatoxins, which release chemical mediators from mast cells. C5a and C5b67 act as chemotactic factors with neutrophils and macrophages. The mean concentrations of C3a and C5a in middle ear effusions in humans are significantly greater than those in corresponding sera.[7] The Fc portion of immunoglobulin has an affinity for neutrophils. Therefore, immune complexes are phagocytosed by neutrophils as demonstrated in the present study, and ultimately undergo cytolysis themselves, releasing

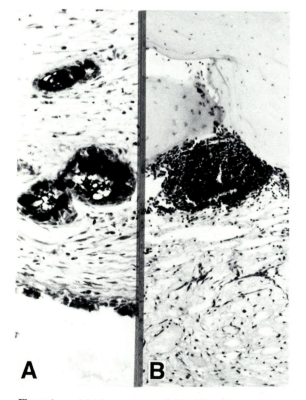

Figure 1 *A*, Middle ear mucosa of chinchilla with chronic otitis media with effusion. *B*, A lymphoid follicle and a large mucous gland can be seen in the epithelial layer.

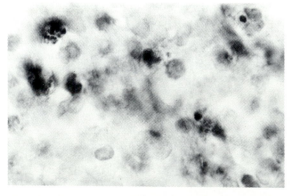

Figure 2 Neutrophils have phagocytosed immune complexes in the middle ear effusion in immune complex mediated otitis media with effusion (immune peroxidase method).

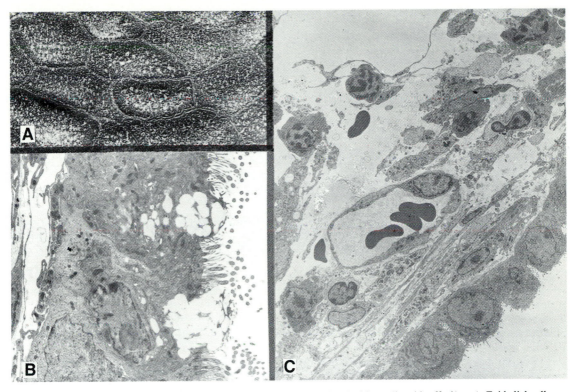

Figure 3 Middle ear mucosa of chinchilla with immune complex mediated otitis media with effusion. *A*, Epithelial cells are swollen. *B*, Infiltration of lymphocytes and plasma cells. *C*, In the subepithelial layer blood capillaries are dilated. Active secretion can be seen in goblet cells.

various lysosomal enzymes. In these cases granulocyte protease activates the alternative pathway of the complement system. The level of granulocyte protease is extremely high in middle ear effusions compared to that in sera.[8]

Immune complexes and other substances in such effusions activate a complement component, leading to the production of inflammation generating fragments, which in turn may activate mast cells. Mast cells release inflammatory mediators, producing vasodilation and mucosal edema as well as neutrophil chemotaxis. These neutrophils then ingest the immune complexes and in turn release granulocyte proteases to produce tissue injury. Therefore, the vicious cycle involving these substances may maintain the inflammatory condition in the middle ear when immune complexes are stagnant or are produced continuously in the tympanic cavity.

This sequence of events is supported by evidence of otitis media maintained for 3 weeks in seven of the 17 animals in this study boosted by intratympanic and intradermal injections with antigen. In this model larger mucous glands and more goblet cells in the middle ear mucosa were seen than in the short term model. In a failed long term model in which the effusion eventually disappeared, the circulating IgG antibody titer was significantly lower than in the long term model. We suspect that immune tolerance was induced in the failed long term model. Our study revealed the formation of lymphoid follicles in the tympanic mucosa of the long term model. However, it is not known whether these newly formed lymphoid follicles serve gut associated lymphoid tissue or bronchus associated lymphoid tissue.

REFERENCES

1. Tsuruta Y, Kohashi K, Ohkura Y. Determination of histamine in plasma by high speed liquid chromatography. J Chromatogr 1978; 146:490–493.
2. Inagawa T. Assay of prostaglandin E_2. J Med Technol (Jpn) 1982; 26:135–147.
3. Ryan AF, Cleveland PH, Hartman M, Catanzaro A. Humoral and cell mediated immunity in peripheral blood following introduction of antigen into the middle ear. Ann Otol Rhinol Laryngol 1982; 91: 70–75.
4. Ryan AF, Catanzaro A, Wasserman SI, Harris JP. Secondary immune response in the middle ear: immunological, morphological and physiological observations. Ann Otol Rhinol Laryngol 1986; 95:242–249.

5. Maxim PE, Veltri RW, Sprinkle PM. Chronic serous otitis media: an immune complex disease. Trans Am Acad Ophthalmol Otolaryngol 1977; 84:234–238.
6. Palva T, Lebtinen T, Rinne J. Immune complexes in middle ear fluid in chronic secretory otitis media. Ann Otol Rhinol Laryngol 1983; 92:42–44.
7. Mogi G, Bernstein JM. Immune mechanisms in otitis media with effusion. In: Bernstein JM, Ogra PL, eds. Immunology of the ear. New York: Raven Press, (in press).
8. Carlsson B, Lundberg C, Ohlsson K. Granulocyte protease in middle ear effusions. Ann Otol Rhinol Laryngol 1982; 91:76–81.

EXPERIMENTAL OTITIS MEDIA WITH EFFUSION: LOCAL IMMUNITY OF A MIDDLE EAR

KOJI HOZAWA, M.D. and TOMONORI TAKASAKA, M.D.

Even though few immunocytes can be observed in the submucosal connective tissue of the normal middle ear mucosa, many immunocytes, such as lymphocytes, macrophages, and plasma cells, appear in the inflamed middle ear mucosa. Recent immunochemical analysis of middle ear effusions has revealed the latent potential of the middle ear in producing specific antibody locally.[1] Thus the middle ear is now considered to possess its own local immune system. By virtue of monoclonal antibody against cell surface antigen, both Leu 4 and Leu 12 positive B lymphocytes were shown to be present in inflamed middle ear mucosa. Some lymphocytes also expressed HLA-DR antigen on the cell surface, indicating that a humoral as well as a cellular immune response can take place in the middle ear. Plasma cells were observed scattered around the lymphocyte accumulations. Our immunoelectron microscopic studies demonstrated IgG on the surface of B lymphocytes as well as rough endoplasmic reticulum and a Golgi complex of mature plasma cells, indicating that the differentiation from B lymphocytes to plasma cells occurred in the middle ear. In other words, the humoral immune system was activated in the middle ear. In the present study animal experiments were carried out to clarify the factors essential for activation of the latent humoral immune system in the middle ear.

MATERIALS AND METHODS

Forty-eight healthy guinea pigs were examined histopathologically after various types of immunologic stimulation. The animals were divided into four groups according to the methods of immunization—(1) nonsensitized group, (2) intrabullar injection group, (3) intradermal injection group, and (4) intradermal as well as intrabullar injection group. Horseradish peroxidase (Sigma type VI) was used as an antigen, and 0.1 ml of horseradish peroxidase solution (1 mg per milliliter of physiologic saline) was injected into the tympanic cavity in the second group of animals. The animals in the third group received an intradermal injection with a mixture of 0.5 ml horseradish peroxidase solution and 0.5 ml of Freund's complete adjuvant once a week for 3 weeks. The animals in each group were rechallenged by an intraperitoneal, intranasal, or intrabullar injection with the same antigen. After an adequate interval the animals were sacrificed under anesthesia, and the eustachian tube and the middle ear mucosa were studied by immunofluorescence and Leduc's immunoelectron microscopic method.[2]

RESULTS

The serum level of antibody against horseradish peroxidase and the cytologic profile of infiltrated cells indicated that local immunity of the middle ear was acquired only through the general intradermal immunization and was enhanced by the additional intrabullar challenge (Table 1). The intratympanic injection was the only effective stimulus for producing persistent middle ear effusions. When horseradish peroxidase was injected into the tympanic cavity in animals that had already acquired local immunity, a specific immune response took place and the middle ear effusion tended to persist

TABLE 1   Serum Levels of Specific Antibodies Against Horseradish Peroxidase and Cytologic Profile of Cells Infiltrating Middle Ear Mucosa

	Control (Unsensitized) Group	Local Stimulation Group*	General Immunization Group[+]	General Immunization and Additional Local Stimulation Group
Serum level of antibody against horseradish peroxidase	-	-	2^5	2^6
Cytologic profile of infiltrated cell in membrane	Fibrocyte	Polymorphonuclear leukocytes	A few plasma cells producing antibody against horseradish peroxidase	Many plasma cells producing antibody against horseradish peroxidase. Macrophages containing horseradish peroxidase within cytoplasm. A few lymphocytes.

* Intratympanic injection of 0.1 ml of horseradish peroxidase solution, 1 mg/ml.
[+] Intradermal injection of 0.5 ml of horseradish peroxidase solution with 0.5 ml of Freund's complete adjuvant once a week for 3 weeks.

for up to 2 weeks, whereas in animals without specific local immunity, only a nonspecific inflammatory response was observed and the middle ear effusion disappeared within 3 days. Intranasal injection with a nebulized vapor failed to bring the antigen into the middle ear. Circulating immune complexes, which are formed following intraperitoneal injection in generally sensitized animals, could not be a cause of otitis media.

Intradermal Injection Group

In the intradermal injection group a few plasma cells were observed beneath the mucosal lining, which produced specific antibody against horseradish peroxidase. Immunofluorescence study revealed that this antibody mainly consisted of IgG. The inoculation of horseradish peroxidase into the middle ear in these animals resulted in an inflammatory change mediated by an antigen-antibody reaction; immune complex deposition was observed in the basement membrane of the middle ear mucosa as well as in submucosal capillary walls.

Intradermal and Additional Intrabullar Injection Group

The number of plasma cells increased significantly after the additional intratympanic injection of horseradish peroxidase into the generally sensitized animals. Plasma cells producing specific antibody against horseradish peroxidase were distributed throughout the thickened middle ear mucosa. However, this phenomenon could not be observed in the osseous portion of the eustachian tube. The specific antibody against horseradish peroxidase was

mainly IgG and partially IgA, with very little IgM. Other lymphoid tissues in these animals, such as the spleen and cervical lymph nodes, contained specific antibody producing plasma cells, but no specific antibody against horseradish peroxidase was observed in lung or intestinal lymphoid tissue. A few macrophages were observed among these lymphocytes in the middle ear mucosa in which horseradish peroxidase appeared within the cytoplasm. These macrophages and plasma cells persisted in the submucosal connective tissue of the middle ear for at least 3 months after injection.

Injection of horseradish peroxidase into the middle ear in conjunction with such local immune system produced proliferation of plasma cells and infiltration of neutrophils as well as macrophages, which phagocitized the immune complexes. Lymphocytes also infiltrated the middle ear mucosa within 7 days after injection to form lymph follicle-like structures. Leduc's method revealed some to be immature plasma cells, showing antibody against horseradish peroxidase on the nuclear membrane and perinuclear cistern. Some were mature plasma cells showing antibody against horseradish peroxidase in the rough endoplasmic reticulum and Golgi complex. Differentiation from lymphocytes to mature plasma cells was observed in human middle ear mucosa, which could be reproduced in the animal model.

Submucosal Vascular Networks

In the generally sensitized group, injected horseradish peroxidase formed immune deposits on the submucosal vascular walls, leading to vasculitis and vascular dilation. Following the fifth day after injection, mitotic figures were frequently observed in the endothelial cells of submucosal capillaries, which brought about formation of new capillary networks with a high columnar endothelium. Lymphocytes were observed inside and outside these new capillary networks.

DISCUSSION

Our study revealed that general sensitization is the essential factor in order for the middle ear to acquire local immunity (Fig. 1). Several antihorseradish peroxidase antibody producing plasma cells were observed in the submucosal connective tissue of the generally sensitized animals, but intratympanic injection of horseradish peroxidase into these animals resulted in immune deposits on the submucosal vascular walls, indicating that specific antibody was derived mainly from the serum rather than being a local product. However, this additional stimulation enhanced the local immune system of the middle ear, producing a significant increase in the number of antihorseradish peroxidase antibody producing plasma cells. Lim[3] reported that horseradish peroxidase injected into the bulla was absorbed by the middle ear mucosa and transported into draining lymph nodes. We found premature antihorseradish peroxidase antibody producing cells in the cervical lymph nodes. The source of lymphocytes in the middle ear mucosa remains obscure.

However, the cervical lymph nodes may be a source of IgG producing plasma cells in the middle ear.

High columnar endothelial cell venules recently have been considered to have receptors for the recognition of circulating lymphocytes because of their ultrastructural similarity to postcapillary venules in lymphoid tissue.[4] In our experiment the mitotic figures in endothelium were evident after intratympanic stimulation of generally sensitized animals, and the high columnar endothelial capillary networks were newly formed; this process may regulate lymphocyte migration into the middle ear.

From the epidemiologic point of view, most of the patients with otitis media with effusion have had earlier episodes of upper respiratory tract infection or acute otitis media.[5] Our experimental results suggest that such preceding infections should be taken into account because sensitization or local stimulation activates a special local immune system in the middle ear.

REFERENCES

1. Meurman OH, Sarkkinen HK, Puhakka HJ. Local IgA class antibodies against respiratory viruses in middle ear and nasopharyngeal secretions of children with secretory otitis media. Laryngoscope 1980; 90:304–311.
2. Leduc EA, Avrameas S, Bougeille M. Ultrastructural locali-

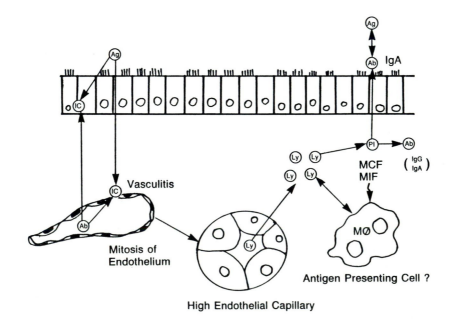

Figure 1 Schema showing how the local immune system was established in the middle ear.

zation of antibody in differentiating plasma cells. J Exp Med 1968; 127:109–118.

3. Lim DJ. Functional morphology of the lining membrane of the middle ear and eustachian tube; an overview. Ann Otol Rhinol Laryngol 1974; 83(Suppl 11):5–11.

4. Bernstein JM, Tsutsumi H, Ogra PL. The middle ear mucosal immune system in otitis media with effusion. Am J Otolaryngol 1985; 6:162–168.

5. Giebink GS. The microbiology of serous and mucoid otitis media. Pediatrics 1979; 63:915–919.

ANTIBODY PRODUCTION IN ACUTE AND CHRONIC IMMUNE MEDIATED OTITIS MEDIA WITH EFFUSION

ALLEN F. RYAN, Ph.D., JEFFREY P. HARRIS, M.D., Ph.D., ELIZABETH M. KEITHLEY, Ph.D., PATRICIA SHARP, B.S., ANTONINO CATANZARO, M.D., and SHARON BATCHER, B.S.

A number of clinical investigations have reported the presence of specific secretory IgA in the middle ear effusions of patients with otitis media with effusion.[1,2] These data suggest that mucosal immunity operates in the middle ear cavity during disease. However, the tympanum represents a unique site for the expression of mucosal immunity. There are few resident lymphocytes in the normal middle ear mucosa and no local accumulations of lymphoid tissue.[3] Any local immune response in the middle ear must be constituted de novo in response to antigenic challenge of the tympanum. This could occur through rapid proliferation of the small number of resident submucosal lymphocytes or by seeding with lymphocytes from distant sites. In particular, the middle ear mucosa could participate in a common mucosal defense system in which IgA committed lymphocytes sensitized at one mucosal location seed mucosae at distant sites.[4]

We have reported that an acute secondary immune response in the middle ear cavity of the guinea pig results in effusion, inflammation, and local antibody production.[5] However, this response is dominated by IgG,[5,6] a fact inconsistent both with mucosal immunity and observations in patients with otitis media with effusion. The role of IgG in our animal model may have been enhanced by the experimental protocol employed to generate immune mediated otitis media with effusion. For example, the role of IgG may have been enhanced by the acute nature of the immune response, which lasted only 1 to 2 weeks. Since the middle ear mucosa is quite rudimentary, it may require more time in order to develop a mature mucosal character, including

IgA based immunity. Also, the intradermal immunization protocol probably sensitized mostly IgG committed lymphocytes. Without a circulating pool of IgA committed B cells, the response to middle ear challenge might be expected to be dominated by IgG.

The otitis media with effusion produced by the secondary immune response in the middle ear lasted for only 1 or 2 weeks.[5] This raises the question of whether the generation of effusion and inflammation during immune response is self-limiting. In our previous study we used a single antigenic challenge to elicit immune mediated otitis media. However, antigens in patients could be self-replicating or could be confined to the middle ear by tubal dysfunction and thus persist in the middle ear for long periods. It is not clear whether a response to such a persistent antigen challenge could contribute to the pathogenesis of chronic otitis media with effusion.

In order to investigate further the possible role of immunity in otitis media with effusion, two experiments were conducted. First, the characteristics of acute and chronic middle ear immune responses were compared. Second, a systemic sensitization protocol that increases the proportion of IgA committed lymphocytes in the circulation was employed prior to middle ear challenge.

MATERIALS AND METHODS

An acute secondary immune response in the middle ear was produced by methods described elsewhere.[5] Briefly, Hartley guinea pigs were immunized by intradermal injection of 1 mg of keyhole limpet hemocyanin (KLH) as an alum precipitate. Three weeks later one middle ear was challenged with 1 mg of the associated form of KLH. The opposite ear was injected with saline as a control. Groups of six animals each were sacrificed at intervals of 1, 3, 7, 14, and 21 days after challenge. The middle ears were washed to recover effusion and cells. Washes were assayed for anti-KLH antibody by enzyme linked immunosorbent assay (ELISA) using polyclonal rabbit antisera against guinea pig IgG, IgG1, IgG2, IgA, and IgM, and were cultured for bacteria. Animals positive for microorganisms were replaced. The bullae were fixed in acid formalin, decalcified, embedded in paraffin, and sectioned. Sections were reacted against the biotinylated antisera just listed or against biotinylated KLH, followed by streptavidin horseradish peroxidase, and were then developed with 2-amino-9-ethylcarbazole for immunohistochemical identification of plasma cells and free immunoglobulin.

A chronic middle ear immune response was produced in 12 animals by repeated intratympanic injection of KLH, 300 μg in 50 μl, twice per week for 6 weeks.[7] Six of the 12 were naive animals, and six had been sensitized 3 weeks earlier by intradermal injection of KLH-alum. Three days after the final challenge the animals were sacrificed, and the middle ears were analyzed as already described.

An additional six animals were sensitized by a protocol to increase the number of circulating lymphocytes committed to IgA.[8] Intraperitoneal injection of KLH with complete Freund's adjuvant was followed 1 week later by an intraperitoneal booster injection of KLH in incomplete Freund's adjuvant. One week later 1 mg of KLH was injected directly into the duodenum, and 1 mg was injected into both middle ear cavities. The animals were sacrificed 10 days later and the middle ears were prepared for immunohistochemical examination.

Immunohistochemical examination results were quantitated in three to five animals of each group for which immunohistochemical staining was intense. The number of positive plasma cells in a standard area (one microscopic field at 400×) was counted for sections reacted against antiguinea pig IgG, IgA, or IgM. The percentage of cells producing each isotype was calculated and averaged.

RESULTS

Acute Secondary Immune Response in the Middle Ear

As we have previously reported,[5] a secondary immune response in the middle ear cavity, elicited by a single challenge dose of antigen, resulted in an acute episode of otitis media with effusion, including mucosal hyperplasia and edema as well as leukocytic infiltration. Most of the cells infiltrating the middle ear lumen were neutrophils. ELISA of the middle ear effusions showed a gradual increase in anti-KLH IgG, reaching a maximum 1 to 2 weeks after challenge. The levels of anti-KLH IgG in the effusion did not exceed that in serum, however. Little or no IgA or IgM was detected at any time (Fig. 1). Immunohistochemical examination demonstrated many plasma cells producing IgG, especially of the IgG2 subclass, but only a few cells producing IgA or IgM (Table 1). Plasma cells producing specific immunoglobulin against KLH were also demonstrated.

Chronic Middle Ear Immune Response

Repeated challenge of the middle ear cavity produced chronic otitis media with effusion. Similar results were observed regardless of whether the animals had been sensitized intradermally prior to the middle ear challenges. Effusion persisted in the middle ear throughout the period of antigenic challenge and for a few days after the final challenge. The inflammatory response observed in the middle ear was similar to that seen in the "acute" animals. However, there was more osteoneogenesis, and the mucosa showed an increase in ciliated and secretory cells. Occasional glandlike structures were observed in the submucosa. The cells infiltrating the tympanic lumen were primarily monocytes-macrophages and neutrophils.

ELISA of middle ear effusions showed large amounts of anti-KLH IgG as well as substantial quantities of anti-KLH IgA (see Fig. 1). The amount of specific IgA in the middle ear greatly exceeded that seen in serum. Immunohistochemical testing showed many plasma cells producing IgG, with IgG2 predominating. However, a moderate number of IgA

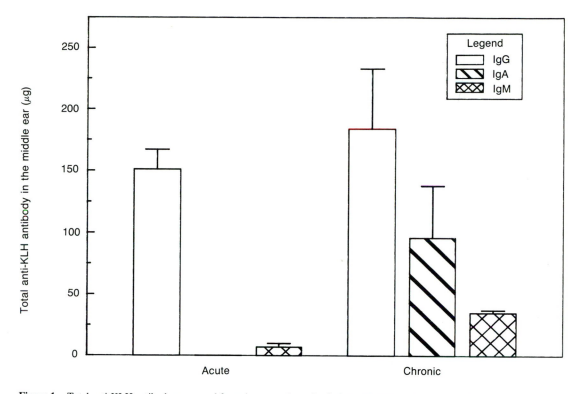

Figure 1 Total anti-KLH antibody recovered from the tympanic cavity during acute versus chronic secondary immune response in the middle ear. Each value represents the mean (vertical bar = standard error) of ELISA measures from six subjects. Note the higher level of anti-KLH IgA ($p < 0.01$, Student's t test) in the chronic immune response.

producing cells were noted. Few cells producing IgM were detected (see Table 1).

Middle Ear Challenge of Duodenally Immunized Animals

Challenge of the middle ear following immunization of the peritoneum and duodenum resulted in middle ear effusion and inflammation, which were comparable to that seen after intradermal sensitization and middle ear challenge in all animals. However, the number of leukocytes infiltrating the middle ear lumen was much greater in the gut immunized animals. Immunohistochemical testing of the middle ear mucosa revealed many IgG producing plasma cells 10 days after challenge. However, IgA producing cells were also commonly observed. IgM producing cells were infrequently encountered (see Table 1).

DISCUSSION

We have shown that IgA plays a role in experimental middle ear immune responses under the appropriate conditions. This increases our understanding of immune mechanisms in the middle ear during otitis media with effusion in humans, in which IgA can play an important role. Second, we have demonstrated that a chronic immune response results in chronic otitis media with effusion in the absence of bacterial infection and negative middle ear pressure. This suggests that immune responses may contribute to the pathogenesis of chronic otitis media in humans.

That sensitization of IgA committed lymphocytes via the gut increased the number found in the

TABLE 1 Percentage Distribution of Plasma Cells in the Middle Ear Mucosa During Secondary Immune Response

Isotype	Acute (n = 4)	Chronic (n = 5)	Duodenum (n = 3)
IgG	93.3	78.5	72.2
IgA	4.6	19.6*	26.6*
IgM	2.1	1.9	1.2

* Significantly different from acute ($p < 0.05$, Mann-Whitney U test).

middle ear after challenge suggests that the middle ear mucosa participates in the circulation of IgA committed lymphocytes between distant mucosae. The middle ear therefore appears to be linked to a common mucosal defense system, as has been proposed for several other mucosal sites.[4,9] However, duodenal immunization did not decrease the incidence or severity of otitis media following middle ear challenge.

Mogi[10] recently reported a similar study of immune mediated otitis media with effusion in a chinchilla model. However, he found that immunization in the gut did not increase IgA secreting plasma cells in the middle ear and that it produced a decrease in immune mediated otitis media. The duodenal immunization protocol used by Mogi was somewhat different from that employed in the present study, which may explain the disparity in results.

When repeated challenge of the middle ear cavity produced a chronic immune response, increased local production of IgA was also observed. This could reflect an increase in seeding of the mucosa from distant mucosal sites. Alternatively, preferential proliferation of lymphocytes committed to IgA may occur in the middle ear. Either of these possibilities could be related to changes in the character of the middle ear lining during a chronic immune response. The normal middle ear lining is only a rudimentary mucosa. During chronic inflammation the mucosa develops more of the characteristics of mucosae at other sites, including an increased population of ciliated and secretory epithelial cells and a substantial submucosa. This environment could preferentially stimulate either the proliferation of IgA committed lymphocytes or the entrance of IgA committed lymphocytes into the middle ear from the circulation.

It is also possible that during repeated challenge of the middle ear, antigen exiting from the middle ear cavity via the eustachian tube gains access to mucosal lymphocytes in the upper airway or gut. This could increase the number of circulating IgA committed B cells that are sensitized to KLH.

In any event our data suggest that route of sensitization and the duration of immune response are important factors in determining the character of middle ear immunity.

In earlier studies of acute immune mediated otitis media with effusion we found that a single antigenic challenge produced acute otitis media, which resolved in 1 to 2 weeks.[5,6] The response to persistent antigen challenge observed in the present study demonstrates that immune mediated otitis media with effusion is not self-limiting. Immune mediated effusion persisted in the middle ear cavity for several weeks in the absence of bacterial infection and, since an opening was maintained in the tympanic membrane by repeated injection, without the existence of negative pressure in the middle ear. This provides evidence that the inflammation associated with the immune response has the potential for contributing to the pathogenesis of chronic as well as acute otitis media with effusion.

Study supported by grant NS14389 from the NIH/NINCDS and by the Duaei Hearing Research Fund.

REFERENCES

1. Bernstein JM, Tomasi TB, Ogra P. The immunochemistry of middle ear effusions. Arch Otolaryngol 1974; 99:320–326.
2. Liu YS, Lim DJ, Lang RW, Birck HG. Chronic middle ear effusions: immunochemical and bacteriological investigation. Arch Otolaryngol 1975; 101:278–286.
3. Lim DJ. Functional morphology of the lining membrane of the middle ear and eustachian tube. Ann Otol Rhinol Laryngol 1974; 80(Suppl 11):1–22.
4. Bienenstock J. Review and discussion of homing of lymphoid cells to mucosal membranes: the selective localization of cells in mucosal tissue. In: Strober W, Hanson LA, Sell KW, eds. Recent advances in mucosal immunity. New York: Raven Press, 1982:35.
5. Ryan AF, Catanzaro A, Wasserman SI, Harris JP. Secondary immune response in the middle ear: physiological, anatomical and immunological observations. Ann Otol Rhinol Laryngol 1986; 95:242–249.
6. Ryan AF, Catanzaro A. Passive transfer of immune-mediated middle ear effusion and inflammation. Acta Otolaryngol (Stockh) 1983; 95:123–130.
7. Ryan AF, Harris JP, Wasserman SI, Catanzaro A. Immunologically mediated models of chronic otitis media with effusion. In: Sade J, ed. Acute and secretory otitis media. Amstelveen, The Netherlands: Kugler, 1986:236.
8. Pierce NF, Gowans JL. Cellular kinetics of the intestinal immune response to cholera toxoid in rats. J Exp Med 1975; 142:1550–1563.
9. Roux MA, McWilliams M, Phillips-Quagliata JM, Weisz-Carrington P, Lamm ME. Origin of IgA-secreting plasma cells in the mammary gland. J Exp Med 1977; 146:1311–1321.
10. Mogi G. Experimental OME with emphasis on mucosal immunity. In: Veldman J, ed. Immunobiology in otology, rhinology and laryngology. Amstelveen, The Netherlands: Kugler, 1987:25.

SUPPRESSION OF IMMUNE MEDIATED OTITIS MEDIA BY MUCOSA DERIVED SUPPRESSOR T CELLS

HIDEYUKI KAWAUCHI, M.D., SHIGEHIRO UEYAMA, M.D., ISSEI ICHIMIYA, M.D., YUICHI KURONO, M.D., and GORO MOGI, M.D.

It has been established recently that an antigen-antibody reaction or immune complex formation in the middle ear cavity, followed by complement activation, can be a pathogenic mechanism in otitis media with effusion.[1-3] On the other hand, the results of many studies support the idea that the tubotympanum is protected against microbial infections at the mucosal surfaces by the secretory immune system, of which the major immunoglobulin is secretory IgA.[4,5] It is well known that there are important regulatory interactions between systemic humoral immunity and the mucosal immune system.[6,7] The oral administration of thymus dependent antigens has been proven to induce the formation of regulatory T cells in Peyer's patches,[6] which suppresses IgG-IgM production and enhance IgA production. In the present study we investigated the effects of these mucosa derived suppressor T cells on the induction of IgG immune mediated otitis media with effusion in mice.

MATERIALS AND METHODS

Animals

C3H/HeN (lipopolysaccharide responsive) female mice bred in a specific pathogen free environment were purchased from a local breeder (Kyudo Experimental Animal Co., Kumamoto, Japan) and maintained in the animal facility of the Medical College of Oita until sacrifice. The mice were used for experiments at 8 weeks of age.

Antigen

Crystallized ovalbumin (grade III) purchased from the Sigma Chemical Co. (St. Louis, MO) was used as a thymus dependent antigen.

Induction of Immune Mediated Otitis Media with Effusion in Mice

C3H/HeN female mice were immunized intraperitoneally with 500 μg of ovalbumin emulsified in complete Freund's adjuvant. Twenty days after systemic immunization 30 μg of ovalbumin distilled in 0.8 percent hydroxypropylcellulose solution was inoculated into the left tympanic cavity through the inferior bullae. The antigen inoculations were performed aseptically under a surgical microscope. A microhole was made into the inferior bullae by use of a hand drill after exposure, and 20 μl of hydroxypropylcellulose solution containing crystallized ovalbumin was slowly injected by insertion of a fine tipped glass capillary tube, using a microinjector. The mice were killed 4 days after the inoculation of antigens into the tympanic cavity.

Induction of Mucosa Derived Suppressor Cells and Their Transfer

C3H/HeN mice were administered 40 mg of crystallized ovalbumin distilled in saline by gastric intubation with a steel syringe. Three days after the gastric intubation of antigens, Peyer's patches and spleen cells were harvested aseptically. These cells from antigen fed mice were transferred to the recipient mice 1 day before immunization. To serve as controls, donor mice were fed with saline. The effects of the transferred cells on antibody production were determined by the titration of serum antibody levels and plaque forming cells in the spleen. Antibody titers in sera were measured by the ELISA technique using horseradish peroxidase conjugated goat antimouse IgG (Fc fragment specific; Cappel, Cochranville, PA). The plaque forming cell assay was carried out according to the method of Richman et al[6] with a minor modification.

Evaluation of Inflammatory Reactions in Middle Ear

To evaluate the extent of the inflammatory reaction in the middle ear, the tympanic membranes were observed before sacrifice and middle ear effusions were removed under a surgical microscope. ELISA and cytologic study of the middle ear effusions were also performed. After sacrifice of the mice the bullae were fixed with 10 percent neutral buffered formalin solution, decalcified with 10 percent EDTA tris buffer (pH 6.93), embedded in paraffin, sectioned at 5 μm, and stained by routine hematoxylin-eosin staining to evaluate the histologic findings in the middle ear mucosa.

Enrichment and Elimination of T Cells

Peyer's patch or spleen cells from antigen fed donors were enriched for T cells by passage over a nylon wool column before adoptive transfer. Eliminationn of T cells in Peyer's patch or spleen cells was carried out by the treatment of these cells with a 1:200 dilution of anti-Thyl.2. monoclonal antibody (Becton-Dickenson) and a 1:10 dilution of rabbit complement (Cedarlane Low-Tox-M rabbit). Viable cells were counted after treatment and adjusted to the desired concentration before adoptive transfer.

RESULTS

Effect of Peyer's Patch Cells from Crystallized Ovalbumin Fed Mice on Induction of Immune Mediated Otitis Media

To induce immune mediated otitis media, mice were sensitized intraperitoneally with 500 μg of crystallized ovalbumin in complete Freund's adjuvant 20 days before delivery of the challenge of ovalbumin to the middle ear. As shown in Figure 1, the circulating anti-ovalbumin IgG titers increased 3 weeks after immunization in the control mice, which had undergone transfer with Peyer's patch cells from saline fed donors. On the other hand, anti-ovalbumin IgG antibody titers in the sera of mice that had undergone transfer with Peyer's patch cells from ovalbumin fed donors were significantly decreased, as compared to those in control mice. In addition, these Peyer's patch cells derived from ovalbumin fed donors suppressed the IgG plaque forming cell response in the spleens of recipients when they were transferred to recipient mice.

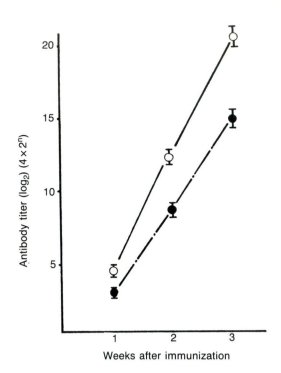

Figure 1 Kinetics of antiovalbumin IgG antibody in sera of mice transferred with Peyer's patch cells from ovalbumin fed donors (●) and from saline fed donors (○).

Analysis of the plaque forming cell response was carried out as follows: Recipient mice were immunized intraperitoneally with crystallized ovalbumin in complete Freund's adjuvant twice at 14 day intervals. Ten days after the secondary immunization, spleen cells were harvested for the plaque forming cell assay to demonstrate antigen specific IgG and IgA producing B cells. The number of IgG plaque forming cells in the spleens of recipients transferred with Peyer's patch cells from ovalbumin fed donors (12,600±673 plaque forming cells per 10^8 spleen cells) was significantly smaller than that in control mice (28,900±1,930), while the number of IgA plaque forming cells (840±49) exceeded that in control mice (240±37). These data reconfirmed the suppressive effect of Peyer's patch cells from ovalbumin fed mice on the IgG antibody response. Table 1 shows the results of the experiment to see whether Peyer's patch cells from ovalbumin fed donors can suppress immune mediated otitis media.

Nine of 10 control mice developed otitis media with effusion whereas otitis media was demonstrated in three of 10 mice transferred with Peyer's patch cells from ovalbumin fed donors. This information suggests that IgG immmune mediated otitis media with effusion can be suppressed to some extent by

TABLE 1   Effect of Adoptive Transfer of Peyer's Patch Cells from Ovalbumin Fed Donors on Induction of Immune Mediated Otitis Media with Effusion in Mice

Transferred Cells (2 × 10⁷)	Induction of Otitis Media with Effusion
Normal Peyer's patch cells (N = 10)	9/10
Peyer's patch cells of ovalbumin fed mice (N = 10)	3/10

Peyer's patch cells from antigen fed mice. In the tympanic cavities of mice that developed otitis media, middle ear effusions and inflammatory cell infiltrates were seen. The effusions were observed through the tympanic membrane under a microscope. Cells infiltrating into the tympanic cavity included substantial numbers of neutrophils and a few macrophages and lymphocytes. Histologically the thickness and edema of the mucosa and inflammatory cell infiltrations in the submucosal layer were observed in the peripheral portion and around the tympanic orifice of the eustachian tube. However, no inflammatory reactions were seen in the tympanic cavity in nonpresensitized mice.

Suppressor T Cells in Peyer's Patches Are Essential for Suppression of Immune Mediated Otitis Media

In this experiment we examined the phenotype of Peyer's patch cells essential for the suppression of immune mediated otitis media. Recipient mice were transferred with 2×10^7 fractionated spleen cells from ovalbumin fed donors, because it has been shown that suppressor cells in Peyer's patches migrate to the spleen.[6] Spleen cells of ovalbumin fed donors were fractionated into T cell and non-T cell populations and transferred to recipient mice 1 day before systemic immunization. When splenic T cells from the ovalbumin fed mice were transferred, antiovalbumin IgG antibody production was suppressed, but it was not suppressed when splenic non-T cells were transferred (Fig. 2).

When splenic non-T cells from ovalbumin fed donors were transferred, otitis media was demonstrated in eight of 10 mice as well as in nine mice transferred with splenic T cells from saline fed donors (Table 2). By contrast, otitis media was demonstrated in only one of 10 mice when splenic T cells from ovalbumin fed donors were transferred. This finding demonstrates that mucosa derived suppressor T cells are essential for the suppression of immune mediated otitis media.

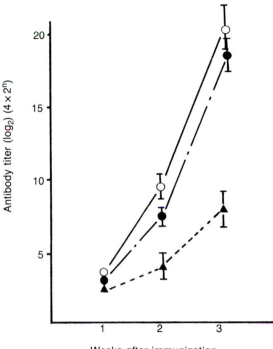

Figure 2 Kinetics of antiovalbumin IgG antibody in sera of mice transferred with splenic T cells from saline fed donors (○), splenic T cells from ovalbumin fed donors (▲), and splenic non-T cells from ovalbumin fed donors (●).

DISCUSSION

Although the etiologic factors responsible for otitis media with effusion have been investigated extensively, there is still controversy concerning its pathogenesis. Over the past decade studies have demonstrated that an immune reaction may be in-

TABLE 2   Effect of Adoptive Transfer of IgG Specific Splenic Suppressor T Cells on Induction of Immune Mediated Otitis Media with Effusion in Mice

Transferred Cells (2 × 10⁷)	Induction of Otitis Media with Effusion
Splenic T cells of saline fed mice (n = 10)	9/10
Splenic T cells of ovalbumin fed mice (n = 10)	1/10
Splenic non-T cells of ovalbumin fed mice (n = 10)	8/10

volved in inflammatory diseases of the middle ear. Thus eustachian tube dysfunction and immaturity of the immune surveillance system are considered to be causative factors of otitis media with effusion, which is followed by microbial infections in the middle ear. Once microbial infections occur in the middle ear, nonspecific and specific immune responses are mobilized to eliminate microorganisms. If the nonspecific immune response against microbial antigens fails, an antigen specific immune response occurs in the middle ear. In this process the antigen specific IgG or IgM antibody functions beneficially by way of opsonization or antibody dependent cell cytotoxicity. On the other hand, inevitable type III allergic reactions may occur concomitantly in the middle ear cavity and may contribute to the prolongation of inflammation—namely, chronic otitis media with effusion. IgG immune mediated otitis media in animal models has been reported by several investigators.[2,3]

In the present study we induced immune mediated otitis media in mice, supporting previous findings. It is clear that inflammatory reactions in the middle ears of mice in our experiments were immunologic in origin because we could not demonstrate inflammatory changes in the middle ears of nonsensitized mice. In addition, crystallized ovalbumin specific IgG antibody activity was significant in middle ear effusions as well as in sera. The question is whether these immunologic events contributing to middle ear inflammation can be controlled.

With this question in mind we attempted successfully to prevent immune mediated otitis media in mice by immunologic procedures with mucosa derived IgG specific suppressor T cells. Our results indicate that the suppression of otitis media in recipient mice can be attributed to the decreasing IgG antibody titer in the sera of mice that were transferred with mucosa derived suppressor T cells. Our results strongly suggest that mucosal immunization can be effective in preventing otitis media with effusion because mucosa derived regulatory T cells are beneficial not only in augmenting mucosal immunity (IgA response) but also in preventing IgG immune mediated inflammatory reactions in the middle ear.

REFERENCES

1. Mravec J, Lewis DM, Lim DJ. Experimental otitis media: an immune-complex-mediated response. Otolaryngology 1978; 86:258–268.
2. Ryan AF, Catanzaro A, Wasserman SI, Harris JP. Secondary immune response in the middle ear: immunological, morphological and physiological observations. Ann Otol Rhinol Laryngol 1986; 95:242–249.
3. Mogi G. Experimental OME with emphasis on mucosal immunity. Proceedings of second international academic conference on immunobiology in otology, rhinology and laryngology. Amsterdam: Kugler Publications, 1986:253–263.
4. Mogi G, Honjo S, Maeda S, Yoshida T, Watanabe N. Secretory immunoglobulin A (SIgA) in middle ear effusions. A further report. Ann Otol Rhinol Laryngol 1974; 82:92–101.
5. Bernstein JM, Tomasi TB Jr, Ogure PL. The immunochemistry of middle ear effusions. Arch Otolaryngol 1974; 99:320–326.
6. Richman LK, Graeff AS, Yarchoan R, Strober W. Simultaneous induction of antigen-specific IgA helper T cells and IgG suppressor T cells in the murine Peyer's patches after protein feeding. J Immunol 1981; 126:2079–2083.
7. Challacombe SJ, Tomasi TB Jr. Systemic tolerance and secretory immunity after oral immunization. J Exp Med 1980; 152:1459–1472.

EFFECTS OF OTITIS MEDIA WITH EFFUSION ON PASSAGE OF ANTIBODY INTO THE INNER EAR

ELIZABETH M. KEITHLEY, Ph.D., ALLEN F. RYAN, Ph.D., and
JEFFREY P. HARRIS, M.D., Ph.D.

It has been suggested that substances present in the middle ear during otitis media with effusion pass into the inner ear where they may cause impairment of function, ultimately resulting in sensorineural hearing loss. Of interest in this regard is the possibility that antigen and antibody in middle ear effusion gain access to the inner ear where they may either form damaging immune complexes or initiate an immune response, which may be deleterious to the inner ear structures.

Using a model of acute immune mediated middle ear effusion,[1] we previously investigated the capacity of antigen and antibody to gain entrance to the perilymph. The present study was designed to determine whether the round window membrane becomes more or less permeable to antibody when the middle ear is in a chronically inflamed state. An immunohistochemical test was used to localize plasma cells, which may be involved in the production of IgG found in the perilymph.

METHODS

Chronic otitis media with effusion was created in three guinea pigs by systemically sensitizing them with subcutaneous injections of 1 mg of keyhole limpet hemocyanin (KLH) in complete Freund's adjuvant followed by a booster of 1 mg of antigen in incomplete Freund's adjuvant 10 days later. Three weeks after the initial sensitization the right middle ear was challenged with soluble KLH (1.0 mg per 100 μl) by injection through the tympanic membrane. Although this procedure is the standard technique used for acute otitis media, chronic otitis media with effusion was created by repeated injections (twice per week for 6 weeks) of antigen (0.3 mg per 30 μl).

Six weeks after the initiation of inflammation, I^{125} labeled anti-KLH IgG (100 Ci, 0.6 mg per 0.1 ml) was injected through the tympanic membrane into the right middle ear, as was done previously in normal ears and in those with acute otitis media with effusion.[2] An additional guinea pig with normal middle ears was injected with I^{125} IgG in order to compare with the results previously obtained. Twenty-four hours later the bullae were opened using a postauricular approach, the middle ears were flushed with saline to eliminate contamination of the samples, and perilymph was collected through a microhole drilled in the cochlear capsule. Perilymph samples were also collected from the noninjected side to assess the background level of radioactivity in the perilymph. This activity presumably derived from the circulation. Gamma counts (counts per minute per microliter) were measured for the injected and noninjected ears.

Following the perilymph sampling procedure the animals were perfused intracardially with warm saline followed by acid-formalin.[3] The cochleas were decalcified in 4 percent ethylenediaminetetraacetic acid (4° C) for 5 to 6 weeks and embedded in Paraplast Plus. Six micron thick sections were

prepared using a direct immunohistochemical assay. They were incubated with either biotinylated goat antiguinea pig IgG (fc) (Cappel Laboratories, Cochranville, Pa.) or rabbit antiguinea pig IgA (ICN ImmunoBiologicals, Lisle, Il.). Both antibodies were tested in an enzyme linked immunosorbent assay and found not to cross react with other antibody isotypes. Streptavidin-horseradish peroxidase and 2-amino-9-ethylcarbazole in addition to 0.06 percent hydrogen peroxide were employed to visualize specific antibody binding in the tissue. Sections were counterstained with hematoxylin and cover-slipped using Dako mounting medium. Adjacent sections were stained with hematoxylin and eosin.

RESULTS

Following 6 weeks of antigen challenge, the middle ear contained persistent effusion, mucosal hyperplasia, fewer leukocytes than in the "acute" middle ears, and high levels of anti-KLH antibody.[4] The round window membrane contained dilated blood vessels and leukocyte infiltrations in the middle fibrous layer similar to that described following acute otitis media with effusion.[5] Leukocytes were most prominent at the margin of the membrane where it attached to the bone. In the "chronic" animals numerous plasma cells were also observed in the scala tympani adhering to the round window membrane. However, there was not an active inflammatory response within the perilymphatic space.

Specific immunohistochemical staining of the plasma cells in the round window membranes from the ears with chronic otitis media with effusion revealed many cells labeled with anti-IgG (Fig. 1). In contrast, only a few cells were labeled with anti-IgA.

Radioactive IgG levels in the perilymph from the ears with chronic otitis media were not significantly different from those measured in the perilymph samples from the opposite noninjected inner ears (Table 1). Gamma counts in the normal ear fell within the range seen previously for normal ears.[5]

DISCUSSION

Although the round window membrane has been shown to be permeable to small molecules such as antibiotics,[6] the results of experiments examining the capacity of large molecules to pass through the membrane have been more variable. Radiolabeled albumin was shown to gain access to peri-

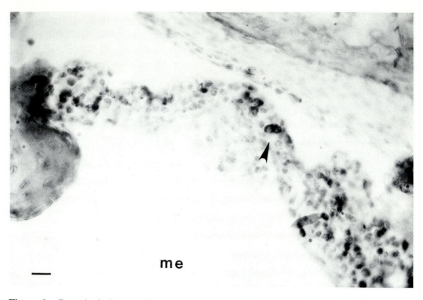

Figure 1   Round window membrane (dorsal margin) from a guinea pig with chronic immune mediated middle ear inflammation. IgG bearing plasma cells are labeled immunohistochemically with antibody to guinea pig IgG. Arrow, two of the labeled cells. me, middle ear. Bar = 20 μm.

lymph in normal and inflamed middle ears.[7] Horseradish peroxidase, on the other hand, was seen in one study to pass through an inflamed round window membrane but not through a normal one.[8] In another similar study the opposite was seen.[9] Horseradish peroxidase crossed the normal round window membrane but only to enter the inflamed round window membrane. KLH, a very large molecule, did not gain access to the inner ear following injection into a noninflamed middle ear (unpublished observations).

In order to examine whether antibody from middle ear effusions could gain access to the inner ear, we measured (by enzyme linked immunosorbent assay) specific anti-KLH antibody in perilymph samples from guinea pigs with acute otitis media with effusion and found elevated values relative to normal.[2] Because these were shown not to be derived from the serum, it was concluded that the antibody had originated in the middle ear. To determine the route of entry, I^{125} IgG was injected into normal or acutely inflamed middle ears, and autoradiographic sections of the inner ear were prepared. It was shown that the oval window was not permeable to IgG, whereas the round window membrane had label on both sides, indicating that at least some of the antibody in the perilymph may pass through the round window membrane from the middle ear.[5]

In the same study, in which radiolabeled IgG was injected into the middle ear space of normal and acutely inflamed middle ears, perilymph samples showed a small but statistically significant difference between the injected and noninjected ears (see Table 1).[5] This indicates that some middle ear antibody

TABLE 1   Radiolabeled IgG in Perilymph 24 Hours After Injection into the Middle Ear

| | No I^{125} IgG | 100 μl I^{125} IgG | | |
	Normal Middle Ear	Normal Middle Ear	Acute Middle Ear	Chronic Middle Ear
Median*	16	65	41	17
Range	0–37	29–125	9–114	4–28
n	14	6	10	3

* gamma counts per minute per μl of perilymph.
Rank sum:
   Normal vs. no injection, p<0.01.
   Acute vs. no injection, p<0.01.
   Chronic vs. no injection, not significant.

does cross the round window membrane to the perilymph. It is of interest that the variability was greater in the "acute" group than in the normal group. Five of the six ears in the normal group yielded counts above the background level, although only five of the 10 ears with acute otitis media with effusion produced counts above the background level. Given the present data indicating no passage into perilymph in an ear with chronic otitis media with effusion, it seems that the round window membrane becomes less permeable to IgG as the duration of otitis media increases. This finding is possibly related to the increased thickness that develops with increasing granulation tissue.

From the data generated in this study it appears that there may be yet another source of perilymph antibody—the IgG bearing plasma cells infiltrating the round window membrane in animals with otitis media with effusion. Their presence around the vessels in the membrane suggests that they emigrated from the systemic circulation. Because these animals were systemically sensitized to the KLH antigen, a clone of antigen specific B cells exists at the time of middle ear challenge. These cells may be recruited to the round window membrane vessels through a generalized middle ear inflammatory response following challenge by the sensitizing antigen. This response may act to protect the inner ear by binding antigens in the middle ear effusion, which otherwise may be able to pass through the membrane. Conversely, in chronic effusions, what was previously a protective mechanism may now result in the generation of immune complexes that go on to ultimately damage the round window membrane and inner ear.

Study supported by the Research Service of the Veterans Administration and by NIH-NINCDS grants NS14389 and NS18643.

REFERENCES

1. Ryan AF, Catanzaro A, Wasserman SI, Harris JP. Secondary immune response in the middle ear: immunological, morphological and physiological observations. Ann Otol 1986; 95:242–249.
2. Harris JP, Ryan AF. Effect of middle ear immune response on inner ear antibody levels. Ann Otol 1985; 94:202–206.
3. Curran RC, Gregory J. Effects of fixation and processing on immunohistochemical demonstration of immunoglobulin in paraffin sections of tonsil and bone marrow. J Clin Pathol 1980; 33:1047–1057.
4. Ryan AF, Harris JP, Keithley EM, Sharp P, Catanzaro A, Batcher S. Antibody production in acute and chronic immune mediated otitis media with effusion. In: Lim DJ, Bluestone CD, Klein JO, Nelson JD, eds. Recent advances in otitis media with effusion. Proceedings of the Fourth International Symposium. Toronto: BC Decker, 1988:199.
5. Harris JP, Keithley EM, Ryan AF. Passage of antibody from the middle ear into the inner ear. In: Sade J, ed. Acute and secretory otitis media. Amsterdam: Kugler, 1986:251–256.
6. Harada T, Iwamori M, Nagai Y, Nomora Y. Ototoxicity of neomycin and its penetration through the round window membrane into the perilymph. Ann Otol 1986; 95:404–408.
7. Goycoolea MV, Paparella MM, Goldberg B, Carpenter AM. Permeability of the round window membrane in otitis media. Arch Otolaryngol 1980; 106:430–433.
8. Saijo S, Kimura RS. Distribution of HRP in the inner ear after injection into the middle ear cavity. Acta Otolaryngol 1984; 97:593–610.
9. Scharchern PA, Paparella MM, Goycoolea MV, Duvall AJ. The permeability of the round window membrane during otitis media. Assoc Res Otolaryngol, 1987; 10:79.

PREVENTION AND MEDICAL MANAGEMENT

SPECIAL LECTURE:
RECENT DEVELOPMENTS OF BACTERIAL VACCINES RELATED TO THE PREVENTION OF OTITIS MEDIA

JOHN B. ROBBINS, M.D., RACHEL SCHNEERSON, M.D., and SHOUSUN C. SZU, Ph.D.

Pneumococci, *Haemophilus influenzae*, and *Staphylococcus aureus* are the three bacteria most frequently isolated in cases of otitis media in infancy and childhood. There are both similarities and differences in the pathogenesis and virulence factors of these three pathogens that influence the development of vaccines for the prevention of otitis media. It has been established by Giebink et al[1] in animal models and in infants and children by Teal and Klein[2] and Makela et al[3] that active immunization by parenteral injection with certain capsular polysaccharides (nonliving antigens) can prevent otitis media. This important principle has directed the research of several laboratories in developing anticapsular polysaccharide vaccines and in characterizing the immunochemical and functional properties of the human response to these protective antigens.

PNEUMOCOCCI

Pneumococci, isolated from otitis media, are invariably encapsulated with polysaccharides. There are now 85 recognized capsular polysaccharide types of pneumococcus; about 10 to 15 of these compose over 90 percent of the isolates from patients.[4,5] Most of those capsular types also cause invasive diseases in infants and children, as well as adults. Pneumococci without capsular polysaccharides may be considered nonpathogenic. Four capsular polysaccharide types—6, 14, 19, and 23—cause the majority of cases of pneumococcal otitis media in infants and children and represent a considerable proportion of the types causing serious disease in individuals of all ages, including adults, who have immunosuppressive conditions.[6] These types do not induce protective levels of antibody in infants and young children and are those most frequently isolated from cases of vaccine failure among adults immunized with the 23-valent pneumococcus vaccine.[3-8]

Austrian et al[4] have brought attention to an important principle that has emerged from the study of capsular polysaccharide vaccines in humans. There is an inverse relation between the disease potential of some capsular polysaccharides and their virulence.[9] Types 3 and 9 can be cited as representatives of capsular polysaccharide types that induce protective levels of antibodies in infants and children.[5] In addition to this age related immunogenicity, capsular polysaccharides possess an additional immunologic property that limits their usefulness as vaccines in infants and children. Reinjection of polysaccharides does not elicit a booster response;[7,10,11] a single injection elicits the maximal response that is characteristic of the age of the recipient. The latter property has been termed "T cell independence" for convenience.

Otitis media is considered an infection of secretory tissue, yet serum capsular antibodies have been shown to protect against otitis media caused by pneumococcus in experimental animals and infants and children.[1-3] These data indicate that the capsular polysaccharide is a virulence factor for pneumococcus that causes otitis media as well as pneumonia and other invasive diseases, and that sufficient levels of vaccine induced serum antibodies to this surface antigen confer type specific immunity to otitis media. That serum antibodies, specific to the capsular polysaccharides, can prevent otitis media has been surprising to some who consider otitis media a disease of the secretory tissue, a process that should not involve the participation of serum antibodies. Serum antibodies could exert their protective effect by two mechanisms: reducing acquisition of carriage of virulent pneumococcal types,[12] and activating complement dependent resistance mechanisms, such as phagocytosis, in the affected tissues.[13] It is probable that both mechanisms are operative.

Two approaches to provide vaccines that will prevent otitis media due to pneumococci in children are under way. The first is to both enhance the immunogenicity of and confer the property of T cell dependence to pneumococcal polysaccharides. The second approach is to use other components of the pneumococcus that could serve as protective antigens. It is hoped that the latter approach could provide a species specific protective antigen that might reduce the number of components necessary in a vaccine to confer type specific immunity in order to prevent pneumococcal otitis media.

Several components have been discussed as potential species specific antigens for pneumococcus. One promising approach, that of using the cell wall polysaccharide of pneumococcus, has been studied recently in our laboratory.[14] The use of the cell wall polysaccharide as a vaccine was prompted by two observations:

1. Monoclonal antibodies to phosphocholine conferred protection against lethal infection with pneumococci in mice.[15] Phosphocholine is a component of the cell wall polysaccharide that is present on all pneumococci but rarely is encountered in other streptococcal species.[16]
2. Monoclonal antibodies that were specific for phosphocholine and conferred protection in the mouse model also reacted with the cell wall polysaccharide.[17,18]

Therefore, it seemed logical that the phosphocholine component of the cell wall polysaccharide could be a protective antigen. Unfortunately our experimental results with antibodies to the cell wall polysaccharide, both those with phosphocholine specificity and antibodies reactive with the backbone of the cell wall polysaccharide, showed no protection in the mouse model against invasive pneumococcal infection.[14] Other components that are under investigation are the hemolysin (pneumolysin) of pneumococci and other, heretofore poorly understood protein components of the organism.[19,20]

The approach (that of inducing type specific antibodies in infants) using capsular polysaccharide-protein conjugates to induce protective levels of type specific antibodies has been more promising. A variety of methods has been employed to prepare semisynthetic vaccines composed of a polysaccharide and a carrier protein that are both T independent and medically relevant. For example, pneumococcus type 6A or 6B — tetanus toxoid conjugates, prepared in our laboratory by the methods used for *H. influenzae* type b and other polysaccharides of pathogenic bacteria, have been shown to be considerably more immunogenic than type 6 polysaccharide alone.[21] Clinical experiments are under way to assess the serologic properties of these new vaccines.[22-24]

HAEMOPHILUS INFLUENZAE

H. influenzae may exist as encapsulated or unencapsulated bacteria in the nasopharynx. Isolates from the middle ear show that only about 5 percent of *H. influenzae* organisms express the type b capsular polysaccharide, the virulence factor necessary for this bacterial species to cause invasive diseases such as meningitis and epiglottitis. The type b capsular polysaccharide, as are the pneumococcal polysaccharides associated with serious disease in infants and children, is nonimmunogenic in the age group that suffers the highest attack incidence of invasive diseases caused by this organism.

Considerable difficulty was encountered during attempts to modify polysaccharides by methods that are clinically acceptable.[25-28] When they are covalently bound to a carrier protein, such as diphtheria or tetanus toxoids, the immunogenicity of type b and other polysaccharides is considerably enhanced and they assume T dependent properties.[15-17] Preliminary evidence indicates that in regard to their increased immunogenicity and T cell dependence, *H. influenzae* type b–tetanus toxoid conjugates can confer protection against invasive disease in infants.[29] It is probable that these polysaccharide-protein conjugate vaccines will be in routine use in the next several years, and it is likely that this immunization procedure will eliminate *H. influenzae* type b as a cause of otitis media.

What about the other 95 percent of the *H. influenzae* ear isolates? A certain proportion have been shown by genetic methods to be derived from type b strains. It is known that repeated passage in vitro of type b strains can result in the development of organisms that have lost the capacity to express this capsule. This loss of type b capsule expression correlates with their decreased invasiveness. Thus, we could predict that immunization with effective type b polysaccharide conjugate vaccines would reduce even more the proportion of *H. influenzae* that cause purulent otitis media. The remainder of the organisms, perhaps about 60 to 80 percent of *H. influenzae*, seem not to be genetically related to the type b strains.

A search for antigens common to these *H. influenzae* strains that could exert protective immunity is under way. Several candidates appear promising. Among them are the surface appendages called pili or fimbriae, which can serve as attachment factors for this bacterial species to mucosal cells.[30-32] Antibodies to these pili could serve as an antiattachment factor and may play a role both in the prevention of otitis media as well as in systemic disease caused by this organism by inhibiting attachment. Other components that could serve as protective antigens are the outer membrane proteins of these bacteria, and work is under way to define what could be protective antigens that are widely shared among unencapsulated *H. influenzae.*[33-35]

STAPHYLOCOCCUS AUREUS

Until recently little was known about acquired immunity to these bacterial species. *S. aureus* can cause a variety of clinical diseases by different mechanisms. Yet invasive disease due to this organism has never been associated with a virulence factor whose activity correlated with invasiveness and that could be neutralized by the presence of an immune factor.[36] Progress in characterizing the structures of *S. aureus* involved in the pathogenesis of and immunity to invasive diseases caused by this organism has been hindered because there is no animal model for bacteremia caused by this pathogen.

Recently it has been discovered that *S. aureus* organisms isolated from the blood of patients possess heretofore unrecognized capsular polysaccharides.[37,38] Two capsular polysaccharides of *S. aureus* have been discovered previously, their effectiveness in an in vitro system characterized, and their structure elucidated. Previously described capsular polysaccharides of *S. aureus* have never been identified in isolates from patients with bacteremia. The newly discovered capsular polysaccharides have some properties that may explain their obscurity to date:

1. The colonial morphology of these capsular types is not distinctive from noncapsular variants.[39]
2. These capsular polysaccharides are cell associated, and their isolation, serologic classification, and structure elucidation have posed greater difficulties than other capsular polysaccharides of other invasive pathogens. The morphology of these capsules, as defined by electron microscopy, is similar to that of other encapsulated bacteria.[40,41]
3. Compositional analysis of five of the 11 known capsular types revealed all to contain aminouronic acids, which are difficult to analyze because of their unusual stability (resistance to hydrolysis).

Surveillance studies have shown that two types, types 5 and 8, compose about 70 percent of disease isolates. Recently three additional types have been isolated and typing sera prepared. With these serologic reagents it is now possible to identify about 90 to 95 percent of the isolates from bacteremia. In vitro studies show that organisms that possess these capsular types resist phagocytosis and that type specific (capsular polysaccharides) antibody enhances this protective activity.

Ordinarily *S. aureus* is a common inhabitant of the skin and respiratory flora. Decreased host resistance, usually induced by chemotherapeutic drugs and surgery, predisposes to bacterial infection with *S. aureus*. Plans are under way to prepare immune sera from volunteers immunized with *S. aureus* polysaccharide-protein conjugates and to evaluate their protective effect. The results of these clinical experiments, now being drafted, will be important in the design of future studies to see whether immunity to otitis media with *S. aureus* can or should be induced by active immunization of infants.

SUMMARY

Capsular polysaccharides serve as both virulence factors and protective antigens for bacteria that cause otitis media in infants and children. The development of chemical methods to bind these age related and T independent antigens to medically relevant proteins by clinically acceptable methods has been accomplished. These new semisynthetic vaccines composed of *H. influenzae* type b bound to diphtheria or tetanus toxoids or the outer membrane proteins of group B meningococci, have been shown to induce protective levels of antibodies in infants. Conjugates of pneumococcal type 6 polysaccharide and tetanus toxoid have been evaluated in adults, and the results are promising.

It can be expected that polysaccharide-protein conjugates will be evaluated for their effectiveness in preventing otitis media in infants in the near future. Other components of bacteria, which could provide more extensive coverage than the type specific immunity expected from conjugates, are being sought. In addition, noncapsular antigens that are widely shared through the *Haemophilus* species are being investigated in order to provide immunity to otitis media caused by unencapsulated *H. influenzae.*

New information about heretofore unrecognized capsular polysaccharides of *S. aureus* is being accumulated. Two types account for about 70 percent of the isolates from patients with bacteremia, and antibodies to these polysaccharides enhance in vitro phagocytosis of pathogenic strains. This information will be extended to investigate otitis media due to this pathogenic species.

REFERENCES

1. Giebink GS, Schiffman G, Petty K, Quie PG. Modification of otitis media following vaccination with the capsular polysaccharide of Streptococcus pneumoniae in chinchillas. J Infect Dis 1978; 138:480–487.
2. Teale DW, Klein JD. Greater Boston collaborators study group: use of pneumococcal vaccine for prevention of recurrent acute otitis media in infants in Boston. Rev Infect Dis 1981; 1:S113–S123.
3. Makela PH, Herva E, Sibakov M, Henrichsen J, Luotonen L, Leinonen LM, Timonen M, Koskela M, Pukander J, Gronroos P, Pontynen S, Karma P. Pneumococcal vaccine and otitis media. Lancet 1980; ii:547–551.
4. Austrian R, Howie UH, Ploussard JH. The bacteriology of pneumococcal otitis media. Johns Hopkins Med J 1977; 141:104–111.
5. Robbins JB, Austrian R, Lee CJ, Rastogi SC, Schiffman G, Henrichsen J, Makela PH, Broome CV, Facklam RR, Tiesjema RH, Parke JC Jr. Considerations for formulating the second-generation pneumococcal capsular polysaccharide vaccine with emphasis on the cross-reactive types within groups. J Infect Dis 1983; 148:1136–1159.
6. Bolan G, Broome CV, Facklam RR, Flikaytis BD, Fraser DW, Schlech WF. Pneumococcal vaccine efficacy in selected populations in the United States. Ann Intern Med 1986; 104:1–6.
7. Sell SH, Schiffman G, Vaughn WK, Wright PF. Pneumococcal polysaccharide vaccine: preliminary report of a clinical trial in infants. In: Parker MT, ed. Pathogenic streptococci. Chertsey, Surrey: Reedbooks Ltd., 1978.
8. Douglas RM, Paton JC, Duncan SJ, Hansman DJ. Antibody response to pneumococcal vaccination in children younger than five years of age. J Infect Dis 1983; 148:131–137.
9. Austrian R. Some observations on the pneumococcal vaccine and on the current status of pneumococcal disease and its prevention. Rev Infect Dis 1981; 3:51–57.
10. Heidelberger M. Persistance of antibodies in man after immunization. In: Pappenheimer DM, ed. Nature and significance of antibody response. New York: Columbia University Press, 1953:24.
11. Kayhty H, Karanko V, Peltola H, Helena Makela P. Serum antibodies after vaccination with Haemophilus influenzae type b capsular polysaccharide. No evidence for tolerance or memory. Pediatrics 1984; 74:857–865.
12. Hodges RG, MacLeod CM. Epidemic pneumococcal pneumonia. V. Final consideration of the factors underlying the epidemic. Am J Hyg 1946; 44:237–248.
13. Winkelstein JA, Shin HS, Wood WB Jr. Heat labile opsonins to pneumococcus. III. The participation of immunoglobulin and of the alternate pathway of C3 activation. J Immunol 1972; 108:1681–1689.
14. Szu SC, Schneerson R, Robbins JB. Rabbit antibodies to the cell wall polysaccharide of streptococcus pneumoniae fail to protect mice from lethal infection with encapsulated pneumococci. Infect Immun 1986; 54:448–453.
15. Briles DE, Forman C, Hudak S, Claflin JL. Antiphosphorylcholine antibodies of the T15 idiotype are optimally protective against Streptococcus pneumoniae. J Exp Med 1982; 156:1177–1185.

16. Sørensen UBS, Henrichsen J. Cross-reactions between pneumococci and other streptococci due to the C-polysaccharide and the Forssman antigen. J Clin Microbiol 1987; 25:1854–1859.
17. Yother J, Forman C, Gray BM, Briles DE. Protection of mice from infection with Streptococcus pneumoniae by anti-phosphocholine antibody. Infect Immun 1982; 36:184–188.
18. Szu SC, Clarke S, Robbins JB. Protection against pneumococcal infection in mice conferred by phosphocholine-binding antibodies: specificity of phosphocholine binding and relation to several types. Infect Immun 1983; 39:993–999.
19. Paton JC, Lock RA, Hansman DL. Effect of immunization with pneumolysin on survival time of mice challenged with Streptococcus pneumoniae. Infect Immun 1983; 40:548–552.
20. McDaniel LS, Scott G, Kearney JF, Briles DE. Monoclonal antibodies against protease sensitive antigens can protect mice from fatal infection with Streptococcus pneumoniae. J Exp Med 1984; 160:385–397.
21. Schneerson R, Robbins JB, Parke JC Jr, Sutton A, Wang Z, Schlesselman JJ, Schiffman G, Bell C, Karpas A, Hardegree MC. Quantitative and qualitative analyses of serum Haemophilus influenzae type b, pneumococcus type 6A and tetanus toxin antibodies elicited by polysaccharide-protein conjugates in adult volunteers. Infect Immun 1986; 52:501–518.
22. Anderson PW, Pichichero ME, Insel RA. Immunization of two-month old infants with protein-coupled oligosaccharides derived from the capsule of Hemophilus influenzae type b. J Pediatr 1985; 107:346–351.
23. Barkin JM, Zahradnik J, Samuelson J, Gordon L. Safety and immunogenicity of Hemophilus influenzae type b polysaccharide and polysaccharide diphtheria toxoid conjugate vaccines in children 15 to 24 months of age. J Pediatr 1987; 110:509–514.
24. Einhorn MS, Weinberg GA, Anderson EL, Granoff PD, Granoff DM. Immunogenicity in infants of Haemophilus influenzae type B polysaccharide in a conjugate vaccine with Neisseria meningitidis outer-membrane protein. Lancet 1986; ii:299–302.
25. Schneerson R, Barrera O, Sutton A, Robbins JB. Preparation, characterization and immunogenicity of Haemophilus influenzae type b polysaccharide-protein conjugates. J Exp Med 1980; 152:361–376.
26. Anderson P. Antibody responses to Haemophilus influenzae type b and diphtheria toxin induced by conjugates of oligosaccharides of the type b capsule with the nontoxic protein CRM 197. Infect Immun 1983; 39:233–238.
27. King SD, Wynter H, Ramlal A, Moodie K, Castle D, Kuo JSC, Barnes L, Williams CL. Safety and immunogenicity of a new Haemophilus influenzae type b vaccine in infants under one year of age. Lancet 1981; ii:705–708.
28. Chu CY, Schneerson R, Robbins JB, Rastogi SC. Further studies on the immunogenicity of Hemophilus influenzae type b and pneumococcal type 6A polysaccharide-protein conjugates. Infect Immun 1983; 40:245–256.
29. Pelotola H, et al. Personal communication.
30. Pichichero ME, Anderson EP, Loeb M, Smith DH. Do pili play a role in pathogenicity of Haemophilus influenzae type b? Lancet 1982; ii:960–962.
31. Tosi MF, Anderson DC, Barrish J, Mason ED Jr, Kaplan SL. Effect of piliation on interactions of Haemophilus influenzae type b with human polymorphonuclear leukocytes. Infect Immun 1985; 47:780–785.
32. Loeb MR, Smith DH. Outer membrane protein composition in disease isolates of Haemophilus influenzae: patho-

genic and epidemiological implications. Infect Immun 1980; 30:709-717.

33. Barenkamp SJ, Munson RS Jr, Granoff DM. Outer membrane proteins and biotype analysis of pathogenic nontypable *Haemophilus influenzae*. Infect Immun 1982; 36:535-540.

34. Hansen M, Musher DM, Baugh RE. Outer membrane proteins of nontypable *Haemophilus influenzae* and reactivity of paired sera from infected patients and their homologous isolates. Infect Immun 1985; 47:843-846.

35. Murphy TF, Bartos LC, Rice LA, Nelson B, Dudas KC, Apicella MA. Identification of a 16,000-dalton outer membrane protein on nontypable *Haemophilus influenzae* as a target for human serum bactericidal antibody. J Clin Invest 1986; 78:1020-1027.

36. Karakawa WW, Vann WF. Capsular polysaccharides of Staphylococcus aureus. Sem Infect Dis 1982; 4:285-293.

37. Arbeit RD, Karakawa MM, Vann WF, Robbins JB. Predominance of two newly described capsular polysaccharide types among clinical isolates of *Staphylococcus aureus*. Diag Microbiol Infect 1984; 2:85-91.

38. Karakawa WW, Vann WF, Sutton A, Schneerson R. Polyclonal and monoclonal anti-type 8 and type 5 capsular polysaccharides induce enhanced type-specific phagocytosis of Staphylococcus aureus (in press).

39. Karakawa WW, Fournier JM, Vann WF, Arbeit R, Schneerson R, Robbins JB. Methods for the serological typing of the capsular polysaccharides of *Staphylococcus aureus*. J Clin Microbiol 1985; 22:445-447.

40. Sompolinsky D, Samra Z, Karakawa WW, Vann WF, Schneerson R, Malik Z. Encapsulation and capsular types in isolates of *Staphylococcus aureus* from different sources and relationship to phage types. J Clin Microbiol 1985; 22:828-834.

41. Hochkeppel HK, Braun DG, Vischer W, Imm A, Sutter S, Staebubli U, Guggenheim R, Kaplan EL, Boutonnier A, Fournier JM. Serotyping and electron microscopy studies of Staphylococcus aureus clinical isolates with monoclonal antibodies to capsular polysaccharide types 5 and 8. Infect Immun 1982; 25:526-530.

CEFUROXIME AXETIL VERSUS CEFACLOR IN TREATMENT OF ACUTE OTITIS MEDIA

MARGARET A. KENNA, M.D., CHARLES D. BLUESTONE, M.D.,
PATRICIA FALL, R.N., B.S.N., C.P.N.P., JANET S. STEPHENSON, B.S., R.M.,
MARCIA KURS-LASKY, M.S., FREDERICK P. WUCHER, M.D., MARK M. BLATTER, M.D.,
and KEITH S. REISINGER, M.D.

Acute otitis media is a common disease in the pediatric age group.[1] Oral antimicrobial therapy is the standard treatment and is generally based on clinical signs and symptoms, as well as a knowledge of the usual bacterial pathogens, *Streptococcus pneumoniae*, *Haemophilus influenzae* (nontypable), and *Branhamella catarrhalis*.[2] Treatment failures with the more commonly utilized antimicrobial drugs are increasing, however, secondary to resistance caused by beta-lactamase production. In some studies 20 percent of *H. influenzae* and 75 to 80 percent of *B. catarrhalis* produce beta-lactamase.

Cefuroxime, a second generation cephalosporin with increased resistance to beta-lactamase, has been very effective and safe in the treatment of meningitis, acute mastoiditis, and acute sinusitis in children. However, it has been available only in a parenteral form, which is not absorbed when given orally.[3]

We studied cefuroxime-axetil, an esterified prodrug form of cefuroxime, which renders it orally absorbable, and compared it with cefaclor for the treatment of acute otitis media with effusion in a pediatric population.

METHODS

All children aged 7 months to 12 years with a possible diagnosis of acute otitis media were evaluated by one of three pediatricians (F.W., M.B., K.R.), all of whom are validated otoscopists. The diagnosis was made if the child had fever, irritability, or otalgia, and middle ear effusion documented by pneumatic otoscopy and tympanometry. After written consent was obtained from the parent(s), and oral assent if the child was 7 years old or older, tympanocentesis of the affected ear(s) was performed using sterile technique. The external ear canal was first cleaned of cerumen and then a culture was taken. Seventy percent alcohol was instilled into the ear canal for 1 minute and then removed by aspiration. Tympanocentesis was performed through the inferior portion of the tympanic membrane. Middle ear fluid was sent for culture and antibiotic susceptibility tests.

The child was randomized to receive either cefuroxime-axetil tablets (125 or 250 mg) or cefaclor suspension (250 mg per 5 milliliter). Children assigned to the cefuroxime group received 125 mg cefuroxime-axetil tablets every 12 hours if they were less than 2 years of age at enrollment and 250 mg cefuroxime-axetil tablets every 12 hours if they were 2 years of age or older. Patients assigned to the cefaclor group received 40 mg per kilogram per day divided equally into three daily doses given 8 hours apart with a maximal dosage of 1 g per day.

At entry, and again at the completion of therapy, a complete blood count with a differential, blood urea nitrogen determination, urinalysis, and liver function studies (SGOT, SGPT, alkaline phosphatase, LDH, total protein) were carried out. In all instances of abnormal laboratory values clinical correlation and medical follow-up were carried out.

The patients were reassessed clinically at days 3 to 5 and 10 to 14. Repeat tympanocentesis was performed at day 3 to 5 if the patient had persistent or recurrent fever or otalgia. Compliance was monitored by urine checks at the day 3 to 5 visit, and the amount of study medication left was measured after the 10 day course. All possibly related adverse events were recorded.

Children were excluded if they had tympanostomy tubes in place, prior ear surgery (excluding tubes), cholesteatoma, tympanic membrane retraction pockets, sleep apnea, severe systemic disease (acute or chronic), cleft palate, or Down's syndrome.

RESULTS

One hundred fifty-one children were initially randomized, 95 to cefuroxime-axetil and 56 to cefaclor. One hundred forty-two met the criteria for final evaluation, 88 in the cefuroxime-axetil group and 54 in the cefaclor group. Of the 88 patients who received cefuroxime-axetil, 47 (53 percent) had unilateral acute otitis media; of the 54 patients who received cefaclor, 31 (57 percent) had unilateral disease.

In the cefuroxime group, 43 percent were aged 7 to 23 months and 55 percent were aged 2 to 6 years (Table 1). Two patients in the cefaclor group were nonwhite; all other patients were white.

The most common pathogens isolated in both groups were S. pneumoniae, H. influenzae, and B.

TABLE 1 Age of Subjects Related to Treatment Received

	Cefuroxime	Cefaclor	Total (% Total Subjects)
7–23 mo	38*	25	63 (44%)
2–06 yr	48	23	71 (50%)
7–12 yr	2	6	8 (6%)
Total	88	54	142

* Number of patients.

catarrhalis; 6 percent of the cefuroxime-axetil group and 17 percent of the cefaclor group had sterile cultures. Beta-lactamase was produced by 27 percent of the H. influenzae and by 68 percent of the B. catarrhalis in the cefuroxime group. In the cefaclor group 25 percent of the H. influenzae and 83 percent of the B. catarrhalis produced beta-lactamase (Table 2).

One hundred twenty-one patients had at least one follow-up visit (68 cefuroxime-axetil and 53 cefaclor). Clinical improvement was noted in 96 percent of the cefuroxime group and in 94 percent of the cefaclor group. Of the 106 patients who underwent a check-up at 10 to 14 days, 58 percent of the cefuroxime-axetil group and 55 percent of the cefaclor group had no middle ear effusion.

There were three initial treatment failures in each group. In the cefuroxime group the initial organism was not isolated on reaspiration in two of the three subjects who underwent reaspiration; however, in two patients in the cefaclor group the initial organism isolated at the time of the second aspiration was S. pneumoniae in one patient and H. influenzae (beta-lactamase negative) in the other (Table 3). Of the patients who underwent a check-up at 10 to 14 days, 39 percent of the cefuroxime-axetil

TABLE 2 Bacteriology of Initial Middle Ear Isolates From 142 Subjects Related to Treatment Received

	Cefuroxime (n=88)	Cefaclor (n=54)	Total (% of Subjects)
S. pneumoniae	34*	17	51 (36%)
H. influenzae	26 [7%]+	16 [4%]	42 (30%)
B. catarrhalis	19 [13%]	6 [5%]	25 (18%)
S. pyogenes	6	3	9 (6%)
S. aureus	0	1	1 (1%)
"Other"	38	27	65 (46%)
No growth	5	9	14 (10%)

* Number of patients.
+ In brackets, the number of isolates that produced beta-lactamase.

TABLE 3   Microbiology of Initial and Repeat Middle Ear Aspirates in Three Subjects in Each Treatment Group Who Were Treatment Failures

Treatment Group	Microbiology at Entry Tap	Microbiology at Retap
Cefuroxime axetil	S. pneumoniae	Alpha strep., S. epidermidis
	H. influenzae (beta-lac. pos.)	Proprionobacterium acnes
	S. pneumoniae and S. epidermis	No retap
Cefaclor	S. pneumoniae (both ears)	S. pneumoniae, alpha streptococcus (left), sterile (right)
	H. influenzae (beta-lac. neg.) both ears	H. influenzae (beta-lac. neg.) both ears
	S. epidermidis (left) and H. influenzae (beta-lac. pos.)	S. epidermidis (left) S. epidermidis

TABLE 4   Side Effects According to Treatment Group

Treatment Group	No Effect	Side Effects Present					Total*
		Gastrointestinal	Rash	Rash/Diarrhea	Other	Total	
Cefuroxime	56 (76%)	11	1	0	6	18 (24%)	74
Cefaclor	47 (85%)	4	3	1	0	8 (15%)	55
Total	103	15	4	1	6	26	129

* Excludes subjects unable to take drug.

group and 35 percent of the cefaclor group had a recurrence of acute otitis media within 90 days.

There was a 24 percent incidence of side effects in the cefuroxime group and a 15 percent incidence in the cefaclor group. Most were mild and gastrointestinal in nature. All side effects cleared after discontinuation of the medication (Table 4). Several infants and young children found the cefuroxime-axetil formulation unpalatable when the tablet was crushed and did not finish a 10 day course of medication. These children were not included in the side effect calculations.

Cefuroxime-axetil was found to be safe and as effective as cefaclor in the treatment of acute otitis media with effusion in our pediatric population.

This study was supported in part by Glaxo, Inc.

REFERENCES

1. Teele DW, Klein JO, Rosner B, Bratton L, Fisch GR, Mathiew OR, Porter PJ, Starobin SG, Tarlin LD, Younes RP. Middle ear disease and the practice of pediatrics. JAMA 1983; 249:1026–1029.
2. Bluestone CD, Klein JO. Otitis media with effusion, atelectasis, and eustachian tube dysfunction. In: Bluestone CD, Stool SE, eds. Pediatric otolaryngology. Philadelphia: WB Saunders, 1983:356.
3. Nelson JD. Cefuroxime: a cephalosporin with unique applicability to pediatric practice. Pediatr Infect Dis 1983; 2:394—396.

CEFIXIME VERSUS CEFACLOR IN TREATMENT OF ACUTE OTITIS MEDIA WITH EFFUSION

MARGARET A. KENNA, M.D., CHARLES D. BLUESTONE, M.D.,
PATRICIA FALL, R.N., B.S.N., C.P.N.P., JANET S. STEPHENSON, B.S., R.M.,
MARCIA KURS-LASKY, M.S., FREDERICK P. WUCHER, M.D., MARK M. BLATTER, M.D.,
and KEITH S. REISINGER, M.D.

Acute otitis media with effusion is a common disease in the pediatric population and oral antimicrobial therapy is the standard treatment. However, because medical therapy for otitis media is generally based on clinical signs and symptoms, some patients continue to have otalgia, fever, and middle ear fluid after 10 days' therapy with an appropriate antimicrobial drug.

Two of the most common bacterial organisms found in acute otitis media, nontypable *Haemophilus influenzae* and *Branhamella catarrhalis*, often produce beta-lactamase,[1] resulting in resistance to some of the currently utilized antimicrobial drugs.

Cefixime, a new oral cephalosporin, is stable to beta-lactamase and is more potent in vitro than cefaclor, cephalexin, and amoxicillin against a wide variety of gram negative bacilli.[2,3] We studied the safety and effectiveness of cefixime and compared it with cefaclor for the treatment of acute otitis media in a pediatric population.

METHODS

Children aged 7 months to 12 years with a possible diagnosis of acute otitis media were evaluated by one of three pediatricians (M.B., K.R., or F.W.). The diagnosis was made if the child had fever, irritability, or otalgia and middle ear effusion was documented by pneumatic otoscopy and tympanometry. After written informed consent was obtained from the parent(s), and oral assent if the child was 7 years of age or older, tympanocentesis of the affected ear(s) was performed. The ear canal was cleaned of cerumen and a culture of the ear canal was obtained. The ear canal was then filled with 70 percent alcohol for 1 minute, after which the alcohol was removed by aspiration. Tympanocentesis was performed through the inferior portion of the tympanic membrane. Middle ear aspirates were sent for culture and antibiotic susceptibility tests. The child was then randomized to receive either cefix-

ime, 8 mg per kilogram once daily (QD); cefixime, 8 mg per kilogram divided into two daily doses (BID); or cefaclor, 40 mg per kilogram divided into three daily doses. The patients were reassessed clinically 3 to 5 days and 10 to 14 days after entry. Repeat tympanocentesis was performed if the patient had persistent or recurrent fever or otalgia up to 72 hours following entry into the trial. Compliance was monitored by evaluation of a patient diary and by measurement of the amount of study medication left after the 10 day course. All possibly related adverse events were recorded. At entry, and again at the 10 to 14 day visit, a complete blood count with a differential, blood urea nitrogen determination, and creatinine, alkaline phosphatase, total bilirubin, SGOT, and SGPT levels were obtained. Children were excluded from eligibility if they had known hypersensitivity to cephalosporins or accelerated hypersensitivity to penicillin, tympanostomy tubes, severe acute or chronic systemic disease, sleep apnea, prior major ear surgery, cleft palate, or Down syndrome.

Randomization to the cefixime QD group was discontinued after 10 patients because of a possible increase in side effects in this group. No comparable increase was seen in either the cefixime BID group or the cefaclor group.

RESULTS

One hundred thirty-five patients entered the study. Sixty-three received cefixime, 8 mg per kilogram twice daily; 10 received cefixime, 8 mg per kilogram daily; and 62 received cefaclor, 40 mg per kilogram three times daily. Of the 135 subjects, 129 patients met the criteria for final clinical evaluation: 60 cefixime BID, 10 cefixime QD, and 59 cefaclor. In the cefixime BID group, 30 were males and 30 were females. Of the cefixime QD group, 6 were males and 4 were females; in the cefaclor group, 31 were males and 28 were females. Unilateral acute otitis media was recorded in 55 percent of the cefixime BID group, 50 percent of the QD group, and 59 percent of the cefaclor group. The age of subjects was not significantly different among the treatment groups (Table 1). All patients were Caucasian.

TABLE 1   Age Distribution of Patients at Entry

Age	Cefixime (BID)	Cefixime (QD)	Cefaclor	Total
7–23 mo	28*	5	24	57 (44%)
2–6 yr	30	5	34	69 (54%)
7–12 yr	2	0	1	3 (2%)
Total	60	10	59	129

* Number of patients.

The middle ear pathogens most commonly isolated in all the groups were *Streptococcus pneumoniae*, *Haemophilus influenzae*, and *Branhamella catarrhalis*. In the cefixime BID group, 32 percent of the *H. influenzae* and 93 percent of the *B. catarrhalis* were beta-lactamase producing; in the cefixime QD group, 50 percent of the *H. influenzae* and 100 percent of the *B. catarrhalis* produced beta-lactamase; and in the cefaclor group, 19 percent of the *H. influenzae* and 56 percent of the *B. catarrhalis* were beta-lactamase positive (Table 2).

Ninety-seven percent of the patients with at least one follow-up visit reported no clinical symptoms. At the end of treatment there was no middle ear effusion in 74 percent of the cefixime BID group, 60 percent of the cefixime QD group, and 60 percent of the cefaclor group. Recurrence of acute otitis media within 90 days was noted in 44 percent of the cefixime BID group, 40 percent of the cefixime QD group, and 38 percent of the cefaclor group. There were four initial treatment failures, two in the cefixime BID group and two in the cefaclor group. Three of these patients underwent a second tympanocente-

sis. In two, one of the original organisms was reisolated, diphtheroids in one patient and *Pseudomonas aeruginosa* in the other. In the third patient no organism was isolated on either entry or follow-up tympanocentesis.

Adverse events, mainly gastrointestinal disturbances, were recorded in 21 percent of the cefixime BID patients, 50 percent of the cefixime QD patients, and 11 percent of the cefaclor patients. One patient in the cefaclor group who developed a rash discontinued the drug; all other patients were able to finish the full 10 day course. All side effects resolved after stopping the antimicrobial.

In our study cefixime appeared safe and effective when compared with cefaclor in the treatment of acute otitis media with effusion in the pediatric age group. Although both the daily and twice daily dosages were effective, there was a higher incidence of transient side effects in the once daily dosage group. We entered only 10 patients in this phase of the study, however, and this incidence of side effects might be different in a larger study population.

This study was funded by the American Cyanamid Company (Lederle Laboratories).

REFERENCES

1. Bluestone CD, Klein JO. Otitis media with effusion, atelectasis, and eustachian tube dysfunction. In: Bluestone CD, Stool SE, eds. Pediatric otolaryngology. Philadelphia: WB Saunders, 1983:356.
2. Neu HC, Chin N, Labtha Vikul P. Comparative in vitro activity and beta-lactamase stability of FR 17027, a new orally active cephalosporin. Antimicrob Agents Chemother 1984; 26:174–180.
3. Shimada K, Yokota T, Saito A, Shimado J, Kumazawa J. Antibacterial activity and tissue levels of FK 027, a new generation oral cephalosporin. Presented at 24th Interscience Conference on Antimicrobial Agents and Chemotherapy, October 1984.

TABLE 2   Bacteriology of Initial Middle Ear Isolates from 129 Subjects Related to Treatment Received

	Cefixime (BID)	Cefixime (QD)	Cefaclor	Total (% of Subjects)
S. pneumoniae	21*	5	23	51 (40%)
H. influenzae	19 [6]+	4 [2]	16 [3]	39 (30%)
B. catarrhalis	15 [14]	1 [1]	9 [5]	25 (19%)
S. pyogenes	2	0	2	4 (3%)
S. aureus	2	0	0	2 (2%)
"Other"	23	6	24	53 (41%)
No growth	1	0	4	5 (4%)

* Number of patients.
+ Numbers in brackets indicate beta-lactamase production.

PENETRATION OF TRIMETHOPRIM AND SULFAMETHOXAZOLE INTO THE MIDDLE EAR IN EXPERIMENTAL OTITIS MEDIA

DANIEL M. CANAFAX, Pharm.D., G. SCOTT GIEBINK, M.D., GARY R. ERDMANN, Ph.D., ROBERT J. CIPOLLE, Pharm.D., F.C.C.P., and STEVEN K. JUHN, M.D.

Children with acute otitis media are given various antimicrobial drugs as standard therapy because bacteria play an etiologic role in the pathogenesis of this disease.[1] Unfortunately not all these patients respond to antimicrobial treatment, and many children develop recurrent infections. Our group of investigators studied penicillin penetration into experimental middle ear effusions and found less of this antimicrobial drug present than in the serum.[2] In addition, the middle ear effusion (MEE) concentrations produced were below the minimal bactericidal and inhibitory concentrations for commonly isolated middle ear bacterial pathogens for a significant period of time.

We suspect that a factor contributing to otitis media recurrence is the failure to achieve and maintain adequate antimicrobial drug concentrations in the middle ear effusion. To test this hypothesis the serum and middle ear effusion pharmacokinetics of trimethoprim and sulfamethoxazole was studied in the chinchilla otitis media model.

MATERIALS AND METHODS

Two sequential studies of the pharmacokinetic behavior of trimethoprim and sulfamethoxazole were performed in the chinchilla model of serous otitis media.

Study I

The pharmacokinetics of trimethoprim and sulfamethoxazole was evaluated in eight healthy chinchillas (400 to 700 g). Two animals each were sampled after trimethoprim and sulfamethoxazole doses of 2.5 and 12.5, 5 and 25, 10 and 50, and 20 and 100 mg per kilogram, respectively. An additional five animals each were studied after 5 and 25 and 10 and 50 mg per kilogram trimethoprim and sulfamethoxazole doses. Blood samples were taken, after ketamine anesthesia (20 mg per kilogram intra-

muscularly), by cardiac puncture at 0, 0.5, 1, 2, 4.5, 7, and 12 hours after the dose for each animal.

Study II

In nine healthy chinchillas (400 to 700 g) the eustachian tubes were obstructed by Silastic sponges 10 to 14 weeks prior to the study. At the time of study 14 of the 18 ears had developed effusions. Sample specimens were taken from the animals on the first study day and on the seventh day after the administration of trimethoprim, 10 mg per kilogram, and sulfamethoxazole, 50 mg per kilogram intramuscularly, every 12 hours. Blood samples were drawn at 1, 2, 5, 8, and 12 hours after the first and last doses for each animal. The middle ear effusion was aspirated through the epitympanic bulla and was cultured on sheep's blood agar.

Trimethoprim and Sulfamethoxazole Liquid Chromatograph Determinations

The trimethoprim and sulfamethoxazole serum and effusion concentrations were analyzed using a Hewlett Packard 1090L liquid chromatograph.[3] The assay sensitivity was 0.1 ng per milliliter with a coefficient of variation equal to 5.2 percent.

RESULTS

Study I

Figure 1 shows the trimethoprim and sulfamethoxazole serum concentration data for the four different dosages studied in single animals. Table 1 summarizes the pharmacokinetic parameters calculated from this pilot study. These data suggest that a trimethoprim and sulfamethoxazole dose of 10 and 50 mg per kilogram best replicated the serum concentrations seen in humans given standard doses.[4]

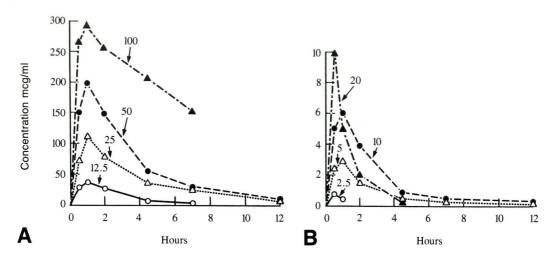

Figure 1 Serum concentration-time curves for sulfamethoxazole (*A*) and trimethoprim (*B*) in single chinchillas given four different doses (mg per kilogram) of each drug.

TABLE 1 The Pharmacokinetics of Trimethoprim and Sulfamethoxazole in Eight Chinchillas Demonstrated by the Mean ± SD Half-life and Maximal Serum Concentration (C_{max})

Drug	Dose (mg/kg)	Half-life (Hours)	Cmax (mcg/ml)
Trimethoprim	2.5	0.4 ± 0.1	1.8 ± 0.4
	5	2.7 ± 1.1	4.2 ± 1.0
	10	4.3 ± 0.4	6.4 ± 5.0
	20	1.2 ± 0.7	18.8 ± 7.0
Sulfamethoxazole	12.5	1.5 ± 0.4	67 ± 12
	25	2.6 ± 0.9	110 ± 85
	50	6.9 ± 4.0	200 ± 99
	100	5.9 ± 1.6	315 ± 7

An additional five animals were given trimethoprim and sulfamethoxazole doses of 5 and 25 mg per kilogram, and the mean ± SD half-life and maximal serum concentration (C_{max}) values were 3.0 ± 0.9 hours and 3.2 ± 1.0 mcg per milliliter for trimethoprim and 3.6 ± 1.7 hours and 136 ± 23 mcg per milliliter for sulfamethoxazole. The five animals given trimethoprim and sulfamethoxazole doses of 10 and 50 mg per kilogram had mean ± SD half-life and C_{max} values of 3.9 ± 0.6 hours and 8.2 ± 4.0 mcg per milliliter for trimethoprim and 5.7 ± 2.8 hours and 238 ± 77 mcg per milliliter for sulfamethoxazole.

Study II

Figure 2 demonstrates the serum and middle ear effusion concentrations achieved after giving trimethoprim and sulfamethoxazole in a single animal. Table 2 shows the half-life and C_{max} values produced by trimethoprim and sulfamethoxazole doses of 10 and 50 mg per kilogram. A slight increase in the half-life but no significant serum accumulation was observed after 7 days. It was noted, however, that the different trimethoprim and sulfamethoxazole half-lifes produced very different ratios of these two drugs; these ratios are thought to be important in the therapeutic benefit of this drug combination.

The calculated area under the serum and middle ear effusion trimethoprim and sulfamethoxazole concentration-time curves (AUC) is shown in Table 2. This evaluation demonstrates a slight serum accumulation of both drugs from day 0 to day 7. The middle ear effusion trimethoprim AUC value does increase (39 percent), suggesting that middle ear effusion antimicrobial drug concentrations require a few doses to achieve eventual steady state concentrations. This accumulation is different for trimethoprim and sulfamethoxazole, again showing the changing drug ratios.

The ratio of serum and middle ear effusion maximal and AUC values increased slightly at steady state (Table 2). Trimethoprim penetrated better into the middle ear effusion than sulfamethoxazole, a property that altered the trimethoprim-sulfa-meth-

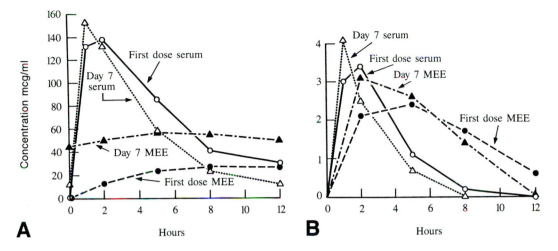

Figure 2 Serum and middle ear effusion concentration-time data from a single chinchilla given sulfamethoxazole, 50 mg per kilogram (*A*), and trimethoprim, 10 mg per kilogram (*B*).

TABLE 2 Pharmacokinetic Parameters (Mean ± SD) Calculated from Serum and Middle Ear Effusion Concentrations after Trimethoprim and Sulfamethoxazole Doses of 10 and 50 mg per kg

	Half-life, hr (N)	Cmax, mcg/ml (N)	AUC (hr-mcg/ml) Serum (N)	AUC (hr-mcg/ml) Middle Ear Effusion	Cmax Middle Ear Effusion / Cmax (Serum) (N)	AUC Middle Ear Effusion / AUC (Serum) (N)
Trimethoprim						
Day 0	1.4 ± 0.4 (9)	2.7 ± 0.7 (9)	9.0 ± 4 (9)	14.4 ± 5 (9)	0.8 ± 0.5 (11)	1.7 ± 0.6 (8)
Day 7	3.9 ± 4.1 (7)	2.9 ± 0.9 (8)	11.1 ± 8 (8)	20 ± 10 (6)	1.1 ± 0.8 (8)	2.1 ± 1.2 (6)
Sulfamethoxazole						
Day 0	4.3 ± 2.1 (9)	141 ± 17 (9)	873 ± 423 (8)	687 (1)*	0.38 ± 0.3 (11)	0.94 (1)*
Day 7	5.0 ± 3.8 (7)	156 ± 29 (8)	971 ± 631 (8)	716 ± 461 (6)	0.54 ± 0.3 (8)	0.76 ± 0.2 (5)

* Only one of nine animals produced data that could be analyzed for AUC.

oxazole middle ear effusion concentration ratio and may affect antibacterial activity.

Most strains of *Streptococcus pneumoniae* are susceptible to trimethoprim (MIC = 1.0 mcg per milliliter) and sulfamethoxazole (MIC = 32 mcg per milliliter).[5] Eight of nine trimethoprim treated animals (89 percent) spent at least 4 hours after each dose with middle ear effusion concentrations of trimethoprim less than 1.0 mcg per milliliter. In three of nine (33 percent) sulfamethoxazole treated animals middle ear effusion concentrations never exceeded 32 mcg per milliliter, and seven of nine animals (78 percent) spent at least 4 hours with middle ear effusion concentrations less than 32 mcg per milliliter.

DISCUSSION

On the basis of these results in an animal model of acute purulent otitis media that parallels human disease, it is likely that subtherapeutic antimicrobial concentrations occur in middle ear effusions in some patients. Even in the ideal case, shown in Figure 2, effusion concentrations just exceed usual MIC values.

Perhaps the most revealing finding from this study is the changing trimethoprim-sulfamethoxazole ratio after the antimicrobial dose is given. This occurs in both the serum and middle ear effusion as a result of faster trimethoprim clearance from both fluids. The ideal ratio of 1:19 is exceeded by 2 to 10 times, depending on the method of ratio calculation. The result would be less trimethoprim antibacterial activity, which is thought to be the more important therapeutic component.

The slight trimethoprim and sulfamethoxazole accumulation in middle ear effusions needs to be taken into account in future studies by pretreating animals with the test antimicrobial drug for several days. The clinical significance of this finding may be that missed antimicrobial doses result in less than optimal middle ear effusion drug concentrations.

The highly variable middle ear effusion drug concentrations seen in animals could allow the production of resistant bacteria or leave unkilled bacteria to cause future episodes of acute otitis media. These events may even account for chronic effusion in some patients. Future studies will be directed at these questions to better define the role of subtherapeutic antimicrobial concentrations in otitis media.

Study supported in part by NIH grant 5P5O-NS-14538.

REFERENCES

1. Klein JO. Microbiology of otitis media. Ann Otol Rhinol Laryngol 1980; 89(Suppl 68):98–101.
2. Juhn SK, Edlin J, Jung TTK, Giebink GS. The kinetics of penicillin diffusion in serum and middle ear effusions in experimentally induced otitis media. Arch Otorhinolaryngol 1986; 243:183–185.
3. Erdmann GR, Canafax DM, Giebinks GS. High performance liquid chromatographic analysis of trimethoprim and sulfamethorazole in microliter volumes of chinchilla middle ear effusion and serum. J Lig Chromatography (In press).
4. Patel RB, Welling PG. Clinical pharmacokinetics of cotrimoxazole. Clin Pharmacokinet 1980, 5:405–423.
5. Kucers A, Bennett NM. Trimethoprim and cotrimoxazole. In: Kucers A, Bennett NM; eds. The use of antibiotics: a comprehensive review with clinical emphasis. 3rd ed. London: W Heinemann, 1979:687.

MEDICAL MANAGEMENT OF CHRONIC SUPPURATIVE OTITIS MEDIA WITHOUT CHOLESTEATOMA

MARGARET A. KENNA, M.D. and CHARLES D. BLUESTONE, M.D.

Chronic suppurative otitis media without cholesteatoma is defined as otorrhea through a perforated tympanic membrane lasting longer than 6 weeks that is unresponsive to medical management with oral antimicrobial therapy and ototopical drugs. In the pediatric population the condition is not infrequent and occurs in patients with both tympanic membrane perforation and tympanostomy tubes.[1]

Tympanomastoid surgery has been the standard treatment for patients who have failed to benefit from medical therapy. There are problems with this approach, including the potential toxicity of ototopical drugs, the lack of antimicrobial drugs that are effective in oral doses against the usual causative organisms (especially *Pseudomonas aeruginosa*), the occurrence of chronic suppurative otitis media in young children with tympanostomy tubes, and the failure of surgery, with continued otorrhea. The use of surgical therapy has been based on the assumption that the histopathologic changes associated with chronic suppurative otitis media are irreversible. A recent report, however, suggests that some patients with this disorder can be treated successfully with medical therapy alone[2] and that some of the pathologic changes are reversible. Previously we reported 36 children with chronic suppurative otitis media.[3] Here we present an updated report of the first 36 patients and data relating to 30 additional patients with chronic suppurative otitis media.

METHODS

Children aged 6 months to 18 years with chronic suppurative otitis media without cholesteatoma unresponsive to intensive medical management for at least 6 weeks were eligible for the study. The patients were referred by Children's Hospital of Pittsburgh staff physicians and by outside referring physicians. Children were excluded if they had any evidence of intratemporal or intracranial suppurative complications or cholesteatoma. All parents gave informed consent, and tympanomastoid surgery was offered as an option. All patients underwent otomicroscopic examination at entry, under general anesthesia if necessary, with culture and susceptibility testing of bacterial isolates of middle ear fluid. After careful cleansing of the external auditory canal, middle ear fluid was obtained through the patent tube or perforation with a sterile 18 or 20 gauge spinal needle attached to a sterile Alden-Senturia trap (Storz, St. Louis, MO). Daily aural toilet, using suction debridement, was performed using the otomicroscope. Granulation tissue was removed and sent for histopathologic review. Antimicrobial drugs were administered intravenously according to the culture and susceptability test reports. At entry all children underwent a complete audiologic examination, complete blood count with differential, and blood urea nitrogen, creatinine, and fasting blood glucose tests. Other laboratory studies, radiographs, and consultations were obtained as needed.

Sixty-six children were enrolled in the study between July 1, 1983, and December 31, 1986. There were 38 males and 28 females aged 11 months to 17 years (Table 1). There were 60 white children, 5 black children, and 1 biracial child. The duration of drainage ranged from 6 weeks to 6 years, with a mean of 4.38 months and a median of 4 months. Otorrhea was unilateral in 41 patients and bilateral in 25. Of the 60 patients, 39 had drainage through tympanostomy tubes and 26 through perforations; 1 patient had drainage through both a tube and a perforation in the same ear. Seven children had had otologic surgery (other than tympanostomy tube placement) in the affected ear. Four had undergone tympanomastoidectomy and three had undergone tympanoplasty.

RESULTS

In 59 patients (89 percent) complete resolution of otorrhea occurred with medical management alone; seven patients required tympanomastoid surgery in addition to medical management. In the latter patients the findings were as follows: two children had occult cholesteatoma, two had middle ear and mastoid cavities completely filled with granulation tissue, one had only hyperplastic middle ear and mastoid mucosa, one had a cholesterol granuloma and an aditus ad antrum block, and one had extensive osteitis of the mastoid. Six patients required more than one admission for recurrent or persistent otorrhea. Three of these patients had perforations and three had tubes. In all patients with tympanostomy tubes in place the tubes had been removed and replaced in an effort to stop the otorrhea; these three children were all younger than 18 months of age. One had choanal atresia and a cleft palate. Of the 66 patients, 21 percent had a congenital anomaly or systemic disease that might have contributed to the development of the middle ear disease (Table 2).

The duration of treatment ranged from 3 to 35 days, with a mean of 8.8 days. Many different antimicrobial drugs were used in the treatment of the 66 patients. A semisynthetic penicillin used alone was the most common treatment. A single antimicrobial drug was used in 51 patients, and two antimicrobial drugs were used concurrently in 15 patients.

Microbiologic Findings

Thirty-one organisms were isolated from 91 ear cultures in the 66 patients (Table 3). The bacterial organism most commonly isolated was *Pseudomonas aeruginosa*, found in 64 percent of the ears cultured. *Staphylococcus aureus* was isolated from 20 percent of the ears and diphtheroids from 18 percent.

TABLE 1 Ages and Sex of 66 Children with Chronic Suppurative Otitis Media Without Cholesteatoma

Ages (Yr)	Male	Female	Total
<1	2*	0	2
1–2	15	8	23
3–6	7	7	14
7–10	9	8	17
11–17	5	5	10
Total	38	28	66

* Number of patients.

TABLE 2 Associated Anatomic-Medical Condition in 14 Patients with Chronic Suppurative Otitis Media

Condition	Number of Patients
Down syndrome	2
Cleft palate	2
Abnormal facies and delay	2
Microcephaly	2
Cri du chat, bifid uvula	1
Bilateral choanal atresia and cleft lip	1
Hypogammaglobulinemia	1
Lipodystrophy	1
Albinism	1
Hypothyroidism	1

TABLE 3 Microbiology of Middle Ear Aspirates from 66 Infants and Children (91 Ears) with Chronic Suppurative Otitis Media

Microbiologic Species	Number of Isolates
Pseudomonas aeruginosa	58
Staphylococcus aureus	18
Diphtheroids	16
Staphylococcus epidermidis	7
Streptococcus pneumoniae	7
Haemophilus influenzae, nontypable	6
Alpha-hemolytic streptococcus	5
Streptococcus pyogenes, group A	4
Pseudomonas maltophilia	3
Proteus mirabilis	3
Nonhemolytic streptococcus	3
Candida albicans	3
Escherichia coli	2
Enterococcus	2
Pseudomonas cepacia	2
Branhamella catarrhalis	2
Acinetobacter calcoaceticus	2
Eikenella corrodens	1
Moraxella sp.	1
Alcaligenes odorans	1
Haemophilus influenzae, type b	1
Citrobacter freundii	1
Serratia marcescans	1
Enterobacter cloacae	1
Micrococcus sp.	1
Klebsiella pneumoniae	1
Aspergillus fumigatus	1
Yeast (not specified)	1
Peptostreptococcus	1
Bacillus sp. (not specified)	1

Audiometric Findings

All children underwent behavioral testing, with both air and bone conduction threshold testing when it was possible. In addition six patients underwent auditory brainstem response testing. During medical treatment no patient had a worsening of hearing. The seven patients who underwent tympanomastoid surgery showed essentially no change in hearing status. Nine patients had varying degrees of mental retardation, which made accurate behavioral testing more difficult, but there appeared to be no significant differences between pre- and post-treatment audiograms.

Radiographic Studies

Mastoid radiography was performed in all the first 36 patients. In no patient was the treatment strategy changed because of these films. Mastoid radiographs were more helpful in confirming the diagnosis than in making it. Specifically, even in retrospect the occult cholesteatoma found at surgery in one child in the first group was not suspected or seen in the plain radiographs.

In the second group of 30 patients, mastoid roentgenography was done in only eight patients usually to confirm the chronicity of chronic suppurative otitis media or to better delineate disease on the contralateral side; treatment was not altered because of radiographic studies.

Three patients in the first group and nine patients in the second group underwent computed tomographic scanning. In four of these patients tympanomastoid surgery was carried out after the failure of medical therapy. In only one of these patients was the underlying disease, cholesteatoma, suggested by the computed tomographic scan. In the other patients the computed tomographic findings, usually read as being consistent with mastoiditis, did not distinguish the group who required surgery (and therefore had failed medical therapy) from the patients who were successfully treated with medical therapy.

Other Studies

Some patients underwent a limited immune work-up when the disease did not initially respond to medical management. In eight children quantitative serum immunoglobulin concentrations were measured, and in six cases they were normal. One child had a low IgA level without other laboratory or systemic abnormalities. The other patient, an 11

month old white male, had a low total IgA level as well as an abnormal T cell helper-suppressor ratio. This child also had sustained chronic and recurrent systemic illnesses, including chronic suppurative otitis media (which did not clear with surgery), gastroenteritis, recurrent pneumonia, and generalized failure to thrive. Two children had skin tests for allergy, with one positive result and one negative.

Follow-Up

The follow-up period ranged from 3 months to 3.5 years, with a mean of 1.4 years. During this time one patient from the first group of 36 patients required tympanomastoid surgery for refractory otorrhea. This patient had bilateral cleft palate and was found to have cholesteatoma at the time of surgery.

Thirteen patients had at least one episode of acute otitis media with otorrhea in the originally affected ear. All responded to prompt treatment with aural toilet, oral antimicrobial therapy, and topical therapy and did not require intravenous antimicrobial therapy. As of March 31, 1987, four patients had not returned for follow-up after discharge from the hospital.

DISCUSSION

Further study of the initial 36 patients, in addition to the 30 additional patients, provided some interesting insights into chronic suppurative otitis media without cholesteatoma. The incidences of success with intensive medical therapy in the first and second groups were 89 percent and 90 percent, respectively. The findings at surgery in the patients who failed to benefit from medical therapy were also similar, and the number of patients from each group with pre-existing congenital anomalies, underlying chronic medical problems, or both was similar (19 percent, group I; 23 percent, group II).

There were some interesting differences. In the first group the mean duration of otorrhea was 6 months, whereas in the second group it was 4 months. This likely reflects the earlier referral of patients with chronic suppurative otitis media because of our encouraging results with the first group of patients. The children in group II were also slightly younger than those in the first group; in group I 28 percent of the patients were 2 years of age or younger, whereas in group II, 49 percent of the patients were 2 years of age or younger. Again this might reflect earlier referral. In group I 61 percent had tympanic membrane perforations and 39 percent had tympanostomy tubes. In group II 83 percent had otorrhea through tympanostomy tubes and only 17 percent through perforations.

The patients who failed to benefit from medical therapy and eventually required tympanomastoid surgery were, on the average, 6 years older than the patients who did not undergo surgery, with only one exception—the 11 month old patient with probable hypogammaglobulinemia and immune deficiency. This may be an indicator of the chronicity of the disease.

One advantage of medical therapy is the avoidance of surgery, with the attendant risks of facial nerve injury, hearing loss, and even continued otorrhea. Surgery in very small children may be questioned because of the small size of the mastoid and the position of the facial nerve. The immune system of a small child is still developing, making recurrent disease a definite possibility; medical therapy "buys time," allowing the immune system to mature.

What should be the plan if medical therapy fails? In a small child removal of the tympanostomy tube can be attempted. In our patients this had usually been tried before the child's referral to us, but either drainage continued through the new tube or the child developed recurrent and symptomatic middle ear disease requiring reinsertion of the tube, with subsequent recurrent otorrhea. Tympano-mastoidectomy would be the obvious alternative in an older child with granulation tissue and aditus block.

If the middle ear and mastoid are fairly clear of granulation tissue but there is continued otorrhea through a large perforation, tympanoplasty can be performed in an attempt to restore the integrity of the middle ear—mastoid—eustachian tube physiology. Surgery remains the treatment of choice if suppurative complications or cholesteatoma is present.

We believe that the success of medical therapy utilizing vigorous systemic and local care gives support to the possibility that many of the histopathologic changes associated with chronic suppurative otitis media are reversible, especially when it is treated early.

REFERENCES

1. Gates GA, Avery C, Priltoda TJ, Holt GR. Post-tympanostomy otorrhea. Laryngoscope 1986; 96:630–634.
2. Haverkos HW, Caparosa R, Yu VL, Kamerer D. Moxalactam therapy: its use in chronic suppurative otitis media and malignant external otitis. Arch Otolaryngol 1982; 108:329–333.
3. Kenna MA, Bluestone CD, Reilly JS, Lusk RP. Medical management of chronic suppurative otitis media without cholesteatoma in children. Laryngoscope 1986; 96:146–151.

DOUBLE BLIND RANDOMIZED CLINICAL TRIAL ON THE EFFECT OF DIFFERENT TREATMENTS IN RECURRENT ACUTE OTITIS MEDIA

JACOB G. MOL, M.D., C.L.M. APPELMAN, M.D., G.J. HORDIJK, M.D., R.A. DE MELKER, M.D., F.W.M.M. TOUW-OTTEN, Ph.D., and G.J. LEPPINK, Ph.D.

Acute otitis media is a common disease among young children in the Netherlands. According to the latest report of the Dutch Health Council, 90 percent have at least one episode of acute otitis media before the age of 10. Half these children have one or more recurrences. Most are cured without any symptoms, but some have chronic ear disease and long-standing hearing loss.

The aim in our continuing study is to determine whether patients at high risk of developing complications can be treated symptomatically with nosedrops and analgesics or whether therapy with antibiotics or myringotomy is necessary.

We did a retrospective study of the medical histories of patients treated surgically for complications of acute otitis media. They had undergone either mastoidectomy in the acute phase or more exten-sive surgery for chronic ear disease. From 1980 to 1983, 86 children up to 14 years of age were oper-ated upon. Fifty-one also had otolaryngologic problems and other serious diseases or syndromes and were excluded from the study. Only five chil-dren had undergone no surgical interventions, and 30 of the remaining 35 children had not had surgi-cal intervention. The patients had undergone a total of 108 surgical interventions (adenotomy, grommet placement, mastoidectomy). This group is at risk of recurrences and complications of acute otitis me-dia. Thus we decided as the most important criteri-on for our prospective study that all patients must have had at least one period of acute otitis media in the 12 months prior to entry into the study.

The study we designed includes 1,380 children with recurrent otitis media between the ages of 6 months and 12 years. At random they are divided into four groups and receive four different treat-ments. The effect of treatment is measured after 3, 14, and 28 days and after 1 year.

On day 1 a child with earache visits the gener-al practioner. The criteria include earache, infect-ed eardrum, previous acute otits media between 4 weeks and 12 months of age, and a present age be-tween 6 months and 12 years. Excluded from the study are those with perforated eardrum, allergy to penicillin, antibiotic therapy in the previous 4 weeks, or any disease other than an otolaryngologic disease not already noted.

The general practitioner takes a detailed medi-cal history and conducts a physical examination, measures the temperature himself, and stages the acute otitis media from stages I to III. After diag-nosis by the general practitioner the child visits the otolaryngology department of the University Hospi-tal where the diagnosis is confirmed. The children are divided at random into four groups and therapy is given. All children are treated with nosedrops and analgesics. In addition to this symptomatic thera-py, group A children receive a placebo and a sham

myringotomy, group B receive antibiotics and a sham myringotomy, group C receive a placebo and myringotomy, and group D receive antibiotics and myringotomy. After 3 days the general practition-er, who is not aware of the therapy that has been given, judges whether the condition of the child has improved or worsened. If there is still earache or fever, we classify the course as irregular and the code is broken. If the condition of the child has im-proved, the general practitioner is consulted again after 14 days for the same procedure. After 28 days the otolaryngologist performs otoscopy, tympano-metry, and (if the child is 4 years or older) audi-ometry. Then the general practitioner follows the child for another year and notes all the otolaryngo-logic problems of the child and his family to detect prognostic factors for recurrences and complica-tions. After 1 year tympanometry and audiometry are done again.

By comparing all the data we hope to answer the question whether it is justified to maintain a "wait and see" attitude in recurrent acute otitis me-dia or whether more aggressive treatment is need-ed. That selection on the basis of a high probability of complications in our patient group is correct is supported by our findings so far. After the 4 week evaluation nearly 80 percent of our patients have hearing problems and B type tympanometric find-ings. In due time we hope to report the results.

REFERENCES

1. Bluestone C. Otitis media in children: to treat or not to treat. N Engl J Med 1982; 306:1399–1404.
2. Van Buchem F. Therapy of acute otitis media: myringoto-my, antibiotics or neither? Lancet 1981; 24: 883–887.
3. Howie VM, Ploussand JH, Sloyer O. The "Otitis Prone" condition. Am J Dis Child 1975; 129:676.
4. Pukander J, et al. Occurrence and recurrence of acute otitis media among children. Acta Otolaryngol 1981; 94: 479–486.
5. Saah J, et al. Treatment of acute otitis media. JAMA 1982; 248:1071–1072.

EFFECTS OF AMPICILLIN TREATMENT ON THE BIOCHEMICAL AND CYTOLOGICAL PROFILES OF EXPERIMENTAL PURULENT OTITIS MEDIA

SUDHIR P. AGARWAL, M.D., JAMES EDLIN, B.S., STEVEN K. JUHN, M.D., and G. SCOTT GIEBINK, M.D.

Acute otitis media is a common childhood disease. At least 70 percent of all children have one episode by age 5 years. Bacterial infection plays a significant role in the pathogenesis of purulent otitis media, and a variety of antimicrobial drugs are used as standard therapy. In vitro bacterial susceptibility testing of common middle ear bacterial pathogens to a variety of orally administered antimicrobial drugs has been well described, but the optimal dosage and duration of therapy in acute purulent otitis media are empiric and have not been carefully defined by pharmacokinetic in vivo study. It is reasonable to assume that distribution into the middle ear varies among antimicrobial drugs, resulting in variable drug concentrations in the middle ear. Characterization of antimicrobial kinetics in otitis media is of practical value in designing intervention trials to compare the relative efficacies of various antimicrobial drugs in the treatment of acute otitis media.[1] Subtherapeutic concentrations of antimicrobial drugs in the middle ear space, particularly subbactericidal levels, may contribute to the persistence of bacteria in the middle ear cavity and continued middle ear inflammation. This eventually may result in chronic otitis media with effusion, a condition that complicates 6 to 10 percent of all cases of acute otitis media.[2]

Our objective in this study was to determine the effect of ampicillin on the cytologic and biochemical features of middle ear effusion in experimental purulent otitis media and to compare several ampicillin dosages and durations of treatment in the chinchilla animal model.

MATERIALS AND METHODS

Purulent otitis media was produced in 20 healthy chinchillas by direct inoculation of type 7F *Streptococcus pneumoniae* into the middle ear bullae. A small bacterial inoculum (20 colony forming units) was used to reduce the likelihood of dissemi-

nated infection. Ampicillin, 100 mg per kilogram, was given intramuscularly every 24 hours, beginning on the sixth day after bacterial inoculation and continuing for 5 days (group A) and 10 days (group B). Control animals received no treatment during the same period of time. Middle ear effusions were aspirated on the day prior to the initiation of treatment, 2 days after initiation, and at 5 days (group A) and 10 days (group B). Each middle ear effusion sample was subjected to culture on 5 percent sheep's blood agar, a leukocyte count using a Neubauer cell chamber and a differential count on a smear stained with May-Grünwald-Giemsa stain,[3] ampicillin assay using a radial diffusion method,[4] biochemical assays for lysozyme using a radial diffusion method,[3] and protease inhibitor assays using immunochemical methods.[5]

RESULTS

All middle ear effusion cultures in the treatment group were sterile after the beginning of ampicillin therapy. The pharmacokinetics of ampicillin after a single dose (100 mg per kilogram) is shown in Figure 1. Serum levels reached a peak of 36 μg per milliliter and declined rapidly to a level below our detection limit (0.5 μg per milliliter) at 24 hours. By contrast, the effusion peak concentration (10 μg per milliliter) was observed at 2 hours and declined to 1.0 μg per milliliter at 24 hours. Effusion ampicillin levels in the treatment group were found to be in the range of 1.0 to 10 μg per milliliter; this is well above the 0.05 μg per milliliter minimal inhibitory concentration for the *Streptococcus pneumoniae* strain we employed.

Cytologic study of the effusion specimens revealed that polymorphonuclear leukocytes were the predominant cell in both the treatment and control groups. A distinct decrease in the number of polymorphonuclear leukocytes was observed after the initiation of treatment, whereas lymphocyte and

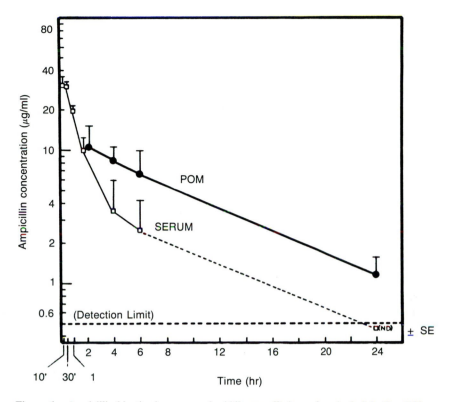

Figure 1   Ampicillin kinetics in serum and middle ear effusions after single injection (100 mg per kilogram). POM, purulent otitis media.

macrophage concentrations remained constant. By contrast, in the control group there was an increase in the number of polymorphonuclear leukocytes, whereas lymphocyte and macrophage numbers remained constant.

Lysozyme activity in middle ear effusion samples from the ampicillin treated animals declined from a pretreatment value of 240 μg per milliliter to 89 μg per milliliter after 5 days of treatment. In the control group lysozyme activity remained unchanged. These results are similar to those in previous experiments in the chinchilla using penicillin.[6]

The concentrations of the protease inhibitors alpha-1-antitrypsin and alpha-2-macroglobulin were determined in the effusion specimens. There was a trend toward increased levels in the treated group compared to those of controls (Figs. 2, 3).

DISCUSSION

These results demonstrate that ampicillin treatment of purulent otitis media causes cytologic as well as biochemical changes in middle ear effusions. Studies of the kinetics of penicillin therapy in an ex-

perimental animal model have been previously reported from this laboratory.[6]

Adequate levels of ampicillin, well above the minimal inhibitory concentration for the pneumococcal strain used to produce purulent otitis media, reached the middle ear, as shown by negative cultures in the treatment group and by the bioassay results. It is not surprising that polymorphonuclear leukocytes were the predominant cell in acute purulent otitis media, since acute inflammatory conditions, regardless of etiology, are heralded by the presence of polymorphonuclear leukocytes. In acute bacterial infections capillary dilation and increased permeability take place, leading to leakage of biologically active chemotactic factors, which induce migration of polymorphonuclear leukocytes to the area of inflammation. Polymorphonuclear leukocyte granules are a major source of lysozyme, a hydrolytic enzyme that aids in the degradation of bacterial cell walls, especially when the cell wall has been weakened by factors such as antibiotics. A decrease in lysozyme activity would be expected with antibiotic therapy and was confirmed in this study.

Protease inhibitors may represent a new biochemical marker for assessing the efficacy of anti-

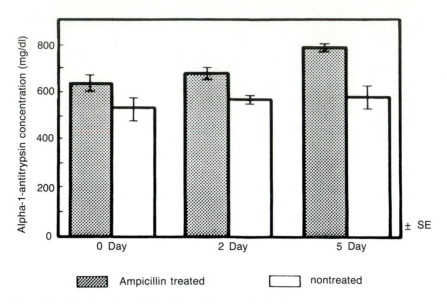

Figure 2   Alpha-1-antitrypsin levels in middle ear effusion in control and ampicillin treated animals.

biotic therapy. The inhibitors alpha-1-antitrypsin and alpha-2-macroglobulin compose about 90 percent of all protease inhibitor function in plasma and complex with various proteases, especially lysosomal proteases, thereby regulating their activity.[5] Polymorphonuclear leukocytes are a storehouse of proteases that may be released into the middle ear. These proteases then can complex with the inhibi-

tors. Polymorphonuclear leukocyte numbers decrease with treatment; therefore less protease is released, resulting in an increase in noncomplexed protease inhibitors. The levels of inhibitors appear to be balanced by several factors, including vascular permeability, degree of inflammation, degradation, and reabsorption.

The establishment of guidelines is needed to de-

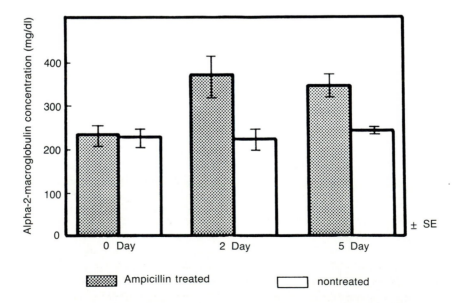

Figure 3   Alpha-2-macroglobulin levels in middle ear effusion in control and ampicillin treated animals.

termine the optimal dosage and duration of anti-biotic therapy for complete resolution of otitis media. Animal models provide a convenient tool to formulate these guidelines. We have presented only a portion of our results on the efficacy of ampicillin treatment in experimental purulent otitis media. Histopathologic examination of the temporal bones from animals in this study is currently being carried out to clarify the efficacy of ampicillin in otitis media treatment.

This research was supported in part by grant 5P5O-NS-I4538 from the National Institute of Neurological and Communicative Disorders and Stroke.

REFERENCES

1. Schentag JJ, Gengo FM. Principles of antibiotic tissue penetration and guidelines for pharmacokinetic analysis. Med Clin North Am 1982; 66:39–49.
2. Howie VM, Ploussard JH, Sloyer JL. The "otitis prone" condition. Am J Dis Child 1978; 129:676–678.
3. Juhn SK, Sipila P, Jung TTK, Edlin J. Biochemical pathology of otitis media with effusion. Acta Otolaryngol 1984; Suppl 14:45–51.
4. Jalling B, Malmborg AS, Lindman A, Boreus LO. Evaluation of a micromethod for determination of antibiotic concentrations in plasma. Europ J Clin Pharmacol 1972; 4:150–157.
5. Hamaguchi Y, Juhn SK, Sakakura Y. Protease inhibitors in middle ear effusions from experimental otitis media with effusion. Am J Otolaryngol (in press).
6. Juhn SK, Edlin J, Jung TTK, Giebink GS. The kinetics of penicillin diffusion in serum and middle ear effusions in experimentally induced otitis media. Arch Otorhinolaryngol 1986; 243:183–185.

EFFECTS OF PENICILLIN, IBUPROFEN, CORTICOSTEROID, AND TYMPANOSTOMY TUBE INSERTION ON EXPERIMENTAL OTITIS MEDIA

TIMOTHY T.K. JUNG, M.D., Ph.D., SOON-JAE HWANG, M.D., DAVID OLSON, B.S., JAE-SUNG LEE, M.D., STANLEY K. MILLER, B.S., DAVID POOLE, M.D., TAE-HYUN YOON, M.D., G. SCOTT GIEBINK, M.D., and STEVEN K. JUHN, M.D.

Otitis media results from the complex interactions of many factors, most important of which are infection and eustachian tube dysfunction. Either infection or eustachian tube dysfunction can cause secretion of inflammatory mediators, which in turn can induce middle ear inflammation and effusion. Thus, the rational treatment of otitis media might include antibiotics for the infection, tympanostomy tube insertion for the eustachian tube dysfunction, and the use of specific inhibitors of inflammatory mediators.

Among the inflammatory mediators in otitis media, arachidonic acid metabolites seem to play an important role in the pathogenesis of otitis media.[1,2] Arachidonic acid metabolites that cause inflammation include prostaglandins (PGs) in the cyclo-oxygenase pathway and leukotrienes (LTs) in the lipoxygenase pathway. Since nonsteroidal anti-inflammatory drugs inhibit prostaglandin synthesis and corticosteroids inhibit both the cyclo-oxygenase and lipoxygenase pathways by reducing the available precursor, arachidonic acid, it is reasonable to investigate the effect of these inhibitors of arachidonic acid metabolism on the pathogenesis of otitis media.

When patients with otitis media with effusion were treated with a nonsteroidal anti-inflammatory drug, naproxen, no significant difference was found between the treated and placebo groups.[3] Therapy with corticosteroid, however, was consistently effective in the treatment, at least in the short term.[4-6] In our previous studies of the effect of ibuprofen, corticosteroids, and penicillin on the pathogenesis of experimental pneumococcal otitis media, we also found that another nonsteroidal anti-inflammatory drug (ibuprofen) alone was not effective for the treatment of otitis media, suggesting that lipoxygenase products such as leukotrienes may be more important in the pathogenesis of otitis media than prostaglandins.[7]

The purpose in the present study was to determine the effect of penicillin, ibuprofen, corticosteroid, and tympanostomy tube insertion alone or in combination on a new model of experimental otitis media in chinchillas, to find the role of different arachidonic acid metabolites in the pathogenesis of otitis media, and eventually to find the best mode of therapy for otitis media.

MATERIALS AND METHODS

Forty-eight healthy chinchillas were used in this study. First, immune mediated otitis media was induced by sensitizing the animals with a subcutaneous injection of keyhole limpet hemocyanin (Pacific Bio-Marine Labs, Venice, CA) with complete Freund's adjuvant. Two weeks after initial sensitization, intrabullar injections of keyhole limpet hemocyanin were carried out every 2 days four times. Then purulent otitis media was induced in the animals by inoculating viable type 7F Streptococcus pneumoniae through the dorsal bullae on day 0.[7]

After 3 days the presence of purulent otitis media was verified by otoscopy and tympanometry, and the bullae were aspirated to obtain effusion fluid for culture. The animals then were assigned randomly to eight treatment groups of six animals each. The various treatment regimens were given for 7 days, days 4 to 10 (Table 1). On day 11 the animals were anesthetized by the intramuscular injection of ketamine hydrochloride (40 mg per kilogram) and the dorsal portions of the bullae were opened. Middle ear fluid was aspirated for culture and biochemical assays. Animals were perfused first with normal saline followed by 10 percent buffered formalin solution. Temporal bones were removed and processed as described previously.[7] Every tenth section was stained with hematoxylin and eosin for microscopic examination.

Microbiologic, biochemical, and morphologic factors tested included the results of bacterial culture; the presence or absence of effusion; tympanometry; concentrations of lysozyme, PGE_2, 6-keto-$PGF_{1\alpha}$, and LTB_4 and temporal bone histopathologic study.

Lysozyme concentrations were determined using a lysozyme test kit (Kallestad Co., Chaska, MN). Prostaglandin concentrations were measured by a double antibody radioimmunoassay method,[8] and LTB_4 levels were measured using a radioimmunoassay kit (Amersham Co., Arlington Heights, IL). Data were analyzed using the analysis of variance methods.

RESULTS

Results are summarized in Table 2 and statistical analyses of data are summarized in Table 3.

Culture Results

All ears were culture positive before treatment started. All penicillin treated ears became culture negative and all nonpenicillin treated ears remained culture positive.

Presence of Fluid

Middle ear effusions were present in all ears of the animals treated with ibuprofen or tympanostomy tubes and in 42 to 90 percent of the animals in the other groups (see Table 2). In general, the groups in which penicillin was given had lower num-

TABLE 1 Experimental Design

Experimental Groups	Items Tested in All Groups
Saline control	Bacterial cultures
Procaine penicillin G, 100,000 U/kg/day intramuscularly	Presence of effusion
	Tympanometry
Hydrocortisone (Solu-Cortef), 4mg/kg/day in two doses every 12 hr intraperitoneally	Lysozyme
	PGE_2
Ibuprofen, 30 mg/kg/day in 2 doses every 12 hr orally	6-Keto-$PGF_{1\alpha}$
	LTB_4
Tympanostomy tube insertion	Temporal bone histopathologic features
Penicillin and hydrocortisone	
Penicillin and ibuprofen	
Penicillin and tympanostomy tube	

TABLE 2 Summary of Results

Experimental Groups	No. Ears with fluid at Day 11 (%)	Lysozyme (µg/ml)	6-Keto-PGF$_{1\alpha}$ (ng/ml)	PGE$_2$ (ng/ml)	LTB$_4$ (ng/ml)
1. Control	67	156.0	7.80	0.487	10.93
2. Penicillin	50	50.9	0.70	0.513	2.24
3. Hydrocortisone	90	100.6	3.52	0.565	7.51
4. Ibuprofen	100	118.8	3.25	1.491	11.42
5. Tympanostomy tube	100	155.1	2.18	0.652	8.20
6. Penicillin and hydrocortisone	42	48.8	12.74	0.658	4.36
7. Penicillin and ibuprofen	58	66.4	5.63	0.284	2.96
8. Penicillin and tympanostomy tube	67	66.1	1.25	0.118	7.67

bers of ears with effusion than nonpenicillin treated groups. Significant differences were found in all factors analyzed except between the tympanostomy tube and ibuprofen groups. Tympanometric findings corresponded well with the presence of fluid.

Concentrations of Lysozyme

Lysozyme concentrations in the middle ear effusions were highest in the control group followed by the tympanostomy tube, ibuprofen, hydrocortisone, penicillin plus ibuprofen, penicillin plus tympanostomy tube, penicillin, and penicillin plus hydrocortisone groups, in that order of decreasing amounts (see Table 2). Significant differences in the concentrations of lysozyme were found between treated and control groups, between penicillin and nonpenicillin groups, and between penicillin and tympanostomy tube groups.

TABLE 3 Analysis of Variance

Contrasts	Variables			
	Lysozyme	LTB$_4$	6-Keto-PGF$_{1\alpha}$	PGE$_2$
A	S* ($0.002 < P < 0.005$)	S ($0.02 < P < 0.05$)	NS†	NS
B	NS	NS	S ($0.02 < P < 0.05$)	NS
C	S ($P < 0.001$)	S ($0.01 < P < 0.02$)	S ($0.02 < P < 0.05$)	S ($0.002 < P < 0.005$)
D	NS	NS	NS	NS
E	S ($0.01 < P < 0.02$)	NS	NS	NS
F	S ($0.005 < P < 0.01$)	S ($0.02 < P < 0.05$)	NS	NS

Contrasts

A: Treated (2, 3, 4, 5, 6, 7, 8) versus control (1)
B: "Pure" (3, 4, 5) versus "mixed" (6, 7, 8)
C: "Penicillin" (2, 6, 7, 8) versus "nonpenicillin" (3, 4, 5)
D: Penicillin (2) versus "mixed" (6, 7, 8)
E: Penicillin (2) versus other single treatments (3, 4, 5)
F: Penicillin (2) versus tympanostomy tube (5)

Experimental groups

1: Control
2: Penicillin
3: Hydrocortisone
4: Ibuprofen
5: Tympanostomy tube
6: Penicillin and hydrocortisone
7: Penicillin and ibuprofen
8: Penicillin and tympanostomy tube

* S, significant difference.
† NS, no significance.

Concentration of 6-Keto-PGF$_{1\alpha}$

The largest concentrations of 6-keto-PGF$_{1\alpha}$ were found in the penicillin plus hydrocortisone group followed by the control, penicillin plus ibuprofen, hydrocortisone, ibuprofen, tympanostomy tube, penicillin plus tympanostomy, and penicillin groups, in that order of decreasing amounts (see Table 2). Significant differences were noted between "pure" and "mixed" treatment and between penicillin and nonpenicillin groups (see Table 3).

Concentration of PGE$_2$

Concentrations of PGE$_2$ were highest in the ibuprofen group followed by penicillin plus hydrocortisone, tympanostomy tube, hydrocortisone, penicillin, control, penicillin plus ibuprofen, and penicillin plus tympanostomy tube groups, in that order of decreasing amounts (see Table 2). A significant difference was noted between the penicillin and nonpenicillin groups (see Table 3).

Concentrations of LTB$_4$

Concentrations of LTB$_4$ were highest in the ibuprofen group followed by the control, tympanostomy tube, penicillin plus tympanostomy tube, hydrocortisone, penicillin plus hydrocortisone, penicillin plus ibuprofen, and penicillin groups (see Table 2). Significant differences were found between treated and control groups, between penicillin and nonpenicillin groups, and between penicillin and tympanostomy tube groups (see Table 3).

Histopathology of Temporal Bones

The histopathologic features of temporal bones from each treatment group were studied. Specifically, the presence or absence and the degree of effusion, leukocytes, granulation tissue, osteoneogenesis, hemorrhage in the middle ear space, and hyperemia, edema, leukocytes, metaplasia, and hemorrhage in the middle ear mucosa were studied. The most severe inflammatory changes were found in the ibuprofen, tympanostomy tube, hydrocortisone, and control groups. The greatest amount of resolution of inflammation was seen in the penicillin plus hydrocortisone and penicillin groups. The penicillin plus ibuprofen group showed a moderate degree of inflammation, with a thickened subepithelial space with dilated capillaries and inflammatory cells.

DISCUSSION

In this animal model penicillin therapy was effective in sterilizing middle ear effusions. The presence of fluid paralleled the degree of inflammation. The highest percentages of fluid filled ears were found in the ibuprofen treated and tympanostomy tube groups. Our previous study using a different animal model showed similar findings after ibuprofen treatment.[7] This is probably because of increased production of lipoxygenase products, which cause more inflammation and increased fluid production. Placement of tympanostomy tubes did not prevent the formation of fluid. In fact, animals with tympanostomy tubes fared the same or worse than controls in terms of most of the factors we studied. Ears with tympanostomy tubes had higher lysozyme and LTB$_4$ levels than those in any other groups except controls. The possible reasons for the ineffectiveness of tympanostomy tubes in the treatment of this animal model of otitis media include reflux from the nasopharynx, contamination from the external auditory canal, and the nature of fluid (being an inflammatory exudate rather than a serous transudate caused by the negative pressure). Similar observations in keyhole limpet hemocyanin induced otitis media were noted by Ryan and Catanzaro.[9]

Concentrations of lysozyme in the middle ear effusions seem to be a sensitive indicator of the degree of inflammation, and, as observed, that the most acute inflammatory condition was present in the control and tympanostomy tube groups and the least in the penicillin plus hydrocortisone group.

Concentrations of PGE$_2$ are another indicator of inflammation. Penicillin treatment significantly lowered the levels of PGE$_2$ compared with groups not treated with penicillin. Ibuprofen alone did not block PGE$_2$ synthesis, but the combination of penicillin and ibuprofen did lower the concentration of PGE$_2$.

Concentrations of LTB$_4$ were highest in the ibuprofen group because ibuprofen shunts more precursor to the lipoxygenase pathway. LTB$_4$ is known to be a potent chemotactic agent to polymorphonuclear leukocytes and also a potent inflammatory mediator.[10,11] LTB$_4$ concentrations in the middle ear fluid seem to be another sensitive marker for the inflammatory process of otitis media. Penicillin treated animals had significantly lower concentration of LTB$_4$ than animals not treated with penicillin.

This study was supported by NIH-NINCDS grant NS-14538, Loma Linda University BRSG, and the Upjohn Co.

REFERENCES

1. Jung TTK, Juhn SK. Prostaglandins and other arachidonic acid metabolites in the middle ear fluids. Auris Nasus Larynx (Tokyo) 1985; 12(Suppl. I):sl48–sl50.
2. Jung TTK, Juhn SK. Leukotrienes and other lipoxygenase products in middle ear effusions. In: Sade J, ed. Acute and secretory otitis media. Amsterdam: Kugler, 1986:269.
3. Volovitz B, Varsano I, Grossman J. The effects of naproxen sodium therapy on acute otitis media and persistence of middle ear effusion in children. In: Sade J, ed. Abstracts of international symposium on acute and secretory otitis media, Jerusalem, Israel, November 1985:138.
4. Persico M, Podoshin L, Fradis M. Otitis media with effusion. A steroid and antibiotic therapeutic trial before surgery. Ann Otol Rhinol Laryngol 1978; 87:191–196.
5. Schwarz RH, Puglese J, Schwarz MD. Use of a short course of prednisone for treating middle ear effusion. A double blind crossover study. Ann Otol Rhinol Laryngol 1980; 89(Suppl 68):296–300.
6. Puhakka HJ, Haapaniemi J, Tushimaa P, et al. Peroral prednisolone in the treatment of middle ear effusion in children: a doubleblinded study. In: Sade J, ed. Abstracts of international symposium on acute and secretory otitis media, Jerusalem, Israel, November 1985:136.
7. Jung TTK, Giebink GS, Juhn SK. Effects of ibuprofen, corticosteroid, and penicillin on the pathogenesis of experimental pneumococcal otitis media. In: Lim DJ, Bluestone CD, Klein JO, Nelson JK, eds. Recent advances in otitis media with effusion. Proceedings of the Third International Symposium. Toronto: BC Decker, 1984:269.
8. Jung TTK, Berlinger NT, Juhn SK. Prostaglandins in squamous cell carcinoma of the head and neck: a preliminary study. Laryngoscope 1985; 95:307–312.
9. Ryan AF, Catanzaro A. Passive transfer of immune-mediated middle ear inflammation and effusion. Acta Otolaryngol (Stockh) 1983; 95:123–130.
10. Goldman DW, Goetzl EJ.Mediation and modulation of immediate hypersensitivity and inflammation by products of the oxygenation of arachidonic acid. In: Ward PA, ed. Immunology of inflammation. New York: Elsevier, 1983:163.
11. Bjork J, Hedquist P, Arfors KE. Increase in vascular permeability induced by leukotriene B_4 and the role of polymorphonuclear leukocytes. Inflammation 1982; 6:189–200.

MANAGEMENT OF ACUTE OTITIS MEDIA WITHOUT PRIMARY ADMINISTRATION OF SYSTEMIC ANTIMICROBIAL AGENTS

ERVIN OSTFELD, M.D., M.Sc., JACOB SEGAL, M.D., D.M.D., MIRIAM KAUFSTEIN, B.Sc., and ILANA GELERNTER, M.Sc.

The widely accepted systemic administration of antimicrobial drugs as the primary therapy of acute otitis media began almost empirically with the advent of penicillin and then increased in acceptance with the development of new generations of antibiotics. The decreased incidence of complications (acute mastoiditis, meningitis, intracranial abscess) during or following the clinical course of acute otitis media in recent decades is the strongest argument supporting the routine use of primary systemic administration of antimicrobial drugs on the basis of a "predicted" bacteriologic forecast.[1] However, objective factors and subjective prejudice have precluded a realistic evaluation of the actual benefits or disadvantages in the primary routine administration—or nonadministration—of antimicrobial drugs in acute otitis media. The incompleteness of our basic knowledge about the objective values of different therapeutic modalities[2] has impaired the decision making process and has resulted in a widely accepted policy of primary routine administration of a wide range of antimicrobial drugs for long (10 days) or short (2 days) periods of time.[1,3,4] This therapeutic method has been challenged by several investigators.[5,6] A critical analysis of published clinical trials has raised doubt about the benefit of antimicrobial drug administration in acute otitis media.[7]

The major flaw in routine primary systemic administration of a "precommanded" regimen of antimicrobial drugs is the relatively high prevalence of unpredictable acute recurrences, long term or frequent otorrhea, and the presence of asymptomatic middle ear effusions following or between acute episodes.

In a prospective consecutive, unselected, unbiased, nonrandomized 2 year longitudinal study, we tried to determine the effect of withholding systemic antimicrobial drug therapy during episodes of acute otitis media on the prevalence of recurrent acute episodes, chronic middle ear effusion and otorrhea, the incidence of tympanostomy tube insertion (for prevention of acute recurrent episodes), and the incidence of complications (mastoid or intracranial).

PATIENTS AND METHODS

During a 2 year period (March 1, 1981, to February 28, 1983) 397 infants and children with proven acute otitis media were treated in a prospective longitudinal, consecutive, unselected, nonrandomized study without primary systemic administration of antimicrobial drugs. The study was not biased by the patient's age, nationality, clinical symptoms, type of middle ear effusion, socioeconomic condition, results of middle ear effusion bacterial cultures, or the need for parents' informed consent.

Patients who had started primary systemic antibacterial drug administration (2 weeks or less) before our examination or who had received antibiotics orally or intravenously for associated medical conditions and who were obligated to continue the initial treatment were considered as a relative nonrandomized control group (296 infants and children). Also included in this category were patients in whom antimicrobial therapy was started after the entering date for the diagnosis of systemic illness.

Infants and children of all ages in whom acute otitis media was suspected were referred by family physicians, pediatricians, nurses, and parents, through our "open door policy," by the hospital's emergency room and pediatric department, and by otolaryngologists.

The diagnosis of acute otitis media at entry and at each subsequent reexamination was based on a decision algorithm integrating overt clinical symptoms, otoscopic indications of inflammation, and evidence of middle ear effusion. The clinical symptoms included one or more of the following: fever, restlessness or otalgia, gastrointestinal manifestations (vomiting or diarrhea), and febrile convulsions. Patients with systemic illness (pneumonia, upper respiratory tract infection, meningitis, spastic bronchitis, Down's syndrome) were not excluded. Patients with otorrhea as a presenting symptom were not enrolled if they did not return with a further episode of acute otitis media and an intact tympanic membrane. Excluded were patients who previously had undergone insertion of tympanostomy tubes or who had had chronic otitis media or external otitis.

The external auditory canal was cleaned by using a number 1 Sprague blunt curet.

The patient's parents received detailed information about the method of therapy without antimicrobial drugs and the reasons we do not recommend primary antibiotic therapy. At the same time our "open door policy" was explained—a readiness to reexamine the infant or child on the same day if there was any doubt or complaint by the parent or the family physician.

Pneumatic otoscopy was performed with a magnifying pneumatic otoscope with an adequately sealed diagnostic head and ear canal speculum by a trained otoscopist. The presence of a middle ear effusion for the diagnosis of acute otitis media was always confirmed by needle aspiration with an Ostfeld tympanotomy collector.[8] Needle aspiration was performed only in patients with overt clinical symptoms. Patients without a proven middle ear effusion were not enrolled. Needle aspiration was performed without disinfection of the external ear canal and made possible rheologic characterization of the type of effusion possible. The effusions were assessed and classified immediately after collection according to appearance and rheologic characteristics as purulent, mucopurulent, mucoid, or serous.[9]

The diagnosis of chronic middle ear effusion was based on confirmation of the presence of an effusion by pneumatic otoscopy (if doubt existed, this was confirmed by needle aspiration) without clinical symptoms, or otoscopic findings of acute otitis media, 1 month or more following or between acute episodes.

Bacteriologic Work-Up

The middle ear effusion from the collecting syringe was plated on blood agar and streaked with one line of *Staphylococcus* (in order to insure rapid isolation of *Haemophilus influenzae)* and incubated aerobically and anaerobically at 35° C. *Streptococcus pneumoniae* was identified by cellular and colonial morphologic studies of sensitivity to optochin. *Haemophilus influenzae* was identified by its characteristic colonies and growth requirements. The streptococcal groups were identified by a bacitracin disc and the Streptex test. *Branhamella* was identified by colony morphology, Gram staining, and the oxidase test. The aerobic gram negative enteric rods were inoculated on a MacConkey agar plate and defined on indole urea and triple sugar agar media. *Staphylococcus epidermidis* and *S. aureus* were identified by use of Veristaph.

Two or more documented episodes of acute otitis media were considered to indicate recurrent disease.

Follow-Up Observations

Patients were reexamined at approximately 10 days and 1 month following each episode of acute otitis media and then at 1 to 3 month intervals for up to 24 months.

Data Analysis

For the bilateral presentation of acute otitis media a test of symmetry between the right and left ears was performed on each "side dependent" parameter. The findings were as follows: type of middle ear effusion (67 percent), *Haemophilus influenzae* (76 percent), *Streptococcus pneumoniae,* (80 percent), sterile cultures (84.5 percent), aerobic gram positive and gram negative cocci (90.4 percent), aerobic gram negative enteric rods (89.2 percent), number of needle aspirations (88.5 percent), recurrent acute episodes (94.2 percent), otorrhea (90.5 percent), and chronic middle ear effusion (93 percent).

The high correlation between the right and left ears in terms of "side dependent" parameters indicates that one ear may be representative of the correlative studies of the "side independent" parameters. Therefore, for each patient one ear was randomly chosen by the computer as the "representative ear." The differences were considered significant if the corrected chi square test value was less than 0.05.

RESULTS

A total of 693 infants and children—Jewish (84 percent) and Arabs (16 percent)—were enrolled in the study. Bilateral acute otitis media was found in 77.5 percent of the patients and unilateral disease in 22.5 percent. Primary systemic antimicrobial drug therapy was administered to 296 patients (42.7 percent); 397 patients (57.3 percent) did not receive any systemic antimicrobial drug therapy. The general compliance in follow-up examinations was 79, 53, 46, 24, and 12 percent at 1, 3, 6, 12, and over 12 months, respectively. Patients who did not receive primary systemic antimicrobial drug therapy had a 57, 52, and 42 percent relative follow-up compliance at 1 to 6 months, 1 year, and over 1 year, respectively, when compared to patients who received systemic antimicrobial therapy ($p < 0.003$).

During the winter 40 percent of the patients received primary systemic antimicrobial therapy and during the summer, 48 percent ($p < 0.035$). The age distribution shows that acute otitis media was most frequent during the first year of life (69 percent; Fig. 1). The differences between the age groups in terms of the frequency of systemic antimicrobial administration was not significant. Presenting symptoms influenced the use of systemic antimicrobial administration (Fig. 2). Patients with fever had higher than statistically expected systemic antimicrobial administration values and those with gastrointestinal symptoms or restlessness had lower values ($p < 0.019$).

Analysis of the presenting pathogenic bacterial growth pattern in middle ear effusions indicates a

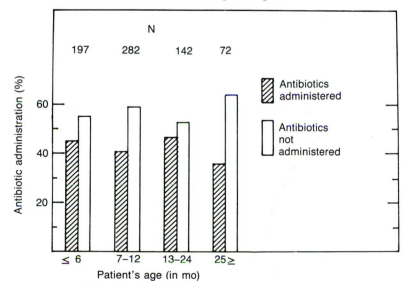

Figure 1 Distribution of patients according to age group and primary systemic antimicrobial drug administration rate. Mo = month.

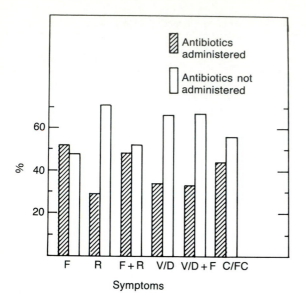

Figure 2 Distribution of patients according to the presenting symptoms and primary systemic antimicrobial drug administration. F = fever; R = restlessness, V/D = vomiting, diarrhea; C = convulsions.

nonstatistical difference between the administered and nonadministered groups (Table 1).

The effect of primary systemic antimicrobial nonadministration on the clinical course of acute otitis media is presented in Table 2. Significantly lower prevalences of acute recurrence episodes, otorrhea, and chronic middle ear effusion were observed in the antimicrobial nonadministered group as well as a lower incidence of tympanostomy tube insertion (for prophylaxis against acute recurrence episodes). The incidence of acute mastoiditis, 0.7

percent, was the same in both groups. Otogenic meningitis was not observed in either group.

DISCUSSION

The aim in this study was to present our clinical experience in the treatment of acute otitis media. This was not an experiment but rather a synthesis of clinical experience as it occurred during a 2 year period. All patients diagnosed as having acute otitis media were included without the interference of any artificial criteria that could distort the original study design. It was our belief that in most instances the primary administration of antimicrobial drugs does not contribute substantially to the final healing process by preventing recurrent acute episodes, otorrhea, or chronic middle ear effusions. Clinical practice has shown that acute otitis media may develop in infants and children given intravenously administered, potent, wide range antimicrobial drugs for associated disease, e.g., pneumonia,[10] and during amoxicillin adminstration for chronic middle ear effusion.[11] Interestingly, amoxicillin administration conferred no more protection against acute episodes than placebo.[11]

This study has certain advantages over previously published works.[4-6] Our study was prospective and longitudinal, the patients being followed for up to 2 years. The study population included all patients with acute otitis media, including 197 infants 6 months of age or younger. Needle aspiration confirmed the presence of middle ear effusions as well as the rheologic characterization of the effusion. The routine performance of needle aspiration made possible a meticulous bacteriologic work-up.

TABLE 1 Distribution of Patients According to Presenting Middle Ear Effusion Pathogenic Bacterial Identification and Primary Systemic Antimicrobial Administrative Rate

Microorganism	Semiquantitative Culture Count	Systemic Antimicrobial Therapy Administered (%)	Not Administered (%)
Haemophilus influenzae	High	34	33
	Low	9	7
Streptococcus pneumoniae	High	26	29
	Low	6	5
Aerobic gram positive and gram negative cocci	High	9	9
	Low	2	—
Aerobic enteric gram negative rods	High	7	7
	Low	4	2
Sterile cultures	—	32	27

All the differences are statistically not significant.

TABLE 2   Effect of Primary Systemic Antimicrobial Nonadministration on Clinical Course in Acute Otitis Media

| Criterion | Systemic Antimicrobial Therapy | | Statistical Significance |
	Administered (%)	Not Administered (%)	
Prevalence of acute recurrent episodes	55	33	p < 0.0001
Prevalence of otorrhea	31	14	p < 0.0001
Prevalence of chronic middle ear effusion	58	42	p < 0.0005
Rate of tympanostomy tube insertion	14	5	p < 0.0001
Acute mastoiditis	3	2	—
Otogenic meningitis	—	—	—

The study population was not randomized, but most of the study parameters, including the bacteriologic data, indicated no difference between the primary systemic antimicrobial administrated group and the nonadministrated group.

Regardless of whether the two groups are comparable, the present study data revealed the following: Primary nonadministration of antimicrobial drugs in acute otitis media did not increase the risk of mastoid or intracranial complications. The clinical course in patients who did not receive primary systemic administration of antimicrobial drugs was acceptable (33 percent prevalence of recurrent acute attacks, 11 percent otorrhea, 42 percent chronic middle ear effusion, and 5 percent tympanostomy tube insertion). There was no clinical indication of handicap or damage in the short or long term in patients who did not receive primary systemic antimicrobial therapy.

The study results indicate that the presenting clinical symptoms influenced the therapeutic decision. In patients with fever there was a greater frequency of primary systemic antimicrobial administration because fever may indicate a high incidence of middle ear bacterial infection. Our results indicate that the presenting clinical symptoms in acute otitis media are not good indicators of middle ear bacterial infection.[12]

Therefore we suggest that the primary choice of management in acute otitis media be needle aspiration drainage of the middle ear and that systemic antimicrobial adminstration be reserved for unresponsive patients.

REFERENCES

1. Bluestone CD. Otitis media in children: to treat or not to treat? N Engl J Med 1982; 306:1399–1404.
2. Feigin RD. Otitis media: closing the information gap. N Engl J Med 1982; 306:1417–1418.
3. Karma P, Palva T, Kouvalainen K, Karja J, Makela PH, Prinssi VP, Ruuskanen O, Launiala K. Finnish approach to the treatment of acute otitis media. Ann Otol Rhinol Laryngol 1987; 96 (Suppl 129):1–10.
4. Meistrup-Larsen KI, Sorensen H, Johnsen NJ, Thomsen J, Mygind M, Sedenberg-Olsen J. Two versus seven days' penicillin treatment for acute otitis media. Acta Otolaryngol (Stockh) 1983; 96:99–104.
5. Diamant M, Diamant B. Abuse and timing of use of antibiotics in acute otitis media. Arch Otolaryngol 1974; 100:226–232.
6. van Buchem FL, Dunk JHM. van't Hof MA. Therapy of acute otitis media: myringotomy, antibiotics, or neither? A double blind study in children. Lancet 1981; 2:883–887.
7. Marchant CD, Shurin PA. Therapy of otitis media. Pediatr Clin North Am 1983; 30:281–296.
8. Ostfeld E. Tympanotomy-collector of middle ear fluid. Laryngoscope 1980; 90:708–710.
9. Ostfeld E, Altmann G. Evaluation of countercurrent immunoelectrophoresis as a diagnostic tool in bacterial otitis media. Ann Otol Rhinol Laryngol 1980; 89:110–114.
10. Ostfeld E, Valdman I, Segal J, Kaufstein M, Gelernter I. Acute otitis media in a mixed Israel population. Poster presentation. Fourth international symposium on recent advances in otitis media, Bal Harbour, Florida, 1981.
11. Mandel EM, Rockette HF, Bluestone CD, Paradise JL, Nozza RJ. Efficacy of amoxicillin with and without decongestant-antihistamine for otitis media with effusion in children. N Engl J Med 1987; 306:432–437.
12. Ostfeld E, Valdman I, Segal J, Kaufstein M, Gelernter I. Clinical and bacteriological correlates in acute otitis media. Poster presentation. Fourth international symposium on recent advances in otitis media, Bal Harbour, Florida, 1981.

RANDOMIZED CONTROLLED TRIAL COMPARING TRIMETHOPRIM-SULFAMETHOXAZOLE, PREDNISONE, IBUPROFEN, AND NO TREATMENT IN CHRONIC OTITIS MEDIA WITH EFFUSION

G. SCOTT GIEBINK, M.D., PAUL B. BATALDEN, M.D., CHAP T. LE, Ph.D.,
JOYCE N. RUSS, R.N., JOANN K. KNOX, RENNER S. ANDERSON, M.D.,
STEVEN K. JUHN, M.D., DAVID J. BURAN, M.D., and ANNE E. SELTZ, M.A., CCC-A.

Several observations suggest that bacteria and their envelope products are etiologic in chronic otitis media with effusion. Bacteria, predominantly *Streptococcus pneumoniae* and nontypable *Haemophilus influenzae*, are cultured from approximately 70 percent of effusion samples from children with acute otitis media and from about 35 percent of chronic effusion samples. In addition, nonviable bacteria, pneumococcal capsular polysaccharide, and endotoxin have been identified in chronic middle ear effusion.

The biochemical composition of middle ear effusion reflects morphologic changes taking place in the middle ear mucosa.[1] The biochemical components of such an effusion include secretory products from epithelial and subepithelial cells, pathogenic microorganisms, and inflammatory cells. The biosynthetic metabolites of arachidonic acid seem to play an active role in the pathogenesis of otitis media with effusion.[2] Further evidence for the role of local inflammatory mediators and bacteria in the pathogenesis of chronic otitis media with effusion is found in the results of medical intervention studies, which indicate that anti-inflammatory and antimicrobial drug treatment causes resolution of chronic otitis media with effusion in some children.

The present study was designed to measure the incidences of response in children with chronic otitis media with effusion to an antimicrobial drug, trimethoprim-sulfamethoxazole, and to two anti-inflammatory drugs, prednisone and aluminum ibuprofen suspension. Nonsteroidal anti-inflammatory drugs, such as ibuprofen, inhibit cyclooxygenase, the enzyme converting arachidonic acid to the cyclic endoperoxides, which are the direct precursors of prostaglandins and thromboxanes. These drugs therefore could be used to block prostaglandin synthesis. The response incidence data provide insight into the relative contributions of arachidonic acid metabolites and viable bacteria in the pathogenesis of chronic otitis media with effusion.

MATERIALS AND METHODS

Between January 1, 1982, and September 30, 1984, the medical records of 16,609 consecutive children returning for ear reexamination following a recent episode of otitis media were screened. Patients were eligible for the study if they met the following criteria: age 10 to 95 months, three or more physician documented otitis media episodes within the previous 18 months, an episode of otitis media diagnosed 10 to 28 days prior to entry, completion of at least 10 days of antibiotic treatment for the most recent acute otitis media episode, and otitis media with effusion documented by otoscopy and tympanometry at entry. Exclusion criteria included a history of adverse reactions to sulfonamides, the presence of tympanostomy tubes, and acute otitis media. Of the 1,567 who were found to have otitis media, 449 had otitis media with effusion and were enrolled after explaining the study design to parents and obtaining their written informed consent.

The middle ear status was evaluated using both pneumatic otoscopy and impedance audiometry. A standard algorithm was used to diagnose middle ear effusion; a separate validation study of 122 ears showed the diagnostic accuracy of the algorithm against myringotomy findings to be 84 percent. Acute otitis media was diagnosed if a middle ear effusion was present according to the algorithm and the tympanic membrane was red; if an effusion was present or uncertain by the algorithm, the tympanic membrane was white, yellow, or orange, and the patient had symptoms of fever, earache, or irritability without other apparent cause; or if there was a tympanic membrane perforation with purulent drainage from the middle ear. Otitis media with effusion was diagnosed when effusion was indicated to be present by the algorithm, the tympanic membrane was not red, and the patient was asymptomatic.

The 449 patients with effusion 10 to 28 days after the diagnosis of otitis media were examined 3 and 6 weeks later, a total observation period of at least 8 weeks. Seventy-six patients had otitis media at all three visits (i.e., chronic otitis media with effusion), and these patients were assigned by random number to one of four study groups: (1) trimethoprim-sulfamethoxazole suspension (Septra, Burroughs Wellcome; 8 mg of trimethoprim and 40 mg of sulfamethoxazole per kilogram per 24 hours divided into two doses for 4 weeks); (2) aluminum ibuprofen suspension (Motrin-A, Upjohn; IND no. 16756, lot numbers 20,479 and 21,582; 24 mg per kilogram per 24 hours divided into four doses for 2 weeks); (3) prednisone tablets (Deltasone, Upjohn; 1.0 mg per kilogram per 24 hours divided into two doses for 7 days, followed by 0.5 mg per kilogram per 24 hours divided into two doses for 4 days, followed by 0.12 mg per kilogram per 24 hours in one dose for 3 days); or (4) no treatment. No other medications, including antihistamines, decongestants, and antipyretics, were prescribed.

Visits were scheduled to determine the middle ear status at 2 and 4 weeks after randomization and monthly thereafter for 12 months. Patients were considered treatment failures and were referred to collaborating otolaryngologists for evaluation and possible surgical insertion of tympanostomy tubes if they continued to have otitis media with effusion in at least one ear at both the 2 and 4 week post-treatment visits or had otitis media with effusion for 10 weeks after a recurrent otitis media episode subsequent to initial resolution. Of the 48 treatment failure patients referred, tympanostomy tubes were placed in 36 (75 percent) within 20 weeks after referral. These patients also were examined at least monthly after surgery for the 12 month study period.

Clinical recurrence of acute otitis media was defined as the appearance of a new middle ear effusion after initial otitis media resolution, or the onset of fever, earache, or irritability in the presence of preexisting otitis media with effusion. At the end of the follow-up period (approximately 12 months) the tympanic membranes in each patient were evaluated using an operating microscope, and pure tone air and bone conduction hearing threshold levels were established.

RESULTS

The median age was 39 months; 32 percent of the subjects were 12 to 23 months of age. Ear involvement at enrollment was bilateral in 58 percent of the subjects, but 100 percent reported that the episodes of otitis media usually were bilateral. Hearing difficulty was reported by 40 percent. Forty-nine percent attended group day care sessions with five or more children for more than 15 hours each week. Nineteen percent had undergone tympanostomy tube placement previously. Subjects had experienced an average of eight episodes of physician documented otitis media prior to the episode that led to enrollment into this study, and otitis media with effusion had persisted for an average of 9.4 weeks prior to randomization. There were no significant differences among the study groups for each of these characteristics.

In this report the findings from the surgically treated group are presented in parallel with those of the study groups for the purpose of illustration only. Statistical comparisons between the surgical group and the study groups are not valid because the surgical group was not assigned by randomization as were the other treatment groups. All the surgical patients were study group failures and represent worst case comparisons with the study groups. For example, the 36 surgical patients experienced an average of 20.1 weeks of continuous otitis media with effusion before surgery, compared with 9.4 weeks for the total group of patients at the time of randomization.

Of the 76 patients randomized, four were excluded from treatment analysis because of refusal or failure to take the assigned medication.

Thirty-four of the 72 patients failed treatment and underwent insertion of tympanostomy tubes. The differences among the treatment groups with respect to time to surgery were not significant. Two patients excluded from treatment analysis also underwent tube insertion. Bilateral tubes were inserted in 33 patients, and unilateral tubes were inserted in three patients. Of these 69 ears, 44 percent contained mucoid effusion, 28 percent contained serous effusion, 6 percent contained seromucoid effusion, and 22 percent contained no discernable effusion. Forty-two tubes (61 percent) extruded during follow-up; the mean time to extrusion was 45 weeks (range, 6 to 54 weeks). The mean time to the first acute otitis media relapse after extrusion was 9.7 weeks (range, 0 to 25 weeks). Overall, 29 of 42 ears (69 percent) with tube extrusion suffered an acute otitis media relapse. Of the 89 episodes of acute otitis media and otitis media with effusion that occurred after tube insertion, 65 percent occurred after tube extrusion in the absence of a tympanic membrane perforation, 25 percent occurred in the presence of a patent tube, 9 percent occurred with an occluded tube, and 1 percent occurred after tube extrusion but with a persisting perforation.

During the first 4 weeks after randomization, the incidence of bilateral resolution of otitis media with effusion was significantly greater in the trimethoprim-sulfamethoxazole and prednisone groups than in the untreated control group (Fig. 1). However, in a similar percentage of patients in all study groups, otitis media with effusion eventually resolved after randomization. The incidence of resolution was much greater in the surgical group. Disease in older patients resolved more rapidly than in younger patients, and in patients who had otitis media with effusion of longer duration before randomization, the effusion took longer to resolve after randomization.

The incidence of relapse in otitis media with effusion (i.e., the percentage of patients who had disease lasting at least 2 weeks after initial resolution) were not significantly different among the study groups, but the incidence was lower in the surgical group (Fig. 2). Patients who had otitis media with effusion of longer duration before randomization relapsed sooner than patients with a shorter duration before randomization. Ears that took a long time to resolve initially again took a long time to resolve if the disease recurred.

Medication compliance measured by a daily diary was 97, 92, and 97 percent for trimethoprim-sulfamethoxazole, ibuprofen, and prednisone, respectively.

Thirty-two of 36 patients who remained in the initial treatment groups after 12 months and 32 of 36 patients who underwent surgical intervention were evaluated audiometrically at the end of follow-up. At this examination ears with otitis media with effusion had a 15 db higher hearing threshold level than ears without, but there were no significant differences in the pure tone average hearing levels among the groups. Overall, 27 percent of the ears showed a mild hearing loss (15 to 30 db), 11 percent showed a moderate loss (30 to 50 db), and 2.5 percent showed a severe loss (greater than 50 db). The pure tone average hearing level at the end of follow-up was significantly higher in patients experiencing a longer duration of otitis media with effusion during follow-up and in patients with more acute otitis media episodes during follow-up.

Among the 36 patients examined who remained in their initial study groups after approximately 12 months of follow-up, tympanic membrane retraction and abnormal membrane mobility were significantly more common findings in the ibuprofen than in the control group. There were no differences among the groups in the frequency of tympanosclerosis, in

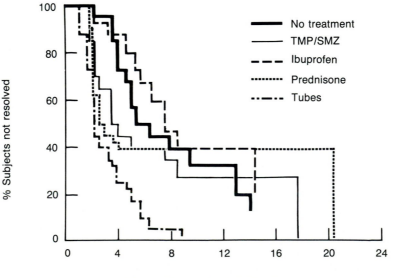

Figure 1 Weeks between randomization or surgery and clinical resolution of otitis media with effusion in both ears, i.e., normal otoscopy and tympanometry.

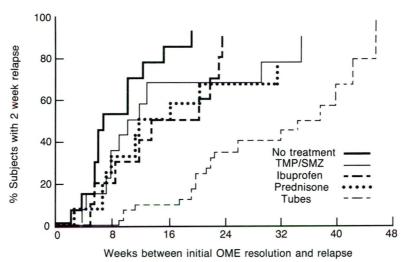

Figure 2 Weeks between the initial resolution of otitis media with effusion in both ears and the first subsequent episode of otitis media (acute otitis media or otitis media with effusion) relapse lasting 2 weeks or more (i.e., documented at two consecutive visits).

membrane color or translucency, or in visualization of fluid.

There were no significant hematologic complications of medical treatment. Serum cortisol values were less than 10 μg per deciliter in 14 of 17 (82 percent) prednisone treated patients tested within 24 hours after stopping treatment. Of 14 patients with low cortisol values, seven had normal values 2 to 4 days after stopping treatment, one had a normal value when retested on day 14, and six had normal values when retested between days 17 and 36 after treatment.

DISCUSSION

In this sample of children with recurring otitis media and chronic otitis media with effusion, neither antimicrobial nor anti-inflammatory drug intervention had a striking immediate or long lasting effect on middle ear disease. Trimethoprim-sulfamethoxazole increased the rate of otitis media with effusion resolution during the first 2 weeks, and the effect was sustained at 4 weeks, suggesting that bacteria inhibited by these drugs were responsible in part, but not entirely, for the chronic disease process. Others have also demonstrated a significantly greater response to trimethoprim-sulfamethoxazole than with no treatment.[3,4]

Prednisone enhanced the resolution of otitis media with effusion in our study, consistent with the hypothesis that biosynthetic metabolites of arachidonic acid contributed significantly to chronic middle ear inflammation. However, the tendency for prednisone treated patients to relapse sooner than control subjects indicates that the short course of treatment did not resolve middle ear histopathologic abnormalities. Some investigators have also reported a significant short term response to corticosteroid drugs,[5-7] whereas others have not found significant improvement.[8,9]

Comparison of the responses to prednisone and ibuprofen in our study revealed a great deal about the relative contribution of different classes of arachidonic acid metabolites to the resolution of chronic middle ear inflammation. Ibuprofen, a nonsteroidal anti-inflammatory drug, is thought to act by inhibiting the activity of cyclo-oxygenase, an enzyme that generates cyclic endoperoxides from arachidonic acid and blocks the biosynthesis of prostaglandin and thromboxane metabolites; it is thought to have no appreciable effect on lipoxygenase, an enzyme that converts arachidonic acid to leukotriene and HETE metabolites. Although prednisone had a short term beneficial effect, ibuprofen had no effect. Therefore, lipoxygenase metabolites, such as the leukotrienes, appear to be more active mediators of chronic otitis media with effusion than are prostaglandin and thromboxane metabolites. These results were mirrored in an experimental animal study conducted in our laboratory in which experimental pneumococcal otitis media responded more effectively to penicillin with methylprednisolone or penicillin alone than to penicillin with ibuprofen.[10]

Although the results in the surgical intervention group are shown only for illustrative purposes, it appeared that tube insertion increased resolution of otitis media with effusion. However, tubes commonly extruded within 1 year, and after extrusion relapse occurred promptly, indicating that prolonged middle ear ventilation alone did not appreciably change the underlying pathologic process. This hypothesis is supported by the observation that audiometric and otomicroscopic results in surgical, control, and drug treated patients were similar at the end of follow-up.

The failure of both medical and surgical interventions to have a long term impact on chronic otitis media with effusion suggests that interventions were either applied too late in the course of the disease, were not applied long enough, or were not appropriate. The short term benefits of trimethoprim-sulfamethoxazole and prednisone and the intermediate benefit of tubes suggest that combinations of these treatments might be more effective, especially since biochemical evidence suggests that the pathogenesis of chronic otitis media with effusion is multifactorial. Clinical and experimental animal trials are in progress to examine this hypothesis.

Study supported in part by grants from the Robert Wood Johnson Foundation, the Upjohn Company, and the Burroughs Wellcome Company and grant 5P50-NS-14538 from the National Institute of Neurological and Communicative Disorders and Stroke.

REFERENCES

1. Juhn SK, Sipila P, Jung TTK, et al. Biochemical pathology of otitis media with effusion. Acta Otolaryngol (Suppl) 1984; 414:45–51.
2. Juhn TTK, Smith DM, Juhn SK, Gerrard J. Prostaglandins and otitis media: studies in the chinchilla. Otolaryngol Head Neck Surg 1980; 88:316–323.
3. Healy GB. Antimicrobial therapy for chronic otitis media with effusion. In: Lim DJ, Bluestone CD, Klein JO, Nelson JD, eds. Recent advances in otitis media with effusion. Proceedings of the Third International Symposium. Toronto: BC Decker, 1984:285.
4. Marks NJ, Mills RP, Shaheen OH. A controlled trial of cotrimoxazole therapy in serous otitis media. J Laryngol Otol 1981; 95:1003–1009.
5. Perisco M, Podoshin L, Fradis M. Otitis media with effusion: a steroid and antibiotic therapeutic trial before surgery. Ann Otol Rhinol Laryngol 1978; 87:191–196.
6. Niederman LG, Walter-Buckholtz V, Jabalay T. A comparative trial of steroids versus placebos for treatment of chronic otitis media with effusion. In: Lim DJ, Bluestone CD, Klein JO, Nelson JD, eds. Recent advances in otitis media with effusion. Proceedings of the Third International Symposium. Toronto: BC Decker, 1984:273.
7. Schwartz RH, Puglese J, Schwartz DM. The use of a short course of prednisone in treating middle ear effusion, a double-blind crossover study. Ann Otol Rhinol Laryngol 1980; 89 (Suppl 68):296–300.
8. Macknin ML, Jones PK. Oral dexamethasone for treatment of persistent middle ear effusion. Pediatrics 1985; 75:329–335.
9. Shapiro GG, Bierman CW, Furukawa CT, Pierson WE, Berman R, Donaldson J, Rees T. Treatment of persistent eustachian tube dysfunction in children with aerosolized nasal dexamethasone phosphate versus placebo. Ann Allergy 1982; 49:81–85.
10. Jung TTK, Giebink GS, Juhn SK. Effects of ibuprofen, corticosteroid, and penicillin on the pathogenesis of experimental pneumococcal otitis media. In: Lim DJ, Bluestone CD, Klein JO, Nelson JD, eds. Recent advances in otitis media with effusion. Proceedings of the Third International Symposium. Toronto: BC Decker, 1984:269.

LONG TERM ANTIBIOTIC TREATMENT OF CHILDREN WITH SECRETORY OTITIS MEDIA: DOUBLE BLIND, PLACEBO CONTROLLED STUDY

JENS THOMSEN, M.D., Ph.D., JØRGEN F. SEDERBERG-OLSEN, M.D., SVEN-ERIC STANGERUP, M.D., VIGGO BALLE, M.D., and RENÉ VEJLSGAARD, M.D.

Secretory otitis media is an extremely frequent disease in children. Surgery is still the prevailing mode of treatment, and the use of myringotomy with insertion of ventilating tubes has increased to almost epidemic proportions.

Nonsurgical treatment of secretory otitis media is limited to a few choices. Antibiotics with and without a decongestant-antihistamine combination are used most frequently, and steroids and mucolytic drugs have been mentioned sporadically as possible treatment modalities. Oral decongestant-antihistamine therapy as well as mucolytic treatment is ineffective by comparison with placebo, whereas the effect of steroids is still a moot point.[1]

The rationale for using antimicrobial therapy for secretory otitis media is based on the observations that secretory otitis media is secondary to bacterial infection of the middle ear space, that the type and frequency of occurrence of pathogenic bacteria recovered from the effusions in secretory otitis are similar to those of bacteria found in acute middle ear infections, and that respiratory pathogens in the nasopharynx may play a role in the development and maintenance of tubal dysfunction, which by and large is responsible for the secretory process in the middle ear space.

A number of uncontrolled clinical trials have reported a varying range of efficacies of antibiotics in the treatment of secretory otitis media. However, one study by Mandel et al[2] seems to fulfill the requirements of a placebo controlled trial, and these authors concluded that amoxicillin treatment increases to some extent the likelihood of resolution.

We conducted a double blind, placebo controlled study of the efficacy of an antimicrobial drug (Spektramox) given for 1 month to children with secretory otitis media. An interim report was given in 1985.[3] A more detailed report is to be published elsewhere.

MATERIAL AND METHODS

Included in the trial from June 1984 to June 1986 were 264 children, 1 to 10 years of age. The inclusion criterion was unilateral or bilateral secretory otitis media, established by tympanometry, of at least 3 months' duration. The patients included were not allergic to penicillin, and informed consent was obtained from the parents.

The patients were allocated to either 1 month of antibiotic treatment or 1 month of placebo treatment. In those with bilateral disease, a ventilating tube was inserted into the right ear, and the left ear was included in the study. In those with unilateral secretory otitis media, the ear in question was included. Tympanometry was performed after the termination of treatment and every month for the next 12 months. A nasopharyngeal culture was carried out before treatment, at the termination of the treatment period, and every month for the following 12 months.

A detailed social, family, and patient history was obtained in all cases and the two groups were comparable with regard to age, sex, family disposition,

social background, and previous otolaryngologic diseases. The mean age was 4.4 years in both the treatment and the placebo groups.

Active medication was given to 131 children (63 boys and 68 girls), and 133 received a placebo (74 boys and 59 girls). There were 159 patients (87 boys and 72 girls) who were younger than 5 years (mean age, 2.88 years), and 105 (50 boys and 55 girls) were between 5 and 10 years of age (mean, 6.82 years). Information about the last three visits for 14 patients is still missing. Since this information will not alter the outcome of the study, the results to be presented are representative.

Antimicrobial Drug

A combination of amoxicillin and potassium clavulanate (Spektramox) was chosen. Clavulanic acid is a potent inhibitor of many beta-lactamase producing bacteria. The rationale behind the choice of this specific combination was that theoretically the antimicrobial therapy was effective against beta-lactamase producing *Haemophilus influenzae* and *Branhamella catarrhalis* as well as amoxicillin susceptible bacteria. A suspension containing 125 mg of amoxicillin and 31.25 mg of clavulanate per 5 ml was used. Children between 1 and 5 years of age received 5 ml three times daily and those aged 6 to 10 years received 7.5 ml three times daily.

RESULTS

Figure 1 depicts the incidence of secretory otitis media as judged by tympanometry. At the termination of the treatment period the incidence in patients who received Spektramox had dropped from 100 to 39 percent, whereas the patients in the placebo group still had secretory otitis media in 69 percent of the ears. This difference is highly significant (p < 0.00001, Mann-Whitney rank sum test). Up to 8 months after treatment there was a strong trend toward normal tympanometric findings in the active group compared with the placebo group. This trend reached significant levels at 3 and 5 months after treatment. At the termination of the study 12 months after treatment, 44 percent of the Spektramox treated patients still had fluid in the ear, while 55 percent of those who received placebos still had secretory otitis media. If the patients are divided according to age, the children younger than 5 years of age displayed an incidence of 31 percent with secretory otitis media compared with 46 percent in those between 5 and 10 years of age treated with Spektramox. There was a tendency for the effect in the younger age

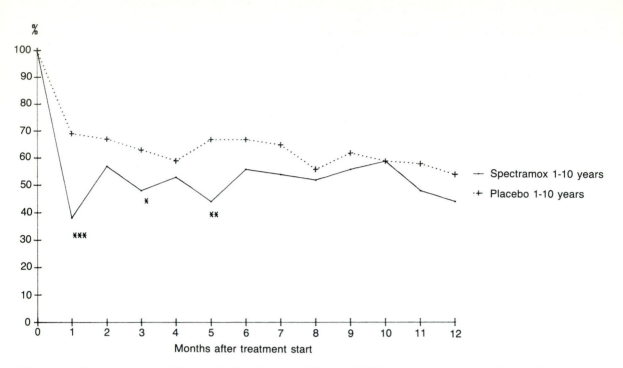

Figure 1 Incidence of secretory otitis media in all patients included in the trial. The ears in patients who received antibiotics have a highly significant lower incidence of secretory otitis media after 1 month of treatment than the ears in patients who received a placebo. The improvement lasted about 6 months.

group to be more prolonged (9 months) than in the older children (7 months); however, this difference was not statistically different.

Bacteriology

In no case did the nasopharyngeal culture display "no growth." In many cases there was more than one type of bacterium. We found that 12 percent of the patients harbored *Staphylococcus aureus*, 18 percent streptococci, 33 percent pneumococci, and more than 50 percent *Haemophilus influenzae*. The incidence of streptococcal infection was reduced from 18 to 4 percent after active treatment, whereas 13 percent of the patients in the placebo group still harbored streptococci. This difference is highly significant. However, after 1 month's further observation the incidence of streptococci was the same in the two groups. The occurrence of pneumococci was reduced in the active group from 34 to 11 percent at treatment termination, a finding that is significantly different from that in the placebo group. However, the difference had disappeared after 1 month of observation, when both groups were back to pretreatment levels. The effect of Spektramox on the presence of *H. influenzae* was less pronounced, with no significant reduction in the active group

when the children were considered as one group. However, in children ages 5 to 10 years there was a significant reduction compared with the response in those younger than 5 years. Again this difference had disappeared 1 month after the cessation of treatment. Three of 132 strains of *H. influenzae* (2.3 percent) were resistant to ampicillin at the beginning of the study, whereas five of 95 (5.3 percent) were resistant at the termination of treatment. We do not yet know whether this increase took place in the active group or occurred randomly in both groups. Later the number of ampicillin resistant strains fell to pretreatment values. However, the strains were most likely not resistant to the drug itself, since clavulanic acid should control the growth of beta-lactamase producing bacteria. In regard to the relation between the presence or absence of pathogens in the nasopharynx and the middle ear tympanometric status, we have not been able to establish any correlation so far.

DISCUSSION

The figures presented in this study justify the conclusion that 1 month of antibiotic treatment has a beneficial effect on middle ear disease in children with secretory otitis media. The effect is striking at the termination of treatment, but the extent to which the effect is long lasting remains an open question, even if the figures tend to support such an effect. Other authors have presented similar results emphasizing the short term effect but deny any long term effect.[2,4,5] We, however, do not deny such an effect but believe that further studies are needed to establish this with certainty.

The most plausible explanation is that the respiratory pathogens in the nasopharynx are reduced in number, thus eliminating or diminishing the inflammation in the eustachian tube and thereby improving middle ear ventilation. A long term effect from a limited period of antibiotic treatment per se is unlikely. However, once the disease process is reversed and the ears have returned to normal aeration, the chances are good that a sizable number of children will remain free from disease. The apparent lack of correlation in this study between the nasopharyngeal flora and tympanometric findings and between in vitro susceptibility and lack of eradication of the bacteria (especially *H. influenzae*) makes it likely that an undetected effect on the middle ear flora also plays a role in resolving secretory otitis media. The lack of correlation also raises the question whether penicillin V might not be as effective as the drug used in this study or other, frequently used broad spectrum antimicrobial drugs.

REFERENCES

1. Cantekin EI, Mandel EM, Bluestone CD, Rockette HE, Paradise JL, Stool SE, Frie JT, Rogers KD. Lack of efficacy of a decongestant-antihistamine combination or otitis media with effusion (secretory otitis media) in children. Results of a double-blind, randomized trial. N Engl J Med 1983; 308: 297-301.

2. Mandel EM, Rockette HE, Bluestone CD, Paradise JL, Nozza RJ. Efficacy of amoxicillin with and without decongestant-antihistamine for otitis media with effusion in children. Results of a double-blind randomized trial. N Engl J Med 1987; 316:432-437.

3. Thomsen J, Sederberg-Olsen J, Stangerup SE, Balle V, Bomholt A, Vejlsgaard R, Tos M. Long-term antibiotc treatment of children with secretory otitis media. A double-blind, placebo controlled study—preliminary report. In: Sadé J, ed. Acute and secretory otitis media. Amsterdam: Kugler Publications, 431.

4. Giebink GS, Batalden PB, Le CT, Russ JN, Knox JK, Anderson RS, Juhn SK, Buran DJ, Seltz AE. Randomized controlled trial comparing trimethoprim-sulfamethoxazole, prednisone, ibuprofen, and no treatment in chronic otitis media with effusion. In: Lim DJ, Bluestone CD, Klein JO, Nelson JD, eds. Recent advances in otitis media. Proceedings of the Fourth International Symposium. Toronto: BC Decker, 1988:240.

5. Schloss MD, Dempsey EE, Rishikof E, Sorger S, Grace M. Double blind study comparing erythromycin-sulfisoxazole (pediazole) T.I.D. to placebo in chronic otitis media with effusion. In: Lim DJ, Bluestone CD, Klein JO, Nelson JD, eds. Recent advances in otitis media. Proceedings of the Fourth International Symposium. Toronto: BC Decker, 1988:261.

CONTROLLED CLINICAL TRIAL FOR PREVENTION OF CHRONIC OTITIS MEDIA WITH EFFUSION

KATHY DALY, M.P.H., G. SCOTT GIEBINK, M.D., BRUCE LINDGREN, M.S., and RENNER S. ANDERSON, M.D.

Several studies have demonstrated that 5 to 10 percent of all children who experience an episode of acute otitis media develop chronic otitis media with effusion.[1-3] A previous study by our group identified three risk factors for chronic otitis media with effusion; bilateral otitis media with effusion, day care attendance, and duration of the disorder for 3 or more weeks.[4] Clinical trials, including a study by our group, have indicated that corticosteroid drugs such as prednisone and antimicrobial drugs such as trimethoprim and sulfamethoxazole have short term effects on the resolution of otitis media

with effusion (OME).[5-7] However, in our previous trial prednisone-treated subjects were more likely than trimethoprim-sulfamethoxazole treated or untreated subjects to have a recurrence of acute otitis media.* In this trial the previously identified risk

---

* From Giebink GS, Batalden PB, Le CT, Russ JN, Knox JK, Anderson RS, Juhn SK, Buran DJ, Seltz AE. A randomized controlled trial comparing trimethoprim-sulfamethoxazole, prednisone, ibuprofen, and no treatment for chronic otitis media with effusion. Presented at the Fourth International Symposium on Recent Advances in Otitis Media, Bal Harbour, Florida, June 1-4, 1987.

factors were used to screen for children in whom resolution was unlikely without treatment. We hypothesized that intervening early in the disease process with a combination of prednisone and trimethoprim-sulfamethoxazole would provide greater short and long term benefits by both resolving otitis media with effusion and preventing the recurrence of acute otitis media in these children.

MATERIALS AND METHODS

The subjects in the study were pediatric patients from a large suburban Minneapolis pediatric clinic who were enrolled between November 1984 and June 1985. Initial eligibility criteria were ascertained from the medical records of children being examined for an ear recheck or a well child visit. Children 6 months to 8 years of age whose immunizations were current, who had experienced three or more episodes of acute otitis media in the preceding 18 months, who had physician documented acute otitis media or otitis media with effusion during the previous 4 weeks, and who had received appropriate antibiotic treatment for the last episode of acute otitis media were eligible for the study. Additional high risk criteria were bilateral otitis media with effusion, day care attendance for 15 or more hours a week with five or more children, or otitis media with effusion for 3 or more weeks. Exclusion criteria included allergy to trimethoprim, sulfonamides, corticosteroids, or amoxicillin; significant underlying disease; concomitant infection; the presence or a history of tympanostomy tube insertions and exposure

to varicella in the previous 4 weeks without a documented history of chicken pox.

At enrollment, subjects were stratified on the basis of three prognostic variables: an age at the first episode of 0 to 6 months or more than 6 months, day care attendance, and a duration of otitis media with effusion of less than 4 weeks or 4 or more weeks. Subjects in each stratum were assigned to treatment with active drug or placebo using an allocation scheme to achieve balanced assignment of these factors in the two study groups. The allocation scheme was unknown to the research nurse and examining physicians. Study group assignment was determined by the study identification number, which was based on the stratum number and the subject's sequence of admission to that stratum.

High risk subjects were enrolled in the double blind, placebo controlled study, and the middle ear status was evaluated at 2, 4, and 6 weeks by a pediatrician and a research nurse practitioner. The results of pneumatic otoscopy and tympanometry were used in a validated algorithm to define the middle ear status. This was not a cross-over study; subjects remained in their original study group for the duration of the study. Subjects were treated with trimethoprim-sulfamethoxazole (8 mg of trimethoprim and 40 mg of sulfamethoxazole per kilogram per day in two divided doses for 14 days) and prednisone (1 mg per kilogram per day in two divided doses for days 1 to 7 and 1 mg per kilogram per day in a morning dose on days 8, 10, 12, and 14) or with placebos for the two drugs. Study drugs were administered according to a stepped protocol in which prednisone was used only if otitis media with effusion did not clear with trimethoprim-sulfamethoxazole (Fig. 1).

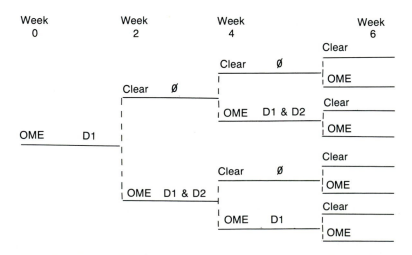

Figure 1 Stepped treatment protocol with trimethoprim-sulfamethoxazole and prednisone. D1, active or placebo trimethoprim-sulfamethoxazole. D2, active or placebo prednisone. Ø, no treatment.

In subjects who experienced acute otitis media during the treatment phase study medication was discontinued, and the subject received amoxicillin (40 mg per kilogram per day in three divided doses for 10 days); the subject re-entered the study after completion of this therapy.

Three measures of compliance with the study medication regimen were used: a medication log, measurement of remaining medication at the subsequent study visit, and a serum assay for sulfamethoxazole.

At the end of the 6 week treatment period, subjects who were free of otitis media with effusion were considered treatment responders, while those with disease in one or both ears were considered treatment failures. Additionally, subjects who experienced 8 continuous weeks of otitis media with effusion during the treatment phase because of one or more recurrences of acute otitis media were considered treatment failures. Treatment responders were examined monthly until they had a recurrence of otitis media with effusion.

The study was approved by the University of Minnesota Committee on the Use of Human Subjects in Research.

RESULTS

During the enrollment period 4,573 medical records were screened to identify eligible children for the study. One hundred forty-seven children with bilateral otitis media with effusion were examined by the research nurse; 42 subjects were ultimately enrolled.

The characteristics of the study groups at baseline were similar. There were no statistically significant differences in the characteristics of the two groups (Table 1), although there were more males in the active drug group than in the placebo group.

Forty-eight percent of the active drug subjects

TABLE 1   Characteristics of Treatment Groups

Characteristic	Active Drug (N = 21), % with factor	Placebo (N = 21), % with factor
Day care	71	67
Family history	50	52
Allergy	5	0
Male	71	48
Nonwhite	0	5
	Mean Value	*Mean Value*
Age (mo)	35	30
Fluid duration (days)	48	41
Age at first episode (mo)	9	8
Number of prior episodes	8	7

and 14 percent of the placebo subjects had resolved otitis media with effusion in both ears at the third visit (Table 2). Placebo treated subjects, however, were much more likely to have experienced an episode of acute otitis media during treatment: 52 percent of placebo treated subjects and 10 percent of active drug treated subjects experienced an episode of acute otitis media. Placebo treated subjects had 4.5 episodes of acute otitis media per person-year of follow-up, compared with 1.9 episodes per person-year in the active drug group.

The percentages of subjects with continuous otitis media with effusion after enrollment were compared in the two study groups. Forty-three percent of the active drug subjects and 85 percent of the placebo treated subjects had continuous otitis media with effusion during the treatment phase. The time until relapse was examined for the subset of subjects in whom the disease resolved during treatment (12 drug and three placebo treated subjects). The median time between resolution and recurrence of otitis media with effusion was 4 to 5 weeks for both groups.

TABLE 2   Response to Treatment for Active Drug and Placebo Groups

	Active Drug (N = 21)	Placebo (N = 21)	P Value
Free of otitis media with effusion at 2 weeks (response to trimethoprim-sulfamethoxazole)	5 (24%)	1 (5%)	0.09*
Free of otitis media with effusion at 6 weeks	10 (48%)	3 (14%)	0.02†
Subjects with acute otitis media during treatment	2 (10%)	11 (52%)	0.01†

* Fisher's exact test.
† Chi square test for association.

Compliance with the study medication regimen was similar in the two groups according to all three measures. The average compliances of placebo and active drug subjects as measured by medication logs were 92 and 85 percent respectively. Measurement of remaining medication revealed that compliance of placebo subjects was 90 percent, while compliance in the active drug group was 88 percent. Compliance was also measured by the presence of sulfamethoxazole in a blood sample drawn after a 14 day course of trimethoprim-sulfamethoxazole. Sera were analyzed using high pressure liquid chromatography. Of 33 assays done in 19 subjects in the active drug group, 27 (82 percent) contained measurable study drug. The mean concentration of sulfamethoxazole in active drug subjects was 33 μg per milliliter; the mean time since the last dose was 20 hours for subjects with measurable drug levels and 60 hours for those who had no detectable drug. Of the 29 assays done in subjects in the placebo group, one had a measurable amount of the study drug; this subject had received active drug because of a pharmacist's error in dispensing medication.

DISCUSSION

This study demonstrated the short term efficacy of a stepped regimen of a corticosteroid (prednisone) and antimicrobial therapy (trimethoprim-sulfamethoxazole) in resolving otitis media with effusion in children at increased risk of developing chronic otitis media with effusion. Long term benefits were not demonstrated; the media duration of otitis media-free time after resolution of the middle ear effusion was only 5 weeks in both treated and untreated subjects. Previous studies have demonstrated the individual effectiveness of these two therapies in resolving otitis media with effusion.[5-7] Because of the study design, it is not possible to determine whether subjects who received prednisone after being unresponsive to the initial 2 week course of trimethoprim-sulfamethoxazole achieved clearance of the otitis media in response to prednisone or in response to an additional 2 weeks of trimethoprim-sulfamethoxazole. In order to compare the relative efficacies of the combined treatment and the individual treatments, three treatment groups would be needed: a group receiving prednisone and trimethoprim-sulfamethoxazole, a group receiving prednisone alone, and a group receiving trimethoprim-sulfamethoxazole alone.

Because treatment responses may have been confounded by gender (there was a preponderance of males in the active drug group), response frequencies were stratified according to gender. Eight of 15 males (53 percent) and two of six females (33 percent) were treatment responders to active drug. Fisher's exact test (one tail p = 0.36) did not reveal an association between gender and the treatment response.

The low incidence of resolution of otitis media with effusion in the placebo group (14 percent) suggests that children with at least two of the identified risk factors for chronic otitis media with effusion (bilateral otitis media with effusion, day care attendance, and middle ear fluid for 3 or more weeks) are unlikely to experience resolution of the disease without treatment. Natural history studies have defined the duration of otitis media with effusion after an episode of acute otitis media. These studies indicate that 20 to 30 percent of the children who experience an episode of acute otitis media still have a middle ear effusion 8 weeks after treatment.[1-3] At the 6 week point in our study, 86 percent of high risk, placebo treated children still had middle ear effusions.

Although the combination of prednisone and trimethoprim-sulfamethoxazole had a short term effect on the resolution of middle ear effusion in high risk children, the duration of otitis media-free time after resolution was not affected by this treatment. Future research should be directed at medical treatments for otitis media with effusion that are effective in prolonging the disease-free period.

Study supported in part by grant 5P50-NS-14538 from the National Institute for Neurological and Communicative Disorders and Stroke and grants from Burroughs Wellcome Company and the Park Nicollet Medical Research Foundation.

REFERENCES

1. Teele DW, Klein JO, Rosner BA. Epidemiology of otitis media in children. Ann Otol Rhinol Laryngol 1980; 89 (Suppl 68):5–6.
2. Marchant CD, Shurin PA, Turczyk VA, Wasikowski DE, Tutihasi MA, Kinney SE. Course and outcome of otitis media in early infancy: a prospective study. J Pediatr 1984; 104:826–831.
3. Schwartz RH, Rodriguez WJ, Grundfast KM. Duration of middle ear effusion after acute otitis media. Pediatr Infect Dis 1984; 3:204–207.
4. Daly K, Giebink GS, Le CT, Lindgren B, Batalden PB, Anderson RS, Russ JN. Determining risk for chronic otitis media with effusion. Pediatr Infec Dis, in press.
5. Healy GB. Antimicrobial therapy of chronic otitis media with effusion. Pediatr Infect Dis 1982; 1:333–338.
6. Schwartz RH. Otitis media with effusion: results of treatment with a short-course of oral prednisone or intranasal beclomethasone aerosol. Otolaryngol Head Neck Surg 1981; 89:386–391.
7. Persico M, Podoshin L, Fradis M. Otitis media with effusion, a steroid and antibiotic therapeutic trial before surgery. Ann Otol 1978; 87:191–198.

ASSESSMENT OF HISTAMINE-GAMMA GLOBULIN CONJUGATE AND NEUROTROPIN COMBINED THERAPY FOR OTITIS MEDIA WITH EFFUSION

KOICHI TOMODA, M.D., Ph.D., KENJI MACHIKI, M.D., NOBUO YOSHIE, M.D., and NOBUO KUBO, M.D.

It has been suggested that type I or type III allergy is related to the pathogenesis of otitis media with effusion. Our purpose was to study the allergic and immunologic incidence of otitis media with effusion by measuring histamine concentration, histaminopexic action (HPA), and histamine receptor, IgE, and complement concentrations in middle ear effusion and sera. In addition, pathologic alterations and the effects of treatment on the disease were evaluated following immunologic treatment.

MATERIALS AND METHODS

The subjects were 35 patients with middle ear effusion: 21 males and 14 females—17 children (5 to 15 years old) and 18 adults (over 16 years old). Fifteen patients had nasal allergy. Twenty patients underwent myringotomy to collect the middle ear effusion. Patients with adenoid hypertrophy or sinusitis were excluded.

The histamine—gamma globulin conjugate (Histaglobin) used for treatment contains human gamma globulin (12 mg/vial) and histamine dihydroxychloride (0.15 μg/vial).[1] It inhibits degranulation and histamine release from the mast cell. Neurotropin, which has been extracted from inflammatory skin tissue in rabbits after inoculation with vaccinia virus, activates the T cell immune reaction.[2] Combined administration of Histaglobin (two vials) and Neurotropin (1.8 mg/1.5 ml) in children and Histaglobin (three vials) and Neurotropin (3.6 mg/3 ml) in adults was carried out subcutaneously five times at weekly intervals. The clinical efficacy of treatment was judged as excellent, good, fair, or poor, as shown in Table 1.

Histamine concentrations were measured by fluorometric assay combined with high performance liquid chromatography.[3] The HPA titer was assayed by the formalin treated sheep erythrocyte agglutination inhibition test.[4] Histamine H_1 receptor in the middle ear mucosa, collected during ear surgery from patients with adhesive or chronic otitis media, was detected by receptor binding assay.[5]

RESULTS

Histamine concentrations in middle ear effusions were significantly higher than in sera (Fig. 1). They were also higher in the patients with nasal allergy than in those without allergy, but there was no significant difference between the values (Table 2); they decreased in the prolonged treatment group after 5 times injection of drug (Fig. 2). Pretreatment titers of HPA in patients' sera were lower than in controls (normal titer, over 1:512). They did not show remarkable changes after treatment of 5 times injection (Fig. 3). There was no significant difference in IgE and complement concentrations between sera and middle ear effusions. The number of histamine H_1 receptors in the membrane fraction of the tympanic mucosa was 18.2 ± 2.3 fmol per milligram of protein and the affinity of H_1 receptors (kd) was 0.94 ± 0.08 nM.

TABLE 1 Clinical Assessment of Treatment

	Clinical Results	Audio Level	Tympanogram	Eustachian Tube Patency
Excellent	−	< 20	B→A	Patent
Good	−	< 10	$\left(\begin{array}{c} B{\to}A \\ B{\to}C \end{array}\right)$	Stenotic
Fair	±	< 5	B→C	Stenotic
Poor	+	0	B→B	Obstructed

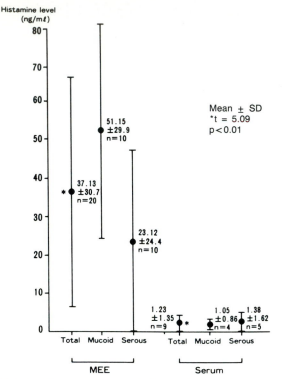

Figure 1 Histamine levels in middle ear effusions (MEE) and sera.

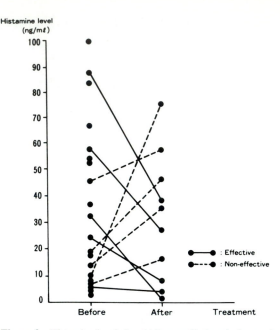

Figure 2 Histamine levels in middle ear effusions before and after treatment.

Nineteen of 35 patients (54.3 percent) showed no accumulation of middle ear effusion and had hearing improvement up to a 2 month follow-up period. The clinical efficacy of the treatment, including excellent and good responses, was significantly greater (p < 0.01) in children (82.3 percent) than in adults (27.7 percent). It was also greater (p < 0.05) in the patients with nasal allergy (80 percent) than in those without allergy (35 percent; Table 3). There were no significant differences in efficacy between any types of effusion, and between those who underwent myringotomy and those who did not. There were no side effects in any of the patients.

DISCUSSION

The measurement of histamine concentrations in middle ear effusions has been reported by Berger et al[6] and Endo et al.[7] Their results showed high levels of histamine as compared to our results. In our study a high-performance liquid chromatography step was added to the conventional Shore technique[8] to distinguish histamine from other substances, such as histidine, serotonin, and spermidine.

The high concentrations of histamine in effusions and the dissociation between serum and effusion levels suggest that histamine is a local product of the middle ear mucosa rather than a transudate from the plasma. Since mast cells with their granules discharged were found in the subepithelial layer of the tympanic mucosa in many cases of otitis media with effusion,[7] it is reasonable to assume that the histamine is released from those mast cells. An

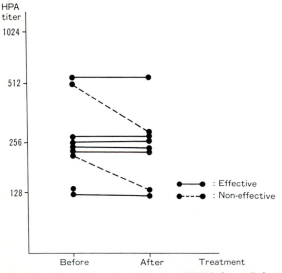

Figure 3 Titers of histaminopexic action (HPA) before and after treatment.

TABLE 2 Comparison of Histamine Levels (ng/ml) in Middle Ear Effusion (MEE) and Sera in Patients With and Without Nasal Allergy (Mean $\pm$ SD)

| | Allergy(+) | | | Allergy(−) | | |
	Mucoid	Serous	Total	Mucoid	Serous	Total
MEE	57.6±30.27 (n=7)	29.5±11.8 (n=3)	49.2±29.1[*] (n=10)	36.0±23.0 (n=3)	20.3±27.7 (n=7)	25.0±27.3[*] (n=10)
Serum	1.23±0.92 (n=3)	0.9 (n=1)	1.15±0.81 (n=4)	0.5 (n=1)	1.5±1.79 (n=4)	1.3±1.65 (n=5)

[*]t=1.81, NS.

TABLE 3 Clinical Efficacy of Treatment

| | No. of Patients (Cumulative %) | | | | |
	Excellent	Good	Fair	Poor	χ^2 Test
Children	7(41)	7(82)	1(88)	2	p<0.01
Adults	3(16)	2(27)	6(61)	7	
Allergic	8(53)	4(80)	2(93)	1	p<0.05
Nonallergic	2(10)	5(35)	5(60)	8	
Total	10(28.5)	9(54.3)	7(74.2)	9	

understanding of the triggering stimuli that activate mast cells to release histamine is needed.

Although an immediate type of hypersensitivity (type I allergy) might be involved in the mechanism of injury, IgE levels were not elevated in the effusions, as reported by Mogi et al.[9] Kurono et al[10] reported that the main role of type I allergy in otitis media with effusion is to induce eustachian tube dysfunction by obstructing the pharyngeal tubal orifice. We postulate that the initiation of injury is a bacterial infection by *Haemophilus influenzae* or *Branhamella catarrhalis* and that immune complexes and endotoxin could activate the production of anaphylatoxin, which may degranulate mast cells and release histamine. The histamine, influencing the permeability of blood vessels, may participate through the receptors in the production of an effusion and edema of the tympanic and tubal mucosa. Additionally it may play an important role in the maintenance of effusion and chronicity of the disease.

Thus, combined therapy with a histamine—gamma globulin conjugate and Neurotropin is a useful treatment for otitis media with effusion, especially in children and patients with associated nasal allergy. We are currently investigating whether this therapy is useful for preventing the recurrence of otitis media with effusion.

REFERENCES

1. Parrot JL, Urquia DA, Laborde C. Captation de l'histamine par le sérum humani normal défant de captation par le sérum d'asthmatique. C R Soc Biol 1951; 145:1045.
2. Koda A, Nagai H, Kurimoto Y, et al. Effect of neurotropin (NPS) on allergic reactions. Folia Pharmacol Japon 1981; 78:319–334.
3. Hasegawa M, Saito Y, Naka F, et al. Seasonal variations of total histamine in patients with seasonal allergic rhinitis. Clin Allergy 1983; 13:277–286.
4. Nakata I, Yamato T, Hamada G. Histaminopexic action (HPA) in the serum of patients with allergic diseases and correlation of the change in HPA values on administration of Histaglobin with the resultant clinical response. Clin Immunol 1983; 15:752–758.
5. Tran VT, Chang RSL, Snyder SH. Histamine H_1 receptors identified in mammalian brain membranes with H-mephyramine. Proc Natl Acad Sci 1978; 75:6290–6294.
6. Berger G, Hawke M, Proops DW, et al. Histamine levels in middle ear effusions. Acta Otolaryngol 1984; 98:385–390.
7. Endo S, Awataguchi T, Suzuki S, et al. Fluorometric assay of histamine levels in middle ear effusions of secretory otitis media. J Otolaryngol Jpn 1985; 88:1541–1547.
8. Shore PA, Burkhalter A, Cohn VH. A method for the fluorometric assay of histamine in tissue. J Pharmacol Exp Ther 1959; 127:182–186.
9. Mogi G, Maeda S, Yoshida T, et al. Radioimmunoassay of IgE in middle ear effusions. Acta Otolaryngol 1976; 82:26–32.
10. Kurono Y, Kato H, Tomonaga K, et al. Role of type I allergy in otitis media with effusion. J Jpn Immunol Allergol Otolaryngol 1985; 3:74–75.

We sincerely thank Mr. Fujio Naka and Mr. Isao Nakata, Institute of Bio-Active Sciences, Nippon Zoki Pharmaceuticals Co. Ltd., Japan, for their help in measuring histamine and HPA titers.

PHARMACEUTICAL TREATMENT OF EXPERIMENTAL OTITIS MEDIA WITH EFFUSION

FUMIHIKO HORI, M.D., HIDEYUKI KAWAUCHI, M.D., MASASHI SUZUKI, M.D., and GORO MOGI, M.D.

Although several pharmacologic investigations have been attempted in efforts to eradicate middle ear effusions in otitis media,[1,2] there is still no conservative therapy that is fully effective, convenient, and safe for this disorder. Disturbance of the mucociliary transport system and release of proteolytic enzymes in the tympanic cavity and eustachian tube are probably the major pathogenetic factors in this disorder. Our study was designed to investigate the therapeutic efficacy of Cepharanthin, a biscoclaurin type of alkaloid (crude drug) extracted from roots of *Stephania cepharanta hayata*, which stabilizes cell membranes, and of s-carboxymethylcysteine (Mucodyne), which restores mucociliary clearance.

MATERIALS AND METHODS

Drugs

Cepharanthin was obtained from the Kakenshoyaku Co. (Tokyo) and Mucodyne was obtained from the Kyorin Pharmacological Co. (Tokyo).

Experimental Design

Seventy-one healthy male chinchillas (weighing 350 to 600 g) with clean external auditory canals and normal tympanic membranes underwent unilateral production of otitis media with effusion, the untreated ear acting as a control. The animals were divided into seven groups. Group 1 animals (N=5) received no medicine. Group 2 (N=5), group 3 (N=5), and group 4 animals (N=5) were given a 1, 2, or 5 mg per kilogram dose of Cepharanthin intraperitoneally daily after the induction of otitis media. Group 5 animals (N=17) received a 2 mg per kilogram dose of Ceparanthin by intraperitoneal injection daily for 7 days before the local antigenic challenge. Group 4 animals (N=17) were given a

100 mg per kilogram dose of s-carboxymethylcysteine orally daily after the induction of otitis media. Group 7 animals (N=17) were given a 200 mg per kilogram dose of s-carboxymethylcysteine orally daily after the induction of otitis media. The dosage was continued in all groups for 14 days following the local antigenic challenge.

Induction of Otitis Media with Effusion

Experimental otitis media with effusion was induced in the chinchillas by immunization with keyhole limpet hemocyanin delivered into the right tympanic cavity following systemic sensitization. Systemic immunization was carried out by injecting the animals intradermally with 1 mg of keyhole limpet hemocyanin in complete Freund's adjuvant. Two weeks later a middle ear challenge with antigens was performed aseptically by the inoculation of 0.1 ml of 0.8 percent hydroxypropylcellulose solution containing 0.3 mg of keyhole limpet hemocyanin into the tympanic cavity through the superior bulla. Then, as a control, hydroxypropylcellulose solution was injected aseptically into the left tympanic cavity.

Observation Scheme

The presence of middle ear effusion was monitored daily by tympanometry and fiberoptic observation of the eardrum. Four days after experimental otitis occurred, the middle ears were aspirated aseptically through the eardrum in nine chinchillas (three untreated animals, three animals treated by a 2 mg per kilogram dose of Cepharanthin, and three animals treated by a 200 mg per kilogram dose of s-carboxymethylcysteine and processed for biochemical analysis. The animals were then killed to permit further studies.

The effusions were divided immediately into cellular and liquid components by centrifugation at 1,000 rpm for 10 minutes. The liquid component was divided into two groups and measured for histamine and prostaglandin E_2.

The histamine content in the effusions was determined by high speed liquid chromatography as described by Tsuruta et al.[3] Effusion specimens were diluted 10 times with distilled water, and 500 μl of these diluted samples was used for analysis. Assay of prostaglandin E_2 was carried out by the radioimmunoassay method described by Inagawa.[4]

The absorption, distribution and disappearance of radioactivity were measured at 0.5 hour and at 1, 6, and 12 hours after a single intraperitoneal injection of ^{3}H-Cepharanthin (5 mg per 50 microcurie per milliliter per kilogram) and after a single oral dose of ^{14}C-s-carboxymethylcysteine (10 mg per 40 microcuries per milliliter per kilogram) on the fourth day after otitis media developed.

Autoradiography was performed by the method of Nagata et al.[5] Radiolabeled Cepharanthin, or s-carboxymethylcysteine was also given intraperitoneally or orally to two different groups of animals, which were sacrificed 6 hours after dosing. The temporal bullae were dissected and fixed in neutral formaldehyde-saline solution. Histologic sections (5 μm) were obtained and were processed by means of the dip method using Sakura NR-M$_2$ emulsion. The specimens were exposed for 6 weeks, developed, stained with hematoxylin and eosin, and observed in a light microscope.

RESULTS

Tympanometry and Fiberoptic Observation

The normal middle ear in the chinchillas was characterized by a type A tympanogram; types B and C usually indicated the presence of effusion.

In all animals in group 1, otitis media with effusion developed 2 or 3 days after the local challenge and subsided spontaneously within 14 days afterward. In none of the group 2 animals, in all the group 3 animals, and in two of the five group 4 animals, otitis media subsided within 10 days after induction of the disease (Fig. 1). Otitis media disappeared on the fourteenth day after induction of the disease in two of the five group 2 animals and in three of the five group 4 animals. In group 5, otitis media was not induced in nine animals (53 percent). In the remaining eight animals the induced disease disappeared within 10 days (Table 1). In four of the 17 group 6 animals and in nine of the 17 group 7 animals, otitis media subsided within 5 or 6 days after induction of the disease (Table 2).

Histamine and Prostaglandin E_2 Concentration

The histamine level of the middle ear effusions in animals treated with Cepharanthin (2 mg per kilo-

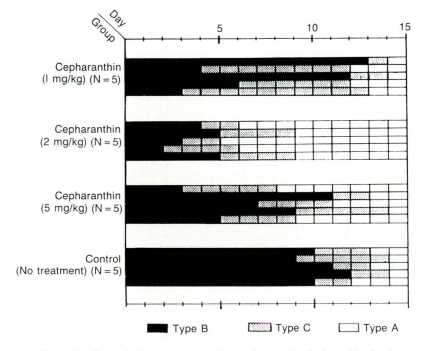

Figure 1 Change in the tympanogram in animal treated by Cepharanthin after induction of otitis media with effusion.

TABLE 1   Results of Cepharanthin Administration Before the Induction of Otitis Media with Effusion

Chinchillas	Induction of Otitis Media with Effusion (%)
Control (no treatment; N=5)	5/5 (100%)
Cepharanthin (2 mg; N=17)	8/17 (47%)

gram) was 40.2±3.5 ng per milliliter, while that of effusions in animals treated with s-carboxymethylcysteine (200 mg per kilogram) was 34.3±3.3 ng per milliliter. The histamine level in three animals treated by Cepharanthin and s-carboxymethylcysteine was not different from that in three untreated animals used as controls. The prostaglandin E_2 level in the effusions in three animals treated with Cepharanthin (2 mg per kilogram) was 4.51±0.7 ng per milliliter, while that in three animals treated with s-carboxymethylcysteine (200 mg per kilogram) was 3.21±0.4 ng per milliliter. The prostaglandin E_2 level in the effusions of three animals treated with Cepharanthin and s-carboxymethylcysteine did not differ from that in three untreated animals used as controls.

Radioactivity in Middle Ear Effusions, Blood, and Bile

It was clear that ^{3}H-Cepharanthin or ^{14}C-s-carboxymethylcysteine was transferred to the middle ear following intraperitoneal or oral administration. Detectable concentrations of these two labeled drugs were found in middle ear effusions as early as 30 minutes after administration, suggesting rapid uptake of the drug into the effusion. After 6 hours the concentration of radioactivity of ^{3}H-Cepharanthin

in the effusion (480±33 CPM) was at a maximum. This concentration was about 10 times that in whole blood (44±11 CPM). The concentration of radioactivity of ^{14}C-s-carboxymethylcysteine in the effusion (323±29 CPM) after 6 hours was at a maximum; this concentration was about six times that of whole blood (54±21 CPM).

Autoradiography

Autoradiography of ^{3}H-Cepharanthin showed that the labeled drug was distributed mainly to the top and base of the epithelial cells, especially those in the area of severe inflammation in the eustachian tube (Fig. 2).

Autoradiography of ^{14}C-s-carboxymethylcysteine showed that the labeled drug was distributed mainly in the mucous layer of the mucociliary cells of the eustachian tube (Fig. 3).

DISCUSSION

Cepharanthin is a crude drug, which is a 606 molecular weight biscoclaurine alkaloid extracted from *Stephania cepharantha hayata*. It has a stabilizing effect on platelet aggregation,[6] inhibits histamine release from mast cells,[7] and inhibits hemolysis induced by snake venom.[8] In addition, Cepharanthin is known to have the capacity to increase the number of peripheral lymphocytes.[9] This drug has been used for the treatment of otitis media with effusion in Japan. However, its pharmacologic efficacy has not been completely proven. In our study it was clear that the maximal pharmacologic efficacy would result by using a suitable concentration in the dose, which was 2 mg per kilogram intraperitoneally. Histamine and prostaglandin E_2

TABLE 2   Effects of S-Carboxymethylcysteine Administration After Induction of Otitis Media with Effusion

	Presence of Middle Ear Effusion (%)		
	Day of Observation		
Chinchillas	5	10	15
Control (no treatment; N=5)	5/5(100)	4/5 (80)	3/5 (60)
S-carboxymethylcysteine (100 mg; N=17)	16/17(94)	14/17(82)	6/17(35)
S-carboxymethylcysteine (200 mg; N=17)	12/17(71)	7/17(41)	4/17(24)

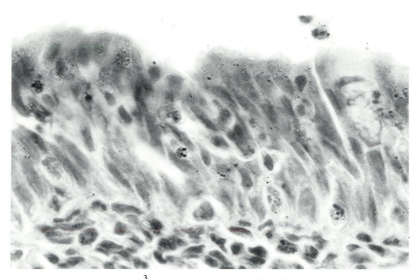

Figure 2 Autoradiography of ^{3}H-Cepharanthin of eustachian tube in induction of otitis media with effusion.

concentrations in the middle ear effusions of chinchillas receiving a 2 mg per kilogram dose were as high as those in nontreated chinchillas. This means that Cepharanthin is not effective in inhibiting histamine and prostaglandin E_2 release from inflammatory cells after inflammation has occurred. However, the findings in radioactivity and autoradiography studies suggest that this drug's effects include membrane stabilization and inhibition of the release of lysosomal enzymes from neutrophils.

Carbocisteine has been used in man for the treatment of mucosal disorders of the upper respiratory tract. Jodice[1] and Taylor and Dareshani[2] have used carbocisteine in man for the treatment of otitis media with effusion. Ohashi et al[10] proved the efficacy of carbocisteine in otitis media in rabbits. It is therefore of interest to know how the drug is distributed following administration. Thus our study was designed to investigate the therapeutic effect of s-carboxymethylcysteine on chinchilla immune mediated otitis media with effusion, which resembles the disease described in humans.

Oral administration of s-carboxymethylcysteine in a dose of 200 mg per kilogram was more effective than a dose of 100 mg per kilogram against experimental otitis media with effusion. This suggests

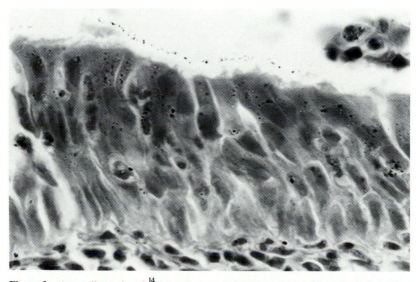

Figure 3 Autoradiography of ^{14}C-s-carboxymethylcysteine of eustachian tube in induction of otitis media with effusion.

that s-carboxymethylcysteine is a dose dependent drug. In view of the finding that experimental otitis media subsided within 5 or 6 days after induction of the disease, s-carboxymethylcysteine was an effective drug for early restoration of the experimental disease. The radioactivity of ^{14}C-s-carboxymethylcysteine in middle ear effusions suggests a rapid uptake of the drug into the effusion, which shows that the drug acts in the middle ear. Autoradiography of ^{14}C-s-carboxymethylcysteine showed that the drug is distributed in the cytoplasm and mucous layer of ciliated cells, suggesting a proteolytic effect and a protecting effect on the ciliated cell. This was also demonstrated in the histologic findings, showing slight damage of the ciliated cells in the eustachian tube.

The results of this study showed the efficacy of Cepharanthin and s-carboxymethylcysteine against experimental otitis media with effusion and suggest that clinical trials of these medicines be carried out.

REFERENCES

1. Jodice S. Indicazioni e vataggi della S Carbossimetilcisteina (Lisomucil) in pathologic ORL. Clin Europ 1974; 13:1–20.
2. Taylor PH, Dareshani N. S-Carboxymethylcysteine syrup in secretory otitis media with effusion caused by long term exposure to SO$_2$. J Otolaryngol Jpn 1980; 88:1051–1055.
3. Tsuruta Y, Okura Y, Kobayaski K. Determination of histamine in plasma by high-speed liquid chromatography. J Chromatogr 1978; 146:490–493.
4. Inagawa T. Assay of prostaglandin E. J Med Technol 1982; 26:135–147 (in Japanese).
5. Nagata T, Shibata O, Nawa T. Simplified methods for mass production of radioautographs. Acta Anat Nippon 1967; 42:162–166 (in Japanese).
6. Kanaho Y, Sato T, Fuji T, et al. In vivo effect of Cepharanthin on platelet aggregation. Jpn Arch Int Med 1983; 30:15–19 (in Japanese).
7. Sugiyama K, et al. Inhibition by Cepharanthin of histamine release from rat peritoneal mast cells. Jpn J Allergol 1976; 25:685–690 (in Japanese).
8. Utsumi K, Miyahara M, Sugiyama K, et al. Effect of biscoclaurin alkaloid on the cell membrane related to membrane fluidity. Acta Histchem Cytochem 1976; 9:59–68 (in Japanese).
9. Makidono A. Effect of anti-leukopenic drugs on the recovery of immunocompetent cells. Acta Med Okayama 1980; 50:475–486 (in Japanese).
10. Ohashi Y, et al. Effects of carbocysteine on the experimental otitis media with effusion caused by long-term exposure to SO$_2$. J Otolaryngol Jpn 1980; 88:1051–1055.

REDUCED NASOPHARYNGEAL CARRIAGE OF BACTERIA IN BREAST FED BABIES

GUSTAV ANIANSSON, M.D., BENGT ANDERSSON, M.D., Ph.D., BERNDT ALM, M.D., PETER LARSSON, OLLE NYLÉN, M.D., Ph.D., HANS PETERSON, M.D., PETER RIGNÉR, M.D., and CATHARINA SVANBORG-EDÉN, M.D., Ph.D.

The human nasopharynx functions as a reservoir for bacteria, e.g., *Streptococcus pneumoniae* and *Haemophilus influenzae*. Nasopharyngeal carriage of these bacterial species occurs in healthy individuals and spread to other sites results, for example, in acute otitis media, meningitis, or pneumonia and septicemia.

The mechanisms that control the persistence and turnover of bacteria in the nasopharynx are poorly understood. The initial contact between bacteria and epithelial surfaces may result in attachment. At other mucosal sites specific attachment of bacteria to epithelial cell receptors promotes bacterial persistance and increases the virulence.[1] Both *Streptococcus pneumoniae* and *Haemophilus influenzae* attach specifically to epithelial cells from the human respiratory tract.[2]

Recently human milk was shown to inhibit this attachment.[3] The inhibitory activity was not associated with the immunoglobulin fraction but with other components of the high and low molecular weight fractions. Free oligosaccharide receptors for pneumococci were identified in the low molecular weight fraction of milk and were shown to inhibit attachment in vitro.[3] These results provided the basis for studying the association between the antiadhesive activity of milk and colonization of the nasopharynx in newborn babies. The present study demonstrates a reduced colonization frequency in breast fed babies compared to infants who receive mixed feeding or who do not receive breast milk.

MATERIALS AND METHODS

Study Population

Three cross sectional samples of infants younger than 1 year of age were obtained in connection with regular visits to well baby clinics. At the age interval of 6 weeks to 3 months, 57 children were sampled; between 4 and 6 months, 27 children were sampled; and between 7 and 11 months, 17 children were sampled (total 101 children). At each visit a nasopharyngeal culture was obtained from the baby and a milk sample from the mother. A detailed history of the feeding pattern was obtained with regard to the number of breast fed meals per day, the type of formula, the introduction of other foods, and the kinds of food used.

The exposure to bacteria was indirectly analyzed through the family size, the age of the siblings, and the form of daycare for the infants and siblings during the study time.

Bacteria

Nasopharyngeal cultures were obtained with a cotton tipped metal swab. After transport to the clinical bacteriological laboratory in modified Stuart's medium, the swabs were used to inoculate three media: blood agar plates, a double layered selective medium containing gentamicin to aid the detection of streptococci, and chocolate agar with nicotinamide adenine dinucleotide and hematin for *Haemophilus influenzae*.[4] Pneumococci were defined by sensitivity to optochin using the disc diffusion method. The bacteria were kept at −70° C in skim milk.

Milk Samples

Milk samples were obtained by the mothers in sterile containers from the contralateral breast while nursing. The milk was centrifuged and the fat removed. Milk was stored at −20° C in aliquots.

Adherence Assay

The attachment of *H. influenzae* and *S. pneumoniae* to human buccal and oropharyngeal epithelial cells, respectively, was tested as previously described.[4] In brief, epithelial cells of healthy donors were mixed with the bacteria. After incubation and elimination of unbound bacterial cells by centrifugation, the number of attached bacteria was determined by interference contrast microscopy as the mean number of bacteria per cell for 40 oropharyngeal epithelial cells.

Adhesion inhibition by milk was tested by preincubation of the bacteria with milk samples at 37° C for 30 minutes. Subsequently epithelial cells were added and the adherence testing proceeded as already described. Adhesion inhibition was given as a percentage of the buffer control.

RESULTS

Of the 101 children enrolled in the study, 53 were girls and 48 were boys. The bacterial recovery from the nasopharyngeal cultures is shown in Table 1. *Staphylococcus aureus* occurred in 50 percent of the youngest children and gradually disappeared with increasing age. By contrast, the frequency of *S. pneumoniae* increased to about 40 percent, *Branhamella catarrhalis* to 44 percent, and *H. influenzae* increased with age to about 12 percent positive at 10 months of age.

Feeding Pattern

The numbers of exclusively breast fed children, of children who received mixed feeding, and of those fed only with other foods are shown in Table 2. At 3 months of age all the children studied received breast milk with or without other foods. Conversely, none was exclusively breast fed at 6 or 10 months of age.

TABLE 1 Nasopharyngeal Cultures, % Positive

Microorganism	Age (months)		
	0–3	4–6	7–11
S. aureus	54	26	8
S. pneumoniae	11	41	53
H. influenzae	2	11	12
B. catarrhalis	18	44	47

TABLE 2 Feeding Pattern

Age (months)	No.	Feeding Pattern* Breast Milk	Feeding Pattern* Mixed Feeding	Feeding Pattern* Other
0–3	57	84	16	0
4–6	27	0	78	22
7–11	17	0	35	65
Total	101	48	36	17

*Percentage of total number of children in each age group.

Colonization in Relation to Breast Feeding

The relation of colonization to breast feeding is shown in Table 3. Since the exclusively breast fed were in the age group of 0 to 3 months, the comparison of nasopharyngeal colonization in breast fed babies and in those with mixed feeding was performed in this age group. The frequency of *S. pneumoniae* and *H. influenzae* was significantly lower in the breast fed babies than in those who received mixed feeding.

Adhesion Inhibition of Milk

The milk from each mother was tested for its capacity to inhibit the attachment of a highly adhering pneumococcal strain (Table 4). The colonization rate was significantly lower in children receiving only inhibitory milk than in those receiving only milk with poor inhibitory activity or mixed feeding.

TABLE 3 Colonization Frequency in Relation to Feeding Pattern

Age (months)	Feeding	Nasopharyngeal Culture % positive for S. pneumoniae
0–3	Breast milk	13
	Mixed feeding	50 p<0.05*
	Other	—
4–6	Breast milk	—
	Mixed feeding	52 n.s.
	Other	17
7–11	Breast milk	—
	Mixed feeding	33 n.s.
	Other	55
Total	Breast milk	5/48 (10%)
	Mixed feeding	17/36 (47%)
	Other	7/17 (41%)

*X^2 = 5.7.

DISCUSSION

Breast feeding protects the infant against infection. Protection may be due to lower exposure to environmental microorganisms, to a reduced microbial colonization of mucosal surfaces with potential pathogenes, or to a direct interference with mechanisms of pathogenesis. The present study provides support for the hypothesis that breast fed babies have a reduced frequency of nasopharyngeal colonization with *Streptococcus pneumoniae* and *Haemophilus influenzae*, compared to age matched children who receive mixed feeding or other foods.

This study was undertaken as a pilot study to define the suitability of the technology and age intervals selected. The results suggested that the age interval of 0 to 3 months was most informative for questions related to breast feeding, whereas all three age intervals were required to evaluate the progression of colonization. An obvious drawback of the pilot study is the fact that the three age groups were separate; in a larger study we will obtain sequential samples from the same individuals at all three ages. It cannot at present be excluded that the differences observed were due to the age factor rather than an effect of breast feeding per se.

The frequency of nasopharyngeal carriage of *S. pneumoniae* and *H. influenzae* as well as *Branhamella catarrhalis* was low during the first 3 months of age. This is in contrast to the colonization frequencies previously reported, e.g., from Papua, New Guinea.[5] The colonization rate at any geographic site is likely to be highly dependent on the extent of exposure and thus indirectly on the living conditions, e.g., the family size. The reduced frequency of colonization in the exclusively breast fed infants may have social explanations. Exclusive breast feeding may reflect the fact that the baby and the mother are in close contact and confined more to the home with less risk of exposure to bacteria. Mixed feeding is likely to occur more often in families where the mother has activities outside the house. This hypothesis was supported by the apparent increase in colonization in babies with siblings in day care (data not shown).

TABLE 4 Feeding Pattern and Breast Milk Quality in Relation to Colonization

Feeding	Colonization Frequency %	Colonization Frequency No.
Inhibitory milk only	7	2/27
Noninhibitory milk or milk plus other	40	12/30

Human milk contains a variety of substances with antibacterial activity. These include immunoglobulin, especially secretory IgA, with antibody activity against several common bacteria, including *H. influenzae* and *S. pneumoniae*, as well as against respiratory viruses and rotavirus. The nonimmunoglobulin component of milk has antibacterial activity as a result of its content of lysozyme, lactoferrin, and peroxidase. Furthermore human milk contains components that interfere with bacterial attachment. Inhibitors of attachment of *S. pneumoniae* and *H. influenzae* are present both as free oligosaccharides corresponding to the cell bound receptors for attaching *S. pneumoniae* and as high molecular weight molecules. Previous studies have attempted to correlate the protective effects of breast feeding against respiratory tract infections without analyzing the microbial flora or the mechanisms of protection in the milk. The lower colonization rate in babies receiving breast milk (observed in this study) and high antiadhesive activity supported the hypothesis that specific interference with attachment reduces in vivo colonization. Provided this can be confirmed in the larger study, it provides a new principle for prophylaxis against infections, i.e., by blocking the binding to mucosal surfaces.

REFERENCES

1. Beachey EH. Bacterial adherence: adhesin-receptor interactions mediating the attachment of bacteria to mucosal surfaces. J Infect Dis 1981; 143:325–345.
2. Andersson B, Dahmen J, Frejd T, Leffler H, Magnusson G, Norri G, Svanborg-Edén C. Identification of a disaccharide unit of a glycoconjugate receptor for pneumococci attaching to human pharyngeal epithelial cells. J Exp Med 1983; 158:559–570.
3. Andersson B, Porras O, Hansson LÅ, Lagergård T, Svanborg-Edén C. Inhibition of attachment of *Streptococcus pneumoniae* and *Haemophilus influenzae* by human milk and receptor oligosaccharides. J Infect Dis 1986; 153:232–237.
4. Porras O, Svanborg-Edén C, Lagergård T, Hansson LÅ. Method for testing adherence of *Haemophilus influenzae* to human buccal epithelial cells. Eur J Clin Microbiol 1985; 4:310–315.
5. Shann F, Germer S, Hazlett D, et al. Aetrology of pneumonia in children in Goro Ka Hospital, Papua, New Guinea. Lancet 1984; 2:537–541.

DOUBLE BLIND STUDY COMPARING ERYTHROMYCIN-SULFISOXAZOLE (PEDIAZOLE) T.I.D. TO PLACEBO IN CHRONIC OTITIS MEDIA WITH EFFUSION

MELVIN D. SCHLOSS, M.D., F.R.C.S.(C)., ELLEN E. DEMPSEY, M.Sc., ELLEN RISHIKOF, M.Sc., SIMON SORGER, and MICHAEL G.A. GRACE, Ph.D., P.Eng.

Chronic otitis media is defined as a middle ear effusion that has persisted for 3 months or longer.[1] In contrast to acute otitis media, chronic effusions are frequently asymptomatic. In younger children suspicion of middle ear disease may rely upon the parent's awareness of changes in behavior or the child's inability to communicate. Older children may describe a hearing loss or complain of a feeling of "fullness" or "popping" in the ears.[2] This hearing loss in infants and children may have severe and life long consequences; the critical period for speech and language is from birth to age 2 years.[3]

When 205 3-year-old children were studied to determine the association between time spent with chronic otitis media and the level of speech development, a negative correlation was observed.[4] Although this association has been well established, it is not known whether this developmental lag persists through later years of life or whether these children are able to catch up to their disease free peers.

In the first half of the 20th century chronic effusions were thought to be sterile; however, in 1958 Senturia[5] was able to identify bacteria in 42 percent of aspirates. In a recent study of 274 children, aged 1 to 16 years, with chronic otitis media, 45 percent of the middle ear aspirates were pathogen positive.[6] Of those positive cultures, approximately 33 percent contained pathogens commonly seen in acute infections: *Streptococcus pneumoniae, Haemophilus influenzae, Streptococcus pyogenes,* or *Staphylococcus aureus*. In 89 middle ear aspirates 67 percent of the culture negative effusions demonstrated endotoxin activity, indicating the potential role of these agents in the etiology of chronic otitis media.[7]

Although the problem and the possible consequences have been defined, the question remains how to manage these chronic middle ear effusions. A middle ear effusion that has persisted for at least 3 months should be considered chronic and requires active treatment. Up to 3 months, observation may be justified, since middle ear effusions may resolve spontaneously.[8]

Of the many methods of management for chronic otitis media, none has been shown to be effective in well controlled clinical trials, including the frequently used surgical treatment options, such as myringotomy with and without tympanostomy tube insertion and adenoidectomy.[1] Nonsurgical methods of management that have been investigated include antimicrobials, decongestants, antihistamines, and adrenocorticosteroids alone or in combination, as well as middle ear inflation employing the Politzer methodology.[9,10] Clearly, well controlled efficacy trials of all medical and surgical treatments are required. Long term follow-up studies are also needed to understand the natural history of chronic effusions and the long term implications for speech development and learning capacity.

RESULTS

Our double blind, randomized trial of 54 children was designed to compare the efficacy of and tolerance to erythromycin-sulfisoxazole (based on 50 mg per kilogram per day of the erythromycin component for 14 or 28 days given three times daily; Pediazole, Abbott Laboratories) with a placebo in eradicating chronic otitis media. Pneumatic otoscopy, tympanometry, and audiology were used to assess the outcome at days 14 and 28 and months 2 to 6. Pretreatment tympanocentesis, performed in all children, confirmed that 53.7 percent of the effusions were sterile and 35.2 percent of the cultures were positive for *Staphylococcus epidermidis* (Table 1). At day 14, 29.6 percent of the placebo patients were cured, 22.2 percent were improved, 25.9 percent were unchanged, and 22.2 percent were worse. Of the erythromycin-sulfisoxazole patients, 24.0 percent were cured, 52.0 percent were improved, 24.0 percent were unchanged, and none was worse. Tympanometry and audiologic assessments did not differ significantly between the two groups.

It is concluded that erythromycin-sulfisoxazole prevented a worsening of chronic otitis media and significantly improved the patients' status immediately after therapy. This benefit dissipated with time, as demonstrated at follow-up in patients up to 6 months after therapy, and is not considered of value in the long term management of patients with chronic otitis media. Both therapies were well tolerated by patients, with no significant difference between placebo and erythromycin-sulfisoxazole in terms of incidence, type and severity of adverse reactions, or the number of withdrawals due to adverse reactions.

REFERENCES

1. Bluestone CD. Treatment of otitis media. Scand J Infect Dis 1983; 39(Suppl):26–33.

TABLE 1 Frequency of Pathogens Isolated From 54 Middle Ear Aspirates by Treatment Group

Microorganism	Placebo	Erythromycin–Sulfa
S. epidermidis (19)	10	9
H. influenzae (1)	1	—
S. pneumoniae (2)	—	2
Beta hemolytic streptococcus (1)	1	—
Corynebacterium sp. (4)	2	2
Neisseria sp. (3)	2	1
C. parapsilosis (1)	—	1
Sterile (no growth) (29)	15	14
Number of aspirates (54)	28	26

2. Bluestone CD. Diagnosis of chronic otitis media with effusion: description, otoscopy, acoustic impedance measurements and assessment of hearing. Pediatr Infect Dis 1982; 1(Suppl 5):S38–S69.

3. Gibson GC. Screening for hearing loss in children. Can Fam Physician 1982; 27:1387–1390.

4. Teele DW, et al. Otitis media with effusion during the first three years of life—development of speech and language. Pediatrics 1984; 74:282–287.

5. Senturia BH, et al. Studies concerned with tubotympanitis. Ann Otol Rhinol Laryngol 1958; 67:440–467.

6. Riding KH, et al. Microbiology of recurrent and chronic otitis media with effusion. J Pediatr 1978; 93:739–743.

7. DeMaria TF, Prior RB, Briggs BR, Lim DJ, Birck HG. Endotoxin in middle ear effusions from patients with. In: Lim DJ, Bluestone CD, Klein JO, Nelson JD, eds. Recent advances in otitis media with effusion. Proceedings of the Third International Symposium. Toronto: BC Decker, 1984:123.

8. Teele DW, et al. Epidemiology of otitis media in children. Ann Otol Rhinol Laryngol 1980; 68(Suppl 89):5–6.

9. Cantekin EI, et al. Lack of efficacy of a decongestant antihistamine combination for otitis media with effusion ("secretory" otitis media) in children. N Engl J Med 1983; 308:297–301.

10. O'Shea JS, et al. Childhood serous otitis media. Clin Pediatr 1982; 21:150–153.

EFFECT OF POVIDONE-IODINE PREPARATION ON THE INCIDENCE OF POST-TYMPANOSTOMY OTORRHEA

JACK W. ALAND Jr., M.D. and ROBERT L. BALDWIN, M.D.

In the battle against persistent middle ear effusion and recurrent acute otitis media in children, the tympanostomy tube has become the otolaryngologist's most important weapon. Tympanostomy was introduced in 1954 by Armstrong,[1] and since then the popularity of the procedure has grown so that it is now one of the procedures most commonly done in the United States. However, enthusiasm for the procedure must be tempered by the not uncommon occurrence of complications, such as otorrhea.

Post-tympanostomy otorrhea is a perplexing problem. This can be classified as either postoperative, occurring in the first 2 weeks after tube placement, or late, occurring later than 2 weeks after the operation. The incidence of otorrhea after tympanostomy tube placement varies with different studies. McLelland,[2] in a review of 307 patients under age 10 in whom tympanostomy tubes had been inserted, found that 19.9 percent of the ears, or 34.5 percent of the patients, developed drainage at some time while the tubes were in place. Large bore ventilation tubes have been associated with a much higher incidence of otorrhea-41 and 69 percent in two series by Holt et al[3] and Per-Lee,[4] respectively. Some authors have recorded the specific incidence of postoperative otorrhea—that is, drainage occurring within 2 weeks after tube insertion. This has been reported as 3.4 to 12 percent in various studies by Gates et al,[5] Hughes et al,[6] and Herzon.[7]

The etiology of postoperative (early) otorrhea is thought to be different from that of late otorrhea. In particular, postoperative otorrhea is thought to be due to contamination of the middle ear during surgery with bacteria from the ear canal. A second possibility is that tympanostomy, by allowing aeration of the middle ear, provides a better environment for growth of the aerobic bacteria contained in the middle ear effusion.

Believing that contamination of the middle ear by bacteria from the ear canal may cause postoperative otorrhea, Gates and co-workers[5] prepared the ear canal with povidone-iodine before performing tympanostomy in 525 cases. They found that 7.1 percent of the patients developed postoperative otorrhea. Gates then compared these results with those in a study by Balkany et al[8] who did not prepare the ear canal with iodine and who had a 12 percent incidence of postoperative otorrhea. Gates concluded that preparing the ear with iodine was probably of benefit. Since this comparison was made between two studies using different protocols, however, we believed that it would be worthwhile to carry out a prospective study to determine whether preparation of the ear canal with povidone-iodine has any effect on the incidence of postoperative otorrhea.

SUBJECTS AND METHOD

The subjects were 111 consecutive children requiring tympanostomy. All had a diagnosis of either recurrent acute otitis media or persistent otitis media with effusion, unresponsive to medical therapy. All the procedures were done by the same surgeon in a 3 month period between June and September 1986.

In each patient the ear canals were cleaned of cerumen and debris. The right ear canal was filled with povidone-iodine solution for 1 minute and then rinsed three times with sterile saline and suctioned dry. The left ear canal served as an internal control and was not irrigated with povidone-iodine.

The myringotomy incision was made in the anterior inferior quadrant of the tympanic membrane. Any fluid present in the middle ear was noted as to its character (serous, mucoid, or purulent) and then suctioned away. The middle ear mucosa was also examined through the incision and noted as being normal, hyperemic, edematous, or granular. A 1.25 mm internal diameter Sheehy collar button ventilation tube was then inserted into the incision. No pre- or postoperative systemic or topical antibiotic therapy was used in any patient.

The patients were seen in the office 1 week following the procedure and examined for the presence of otorrhea. The patient was determined to have postoperative otorrhea if drainage was seen on the return visit or if the drainage lasted longer than 3 days after operation.

RESULTS

In this study there were 72 boys and 39 girls. The ages ranged from 2 months to 8 years, the mean age being 26 months. There were 89 patients having the first set of tympanostomy tubes placed, 15 patients having the second set, and seven patients having the third or greater set. Four patients underwent adenoidectomy. A total of 14 (12.6 percent) of the patients developed postoperative otorrhea—18 (8.1 percent) of the ears. Thus seven (6.3 percent) of the povidone-iodine prepared ears and 11 (9.9 percent) of the unprepared ears developed otorrhea. This difference was checked by the chi square test and was not found to be statistically significant. Furthermore, the age of the patient and the number of times tympanostomy tubes had been placed had no predictive value in estimating the likelihood of postoperative otorrhea. In the patients in whom mucoid or purulent fluid was found at the time of surgery there was a statistically higher incidence of postoperative otorrhea than in those who had no fluid or serous fluid present ($p < 0.05$; Table 1). Patients with no fluid, or with serous fluid, did not develop otorrhea. We found that 18.9 percent of the patients with mucoid fluid and 28.6 percent with purulent fluid did develop otorrhea. Also the presence of an edematous or granular middle ear mucosa implied that the patient had a significantly higher chance of developing otorrhea than did those with a normal or hyperemic middle ear mucosa, as can be seen in Table 2. This study suggests that preparing the ear canal with povidone-iodine has no effect on the incidence of postoperative otorrhea.

DISCUSSION

Gates believed that preparing the ear canal with povidone-iodine was effective in reducing the number of patients with postoperative otorrhea. However, Gates' study had no control group. Gates compared the 7.1 percent of the patients in his study who developed postoperative otorrhea with the 12 percent of the patients who developed postoperative otorrhea in the Balkany study. However, in the Balkany study approximately one third of the pa-

TABLE 1 Middle Ear Fluid Found at Operation and Number of Ears with Postoperative Otorrhea

| Fluid Present | Ear | | Total | No. with Postoperative Otorrhea (%) |
	Right	Left		
None	63	61	124	0
Serous	6	2	8	0
Mucoid	35	39	74	14 (18.9)
Purulent	6	8	14	4 (28.6)

TABLE 2 Middle Ear Mucosa Found at Operation and Number of Ears with Postoperative Otorrhea

Mucosa	Ear Right	Left	Total	No. with Postoperative Otorrhea (%)	
Normal	55	54	109	1	(0.9)
Hyperemic	6	10	16	1	(6.2)
Edematous	25	20	45	7	(15.6)
Granular	24	26	50	9	(18.0)

tients received postoperative topical neomycin-polymyxin-cortisone therapy. In the Gates study most of the patients received these drops postoperatively. Also in the Balkany study postoperative otorrhea was defined as occurring within 4 weeks, but in the Gates study the patients were said to have otorrhea if drainage was seen in the ear canal at the postoperative visit, up to 7 weeks after surgery. Therefore, because of the differences in experimental design, no inferences can be drawn by comparing the Gates study to the Balkany study, and thus it was thought that a controlled trial was necessary.

The type of fluid present at the time of surgery did correlate with the incidence of postoperative otorrhea, and this was statistically significant, since no patients with dry middle ears or serous fluid present at surgery developed otorrhea. An edematous or granular appearance of the middle ear mucosa at surgery was also associated with a significantly higher incidence of postoperative otorrhea, but this is to be expected, since the ears with edematous or granular mucosa were generally filled with mucoid or purulent fluid.

Although Balkany and Gates found that younger children had a higher incidence of postoperative otorrhea, this correlation was not found in our study. There was also no correlation between the number of times a patient had had tubes placed previously and the incidence of postoperative otorrhea. We conclude the following:

1. There is no evidence that preparing the ear canal with povidone-iodine before performing tympanostomy has any effect on the incidence of postoperative otorrhea.

2. Children with mucoid or purulent fluid in the middle ear at the time of surgery are more likely to have postoperative otorrhea than children with serous fluid or no fluid.

3. The age of the patient appears to have no predictive value in regard to the incidence of postoperative otorrhea.

REFERENCES

1. Armstrong BW. A new treatment for chronic secretory otitis media. Arch Otolaryngol 1954; 58:653–654.
2. McLelland CA. Incidence of complications from use of tympanostomy tubes. Arch Otolaryngol 1980; 106:97–99.
3. Holt JJ, Harners SG. Effects of large-bore middle ear ventilation tubes. Otolaryngol Head Neck Surg 1980; 88:581–585.
4. Per-Lee JH. Long term middle ear ventilation. Laryngoscope 1981; 91:1063–1072.
5. Gates GA, et al. Post-tympanostomy otorrhea. Laryngoscope 1986; 96:630–634.
6. Hughes LA, Warder FR, Hudson WR. Complications of tympanostomy tubes. Arch Otolaryngol 1974; 100:151–154.
7. Herzon FS. Tympanostomy tubes. Arch Otolaryngol 1980; 106:645–647.
8. Balkany TH, et al. A prospective study of infection following tympanostomy and tube insertion. Am J Otol 1983; 4:288–291.

SURGICAL MANAGEMENT

EFFICACY OF MYRINGOTOMY WITH AND WITHOUT TYMPANOSTOMY TUBE INSERTION FOR CHRONIC OTITIS MEDIA WITH EFFUSION: FIRST YEAR RESULTS IN TWO RANDOMIZED CLINICAL TRIALS

ELLEN M. MANDEL, M.D., HOWARD E. ROCKETTE, Ph.D., CHARLES D. BLUESTONE, M.D., JACK L. PARADISE, M.D., and ROBERT J. NOZZA, Ph.D.

At the Third International Symposium in 1983 we reported the first year's experience in a trial of the efficacy of myringotomy alone (M) and of myringotomy with tympanostomy tube insertion (M&T) in children with chronic asymptomatic middle ear effusions.[1] Because of the possibility that the results were in part attributable to problems of study design, the protocol was revised and another group of children was enrolled in the study. Despite the revised design, the first year results of the second trial were similar to those of the original trial, in effect confirming its findings. The original trial will hereafter be referred to as M&T–I, and the trial with the revised protocol will be referred to as M&T–II. Subjects in both trials were observed for 3 years, but only the first year results are reported here.

M&T–I

Subjects and Methods

Children between the ages of 7 months and 12 years who had documented asymptomatic otitis media with effusion that had been present for at least 2 months and had not responded to combined antimicrobial and decongestant-antihistamine treatment were eligible for the study. Children were excluded if they had any major disorder or illness, including, among others, cleft palate, Down's syndrome, sensorineural hearing loss, asthma, and seizure disorder. Also excluded were children who had undergone tonsillectomy, or adenoidectomy or tympanostomy tube insertion.

Following entry but before assignment to treatment the subjects were divided into two groups:

1. Those who had either "significant" hearing loss (defined arbitrarily as a pure tone average greater than 20 dB bilaterally or 40 dB unilaterally, or a speech awareness threshold more than 20 dB above the age appropriate level[2]), or otalgia or vertigo unresponsive to medical treatment.
2. Those who had neither significant hearing loss nor the specified symptoms.

Because it was considered ethically questionable to assign children with significant hearing loss or persistent symptoms to a nontreatment control group, such children were randomly assigned to undergo either myringotomy or myringotomy with tympanostomy tube insertion, whereas children without significant hearing loss or symptoms were randomly assigned to undergo either myringotomy, myringotomy with tube insertion or no surgery (NS). The assignments were carried out after the subjects had been stratified according to age and duration of disease, with the duration estimated on a "best guess" basis from historical information and prior medical records. Following initial treatment all subjects were reevaluated at monthly intervals.

A standardized history was obtained for each subject, and the findings of a standardized ear, nose, and throat examination were recorded. The diagnosis of otitis media at entry and at each subsequent examination was based on a previously described decision tree algorithm, which combined otoscopic findings obtained by a "validated" otoscopist with the results of tympanometry and middle ear muscle reflex testing.[3] Hearing acuity was assessed monthly by determining air conduction and bone conduction thresholds at four frequencies, as well as speech reception or awareness thresholds.

Subjects were followed for persistence or recurrence of otitis media with effusion. Additional medical treatment was not prescribed for persistent disease, but recurrent disease (that is, otitis media with effusion observed following a visit at which there was no disease) was treated with an antimicrobial drug and a decongestant-antihistamine combination for 14 days. Acute symptomatic otitis media, purulent rhinitis, and other illnesses for which antimicrobial drugs were indicated were treated accordingly.

The following criteria were used in undertaking repeat treatment and in defining "treatment failure": In M subjects, the presence of otitis media with effusion on three consecutive monthly visits (i.e., over a 2 month period) warranted repeat myringotomy; if a third myringotomy was warranted within a 1 year period, myringotomy and tube insertion were performed instead and the subject was termed a treatment failure. In M&T subjects, the presence of otitis media with effusion on three consecutive monthly visits warranted a repeat myringotomy and tube insertion; if a third such procedure was warranted within 1 year, the subject was termed a treatment failure. For subjects in the NS group, two consecutive monthly visits with both otitis media with effusion and significant hearing loss (i.e., over a 1 month period) warranted performance of myringotomy and tube insertion and categorization as a treatment failure. NS subjects with persistent otitis media with effusion but without significant hearing loss received no further treatment.

RESULTS

Of 109 subjects enrolled in the trial, nine withdrew before the 1 year endpoint without becoming treatment failures. Among the remaining 100 subjects, treatment failure criteria were met within the first year by 13 of the 25 subjects (52 percent) in the NS group, by 20 of 38 subjects (53 percent) in the M group, but by none of the subjects in the M&T group. Because of the unexpectedly high treatment failure incidence in the M and NS groups, and because of the desirability of consistent criteria for treatment failure across study groups, entry into this trial was terminated and the protocol was revised.

M&T–II

Subjects and Methods

The original protocol (M&T–I) permitted the entry of subjects with any degree of conductive hearing loss and classified such loss as either significant or nonsignificant. In the revised protocol (M&T–II), children were excluded whose pure tone average was more than 35 dB bilaterally. Children with lesser degrees of hearing loss were considered ethically acceptable candidates for assignment to any of the three treatment groups, thus eliminating the need for two separate sets of assignments.

The criteria for undertaking surgical procedures and for defining treatment failure were also revised in M&T–II in order to make such criteria uniform for all three treatment groups. For each treatment group, surgical intervention during the first year after the initially assigned treatment consisted of tympanostomy tube insertion and was based uniformly on the time with middle ear effusion. The time until intervention was lengthened to 4 months for bilateral effusion and to 6 months for unilateral effusion.

Results of M&T–II and Comparison with M&T–I

One hundred eleven subjects were enrolled and followed in the M&T–I study. A comparison of subject characteristics in the M&T–I and M&T–II studies shows that the two study populations were similar (Table 1). In both studies half the subjects were in the 2 to 5 year old age group. Similarly, in both studies approximately one-third of the subjects had a middle ear effusion estimated to be of 2 to 3 months' duration at entry, one-third had an effusion estimated to be of 4 months' duration or longer, and in one-third the total duration of effusion could not be estimated but the effusion was known to have been present for at least 2 months. The groups were also similar in sex and race distributions; two-thirds of each group were male and about three-fourths of each group were white. A somewhat higher proportion of subjects in M&T–I than in M&T–II had bilateral effusion at entry.

Table 2 shows the major first year outcome measures for both M&T–I and M&T–II: the percentage of subjects meeting the treatment failure criteria and the percentage of time with middle ear effusion. Subjects who dropped out of the study before completing the full year of follow-up and without meeting the treatment failure criteria were excluded from the treatment failure analyses. Only subjects completing 1 full year in the study were included in the analyses of the percentage of time with otitis media with effusion. Results in the two studies are similar in regard to the percentage of time with otitis media with effusion and the percentage of treatment failures for each treatment mode.

TABLE 1   Subject Characteristics at Entry

	M&T−I (N=109)	M&T−II (N=111)
Age group		
7–23 mo	34 (31.2)*	35 (31.5)
2–5 yr	55 (50.5)	56 (50.5)
6–12 yr	20 (18.3)	20 (18.0)
Estimated duration of otitis media with effusion		
2–3 mo	41 (37.6)	38 (34.2)
4–5 mo	17 (15.6)	24 (21.6)
6–12 mo	15 (13.8)	14 (12.6)
>12 mo	4 (3.7)	0 (0.0)
Unknown but > 2 mo	32 (29.4)	35 (31.5)
Sex		
Male	73 (67.0)	74 (67.0)
Female	36 (33.0)	37 (33.0)
Race		
White	81 (74.3)	80 (72.1)
Black	28 (25.7)	31 (27.9)
Laterality of disease		
Unilateral	33 (30.3)	46 (41.4)
Bilateral	76 (69.7)	65 (58.6)

* Numbers in parentheses are percentages.

TABLE 2   Major Outcomes During First Year

	M&T−I				M&T−II		
	NS	M	M&T		NS	M	M&T
Treatment failure							
%	56.0	52.6	0		67.6	62.9	5.9
N	25	38	37		34	35	34
Time with otitis media with effusion[†]							
%	56.3	56.6	14.6		63.3	60.8	17.5
N	18	36	37		33	35	34

NS, no surgery. M, myringotomy. M&T, myringotomy and tube.
† Only subjects completing 1 full year in the study are included.

DISCUSSION

Analysis of the major outcomes during the first year in the M&T–I and M&T–II studies shows that extending the time until treatment failure in the design of M&T–II did not result in reducing the proportions of subjects in the M and NS groups who became treatment failures or in substantially changing the proportions of time with otitis media with effusion. The results in the M&T–II study lend support to the findings in the M&T–I study: among the children studied with long-standing otitis media with effusion unresponsive to antimicrobial treatment, those who had undergone tympanostomy tube insertion had less time with otitis media with effusion during the first year than those who underwent myringotomy only or no surgical treatment. Moreover, in these children myringotomy without tube insertion offered no statistically significant advantage during the first year over nonsurgical treatment. However, analysis of data from the full 3 year experience of both trials will provide additional information concerning the long term outcome and complications of each treatment modality.

Study funded in part by Maternal and Child Health Research grant MCR—420434 and by NIH Otitis Media Research Center grant NS16337.

REFERENCES

1. Mandel EM, Bluestone CD, Paradise JL, Cantekin EI, Rockette HE, Fria TJ, Stool SE, Marshak G. Efficacy of myringotomy with and without tympanostomy tube insertion in the treatment of chronic otitis media with effusion in infants and children—results for the first year of a randomized clinical trial. In: Lim D, Bluestone CD, Klein JO, Nelson JD, eds. Recent advances in otitis media with effusion. Proceedings of the Third International Symposium. Toronto: BC Decker, 1984:308.
2. Wilbur LA. Threshold measurement methods and special considerations. In: Rintelmann WF, ed. Hearing assessment. Baltimore: University Park Press, 1979:20.
3. Cantekin EI. Algorithm for diagnosis of otitis media with effusion. Ann Otol Rhinol Laryngol 1983; 92 (Suppl 107):6.

LATE RESULTS OF TREATMENT WITH GROMMETS FOR MIDDLE EAR CONDITION

JØRGEN F. SEDERBERG-OLSEN, M.D., ALIX E. SEDERBERG-OLSEN, M.D., and ANDERS M. JENSEN, M.Sc.

In recent years an increasing number of long term sequelae after the treatment of acute and secretory otitis media have been reported.[1-3] Our knowledge of the epidemiology and the changes in the eardrum is still rather limited. Whether active treatment or a more conservative attitude should be recommended is still an open question.

MATERIAL AND METHODS

From November 1975 to October 1978, 262 children (481 ears), age 0 to 9 years, were treated in our clinic for long-standing middle ear conditions. Before and after the intubation period the patients were followed according to previously published guidelines, including visits 3 months and 1 year after grommet extrusion.[4] From February 1986 to February 1987 we conducted reevaluations of 191 patients (73 percent; 103 males and 88 females; 355 ears). The mean duration following the last grommet extrusion was 7½ years (range, 14 to 132 months).

Clinical information about the period following the preceding visit was obtained. Otomicroscopy, including pneumatic otoscopy, was performed. Changes in the eardrum were noted and graded according to guidelines described by Tos et al.[5] These included the degree of attic retraction, the extent and location of atrophy, and tympanosclerosis as well as retraction of the pars tensa. Tympanometry and pure tone audiometry were also carried out.

Seventy-one patients (27 percent) did not participate in the reevaluation; 62 had moved away, 5 refused to appear, 1 died, and in 3 cases we did not succeed in obtaining any contact or information. Seven ears had been intubated again elsewhere—one after discharge at the final examination 1 year after grommet extrusion. Twenty ears were still under observation for various reasons at the time of reevaluation. Thus the final study group consisted of 328 ears in 181 patients. The age distribution at the first visit is presented in Figure 1.

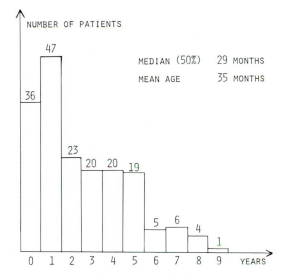

Figure 1 Age distribution of the 181 patients.

RESULTS

The pathologic changes in the eardrum were assessed separately according to location in the area of Shrapnell's membrane and the pars tensa.

Attic Retraction

Attic retraction, type I or II, classified according to the criteria of Tos et al,[5] was found in 18 percent of the ears. Marked type III retractions were found in 2 percent and type IV retractions in 1 percent; 260 ears (79 percent) did not show any retraction. In patients under 2 years of age we found a surprisingly low incidence of severe retractions (Table 1). Significance analysis was not done because the two ears in a person are not statistically independent.

Atrophic Area of Pars Tensa

Markedly atrophic areas of the pars tensa, diffuse atrophy, incudopexy, or retraction pockets were present in 3 percent. Partial atrophic areas were seen in 22 percent, and 278 ears (75 percent) did not show any atrophy. In patients under 2 years of age we again found a low incidence of atrophy, 18 percent compared with 29 percent in the older group. This might be significant if the two ears in the same person were statistically independent.

Myringosclerosis of Pars Tensa

With regard to myringosclerosis, 39 percent showed partial and 8 percent diffuse disease; 175 ears (53 percent) did not show any abnormalities. In patients under 2 years of age we did not find any

convincing difference compared with the elder group (41 percent versus 52 percent).

Myringosclerosis related to an increasing number of grommet insertions was pronounced. Up to four grommets—about 50 percent (40 to 56 percent) and thereafter about 90 percent—had produced myringosclerosis. The grommets preferably were inserted in the anterior area, most often under local anesthesia, but pathologic findings were not necessarily located at that site.

Impedance and Pure Tone Audiometry

A tympanometric profile showed A + C_I in 93 percent and C_{II} + B in 7 percent of the cases. The pure tone audiometry average at 500, 1,000, and 2,000 Hz was estimated to be 15 db or less in 96 percent of the 328 ears (Table 2). In 124 ears (38 percent) there was no evidence of disability and the hearing loss was 10 db or less.

Episodes After Final Examination

It is remarkable that of 308 ears in patients discharged at the final examination 1 year after grommet extrusion, only 83 ears (27 percent) were subject to an episode of otitis media afterward. Myringotomy was performed in 17 ears, twice in a single case. In only one ear was grommet reinsertion carried out. In no case was mastoidectomy necessary.

Continuing Observation

The 20 ears under continuing observation were distributed as follows: nine with severe atrophy of the pars tensa, five with a defect, and two under postoperative observation after myringoplastic sur-

TABLE 1 Pathologic Findings (Attic Retractions) Correlated with Age at First Visit*

Years	Degree	Number of Ears	Percentage
	0	130	
0–1	1–2	16	11%
	3–4	1	1%
	0	114	
2–9	1–2	37	23%
	3–4	10	6%
	Total with final control 308 ears		

* Follow-up, 1 to 11 years. Mean, 7½ years.

TABLE 2 Pure Tone Average (500, 1,000, and 2,000 Hz)

db	No. Ears	Percentage
0– 5	196	60
6–10	86	26
11–15	31	10
16–20	11	3
21–25	3	1
26–30	1	0

gery for defects. Two ears are still intubated. Furthermore, there was one with granulomatous myringitis and one ear showing sensory hearing loss, probably of a congenital nature. In these 20 ears the hearing loss was 20 db or less, except for the single case mentioned. No cholesteatoma or meningitis has been found.

COMMENTS

A relatively restricted therapeutic policy for these conditions is absolutely necessary because of their prevalence.[6] This series is part of a prospective study of ears surgically treated for acute and secretory otitis media in otolaryngologic practice. We found that 230 ears intubated during the same period from the same population 1 year after grommet extrusion showed myringosclerosis and atrophy in another evaluation in 25 and 33 percent compared with 47 and 25 percent in the actual material.[7] This tendency has also been found recently by Tos et al.[8,9] The frequencies of serious atrophic retractions of Shrapnell's membrane and the pars tensa reported by Tos et al[10,11] in 1979–1980 with an observation period of 3 to 8 years correspond to our frequencies when we include the 20 ears under continued observation. The latest report concerning this cohort has caused us to follow carefully all pars flaccida retractions, including types I and II. We expect to find as many as three times the number of serious pars flaccida retractions.[12]

The idea that younger children who have grommets inserted are less apt to develop serious complications[5] is supported by our results. The price seems to be some degree of myringosclerosis, but so far this does not compromise the hearing level dramatically later in life. However, progression of myringosclerosis is a problem and the observation time has not been sufficiently long.[3] Because of this reservation we recommend a conservative attitude toward grommet insertion. Children who prove to have an indication for grommet insertion probably should have this done at a relatively young age. If patients are intubated, we recommend careful observation with otomicroscopy at each visit, especially 3 months and 1 year after grommet extrusion.

REFERENCES

1. Tos M, Bonding P, Poulsen G. Tympanosclerosis of the drum in secretory otitis after insertion of grommets: a prospective comparative study. J Laryngol Otol 1983; 97:489–496.
2. Lildholdt T. Ventilation tubes in secretory otitis media. A randomized, controlled study of the course, the complications, and the sequelae of ventilation tubes. Acta Otolaryngol 1983; Suppl 398.
3. Moeller P. Sekretorisk otitt og tympanosclerose. Thesis, University of Bergen, 1985.
4. Sederberg-Olsen JF, Sederberg-Olsen AE. Therapeutic strategy in secretory middle ear conditions. Proceedings of the International Conference on acute and secretory otitis media, Part 1, Jerusalem, Israel. Amsterdam: Kugler Publications, 1985:413.
5. Tos M, Stangerup S-E, Holm-Jensen S, Sørensen CH. Spontaneous course of secretory otitis and changes of the eardrum. Arch Otolaryngol Head Neck Surg 1984; 110:281–289.
6. Fiellau-Nikolajsen M. Tympanometry and secretory otitis media. Acta Otolaryngol 1983; Suppl 394.
7. Sederberg-Olsen JF, Sederberg-Olsen AE, Jensen AM. Complications of ventilation tubes in ENT specialist practice: tubulationskomplikationer i speciallaegepraksis. Ugeskr Laeger 1986; 146:894–896.
8. Tos M, Stangerup S-E, Andreassen UK. Prevalence and progressions of sequelae after secretory otitis. Ann Otol (in press).
9. Tos M, Stangerup S-E, Larsen P. Dynamics of attic retractions and changes of pars tensa following secretory otitis. A prospective study. Arch Otolaryngol (in press).
10. Tos M, Poulsen G. Attic retractions following secretory otitis. Acta Otolaryngol 1980; 89:478–486.
11. Tos M, Poulsen G. Changes of pars tensa after secretory otitis. ORL J Otorhinolaryngol Relat Spec 1979; 41:313–328.
12. Tos M, Stangerup S-E, Larsen P. Dynamics of eardrum changes following secretory otitis. Arch Otolaryngol Head Neck Surg 1987; 113:380–385.

EVALUATION OF VENTILATING TUBES AND MYRINGOTOMY FOR THE TREATMENT OF OTITIS MEDIA

DOUGLAS FREEMAN, M.D. and CHINH T. LE, M.D.

The widespread use of ventilating tubes and myringotomy for the treatment of otitis media is based on few controlled studies. In January 1984 we started a prospective randomized study in a group of children referred to the otolaryngology clinic for insertion of ventilating tubes. Our research questions were as follows:

1. What are the efficacies and sequelae of myringotomy and ventilating tubes when compared with continuing medical therapy?
2. Can we identify risk factors for children who may benefit from surgical intervention, and can we identify children who could be continued on medical therapy alone?

MATERIALS AND METHODS

The study protocol dictated that all patients must have bilateral middle ear disease of equal severity in each ear and must have "failed" antimicrobial prophylaxis for 3 months prior to study enrollment. Recurrent acute otitis media was defined as six or more documented episodes in the preceding 12 months or four or more episodes in children less than 1 year of age. Persistent middle ear effusion must have been documented by pneumatic otoscopy and tympanometry for three consecutive months. Children with acute otitis media and persistent middle ear effusion were counted with the recurrent acute otitis media group. Patients with Down's syndrome, cleft palate, known immune deficiencies, prior myringotomies, or ventilating tubes were excluded.

After parental consent, patients who fulfilled these criteria were sequentially randomized to receive unilateral ventilating tubes. The contralateral ear was further randomized to receive either myringotomy or no surgery. All surgical procedures were performed by standard techniques, with incisions made in the anterior inferior quadrant and insertion of a Pope Teflon grommet. Pneumatic otoscopy,

tympanometry, and audiometry by pure tone audiography were performed prior to the study, 1 month after the surgical procedure, and thereafter at 3 month intervals up to 2 years. During the study, patients continued to receive standard medical treatment for each episode of otitis and antimicrobial prophylaxis if indicated.

The 2 year evaluation was performed by an otolaryngologist and an audiologist who were not aware of the initial surgical randomization. The statistical significance was calculated by the two tailed paired t test and by the sign test.

RESULTS

We randomized and followed 57 patients: 44 had recurrent acute otitis media; 26 were males and 18 were females. The mean age in this group of children was 20.4 months (range, 9 to 82 months) at the time of surgical randomization. The mean number of episodes of otitis media during the year preceding study enrollment was 7.6 episodes per child. Fifty-one patients with persistent middle ear effusions enrolled in the study after meeting the study criteria, but in 38 patients the effusion cleared either spontaneously or with a second course of medical therapy. Therefore, only 13 patients were randomized; six were males and seven were females. Their mean age was 53.6 months (range, 41 to 78 months), and the mean duration of middle ear effusion was 6.2 months.

Further demographic characteristics of the study population were as follows: 56 children were Caucasians and one was black. All gave a history of middle ear disease in an immediate family member. Seventy-one percent attended day care or kindergarten. Thirty-five percent had one or more smoking parents, and 33 percent had allergic diatheses (defined as allergic rhinitis, atopy, or asthma).

The mean duration of follow-up was 29 months; the mean number of visits per child during the 2 year study was 20 (range, 11 to 37). Seventy-five percent of the patients were followed for 24 months or more. The ventilating tubes remained functional for a mean of 10 months (range, 2 weeks to 24 months). Six patients underwent further surgical procedures on tympanic membranes because of significant ear disease during the study. Three patients had a ventilating tube inserted in the ear that initially did not receive a ventilating tube. Three other patients underwent bilateral insertion of ventilating tubes. Statistics for these patients were included until the time of contralateral tube insertion.

Figure 1 shows the mean number of episodes of otitis media per 6 month interval, before and during the 2 year study for 57 patients. We defined improvement as a greater than 50 percent reduction in the number of episodes of acute otitis media per year, no middle ear effusion for 3 months or more, and a mean decibel hearing loss of less than 20. We observed, in cases with recurrent infections, that the ear that did not receive a ventilating tube improved in 30 of 44 patients (68 percent) during the first year and in 87 percent during the second year.

In paired sample analysis each ventilated ear was compared to its contralateral mate. Table 1 shows the difference in mean reduction of numbers of otitis episodes, negative numbers indicating fewer infections in the ventilated ear. During the first 6 months 33 contralateral ears had more otitis episodes than the paired ventilated ear, 13 had the same number, and 11 had fewer. However, at the end of the second year the trend was reversed: 15 ventilated ears had more infections and 9 had fewer.

The analysis of hearing function is shown in Figure 2. In paired sample analysis the difference of 3.5 in mean decibel loss was significant during the first 6 months but not subsequently (Table 2). Comparing hearing levels for matched pairs, we found that the ventilated ears did better during the first 6 months—14 better versus 5 worse—but tended to be worse by the end of the second year—7 better versus 10 worse. However, this tendency during the second year was not significant.

Table 3 shows the anatomic sequelae diagnosed by an independent otolaryngologist 2 years into the study.

The outcome in ears that did not receive ven-

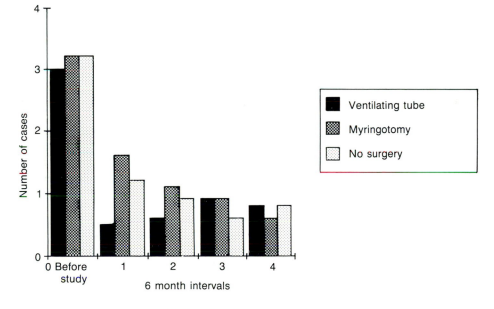

Figure 1 Episodes of acute otitis media.

TABLE 1   Differences in Numbers of Otitis Media Episodes in Ventilating Tube Ear Versus Contralateral Ear

Months into Study	1 to 6	7 to 12	13 to 18	19 to 24
Number of patients	57	55	55	43
Difference in mean reduction (range)	−0.9 (−5 to +2)	−0.3 (−3 to +3)	+0.1 (−3 to +2)	+0.1 (−1 to +2)
p value*	0.0001	0.02	0.18	0.38
95% CI†	−1.3 to −0.5	−0.6 to −0.1	−0.1 to 0.4	−0.1 to 0.4

* Two tailed paired t test.
† Confidence interval.

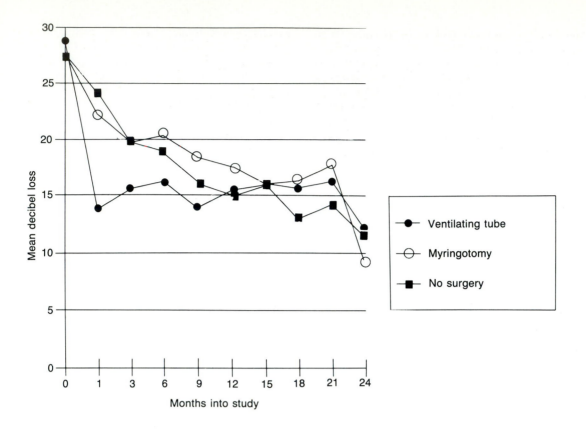

Figure 2 Audiologic function.

TABLE 2 Audiogram Results in Ventilating Tube Ear and Contralateral Ear

	Before Study	Months into Study		
		1 to 6	9 to 15	18 to 24
Number of patients	57	55	55	43
Difference in mean db loss (ventilating tube— contralateral)	+0.7	−3.5	−1.1	+0.7
p value	0.56	0.005	0.20	0.55
95% confidence interval	−1.7 to 3.2	−5.9 to −1.2	−2.8 to 0.6	−1.5 to 2.8

TABLE 3 Anatomic Sequelae

Randomized Tympanic Membrane	Tympanosclerosis	Retraction Atrophy	Chronic Perforation
Ventilating tube	35/63 (56%)	15/63 (24%)	1/63
Myringotomy	5/25 (20%)	8/25 (32%)	0/25
No surgery	2/26 (8%)	1/26 (4%)	0/26

tilating tubes was correlated with possible demographic risk factors for childhood ear disease. These include male sex, a young age, a history of ear disease in the family, the type of feeding in infancy (bottle versus breast), the presence of allergy, smoking by the parents, day care attendance, and a young age at the onset of the first otitis episode. Using multivariable regression analysis, we found that a trend for a worse outcome exists for all these factors, but only the presence of smoking parents had statistical significance. We determined after study enrollment that a child whose parents continued to smoke would have an excess of 1.2 episodes of otitis per year when compared to children whose parents did not smoke ($p < 0.05$).

DISCUSSION

The problem of recurrent or persistent middle ear infections is a difficult one. The standard practice is to insert ventilating tubes after a trial of antimicrobial treatment and prophylaxis, yet there have been few controlled studies on the efficacy of ventilating tubes. To be valid, any claim of ventilating tube benefits must be compared with the amount of improvement the child can obtain with medical therapy alone. In addition, parents and physicians should be aware of the potential long term sequelae of surgical intervention. Unilateral insertion of tubes, with the use of the contralateral ear as its control, is ideal to answer that question. Although previous investigators have used that study design, the majority addressed the problem of the "glue ear" or persistent middle ear effusion in the older child.[1-4]

Many included adenoidectomy with or without tonsillectomy. Most patients were not given a trial of antimicrobial therapy. Most authors failed to use paired sample analysis to take full advantage of their study design. The only study of patients with recurrent acute otitis media had a short duration of follow-up (6 months for the incidence of otitis).[5] We believe that our investigation adequately corrected for these problems.

We found that ventilating tubes reduced the incidence of otitis media for about 1 year and improved hearing for about 6 months. However, the majority of children with recurrent and persistent ear disease significantly improved within 1 year with continuing medical therapy alone. Also tympanic membranes treated with ventilating tubes or myringotomy developed more tympanosclerosis and atrophy. We believe that there is a need for more selective use of surgical intervention for middle ear disease in children.

REFERENCES

1. Brown MJKM, Richards SH, Ambegaokar AG. Grommets and glue ear: a five-year follow-up of a controlled trial. J Roy Soc Med 1978; 71:353–356.
2. Lildholdt T. Ventilating tubes in secretory otitis media. Acta Otolaryngol 1983; Suppl 398:4–27.
3. Bonding P, Tos M. Grommets versus paracentesis in secretory otitis media. Am J Otol 1985; 6:455–460.
4. Maw AR, Herod F. Otoscopic, impedance, and audiometric findings in glue ear treated by adenoidectomy and tonsillectomy: a prospective randomized study. Lancet 1986; 1:1399–1402.
5. Gebhart DE. Tympanostomy tubes in the otitis media prone child. Laryngoscope 1981; 91:849–866.

PERCUTANEOUS TITANIUM IMPLANT FOR OPEN COMMUNICATION TO THE MASTOID AIR CELL SYSTEM

JÖRGEN HOLMQUIST, M.D., Ph.D., TOMAS ALBREKTSSON, M.D., Ph.D., and ANDERS TJELLSTRÖM, M.D., Ph.D.

The establishment of an open communication into the mastoid air cell system through the skin and cortical bone may be useful in certain clinical situations: to house connections to cochlear and middle ear implants, to ventilate a poorly aerated mastoid and middle ear (as in atelectatic ears), or as a route to change middle ear air pressure artificially (for example, a treatment choice in Meniere's disease).[1] The open communication is also useful for continuous recording of mastoid and middle ear air pressure changes.

Because we believed that there is a need for creating open communications to the mastoid air cell system, a special titanium implant was designed and installed on the mastoid in five cases. The surgical technique we used is similar to that used to implant hearing aids.[2] The aim in this communication is to present our surgical technique and our experience with these implants in five cases. Also one patient with a posterior tympanic membrane retraction underwent implantation and is discussed.

SURGICAL TECHNIQUE

The surgical technique used in this study is based on the procedure used in our department for bone anchored hearing aids; a detailed description of this procedure was presented in an earlier report.[2] In order to establish a safe communication to the air cell system, the site for the ventilating implant was 1 cm behind the postauricular fold and 2 to 3 cm cranial to the mastoid tip. A skin incision was made and a 2 by 2 cm area of the bone was exposed. With a 2 mm cutting bur the mastoid cortex was penetrated and generally found to be about 3 mm thick. The hole was widened slightly as much as possible in the direction of an air cell. The hole was further widened with a spiral drill and then threaded with a titanium tap.

In contrast to the normal implant procedure to establish osseous integration, little irrigation was used to avoid saline seeping down into the air cell system. The drilling and threading were done only through the cortical layer, thus minimizing trauma near the mucosa. A hollow ventilating titanium screw was introduced, and a titanium coupling specially designed for a pressure transducer was attached to the implant. The ventilating screw was 4 mm long and the central air channel, 2 mm in diameter. The coupling was kept in place on the screw with an internal abutment screw, which also had an air channel 0.4 mm in diameter and 4 mm in length. A hole was made in the skin to fit this coupling and the skin flap was sutured in place. A small piece of gauze was wound around the skin incision to avoid postoperative hematoma and swelling. The procedure was completed by checking the patency of the coupling screw and the ventilating implant. Figure 1 shows the arrangement schematically.

MATERIAL

In the present study four patients were selected from those scheduled to undergo endolymphatic sac drainage surgery. Three days prior to the sac surgery a titanium implant was installed into the mastoid process. An additional patient had a pure sensorineural hearing loss, probably of congenital origin. These five patients were selected for our study focusing mainly on the methodologic aspects. In addition an implant was installed in a patient with a posterior retraction of the tympanic membrane. For further details see Table 1.

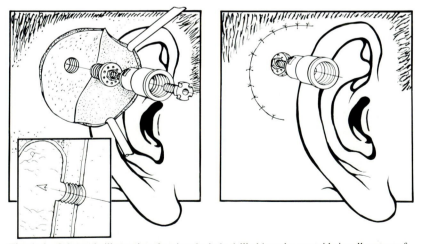

Figure 1 Schematic illustration showing the hole drilled into the mastoid air cell system after raising a skin flap. The bone anchored screw and the coupling cylinder with its screw are demonstrated.

TABLE 1   **Titanium Implants on the Mastoid for Ventilation of the Mastoid Air Cell System**

Identification No.	Age	Sex	Ear	Diagnosis	In Place	Patent
1	54	F	R	Meniere	3 days	3 days
2	50	M	L	Meniere	3 days	3 days
3	58	F	R	Meniere	3 days	3 days
4	35	M	L	Meniere	3 days	3 days
5	30	M	R	Surdit. diagnosis	12 days	12 days
6	42	M	L	Retraction pocket	15 months	7 months

FOLLOW-UP

To demonstrate the presence of the permanent open communication to the mastoid and middle ear, repeated postoperative measurements were carried out. A tympanometer was connected to the ear canal and an air pressure device with a manometer was connected to the implant; a schematic illustration of the set-up is shown in Figure 2.

It was found that in the four patients with endolymphatic sacs the hole was kept patent and functioning until the implant was removed on the third postoperative day. In the patient with profound sensorineural hearing loss the implant was kept open during a 12 day observation period; the screw with the channel was then removed. A typical recording showing the open communication between the implant and the middle ear is presented in Figure 3. So far we have used the implant in only one patient with an atelectatic ear (see case report).

Case Report

A 42 year old man was seen in our clinic repeatedly during a 10 year period while he developed a posterior retraction and a thin monomeric tympanic membrane in the left ear. Tympanometry revealed a negative middle ear air pressure in the range of -300 to -500 mm H_2O. Air-bone gaps varied between 20 and 40 db. He could not autoinflate the left ear. Ventilating tubes were put in at several occasions but had no effect on the retraction. Therefore, it was decided to install a mastoid implant with an open channel. For 7 months the implant was patent. The tympanic membrane retraction did not disappear, but the tympanogram indicated a middle ear pressure within the normal range. A few months later (during the summer season) the implant became blocked. The area around the implant was slightly inflamed and infected. The implant was removed. Healing was uneventful, but the tympanic

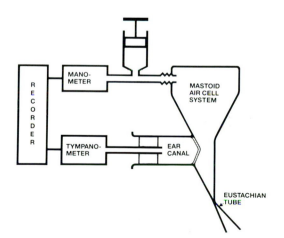

Figure 2   Schematic drawing of the measurement set-up to demonstrate the open communication between the implant and the middle ear. A manometer and an air pressure pump are connected to the implant while a tympanometer recording tympanic impedance changes is attached to the ear canal.

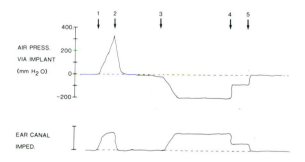

Figure 3   Copy of an original recording demonstrating the open communication. The air pressure changes via the implant are demonstrated in the upper section and the simultaneous impedance changes are shown in the lower section of the figure. At "1" the air pressure via the implant is manually increased. At "2" there is a sudden air pressure drop (possibly spontaneous opening of the eustachian tube). At "3" the air pressure is manually decreased to 200 mm H_2O, and at "4" and "5" the patient is swallowing while the air pressure is returning to the 0 level (atmospheric air pressure).

membrane now has a fixed posterior retraction pocket and the patient has conductive deafness.

DISCUSSION

To date there has been no report of the establishment of a permanent open communication through the skin and cortical bone into the mastoid air cell system in humans. Such a permanent communication would house connections to cochlear implants but also might be used to ventilate the mastoid and middle ear in certain cases.

In this report we present our surgical technique for applying a percutaneous titanium implant on the mastoid. By using ear canal tympanometry the implant's permanent patency and open communication with the tympanic cavity were demonstrated.

As shown in an earlier report,[3] the majority of ears with retractions have subatmospheric intratympanic air pressures. Also it has been demonstrated that ears with retractions have dysfunction of the eustachian tube.[4] Therefore there seem to be indications for the establishment of open communications to the mastoid and the middle ear in an attempt to normalize the subatmospheric air pressure due to poor eustachian tube function. In a recent communication one of us reported the beneficial effect of mastoidectomy in ears with atelectasis.[5] Establishment of an open communication into the mastoid air cell system may be used before such mastoid surgery is done. The case reported here shows that it is possible to ventilate the mastoid air cell system via an implant for a long period of time. Our experience with almost 300 mastoid implants shows that problems around the implant in the skin, as occurred in this case, are extremely rare.[6] Only one of the implants used since 1977 for bone conduction hearing aids has been removed owing to skin infection. The reason the retraction in the reported case persisted despite good aeration of the middle ear may be that it was fixed by adhesions onto the promontory wall. We did not use positive pressure in this case in an attempt to break the adhesions. We will continue to use mastoid ventilation implants in an attempt to aerate a malventilated middle ear cleft in selected cases of atelectasis and hope to report our experience soon.

REFERENCES

1. Densert B. On the relationship between ambient pressure changes and inner ear hydrodynamics. Thesis, Infotryck AB, Malmö, Sweden, 1986.
2. Tjellström A. Percutaneous implants in clinical practice. Crit Rev Biocompat 1985; 1:205–228.
3. Holmquist J, Lindeman P. Tympanometric studies in ears with cholesteatoma and retraction pockets. In: Sadé J, ed. Cholesteatoma and mastoid surgery. Amsterdam: Kugler, 1982:225.
4. Holmquist J, Renvall U, Svendsen P. Eustachian tube function and retraction of the tympanic membrane. Ann Otol Rhinol Laryngol 1980; Suppl 68:65–66.
5. Holmquist J, Lindeman P. Mastoid surgery in atelectatic ears. In: Sadé J, ed. Acute and secretory otitis media. Amsterdam: Kugler, 1986:563.
6. Tjellström A, Yontchev E, Lindström J, Brånemark P-I. Five years' experience with bone-anchored auricular prostheses. Otolaryngol Head Neck Surg 1985; 93:366–372.

TREATMENT OF EUSTACHIAN TUBE DYSFUNCTION— LASER SURGERY AND TWO THERAPEUTIC METHODS

KEIJI HONDA, M.D., MASAHITO TANKE, M.D., and TADAMI KUMAZAWA, M.D.

Adenoidectomy is a well known treatment for hearing loss resulting from otitis media with effusion. However, hearing disturbance persists in some patients even after adenoidectomy.

We report herein our findings in a study of the postnasal spaces in children with recurrent otitis media with effusion. We also report the use of two methods—steroid injection into the mouth of the occluded eustachian tube in otitis media with effusion and silicon fluid injection into the patent eustachian tube—as treatment for these tubal dysfunctions.

CARBON DIOXIDE LASER SURGERY FOR TUBAL TONSIL HYPERTROPHY IN RECURRENT OTITIS MEDIA WITH EFFUSION IN CHILDREN

Our subjects were children 5 to 11 years old in whom either adenoidectomy or tonsilloadenoidectomy had been performed to restore hearing. We examined 177 ears 18 to 20 months after surgery. Thirty ears, or 17 percent were diagnosed as having otitis media with effusion. The diagnosis was confirmed by pneumatic otoscopy together with pure tone audiometry and acoustic impedance methods. We also employed aerodynamic recording and conducted endoscopic examinations.[1]

The mean hearing loss was 22 db at 1,000 Hz. Tympanography showed 7 percent with type A, 70 percent with type B, and 23 percent with type C tympanograms. Of the ears tested by the aerodynamic method, 54 percent were classified as showing good inflation and 46 percent as showing poor exhalation. Analysis of the endoscopic findings revealed (50 percent) tubal tonsil hypertrophy in all cases (Fig. 1).

Because the tubal orifices cannot be observed through the oral cavity, metallic mirrors are indispensable for vaporization. Subjects were operated upon in the supine position under general anesthesia. It is important to protect the patient's eyes as well as the eyes of others in the operating theater.

The laser beam was applied for 0.1 second at an amplitude of 15 watts. Before removing the tracheal tube we performed a paracentesis, removed the effusion by suction, and injected a steroid solution. Six months after surgery hearing had returned almost to normal in most of the patients. The tympanograms, which were obtained 6 months after surgery, and the tubotympanoaerodynamic recordings showed good results in almost every case. Otitis media with effusion was found to have recurred in three ears.

After adenoidectomy, recurrent otitis media has been seen to improve by some investigators, although others have found no improvement. The effect is apparently dependent upon age, the size of the adenoids, and the influence of allergies and sinusitis. Furthermore, our cases suggest that tubal tonsil hypertrophy is one of the factors found in recurrent otitis media with effusion in older children. Thus, it can be inferred that endoscopic examination of the postnasal space is useful in children with recurrent otitis media with effusion after adenoidectomy and that carbon dioxide laser surgery is a reliable therapeutic method in the treatment of this disease.

STEROID INJECTION INTO THE OCCLUDED TUBE IN OTITIS MEDIA WITH EFFUSION

Our subjects were 16 to 78 years old. There

	ADENOID	TUBAL TONSIL	
NORMAL	5 EARS(17%)	0 (0%)	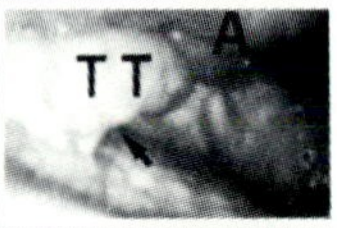
MILD HYPERTROPHY	6 EARS(20%)	7 EARS(23%)	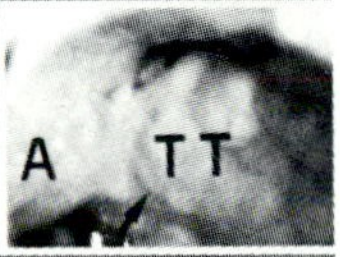
MODERATE HYPERTROPHY	10 EARS(33%)	8 EARS(27%)	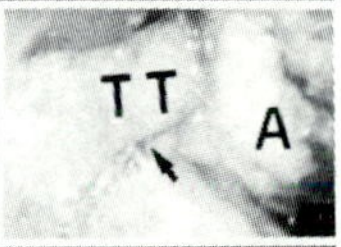
MARKED HYPERTROPHY	9 EARS(30%)	15 EARS(50%)	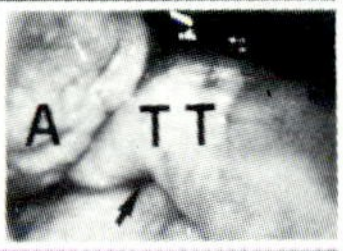

Figure 1 Results of tympanography. A, adenoid. TT, torus tubarius. Arrow, opening of eustachian tube.

were 33 individuals with 39 occluded tubes. Fifty-six percent were males and 44 percent, females. The diagnosis was confirmed by the five methods mentioned earlier.

The mean hearing loss was 27 db at 1,000 Hz before treatment. Tympanography revealed none with type A, 77 percent with type B, and 23 percent with type C tympanograms. With aerodynamic recordings 18 percent of the tested ears were classified as showing good inflation and poor exhalation; 82 percent were classified as showing poor inflation and exhalation. Analysis of the endoscopic findings revealed 67 percent with mild, 18 percent with moderate, and 15 percent with marked hypertrophy.

We used this method to restore hearing in cases in which hearing loss was caused by occlusion of the mouth of the eustachian tube.[2] Initially 0.2 ml of steroid (triamcinolone acetonide, 40 mg per 1 milliliter) was injected into the swollen (edematous) part of the mouth, and injections were performed under endoscopic observation once a week. Six months after steroid injection,the mean hearing loss was 17 db at 1,000 Hz. Tympanography showed 31 percent with type A, 38 percent with type B, and 31 percent with type C tympanograms. The aerodynamic recordings also showed good results in almost every case.

INJECTION OF SILICON FLUID INTO THE PATENT EUSTACHIAN TUBE

The subjects were 18 to 75 years old. Sixty-five percent were males and 35 percent females, a total of 32 individuals with 49 patent eustachian tubes.

With the patient in a sitting position about 0.5 ml of silicon (dimethylpolysiloxane) fluid was injected into the floor of the mouth under endoscopic observation once a week.[3]

The results of tympanography showed 88 percent with type A, 8 percent with type B, and 4 percent with type C tympanograms. The hearing loss in these cases was not remarkable. All aerodynamic recordings showed a patent pattern. Examination of the tubal openings revealed 61 percent with mild, 29 percent with moderate, and 10 percent with marked atrophy. About 6 months after the silicon injection, the number of type B and C cases increased, and half the aerodynamic recordings showed good tubal closure.

This method should be performed only to relieve uncomfortable symptoms, such as autophony and fullness in the ear. The therapist must be careful not to disturb the active opening mechanism and must avoid injection into the artery.

REFERENCES

1. Kumazawa T, Honjo I, Honda K. Aerodynamic evaluation of eustachian tube function. Arch Otorhinolaryngol 1974; 208:147–156.
2. Baker DC Jr, Strauss RB. Intranasal injections of long acting corticosteroids. Ann Otol Rhinol Laryngol 1962; 71:525–531.
3. Pulec JL. Abnormally patent eustachian tubes; treatment with injection of polytetrafluoroethylene (Teflon) paste. Laryngoscope 1967; 77:1543–1555.

EFFECTS OF DIFFERENT TYMPANOSTOMY TUBES (TEFLON AND STAINLESS STEEL) ON THE TYMPANIC MEMBRANE STRUCTURE

OVE SÖDERBERG, M.D., Ph.D. and STEN O.M. HELLSTRÖM, M.D., Ph.D.

Tympanostomy tubes are a well accepted form of treatment of secretory otitis media. However, the use of grommets is associated with complications, for example, otorrhea, tympanosclerosis, and persistent perforations.[1-3]

Recently tympanostomy tubes inserted into the tympanic membranes of healthy rat ears were shown to cause pronounced alterations of the tympanic membrane structure.[4] The changes were located mainly in the connective tissue layer. It was inferred from that study that the material of the tube could be of significance in regard to the extent of the alterations of the tympanic membrane. In the present study the effects on tympanic membrane structure of the use of tympanostomy tubes of Teflon and stainless steel were analyzed and compared.

MATERIALS AND METHODS

In 10 healthy anesthetized rats a tympanostomy tube made of Teflon was inserted into the upper rear quadrant of the right tympanic membrane and one made of stainless steel was inserted into the corresponding part of the contralateral tympanic membrane. The tympanostomy tubes were removed after 2 weeks and the tympanic membranes were left to heal for 3 weeks. The insertion-removal procedure was then repeated four times. Five animals were sacrificed after 3 weeks and the other five animals after 3 months.

The tympanic membranes were dissected out together with adjacent meatal skin and prepared for histologic evaluation, including morphometric measurement of the tympanic membrane thickness. Histologic sections were prepared from five different levels through the two upper quadrants. On each such section the distance from the handle of the malleus to the annulus was determined under the light microscope. This distance was then divided into four equal parts, and the points of division were selected for measurement of the pars tensa thickness. By applying three measuring points at five different levels, the thickness of the pars tensa of each upper quadrant was determined at 15 different points. The significance of the differences in thickness between Teflon and steel tympanostomy tube treated tympanic membranes was tested with a multivariate general linear hypothesis model.[5]

RESULTS

At the insertion-removal procedure it was noted that the Teflon tympanostomy tubes were easier to handle than the steel tubes. Furthermore, the Teflon tubes became clogged less often. Observed by otomicroscopy 3 weeks and 3 months after the last intubation period, the tympanic membranes showed masses of opaque tissue in the intubated quadrants. However, there was no evident difference between tympanic membranes treated with Teflon tubes and steel tubes.

With the light microscope it was noted, in addition to the difference in thickness, that the connective tissue in the lamina propria of the Teflon tube treated tympanic membranes was more regularly organized than that of stainless steel tube treated tympanic membranes.

Morphometric analysis of tympanic membrane thickness supported this observation (Fig. 1). After 3 weeks the scarred posterior half of the tympanic membrane in Teflon tympanostomy tube treated animals was about 18 times thicker, and that of steel

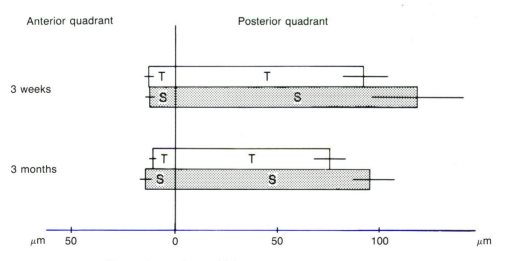

Figure 1 Morphometric measurement of tympanic membrane thickness after repeated insertion of tympanostomy tubes made of Teflon (T) and stainless steel (S) in the posterior half of the tympanic membrane. The anterior halves were left intact. The values are presented as means and their 95 percent intervals of confidence (bars). The thickness of age matched, normal tympanic membrane is about 5 μm.

tube treated animals about 23 times thicker, than the original tympanic membrane. After 3 months the increase in thickness was estimated to be about 15 times for the Teflon tube treated tympanic membranes versus 19 times for the steel tube treated tympanic membranes compared to age matched normal tympanic membranes. With the statistical method of variance analysis used, the difference between Teflon treated and stainless steel treated tympanic membranes was significant at both the 3 week and 3 month intervals.

We can state that tympanostomy tubes inserted into healthy tympanic membranes caused advanced structural changes of the tympanic membrane and that the extent of the alteration differed in relation to the different materials used for tubes. This study also showed that tympanostomy tubes made of Teflon caused less pronounced structural changes than tympanostomy tubes made of stainless steel. The alterations should be compared to the results from an earlier study, which showed the thickness of the tympanic membrane after myringotomy alone to be most identical to that observed in the Teflon group.[4] Furthermore, the data should be compared to data obtained in the use of polyethelene tympanostomy tubes, which caused the tympanic membrane thickness to increase manyfold, about 30

times. Complications related to the use of tympanostomy tubes should be minimized. In view of the present results the side effects of already existing tube materials should be further elucidated and new materials sought.

Study supported by grants from the Swedish Medical Research Council (17X–6578), Ragnar and Torsten Söderbergs Foundation, and the IngaBritt and Arne Lundbergs Research Foundation.

We express appreciation to Richards AB, Sweden, for manufacturing the tympanostomy tubes.

REFERENCES

1. Kokko E. Chronic secretory otitis media in children. Acta Otolaryngol (Stockh) 1974; Suppl 327:1–44.
2. Bluestone CD, Klein JO, Paradise JL, Eichenwald H, Bess FH, Downs MP, Green M, Berco-Gleason J, Ventry IM, Gray SW, McWilliams BJ, Gates GA. Workshop on effects of otitis media on the child. Pediatrics 1983; 71:639–652.
3. Lildholt T. Ventilation tubes in secretory otitis media. Acta Otolaryngol (Stockh) 1983; Suppl 398:1–28.
4. Söderberg O, Hellström S, Stenfors LE. Structural changes in the tympanic membrane after repeated tympanostomy tube insertion. Acta Otolaryngol (Stockh) 1986; 102:382–390.
5. Wilkinson L. SYSTAT: the system for statistics. Evanston, IL: SYSTAT, Inc., 1986.

EARLY AND LATE EFFECTS OF SURGERY FOR OTITIS MEDIA WITH EFFUSION

A. RICHARD MAW, M.S., F.R.C.S.

A previous report to the Third International Symposium on Recent Advances in Otitis Media demonstrated the effects of adenoidectomy and tonsillectomy in children suffering with established otitis media with effusion. There was clearance of the effusion in 40 percent of the cases 12 months after each procedure, with no additional benefit from the combined procedure, compared with adenoidectomy alone.[1]

Subsequently it was shown that there was a commensurate change of impedance measurements from flat type B to A, C1, or C2 curves. A significant pure tone audiometric hearing gain also oc-

curred. The beneficial effects were all more marked 6 months postoperatively in the adenotonsillectomy group, but after 12 months the trend was reversed in favor of adenoidectomy. Because the addition of tonsillectomy conferred no extra long term benefit over adenoidectomy alone, the combined procedure was discontinued after 150 cases had been evaluated.[2]

The present report includes 42 additional cases satisfying the entry criteria of the previous study but allocated randomly into either adenoidectomy or no surgery groups. In all cases the effusions were bilateral. Myringotomy and ventilation tube insertion were performed at random in one ear and the contralateral ear was not submitted to any surgery. The unoperated ear was examined otoscopically for resolution of the effusion, impedance change, and audiometrically measurable hearing gain.

The changes in these three parameters following surgery are presented 1, 2, and 3 years following surgery and are compared with the earlier changes occurring during the first year. The design of this study permits evaluation of the effects of adenoidectomy, adenotonsillectomy, and ventilation tube insertion in isolation. It also demonstrates the natural history of the untreated condition in these children.

MATERIALS AND METHODS

Ethical committee approval for the study was obtained. Five entry criteria were satisfied: age range between 2 and 9 years, a mandatory complaint or report of persistent hearing loss, pneumatic otoscopic confirmation of bilateral middle ear effusions by a validated observer, impedance studies showing only type B, C1, or C2 curves preoperatively, and a hearing loss in each ear in excess of 25 db at one or more frequencies on pure tone audiometry or free field hearing assessment. All the criteria were satisfied on entry and again at the second and third examinations 6 and 12 weeks later, respectively.

Three hundred twenty-two children entered the initial study. One hundred fifty-nine were excluded at the first or second appointment for reasons previously reported.[1] Surgery was carried out by allocation at random into three groups—adenotonsillectomy (47 cases), adenoidectomy (47 cases), and no surgery (56 cases). Thirteen subjects were excluded at operation. Subsequently a further 84 cases satisfying the same entry criteria were evaluated. Forty-two were excluded at the second or third examination, and 42 were then allocated at random into the adenoidectomy and no surgery groups, thus increasing the numbers in these groups to 70 and 75, respectively. Re-examination was undertaken at 6 weeks, at 6 and 9 months, and at 1, 2, and 3 years postoperatively by the same observer without prior knowledge of the previous treatment. Identical impedance and audiometric studies were performed. Not all children attended each follow-up appointment and some would not cooperate with the investigations. In some cases, when the ventilation tube in the operated ear had extruded and there was persistent fluid in the unoperated ear with significant hearing difficulty, reinsertion of a second or subsequent ventilation tube was required—always into the previously operated ear.

RESULTS

Examination of the unoperated ear in the three treatment groups permits assessment of the effects of adenotonsillectomy and adenoidectomy in isolation. It also allows assessment of the effects of ventilation tube insertion. The unoperated ear in the no surgery group reflects the natural history of the untreated condition.

Figure 1 shows the percentage clearance of fluid in the unoperated ear and in the ear treated by ventilation tube insertion and reinsertion when required. Absolute numbers in the three groups are shown, together with actual numbers (in brackets) of children attending and cooperating. Chi squared analysis shows a highly significant clearance of effusion in the unoperated ear in all surgical groups compared with the unoperated ear not submitted to any surgery. After 3 years there is still a significant clearance as a result of adenotonsillectomy but only a trend in ears treated by adenoidectomy or insertion of a ventilation tube. As expected, there is a dramatic clearance of effusion in the ears treated by ventilation tubes compared with other treatments, but the extra benefit is lost after 9 months. Without any treatment there is a slow spontaneous resolution of effusion, although 40 percent are unresolved after 3 years.

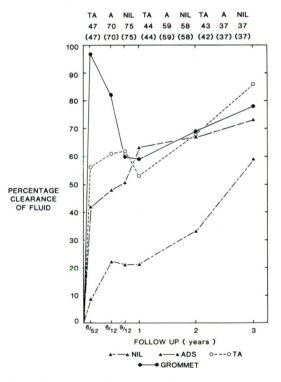

Figure 1 Percentage clearance of middle ear fluid in each treatment group at each follow-up time postoperatively.

Type B impedance curves were present pre-operatively in 98 percent of the cases, with type C1 or C2 curves in the remainder. Figure 2 shows the percentage change from B, C1, or C2 curves to A, C1, or C2 curves, the so-called no peak-peak conversion. There is a significant difference between the untreated ear in the no surgery group and those treated by adenotonsillectomy at 1, 2, and 3 years. There is a significant improvement in the adenoidectomy group but only 1 and 2 years after operation.

In most children six frequency thresholds were estimated by pure tone audiometry. Three frequencies were obtained in younger children and in the youngest a free field assessment was made. The mean of the preoperative thresholds obtained was greater than 30 db in all ears in all groups. Figure 3 shows the change in mean hearing thresholds.

Compared with the unoperated ear in the no surgery group, analysis of variants and paired T tests show a significant hearing gain at each follow-up time as a result of the three surgical procedures. This is most marked during the first 6 to 9 months in ears treated with a ventilation tube alone, although thereafter there is no difference between the groups. By virtue of the study design in patients with recurrence of significant subjective hearing loss following extrusion of the tube and persistence of fluid in both ears, reinsertion was required on one or more occasions. Figure 4 shows the percentage of revision procedures required for reinsertion of a tube

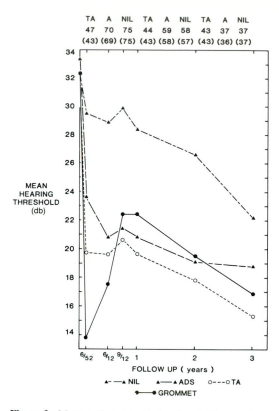

Figure 3 Mean audiometric hearing thresholds in each treatment group at each follow-up time postoperatively.

on one, two, three, or four occasions during the 3 year period. The difference between the two surgical groups and the no treatment group is significant at each time. It is seen that only when a ventilation tube is used alone is there need for a second revision during the first year and a fourth revision during the third year.

DISCUSSION

Previous studies reporting the effects of surgery for otitis media with effusion have invariably investigated the effect of adenoidectomy with or without tonsillectomy, but in combination with insertion of a ventilation tube.[3,4] The present investigation is unique in its assessment of these surgical procedures in isolation. The study shows significant clearance of the effusion as judged by a validated pneumatic otoscopist. There is acceptable correlation between the clinical results and the change in impedance measurements. The impedance changes from flat to peaked curves are slower to occur than the changes seen on otoscopy. All three operative procedures produce significant hearing gain, which continues

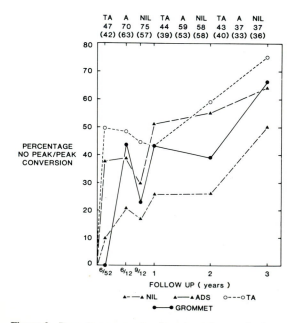

Figure 2 Percentage conversion from no peak to peak of impedance curves in each treatment group at each follow-up time postoperatively.

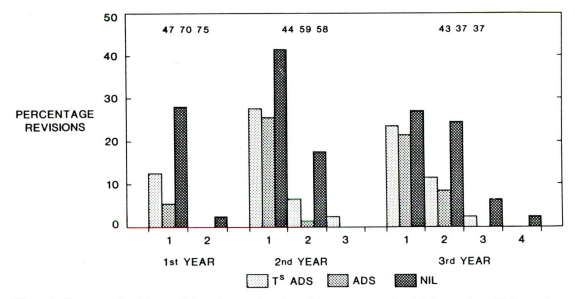

Figure 4 Percentage of revision ventilation tube procedures in each treatment group at each follow-up time with the number of reinsertions required during the first, second, and third years.

to improve with follow-up. After ventilation tube insertion the changes are all more marked during the first 9 months, but thereafter the improvement is similar, irrespective of the surgical procedure employed.

A slow improvement in the state of the unoperated ear in the no surgery group reflects spontaneous improvement in eustachian tube function and resolution of the effusion as the child grows older. However, when on average these children would be aged 8.25 years, the effusions are still present in 40 percent, impedance conversion has not occurred in 50 percent, and there is still a mean hearing loss of 22 db. Ventilation tube reinsertion is required twice as frequently when a tube is used alone than in combination with adenoidectomy or adenotonsillectomy. Only if it is used in isolation is there a need to reinsert a tube on as many as four occasions during this period.

We have previously reported significant development of tympanosclerosis in ears treated by tube insertion.[5] After 1 year 40 percent of the patients were affected to some degree, and after 2 years the incidence of tympanosclerotic change reached 70 percent. In the unoperated ear such changes were almost never found. There was also a progression of the sclerotic change within the tympanic membrane.

CONCLUSIONS

The study demonstrates a significant resolution of effusion as a result of adenoidectomy alone or in combination with tonsillectomy. The improvement is maintained for at least 3 years and is accompanied by significant audiometric hearing gain. There is a slight but statistically insignificant trend in favor of the combined procedure compared with adenoidectomy alone. During the first 9 months of treatment a greater clearance of the effusion and more marked hearing gain can be achieved by use of a ventilation tube, but after 9 months this extra benefit is lost. In this study reinsertion of a tube was required twice as often with a tube alone than in cases in which it was combined with removal of the tonsils or adenoids.

If consideration is given to the relative incidences of mortality and morbidity in treatment with a ventilation tube alone compared with adenoidectomy or adenotonsillectomy, a more acceptable treatment regimen for otitis media with effusion can be suggested on the basis of the present results. There would seem to be little additional benefit from a combination of tonsillectomy with adenoidectomy over adenoidectomy alone. The need for reinsertion of a ventilation tube in patients treated with a tube alone and the induction of tympanosclerotic change in the tympanic membrane also must be considered. Discriminant analysis of some of these data suggests that the results of adenoidectomy may be improved with careful case selection preoperatively.[6] Overall the results give some support to the suggestion that the treatment of choice for established bilateral otitis media with effusion may be adenoidectomy in selected cases, combined with unilateral insertion of a ventilation tube and simple myringotomy and aspiration of the effusion in the contralateral ear. Tube insertion produces immediate but short lived hearing gain, and adenoidectomy effects sustained improvement, which persists following extrusion of the tube.

REFERENCES

1. Maw AR. Chronic otitis media with effusion and adenoidectomy: a prospective randomized controlled study. In: Lim DJ, Bluestone CD, Klein JO, Nelson JD, eds. Recent advances in otitis media with effusion. Third International Symposium Toronto: BC Decker, 1984:299.

2. Maw AR, Herod F. Otoscopic, impedance and audiometric findings in glue ear treated by adenoidectomy and tonsillectomy. A prospective randomized study. Lancet 1986; 1:1399–1402.

3. Widemar L, Svensson C, Rynell-Dagöö B, Schiratzkj H. The effect of adenoidectomy on secretory otitis media. A two-year controlled prospective study. Clin Otolaryngol 1985; 10:345–350.

4. Black N, Crowther J, Freeland A. The effectiveness of adenoidectomy in the treatment of glue ear: a randomized controlled trial. Clin Otolaryngol 1986; 11:149–155.

5. Slack RWT, Maw AR, Capper JWR, Kelly S. A prospective study of tympanosclerosis developing after grommet insertion. J Laryngol Otol 1984; 98:771–774.

6. Maw AR. Adenoidectomy and adeno-tonsillectomy for otitis media with effusion (glue ear) in children: a prospective randomized controlled study. Master's thesis, University of London, 1986.

PATHOGENESIS

SPECIAL LECTURE: PATHOGENESIS OF VIRAL RESPIRATORY TRACT INFECTION

BENJAMIN VOLOVITZ, M.D. and PEARAY L. OGRA, M.D.

Acute viral infections of the upper respiratory tract are generally considered to be benign, self limiting, and not associated with any long term sequelae. However, infections in the bronchopulmonary tree can result in the development of pneumonia, bronchiolitis, and bronchial hypersensitivity. Such infection can result in long term complications with potentially serious impairment of pulmonary function.[1,2] Viral infections account for 40 to 50 percent of the acute episodes of bronchospasm in childhood. The agents that have been associated with episodes of wheezing include respiratory syncytial virus, parainfluenza virus types 1 and 3, influenza viruses, and rhinoviruses, especially in adult asthmatics.[3-5]

Recent epidemiologic studies have provided convincing evidence of a strong association between the acquisition of upper respiratory tract infections with respiratory syncytial virus, and less frequently with other viruses, and the subsequent development of acute otitis media with effusion.[6] The pathogenesis of otitis media with effusion in childhood remains to be determined. However, several important lessons emanating from studies of lower respiratory tract viral disease may be applicable to the understanding of virus induced middle ear disease. This information is briefly reviewed in the following discussion.

The factors that determine the pathogenesis and outcome of viral infections in the respiratory tract are diverse. Many facets of the evolution of bronchopulmonary disease following a viral infection remain to be elucidated. However, available information suggests that the homeostatic mechanism innate in the host's respiratory tract, the characteristics of the virus, and induction of secondary events as a result of the primary host-pathogen interaction determine the eventual expression of disease. A listing of the major determinants is presented in Table 1.[7]

The human respiratory tract is replete with secretory IgA and to a smaller extent with IgM, IgG, and IgE isotypes and immunoglobulin producing cells, T lymphocytes and their subsets. Recent observations have suggested that different strata of respiratory epithelium also contain a wealth of other effector cells that participate in the development of inflammation and the release of pharmacologically active mediators. The relative frequencies of their presence in the bronchopulmonary tree, nasal mucosa, and different segments of the middle ear system are shown in Table 2.

On the basis of recent observations it is clear that immunologic or allergic reactions in the respiratory tract consist of sequences of events involving activation of B and T lymphocytes, macrophages, and (or) other effector cells.[8] These include the activation of mast cells by immunologic stimuli (IgE, immune complexes) and other nonspecific stimuli, resulting in cell degranulation and the release of preformed granule associated mediators, such as histamine, eosinophilic chemotactic factors of anaphylaxis, and neutrophilic chemotactic factors, during the acute phase reaction. These mediators, in association with other membrane derived products generated during the course of mast cell activation (prostaglandins [PGD_2] and leukotrienes [LTC_4, LTD_4, and LTE_4]), interact with target organs such as mucous gland innervation pathways and bronchial and vascular smooth muscles, resulting in increased mucous secretion, vasodilation, and bronchospasm (Fig. 1). As a result of the release of eosinophilic chemotactic factors of anaphylaxis, neutrophilic chemotactic factors, and other mast cell mediators, there is accumulation in varying degrees of neutro-

TABLE 1   Determinants of Pathogenesis in Human Viral Respiratory Tract Infections

Host Respiratory Tract	Pathogen	Secondary Events
Prior antigenic exposure	Nature of virus and virulence determinants	Induction of neoantigens cross reactive with host
Alterations in specific immunocompetence	Route of exposure and tissue tropism	Induction of binding sites for other infectious agents
Immunologic or nonspecific cellular mechanism 　Mast cells 　Macrophage 　Neutrophils 　Eosinophils 　Basophils	Magnitude of replication at site of disease	Alterations in uptake of and immune response to concurrently available environmental macromolecules or pathogens
Abnormal neuroregulatory (neuropeptide) functions	Potential for and level of direct cytotoxicity or tissue injury	
Genetic predisposition	Potential for persistence in infectious form	

TABLE 2   Presence of Inflammatory Cells in the Respiratory Tract Normally and in Pathologic Situations

Cell Type	Bronchopulmonary N*	W	Nasal N	R	Tympanic Membrane	Middle Ear Cleft†	Eustachian Tube
Mast cells	+‡	+++	+	+++	+/−	++	+
Basophils	+	++	+	+++	ND	ND	ND
Eosinophils	+	+	+	++	+/−	+	+/−
Neutrophils	+	+++	+	++	−	++	+
Macrophages-monocytes	+++	+++	+	++	+/−	++	+

* N, Normal control. W, During wheezing. R, During rhinitis.

† During otitis media with effusion.

‡ ND, No data. −, Rare or absent. +/− to +++, Minimal to large number.

phils, eosinophils, or basophils. These cells have been shown to release significant amounts of potent vasoactive or bronchoactive mediators generated during metabolic activation by immune complexes, aggregated immunoglobulin, complement, or mast cell products. Finally, each of these effector cells has been shown to release mediators capable of causing mast cell activation and degranulation, as shown in Figure 1.[8-11]

The role of the immunologic events just described in environmental allergen-induced rhinitis, bronchial asthma, and insect bite allergies is well established. Recent observations have suggested that virus induced bronchospasm may be mediated by similar immunopharmacologic mechanisms. Studies in experimentally induced infections have

demonstrated the release of histamine from peritoneal mast cells after direct exposure to Sendai virus, and of LTB_4–LTC_4 by peripheral monocytes upon stimulation by antigen-antibody complexes.[12-14]

Studies carried out in children with different forms of infection with respiratory syncytial virus (bronchiolitis, pneumonia, or subclinical infection) have shown that most virus infected subjects exhibit transient development of homocytotropic virus specific IgE antibody response. However, only subjects with bronchiolitis or wheezing manifest prolonged cell bound IgE activity, the presence of respiratory syncytial virus IgE in a free form in nasopharyngeal secretions and in association with subsequent episodes of virus induced wheezing.[15] The develop-

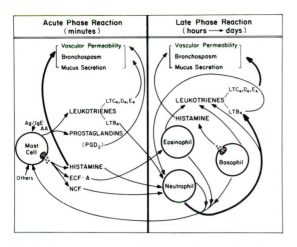

Acute Phase Reaction (minutes)	Late Phase Reaction (hours ⟶ days)

Figure 1 Sequence of reaction initiated by activation of mast cell followed by influx of inflammatory cells responsible for the release of active mediators in the human respiratory tract. AA, arachidonic acid. ECF-A, eosinophil chemotactic factor of anaphylaxis. NCF, neutrophil chemotactic factor.

ment of respiratory syncytial virus IgE and bronchospasm has been correlated with the presence and levels of histamine observed in the nasopharyngeal secretions.[16] Other studies have also demonstrated the presence of respiratory syncytial virus IgE and elevated histamine levels in the serum in patients with respiratory syncytial virus bronchiolitis.[17,18] Virus specific IgE also has been observed after infection with parainfluenza, herpes simplex, and rubella virus. Although rhinoviruses have been associated with otitis media with effusion and exacerbations of bronchospasm, studies carried out in adult volunteers have failed to demonstrate histamine release during experimental infections.[19] It is not known whether rhinovirus induces specific IgE antibody in patients with otitis media with effusion or bronchospasm.

In addition to the release of histamine, there is evidence to suggest the release of generated mediators of bronchospasm during the course of respiratory syncytial virus and other respiratory viral infections.[20] Most respiratory syncytial virus infected patients have been shown to have high levels of LTC_4 in the respiratory tract during active infection. The levels in the respiratory syncytial virus infected wheezing subject appear to be significantly higher than in nonwheezing subjects. Although LTC_4 activity could be generally correlated with the presence of virus specific IgE, some infected wheezing subjects without any detectable IgE activity demonstrated LTC_4 activity in the respiratory tract.[21] These observations suggest that respiratory viral infections may be involved in the activation of mast cells during acute phase reactions, and other effector cells during late phase reactions, in a man-

ner similar to the traditional allergens, such as ragweed pollen, mold spores, and possibly dietary proteins.

The detrimental role of influenza and measles virus infections in potentiating the pathogenesis of respiratory tract infection with *Staphylococcus aureus* and hemolytic streptococcus has been well established during epidemics of these viral infections. Although the precise mechanism underlying such interactions has not been fully characterized, experimentally induced infections have suggested a profound loss of antibacterial function in the host during acute viral respiratory tract infection. Such a decline in antibacterial activity appears to peak during convalescence from viral infection, when viral shedding has declined to low levels and local viral specific immunologic responses and pulmonary macrophage activity have attained peak levels.[7]

In addition to the secondary events just described, recently it has been observed that during acute infection with respiratory syncytial virus the uptake of and immune response to other inhaled antigens concurrently available in the respiratory tract may also be significantly altered. Studies carried out with inhalation of ovalbumin,[22] a food protein, or ragweed,[23] an environmental allergen, during respiratory syncytial virus infection have shown a significant increase in the uptake of these antigens in the sera and the development of a specific IgG antibody response in the serum and of IgE reactivity in the respiratory tract. These observations may explain the broad immunologic hyperreactivity to other food proteins and allergens in allergic patients during certain acute respiratory viral infections.

The information just summarized provides strong evidence for the role of IgE, mast cell preformed mediators, and other products generated by hematopoietic cells and mast cells in the pathogenesis of virus induced respiratory tract disease. In view of the striking similarities in the local immunologic reactivity and the distribution of other effector cellular mechanisms between the lower respiratory tract and the middle ear cleft and eustachian tube (see Table 2), it is possible that viral infection may contribute to the pathogenesis of otitis media with effusion in a manner similar to that of the respiratory tract. In preliminary studies the release of high levels of LTC_4 in the nasopharynx during naturally acquired exposure to ragweed pollen has been demonstrated in sensitive children with allergic rhinitis.[24] The presence and the level of LTC_4 in the nasopharynx were directly related to the degree of eustachian tube dysfunction in these patients. The role of eustachian tube functional impairment during LTC_4 release secondary to exposure to allergens or viral infections of the respiratory tract in the pathogenesis of otitis media with effusion is very tempting to postulate. However, the precise contribution of the viral infection itself, the development of IgE, or the release of pharmacologic mediators in the upper airway in acute or chronic middle ear disease remains to be determined.

Study supported in part by grants from the National Institute of Allergy and Infectious Disease (AI-15939) and the National Institute of Child Health and Human Development (HD-19679).

REFERENCES

1. McIntosh K, Ellis EF, Hoffman LS, Lybass TG, Eller JJ, Fulginiti VA. The association of viral and bacterial respiratory infections with exacerbations of wheezing in young asthmatic children. J Pediatr 1973;82:578–590.
2. Berkovich S, Millian SJ, Snyder RD. The association of viral and mycoplasma infections with recurrence of wheezing in the asthmatic child. Ann Allergy 1970; 28:43–49.
3. Horn MEC, Grett I. Role of viral infection and host factors in acute episodes of asthma and chronic bronchitis. Chest 1973; 63:44S.
4. Henderson FW, Clyde WA Jr, Collier AM, et al. The etiologic and epidemiologic spectrum of bronchiolitis in pediatric practice. J Pediatr 1979; 95:183.
5. Loda FA, Clyde WA Jr, Glezen WP, Senior RJ, Sheaffer CI, Denny FW Jr. Studies on the role of viruses, bacteria, and M. pneumoniae as causes of lower respiratory tract infections in children. J Pediatr 1968; 72:161–176.
6. Sarkkinen H, Ruuskanen O, Meurman O, Putakka H, Virolainen E, Eskola S. Identification of respiratory virus antigen in middle ear fluids of children with acute otitis media. J Infect Dis 1985; 151:444–448.
7. Bienenstock J. Immunology of lung. New York: McGrawHill, 1984.
8. Kay AB. Mediator of hypersensitivity and inflammatory cells in the pathogenesis of bronchial asthma. Eur J Respir Dis 1983; 129S:1–44.
9. Austen KF, Organ RP. Bronchial asthma: the possible role of the chemical mediators of immediate hypersensitivity in the pathogenesis of subacute chronic disease. Am Rev Respir Dis 1975; 112:423–436.
10. Kaliner M. Mechanisms of glucocorticosteroid action in bronchial asthma. J Allergy Clin Immunol 1985; 76:321–329.
11. Kaliner M. Mediators and asthma. Chest 1985; 87S:2–5.
12. Sugiyama K. Histamine release from rat mast cells induced by Sendai virus. Nature 1977; 270:614–615.
13. Ida S, Hooks JJ, Siraganian RP, Notkins AL. Enhancement of IgE-mediated histamine release from human basophils by viruses: role of interferon. J Exp Med 1977; 145:892–906.
14. Ferri NR, Howland WC, Spieglberg HL. Release of leukotrienes C4 and B4 and prostaglandin E2 from human monocytes stimulated with aggregated Ig, IgA and IgE. J Immunol 1986; 136:4188–4193.
15. Welliver RC, Ogra PL. The role of IgE in pathogenesis of mucosal viral infections. Ann NY Acad Sci 1983; 409:321–332.
16. Welliver RC, Wong DT, Sun M, Middleton E Jr. Vaughn RS, Ogra PL. The development of respiratory syncytial virus-specific IgE and release of histamine in nasopharyngeal secretion after infection. N Engl J Med 1981; 305:841–846.
17. Bui RHD, Molinaro GA, Kettering JD, Heiner DC, Imagawa DT, St Geme JW Jr. Virus-specific IgE and IgG4 antibodies in serum of children infected with respiratory syncytial virus. J Pediatr 1987; 110:87–90.
18. Smith TF, Remigio LK. Histamine in nasal secretion and serum may be elevated during viral respiratory tract infection. Int Arch Allergy Appl Immunol 1982; 67:380–383.
19. Eggleston PA, Hendley JO, Gwaltney JM Jr. Mediators of immediate hypersensitivity in nasal secretion during natural colds and rhinovirus infection. Acta Otolaryngol (Stock) 1984; 413S:25–35.
20. Volovitz B, Faden H, Ogra PL. Release of leukotrienes in human respiratory tract during viral infection: implication in virus induced wheezing. J Pediatr 1988; 112:218–222.
21. Volovitz B, Welliver R, Krystofik D, Ogra PL. Role of virus specific IgE in the release of leukotriene C4 (LTC4) in nasopharyngeal secretion of infants with respiratory syncytial virus infection. Pediatr Res 1987; 21:337A.
22. Freihorst JA, Piedra PA, Ogra PL. Effect of respiratory syncytial virus infection on the uptake and immune response to dietary antigens; possible role in potentiation of allergy. Proc Soc Exp Biol, Med (in press).
23. Leibovitz E, Freihorst JA, Piedra PA, Ogra PL. Modulation of systemic and humoral immune response to inhaled ragweed antigen in experimentally-induced infection with respiratory syncytial virus (RSV) (in preparation).
24. Volovitz B, Osur SL, Ogra PL. Leukotriene C4 (LTC4) release in respiratory mucosa during natural exposure to ragweed pollen in ragweed sensitive children. J Allergy Clin Immol (in press).

SPECIAL LECTURE:
BACTERIAL ADHERENCE: ATTACHMENT OF GROUP A STREPTOCOCCI TO MUCOSAL SURFACES

EDWIN H. BEACHEY, M.D. and HARRY S. COURTNEY, Ph.D.

A large body of evidence has accumulated to demonstrate that most natural bacterial infections are initiated by the adhesion of the microorganisms to the mucosal surfaces of the respiratory, gastrointestinal, or urogenital tract.[1] Adhesion prevents the colonizing bacteria from being swept away by mechanical forces and cleansing mechanisms such as sneezing, coughing, peristalsis, or fluid flow. In order to colonize the mucosal surfaces, the organisms must not only adhere, they must multiply at a sufficiently rapid rate to replenish newly exposed epithelial cell surfaces as old epithelial cells along with their adherent bacteria are exfoliated and swept away.

Once the bacteria have overcome the nonspecific mechanical and cleansing forces, they interact with the mucosal surfaces in a highly selective manner, depending on whether a given mucosal surface possesses receptors that recognize adhesive structures on the surface of the invading organisms. If present, these complementary structures interact with each other in a lock-and-key (or induced fit) fashion analogous to the combination of an enzyme with its substrate, or an antibody with its antigen (Fig. 1).[1-6] The terms "adhesin" and "receptor" have been coined to refer to the corresponding molecules on the surfaces of the bacteria and the animal cells, respectively.[2,6] The chemical composition and conformation of several bacterial adhesins and their corresponding receptors on host tissues have been defined to varying degrees for a number of different pathogenic microorganisms.[5] In general, the bacterial adhesins are composed of proteins in the form of fimbriae or fibrillae, and the receptors are composed of carbohydrate moieties of glycolipids or glycoproteins.[5] In certain cases, as is

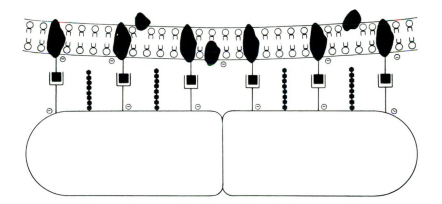

Figure 1   Adhesion of a bacterium bottom via specific adhesins (⊔) to a complementary receptor (■) on the host cell membrane top. The net negative charges (⊖) on both the bacterial and host cell surfaces are overcome by hydrophobic molecules (●) on the surface of the bacterium attracted to hydrophobic phospholipid molecules (⅄) of the host cell membrane. The irregular black structures represent protein and glycoprotein molecules incorporated into the host cell membrane. (Reproduced by permission from Ofek I, Beachey EH. General concepts and principles of bacterial adherence in animals and man. In: Beachey EH, ed. Bacterial adherence. London: Chapman and Hall, 1980:1–29.)

to be described for group A streptococci (*S. pyogenes*), however, the adhesin may be composed of a more complex structure in which several molecules interact with hydrophobic niches of proteins such as fibronectin bound to the surface of epithelial cells.

The only known natural reservoir for *S. pyogenes* is the human host. The organisms reside on the surfaces of the nasopharynx and the skin. In order to survive, the streptococci produce specialized surface macromolecules, which mediate the attachment of the organisms to mucosal surfaces.[7,8] One of these molecules, the lipoteichoic acid (LTA), forms an ionic complex with surface fibrillar proteins such as the M protein.[9,10] This interaction exposes the lipid end of the molecule in such an orientation that it can interact with fatty acid binding sites on the surface of epithelial cells. In this article we shall review the evidence that LTA mediates the attachment of *S. pyogenes* cells to mucosal surfaces, that LTA forms ionic complexes with M protein, the major surface protein of virulent organisms, that the epithelial cell receptor for the LTA mediated binding of streptococci is composed of fibronectin, and that *S. pyogenes* cells bind to the NH$_2$-terminal region of the fibronectin molecule.

THE ATTACHMENT OF *S. PYOGENES* TO EPITHELIAL CELLS

When suspensions of streptococci are mixed with suspensions of oral epithelial cells, the bacteria adhere in a patchy manner to the surface of the epithelial cells.[1] Transmission electron microscopy suggests that attachment is mediated by the surface fibrillar structures radiating from the surface of the streptococci to the epithelial cells.[1] In our search for the streptococcal ligand (adhesin) that mediates the binding, we found that of the purified surface substances tested, including LTA, M protein, C carbohydrate, or a peptidoglycan sonicate, only LTA was capable of inhibiting attachment.[8] As a corollary, treatment of streptococci with antibodies directed against LTA but not against M protein or C carbohydrate also inhibited adherence. Moreover, the inhibitory effect of the anti-LTA could be abolished by absorbing the antiserum with erythrocytes coated with LTA, indicating that the inhibitory effect was specifically directed against LTA exposed on the surface of the streptococci.[8]

FORMATION OF LTA-PROTEIN COMPLEXES

Further studies indicated that the membrane binding of *S. pyogenes* LTA is mediated by the glycolipid region of the molecule.[1] The lipid moiety of the hydrolyzed molecule inhibited the binding of whole streptococci to epithelial cells, whereas the deacylated LTA (dLTA) did not.[8] During transit through the cell wall, some of the LTA molecules appear to become complexed through their polyanionic backbones to clusters of positive charges on surface protein molecules. This orients some of the LTA molecules with their lipid ends protruding from the bacterial surface. LTA is able to form complexes with certain surface proteins, including the M protein.[11] The complexes with M protein are formed equally as well by LTA or dLTA, indicating that the polyanionic backbone rather than the glycolipid moiety is involved in the formation of complexes. Thus, it appears that clusters of positive charges on the M protein molecule or other LTA binding molecules must be important, as has been described for other proteins.[12,13] Having established the primary structure of most of the peptides of one M protein (pep M24),[14,15] and assuming an α-helical coiled-coiled structure of M protein,[16] we have proposed an alignment of the clusters of positive charges on the M protein molecule with the negatively charged backbone of LTA.[11] The concept that the complexes are the result of ionic interaction is supported by experiments in which the positively charged lysyl residues on the M protein were blocked by maleic anhydride. The blocked M protein failed to form either soluble or insoluble complexes with LTA. Deblocking of the lysyl residues with pyridine acetate restored full complexing activity to the M protein.[11]

The idea that some of the LTA molecules expose their lipid ends toward the surface of the bacteria is consistent with recent findings that the surfaces of group A streptococci are hydrophobic.[17,18] Studies of the partition of strains of *S. pyogenes* in a biphasic mixture of water and hexadecane demonstrated that the surface of the streptococci, in fact, were as hydrophobic as oil degrading bacteria.[18]

BINDING OF STREPTOCOCCI TO LIPID BINDING REGION OF FIBRONECTIN ON OROPHARYNGEAL EPITHELIAL CELLS

Having established that LTA forms complexes with LTA binding proteins, in particular M protein, we sought to identify a complementary receptor on human oral epithelial cells. Johansson et al[19] had reported that in patients in the hospital the upper respiratory tract frequently become colonized by gram negative bacteria with a concomitant loss of gram positive flora, and recent studies by Woods et al[20-22] suggested that fibronectin on the surfaces of oropharyngeal epithelial cells forms a barrier against the attachment of certain gram negative bacteria. Accordingly, we investigated the possibility that epithelial fibronectin may serve as a receptor for the binding of group A streptococci.

Fibronectin is a large glycoprotein (molecular weight about 440,000) present in soluble form in plasma and various other body fluids and in insoluble form on the surfaces of various tissue cells and in connective tissues. This glycoprotein has been shown to possess specific binding sites for a number of macromolecules, including collagen, heparin, hyaluronic acid, glycosaminoglycans, proteoglycans, arginine, and glucose.

Using fibronectin purified from human plasma, we were able to show that as little as 1 μg per milliliter of the glycoprotein was capable of inhibiting the attachment of each strain of group A streptococci tested to human buccal epithelial cells.[23] Moreover, the level of fibronectin on these cells as determined by radioimmunochemical methods was directly related to the adhesiveness of the epithelial cells for streptococci.[23] For example, when cell associated fibronectin was reduced by 50 percent by heating at 90° C for 1 minute or by treating the cells with β-mercaptoethanol, we observed a corresponding decrease in the adhesion of streptococci.[23] Conversely, when the level of cell surface fibronectin was increased by preincubating the cells with an excess (150 μg per milliliter) of plasma fibronectin, we observed a corresponding increase in streptococcal binding.[23] Immunoelectron microscopy of the attachment of streptococci to oral epithelial cells indicated that the streptococci attached only to epithelial cells coated with fibronectin, whereas gram negative bacteria such as *Pseudomonas aeruginosa* or *Escherichia coli* attached only to cells lacking immunoreactive fibronectin (Fig. 2).[24]

LTA, but not deacylated LTA, inhibited the binding of fibronectin to streptococcal cells.[23] In contrast, LTA had no effect on binding of fibronectin to staphylococci.[25] Because fibronectin had previously been shown to bind to staphylococci, our results clearly demonstrate that the binding sites on fibronectin for streptococci and staphylococci are different.

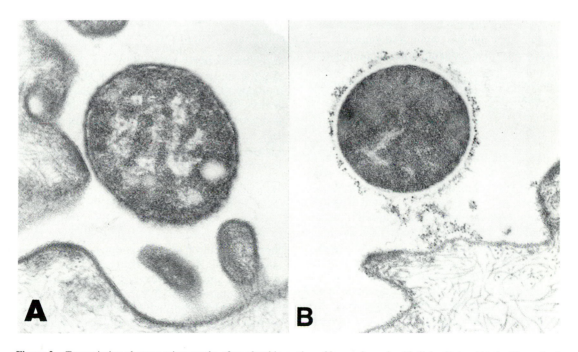

Figure 2 Transmission electron micrographs of an ultrathin section of human buccal epithelial cells incubated with a mixed suspension of *S. pyogenes* and *E. coli* followed by treatment with rabbit antifibronectin and then with ferritin conjugated goat antirabbit IgG. *A*, A cell of *E. coli* is seen associated with a cell devoid of ferritin particles, whereas *B*, a cell of *S. pyogenes* is seen associated with a cell coated with ferritin particles, indicating the presence of fibronectin. The rim of ferritin labeled antibody around the bacterium appears to be due to the acquisition of fibronectin from the surfaces of the epithelial cells during incubation. (Reproduced by permission from Abraham SN, et al. Adherence of *Streptococcus pyogenes, Escherichia coli*, and *Pseudomonas aeruginosa* to fibronectin coated and uncoated epithelial cells. Infect Immunol 1983; 41:1261–1268.)

FORMATION AND RELEASE OF LTA-FIBRONECTIN COMPLEXES FROM STREPTOCOCCAL SURFACE

Although we had demonstrated that LTA forms complexes through its polyanionic backbone with streptococcal surface proteins and through its lipid moiety with fibronectin, we had not shown in a direct way that fibronectin forms complexes with intact LTA on the surface of the bacteria. Therefore, we undertook studies to determine whether such complexes are formed in situ.[25] We took advantage of our previous findings that group A streptococci incubated in the presence of sublethal concentrations of penicillin released their surface LTA; as they lost their surface LTA, the bacteria lost their capacity to bind to oral epithelial cells.[16] We reasoned that if fibronectin binds to LTA, the bound fibronectin should be released along with the LTA in the presence of sublethal concentrations of penicillin.

In order to determine the specificity of the formation of LTA-fibronectin complexes on the surface of group A streptococci, we undertook comparative studies with a strain of S. aureus. The latter organisms are known to possess LTA, but appear to bind fibronectin mainly via a protein moiety that is sensitive to clindamycin.

As expected, the binding of fibronectin to streptococci decreased in the presence of penicillin, and the decrease corresponded to the loss of LTA.[25] Clindamycin had no effect on fibronectin binding to streptococci. In contrast, the binding of fibronectin to staphylococci was reduced by clindamycin but not by penicillin, even though penicillin released equally as much LTA from staphylococci as streptococci.[25] These results are consistent with the idea that LTA is the major receptor for fibronectin on streptococci, whereas a protein moiety is the major receptor for this molecule on staphylococci.

When cells of S. pyogenes coated with [^{3}H] fibronectin were incubated with penicillin, most of the radiolabel was released. Clindamycin had no effect. Neither antibiotic released the bound fibronectin from cells of S. aureus. Anti-LTA, but not preimmune or anti-M protein serum followed by goat anti-rabbit IgG, precipitated almost all the radiolabeled fibronectin released from the streptococci.[25] The immunoprecipitating activity of the anti-LTA was abolished by absorbing the antiserum with erythrocytes coated with LTA, but not by control uncoated erythrocytes. These results indicate that fibronectin is released in complex with LTA from streptococci treated with sublethal concentrations of penicillin and demonstrate for the first time that fibronectin forms complexes with the surface LTA of group A streptococci in situ.

LTA AND STREPTOCOCCAL BINDING REGION OF THE FIBRONECTIN MOLECULE

In an attempt to localize the group A streptococcal binding site within the fibronectin molecule, we cleaved fibronectin with thermolysin and then absorbed the enzymatic digest with cells of S. aureus or S. pyogenes. As can be seen in Figure 3, the S. aureus cells adsorbed three major high molecular weight polypeptides as well as a 28 kDa and a 23 kDa fragment. In contrast, S. pyogenes cells failed to absorb the high molecular weight polypeptides but completely absorbed the 28 kDa fragment and only partially absorbed the 23 kDa fragment.

To identify the region of the fibronectin molecule absorbed by the S. aureus and S. pyogenes cells, we performed Western immunoblots using monoclonal antibodies specific for the cell attachment region and the collagen binding region[27] and polyclonal antibodies prepared in rabbits against a synthetic peptide, S-Fn(25–55), copying an NH$_2$-terminal region of fibronectin.* The high molecular weight polypeptides absorbed by S. aureus reacted only with the antibody directed against the cell attachment site, whereas the 28 kDa fragment reacted only with the NH$_2$-terminus specific antibody (Fig. 3). Neither reacted with the antibody directed against the collagen binding region. These results indicate that whereas both S. pyogenes and S. aureus cells bind to the NH$_2$-terminal region of fibronectin, S. aureus cells bind to an additional site close to the cell attachment region as reported previously.[28,29]

DISCUSSION

It is now clear that LTA plays a central role in the attachment of group A streptococci to mucosal surfaces. The LTA is constantly in transit from the cytoplasmic membrane through the cell wall. During transit, some of the LTA molecules appear to reorient themselves in such a way that their lipid ends are exposed on the surface of the organisms. Because of the capacity of the polyglycerol phosphate backbone of LTA to form ionic complexes with isolated surface proteins, especially M protein, we postulate

---

* H.S. Courtney et al: Manuscript in preparation.

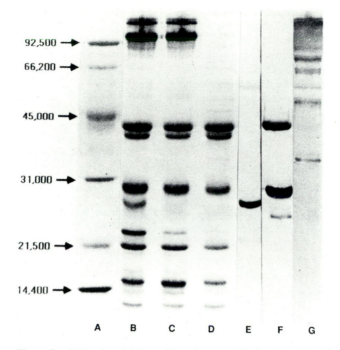

92,500 →
66,200 →
45,000 →
31,000 →
21,500 →
14,400 →

A   B   C   D   E   F   G

Figure 3 SDS gels and Western blots demonstrating the absorption of a 28 kDa NH$_2$-terminal peptide fragment by cells of *S. pyogenes* from a thermolysin digest of fibronectin. Lane A, molecular weight standards. Lane B, thermolysin digest of fibronectin absorbed with cells of *S. pyogenes*; note the complete removal of the 28 kDa band and partial removal of the 23 kDa bands. Lane D, the same digest absorbed with cells of *S. aureus*; note the removal of the high molecular weight bands in addition to the 28 and 23 kDa bands. Lanes A to D stained with Coomassie blue. Lanes E and F are Western immunoblots of the thermolysin digest with polyclonal antibody against a synthetic NH$_2$-terminal peptide (lane E), a monoclonal antibody against the collagen binding region of fibronectin (lane F), and a monoclonal antibody against the cell attachment region of fibronectin (lane G).

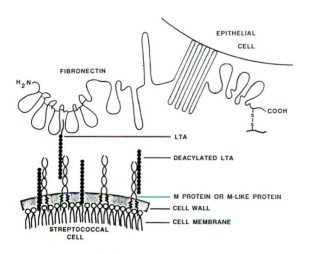

Figure 4 Hypothetical diagram of the LTA and fibronectin mediated interaction of a cell of *S. pyogenes* (bottom left) with an oral epithelial cell (top right). After release from the cytoplasmic membrane, some of the LTA molecules during transit through the cell wall form ionic bands with LTA linking proteins in such an orientation as to expose the lipid ends of the molecule toward the surface where it interacts with hydrophobic niches at the NH$_2$-terminus of the fibronectin molecules. The fibronectin molecule in turn is bound to the epithelial cell, thereby forming a bridge between the host cell and the bacterial cell.

that the LTA is held in place by forming such complexes on the intact surface of the streptococcal cells. In contrast to this form of ionic complexing to bacterial surface proteins, LTA forms complexes with the NH_2-terminal region of fibronectin through its lipid moiety. This permits the LTA anchored to the surface proteins through the negatively charged polyglycerol phosphate backbone to interact with the fatty acid binding sites of fibronectin molecules anchored to mucosal cells, as shown diagrammatically in Figure 4.

This article was adapted from *Reviews of Infectious Disease* by permission. The studies of the authors are supported by research funds from the U.S. Veterans Administration and by research grants AI-10085 and AI-13550 from the U.S. Public Health Service.

We thank Johnnie Smith for expert secretarial assistance in preparing the manuscript.

REFERENCES

1. Beachey EH. Bacterial adherence: adhesin receptor interactions mediating the attachment of bacteria to mucosal surfaces. J Infect Dis 1981; 143:325–345.
2. Jones GW. The attachment of bacteria to the surfaces of animal cells. In: Reissig JL, ed. Microbial interactions. Receptors and recognition. Series B. Vol 3. London: Chapman and Hall, 1977:139–176.
3. Gibbons RJ, van Houte J. Bacterial adherence and the formation of dentalplaques. In: Beachey EH, ed. Bacterial adherence. Receptors and recognition. Series B. Vol 16. London: Chapman and Hall, 1980:60–104.
4. Beachey EH, Eisenstein BI, Ofek I. Bacterial adherence and infectious diseases. In: Current concepts. Kalamazoo: The Upjohn Company, 1982:1–52.
5. Beachey EH, Ofek I. The adherence of bacteria to mammalian tissues. Roche seminar series (monograph), Nutley, NJ: 1987.
6. Ofek I, Beachey EH. General concepts and principles of bacterial adherence in animals and man. In: Beachey EH, ed. Bacterial adherence. London: Chapman and Hall, 1980:1–29.
7. Ofek I, Beachey EH, Jefferson W, Campbell GL. Cell membrane binding properties of group A streptococcal lipoteichoic acid. J Exp Med 1975; 141:990–1003.
8. Beachey EH, Ofek I. Epithelial cell binding of group A streptococci by lipoteichoic acid on fimbriae denuded of Mprotein. J Exp Med 1976; 143:759–771.
9. Swanson J, Hsu KC, Gotschlich EC. Electron microscopic studies on streptococci. I.M. antigen. J Exp Med 1969; 130:1063–1091.
10. Lancefield RC. Current knowledge of typespecific M antigens of group A streptococci. J Immunol 1962; 89:307–313.
11. Ofek I, Simpson WA, Beachey EH. Formation of molecular complexes between a structurally defined M protein and acylated or deacylated lipoteichoic acid of *Streptococcus pyogenes*. J Bacteriol 1982; 149:426–433.
12. Elbein AD. Interactions of polynucelotides and other polyelectrolytes with enzymes and other proteins. In: Meister E, ed. Advances in enzymology. New York: John Wiley, 1974: Vol 40, 29–64.
13. Fischer W, Koch HU, Rosel P, Fiedler F, Schmuch L. Structural requirements of lipoteichoic acid carrier for recognition by the poly ribitol phosphate polymerase from *Staphylococcus aureus*. A study of carrier lipoteichoic acids, derivatives, and related compounds. J Biol Chem 1980; 255:4550–4556.
14. Beachey EH, Seyer JM, Kang AH. Repeating covalent structure of streptococcal M protein. Proc Natl Acad Sci USA 1978; 75:3163–3167.
15. Beachey EH, Seyer JM, Kang AH. Primary structure of protective antigens of type 24 streptococcal M protein. J Biol Chem 1980; 255:6284–6289.
16. Phillips GN, Flicker PF, Cohen C, Manjula BN, Fischetti VA. Streptococcal M protein: α-helical coiled-coil structure and arrangement on the cells surface. Proc Natl Acad Sci USA 1981; 78:4689–4693.
17. Tylewska S, Hjerten S, Wadstrom T. Contribution of M protein to the hydrophobic properties of *Streptococcus pyogenes*. FEMS Microbiol Lett 1979; 6:249–253.
18. Rosenberg M, Perry A, Bayer EA, Gutnick DL, Rosenberg E, Ofek I. Adherence of *Actinetobacter calcoaceticus* RAG1 to human epithelial cells and to hexadecane. Infect Immun 1981; 33:29–33.
19. Johansson WG, Pierce AK, Sanford JP. Changingpharyngeal bacterial flora of hospitalized patients: emergence of gramnegative bacilli. N Engl J Med 1969; 281:1137–1140.
20. Woods DE, Bass JA, Johansson WG, Straus DC. Role of adherence in the pathogenesis of *Pseudomonas aeruginosa* lung infections in cystic fibrosis patients. Infect Immun 1980; 30:694–699.
21. Woods DE, Straus DC, Johansson WG, Bass JA. Role of fibronectin in the prevention of adherence of *Pseudomonas aeruginosa* to buccal cells. J Infect Dis 1981; 143:784–790.
22. Woods DE, Straus DC, Johansson WG Jr, Bass JA. Role of salivary protease activity in adherence of gram-negative bacilli to mammalian epithelial cells in vivo. J Clin Invest 1981; 68:1435–1440.
23. Simpson WA, Beachey EH. Adherence of group A streptococci to fibronectin on human oropharyngeal cells. Infect Immun 1983; 39:275–279.
24. Abraham SN, Beachey EH, Simpson WA. Adherence of *Streptococcus pyogenes, Escherichia coli*, and *Pseudomonas aeruginosa* to fibronectin coated and uncoated epithelial cells. Infect Immun 1983; 41:1261–1268.
25. Nealon T, Beachey EH, Courtney H, Simpson WA. Release of fibronectin lipoteichoic acid complexes from group A streptococci with penicillin. Infect Immun 1986; 51:529–535.
26. Alkan ML, Ofek I, Beachey EH. Adherence of group A streptococci to human skin and oral epithelial cells. Infect Immun 1977;18:555–557.
27. Hasty DL, Courtney HS, Simpson WA, McDonald JA, Beachey EH. Immunochemical and ultrastructural mapping of the gelatin-binding and cell attachment regions of human plasma fibronectin with monoclonal antibodies. J Cell Sci 1986; 81:125–141.
28. Mosher DF, Proctor RA. Binding and factor XIIIa-mediated cross-linking of a 27 kDa fragment of fibronectin to *Staphylococcus aureus*. Science 1980; 209:927–929.
29. Kuusela P, Varto T, Vuento M, Myhre EB. Binding sites for streptococci and staphylococci in fibronectin. Infect Immun 1984; 45:433–436.

OTITIS MEDIA WITH EFFUSION IN ALLERGIC AND NONALLERGIC CHILDREN: COMPARATIVE FOLLOW-UP

ISAAC SHUBICH, M.D. and LUIS F. JUAREZ, M.D.

Otitis media with effusion is prevalent in the pediatric population, as many studies have reported.[1] Middle ear disease of this kind in allergic children is also considered to be an important clinical entity.[2,3]

A 4 year prospective study was designed to follow two groups of children—allergic and nonallergic patients with middle ear effusion in whom surgical treatment as well as medical and immunologic therapy was performed, the objective being thorough clinical evaluation of the patients at the time of treatment and 2 to 4 years thereafter.

MATERIAL AND METHODS

Ninety children completed the evaluation, being followed for at least 2 years after diagnosis and treatment. The ages ranged from 8 months to 8 years, with a median of 3.1 years. The patients were divided into two groups—30 patients (16 males, 14 females) in whom the diagnosis was respiratory tract allergy and 60 patients (39 males and 21 females) in whom no allergy could be identified.

All the children underwent a complete pediatric and otolaryngologic work-up in addition to routine clinical and immunologic examination in those with allergy. Myringotomy and ventilation tube insertion (unilateral or bilateral) were performed in all the patients. The data recorded included the otologic history and previous otoscopic findings, the results of tympanometric and audiologic studies, and evidence of ethmoidal or maxillary sinus disease as well as the status of the adenoids and tonsils.

The follow-up consisted of recording immediate or delayed complications of the surgical procedure, the therapeutic response in new or recurrent episodes of acute otitis media, and the presence of effusion, including the time of clearance and the need for further surgical treatment in each group. Tables 1 and 2 summarize the pretreatment findings.

RESULTS

A total of 56 ears in allergic children and 109 ears in nonallergic children showed no statistically significant differences in immediate or delayed complications due to the ventilation procedure. After the ventilation tubes were extruded (without a significant difference in time span in the two groups), new episodes of acute otitis media and persistence or recurrence of middle ear effusion were compared in the two groups and found not to be of statistical significance ($p < 0.02$ in allergic children). Reinsertion of ventilation tubes was undertaken in three of the allergic children (10 percent) and in five of the nonallergic children (8 percent).

TABLE 1 Middle Ear Effusions in Allergic and Nonallergic Children

Acute Otitis Media	Allergic	Nonallergic	Totals
Previous episodes			
Minimum–maximum	· 3–8	3–6	
Otoscopic findings, (N=90)			
Hyperemic tympanic membrane with or without retraction	1	8	9 (10%)
Tympanic membrane retraction	3	9	12 (12%)
Full middle ear cleft, opacity	23	46	69 (76%)
Unilateral tympanic membrane perforation	3	3	6 (6%)

TABLE 2 Middle Ear Effusions in Allergic and Nonallergic Children (N=90)

	Allergic	Nonallergic
Ethmoidal maxillary sinusitis	19 (63%)	25 (41%)
Without sinusitis	11 (3%)	35 (59%)
	p<0.02 in allergic children	

In regard to medical treatment and the response to immunotherapy, the time of clearance of signs and symptoms in each child was recorded as 1 to 3 weeks, 3 to 5 weeks, and more than 5 weeks. This information was obtained by observation of the response to therapy immediately after the ventilation procedure in all 90 patients. A statistically significant difference for the allergic group (p=0.01) was demonstrated in regard to the duration of the clearance period (Table 3).

DISCUSSION

There is still controversy concerning the role of the middle ear structures in the allergy response in pediatric patients when the upper respiratory tract is affected. Clinical and laboratory studies in animal models seem to demonstrate the existence of different immunologic reactions, mainly of the IgE mediated atopic type and complement type 3 immunologic type.[4-6] However, some studies have failed to consider the role of the primary reaction in the middle ear itself.[7]

Our clinical study shows that both allergic and nonallergic children show prominent middle ear effusions. Both groups have similar histories of acute otitis media episodes, and there is a slight statistically significant difference in regard to ethmoidal-maxillary sinus involvement in allergic children, as expected (see Table 2).

Postmyringotomy complications and the incidences of extrusion and tube reinsertion are not significantly different. Adenoidectomy was a frequent and necessary procedure in both groups, but the response to medical therapy occurred earlier in nonallergic children. The incidence of recurrence of acute otitis media ear effusion seems to be of slight significance in allergic children, but further studies should be done to confirm this impression. Allergic children should be diagnosed and treated carefully and given proper follow-up care, and the therapeutic outcome should be similar to that in their nonallergic peers. A better understanding of the effects of allergy in the middle ear is required.

TABLE 3 Middle Ear Effusions in Allergic and Nonallergic Children: Medical Treatment or Immunotherapy Response

Weeks of Therapy	Allergic (N=30)	Nonallergic (N=60)
1–3 weeks	1 (3%)	19 (32%)
3–5 weeks	6 (20%)	35 (58%)
> 5 weeks	23 (77%)	6 (10%)
	p <0.01 in allergic children	

REFERENCES

1. Hinchcliffe R. Epidemiological aspects of otitis media. In: Glorig A, Gerwin K, eds. Otitis media: proceedings of the national conference. Springfield, IL: Charles C Thomas, 1972:36.
2. Dees SC, Lefkowiz D. Secretory otitis media in allergic children. Am J Dis Child 1972; 124:364–368.
3. Marshal SG, et al. Prevalence of middle ear dysfunction and otitis media with effusion in atopic children. In: Lim DJ, Bluestone CD, Klein JO, Nelson JD, eds. Recent advances in otitis media with effusion. Proceedings of the Third International Symposium. Toronto: BC Decker, 1984:240.
4. Bernstein JM, Reisman RE. The role of acute hypersensitivity in secretory otitis media. Trans Am Acad Ophthalmol Otolaryngol 1974; 78:120–127.
5. Bernstein JM, et al. Otitis media: the immunological factor. In: Sade J, ed. Acute and secretory otitis media: proceedings of the international conference. Part 1. Jerusalem, Israel: Kugler, 1986:203.
6. Miglets A. The experimental production of allergic middle ear effusion. Laryngoscope 1973; 83:1355–1384.
7. Doyle WJ, Takahara T, Fireman P. The role of allergy in the pathogenesis of otitis media with effusion. Arch Otolaryngol 1985; 111:502–506.

CILIARY ACTIVITY DURING EXPERIMENTAL OTITIS MEDIA WITH EFFUSION INDUCED BY LIPOPOLYSACCHARIDE

YOSHIHIRO OHASHI, M.D., YOSHIAKI NAKAI, M.D., HIROSHI IKEOKA, M.D., HIROYUKI KOSHIMO, M.D., YUSUKE ESAKI, M.D., and SHOKO KATO, M.D.

Direct inoculation of bacterial endotoxin, especially that derived from *Haemophilus influenzae*, is an established experimental means for inducing otitis media with effusion in laboratory animals.[1] In these models increased vascular permeability is the mechanism responsible for middle ear effusions. However, any effusion is removed to the pharynx via the eustachian tube if the mucociliary system in the tubotympanum is functioning effectively. Our purpose in this study was to examine the effect of lipopolysaccharide (LPS) on the mucociliary system in the tubotympanum.

MATERIALS AND METHODS

In Vitro Study

Thirty-five Hartley strain guinea pigs (average weight, 250 g) were used. Mucosal samples were obtained from three sites—the bony portion of the eustachian tube, the middle ear close to the tympanic orifice (proximal site), and the middle ear more distal to the orifice (distal site). Each mucosal sample was placed in a sealed chamber containing 3 ml of RPMI 1640.[2] First, the baseline ciliary activity (beats per minute) in the most active cell of each culture was determined at an ambient temperature of 30° C, using the direct and quantitative photoelectric method of Ohashi and Nakai.[3] After determination of the baseline activity, the RPMI 1640 in each chamber was decanted. Fifteen cultures were immediately filled with fresh RPMI 1640. Those remaining were also filled with RPMI 1640 containing varying concentrations (0.1 ng per milliliter, 1.0 ng per milliliter, 10 ng per milliliter, 100 ng per milliliter, 1 μg per milliliter, and 10 μg per milliliter) of *Klebsiella pneumoniae* LPS (Sigma). All cultures were kept at room temperature in an aseptic box. At intervals of 12, 24, 36, 48, 72, 96, 120, 144, and 168 hours after the sampling,

the ciliary activity of the cell whose baseline activity was determined was measured at 30° C by the same photoelectric method. We substituted fresh solution every 24 hours. In this study any change in ciliary activity was expressed as a percentage deviation from the baseline and the baseline set at 100 percent.

In Vivo Study

Thirty Hartley strain guinea pigs (average weight, 250 g) were used. Under Nembutal anesthesia, a 10 μg per milliliter solution of LPS from *K. pneumoniae* (Sigma) was inoculated into the right tympanic bulla of each animal through the tympanic membrane until the solution overflowed from the tympanic membrane. With the same procedure, sterile physiologic saline solution was injected into the left ear of each animal to serve as a control. The three groups of animals were sacrificed by decapitation on the first, third, or seventh day after the procedure. Bilateral mucosal samples were obtained from three sites (eustachian tube, proximal site, and distal site). The samples obtained from five animals of each group were used for the assessment of ciliary activity (beats per minute), and those from the rest were used for electron microscopic examination. The ciliary activity in the most active cell of each sample was examined in a physiologic saline solution at 30° C by our photoelectric method.[3]

RESULTS

In Vitro Study

The ciliary activity in the eustachian tube and that in the proximal site presented similar patterns of reaction to RPMI 1640 and to a variety of concentrations of LPS. The effect of LPS was more dramatic on the ciliary activity in the distal site than on that in the eustachian tube and the proximal site. LPS did not impair the ciliary activity up to 168 hours if the concentration was 1 ng per milliliter or less. An LPS concentration of 10 ng per milliliter did not impair ciliary activity in the eustachian tube or the proximal site up to 168 hours but caused reduced activity in the distal site after extended exposure (more than 96 hours). LPS concentrations of 100 ng per milliliter or more caused cilia dysfunction in the tubotympanum; in particular, 1 μg per milliliter or more of LPS quickly disabled ciliary activity in the distal site.

In Vivo Study

Saline Inoculated Ears (Left Ears)

No effusions were observed in each left ear of 30 animals at the time of sacrifice. The ciliary activities (mean ± SD) in the eustachian tube were 784 ± 65 beats per minute on the first day, 791 ± 46 beats per minute on the third day, and 781 ± 52 beats per minute on the seventh day. The ciliary activities in the proximal and distal sites were 732 ± 35 beats per minute and 822 ± 57 beats per minute on the first day, 753 ± 56 beats per minute and 853 ± 54 beats per minute on the third day, and 743 ± 48 beats per minute and 822 ± 57 beats per minute on the seventh day, respectively. Electron microscopy revealed that fewer than 5 percent of the ciliated cells in the tubotympanum were pathologic at any time.

LPS Inoculated Ears (Right Ears)

First Day. Massive effusions completely filled the tympanic cavities in all animals. The ciliary activities were 406 ± 65 beats per minute in the eustachian tube, 420 ± 26 beats per minute in the proximal site, and 466 ± 70 beats per minute in the distal site. Many pathologic changes were observed in the tubotympanic mucosa. The major findings included compound cilia, vacuolation of ciliated cells, infiltration of polymorphonuclear leukocytes, leakage of erythrocytes, thickening of the subepithelial layer, and sporadic desquamation of epithelial cells (Fig. 1). Over 55 percent of the ciliated cells in the eustachian tube and over 65 percent of those in the tympanic cavity were pathologic.

Third Day. Moderate effusions (average volume, 0.17 ml) in the tympanic cavity were observed. The ciliary activities in the eustachian tube, proximal site, and distal site were 611 ± 62, 561 ± 76, and 484 ± 64 beats per minute, respectively. Several pathologic changes, such as compound cilia, leakage of erythrocytes, vacuolation and cytoplasmic protuberances of epithelial cells, and infiltration of polymorphonuclear leukocytes, were observed under electron microscopy (Figs. 2, 3). Approximately 40, 45, and 55 percent of the ciliated cells in the eustachian tube, proximal site, and distal site, respectively, were pathologic.

Seventh Day. Little fluid could be seen in the tympanic cavity of each animal. The respective ciliary activities in the eustachian tube, proximal site, and distal site were 763 ± 58, 699 ± 62, and 527 ± 55 beats per minute. Electron microscopy showed that fewer than 10 percent of the ciliated cells in the tube and the proximal site were pathologic. However, some pathologic changes were found in the distal site, including sporadic infiltration of polymorphonuclear leukocytes, compound cilia, and vacuolation of ciliated cells; about 40 percent of the ciliated cells had degenerated.

DISCUSSION

Indirect evidence has been accumulating that damaged or inflamed mucociliary tissue in otitis media with effusion might be associated with insufficient clearance in the middle ear. However, our knowledge of the mucociliary system in the tubotympanum is still limited. Only recently has the mucociliary system been considered to play an important role in the defense system of the tubotympanum. Since the mucociliary system is composed of ciliated cells as well as secretory cells and a mucous blanket, mucociliary function is impaired not only because of mucous abnormalities but also because of decreased ciliary activity. It seems necessary to study ciliary activity, a component of mucociliary clearance, to gain a better understanding of the nature of this system.

Our studies have documented this activity directly and quantitatively using our photoelectric method.[4] With the same method we studied the effects of a variety of pathologic agents on ciliary activity in the tubotympanum, including x-ray irradiation,[5-8] infectious pathogens,[9,10] and environ-

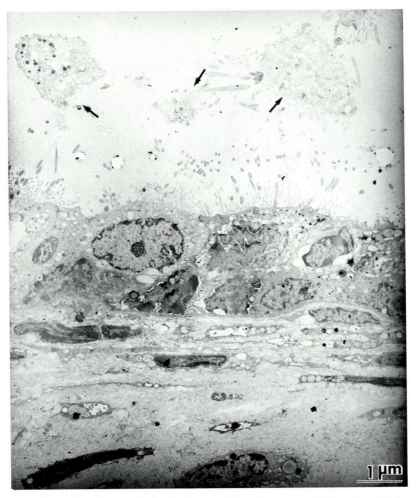

Figure 1 Electron micrograph showing the eustachian tube mucosa on the first day. Cellular debris (arrows) and vacuolation of ciliated cells are seen.

mental pollutants.[11,12] In these studies we established that ciliary activity in the tubotympanum can be reduced by a variety of agents.

In the present study we determined the effect of LPS on ciliary activity in the tubotympanum. With an in vitro study we confirmed that LPS can affect ciliary activity in the tubotympanum in a dose-response fashion. However, the possibility cannot be ruled out that ciliated cells in situ could behave differently when in contact with LPS. Thus we also inoculated the tympanic cavity of guinea pigs with LPS from *K. pneumoniae* and examined the ciliary beating activity as well as the structure of ciliated cells under such conditions. In our in vitro study we found serous effusions on the first and third days, when we confirmed the reduction in ciliary

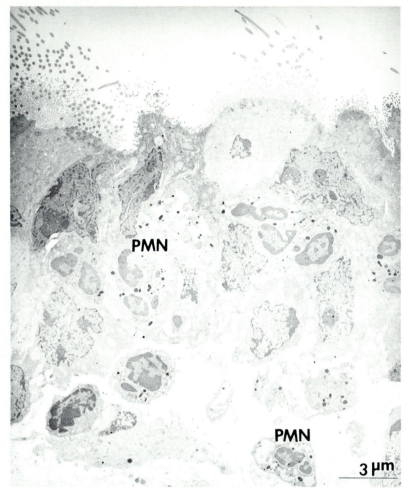

Figure 2   Electron micrograph showing the eustachian tube mucosa on the third day. There is infiltration with many polymorphonuclear leukocytes (PMN) and loss of cilia.

activity and the presence of pathologic ciliated cells in the tubotympanum. It seems apparent that diminished ciliary activity in the tubotympanum is responsible for the accumulation of fluid in the tympanic cavity. On the seventh day little fluid could be found, and ciliary activity in the distal site was reduced but that in the eustachian tube and at the proximal site had returned to normal.

It has been established that serous middle ear effusion formation due to endotoxin or LPS is the result of increased vascular permeability.[1] Past investigation and our present data indicate that two specific pathologic factors are needed for the development and clinical manifestation of otitis media with effusion: middle ear effusion production as a result of increased vascular permeability and failure of effusion transport as a result of impaired mucociliary activity. It may be assumed also that

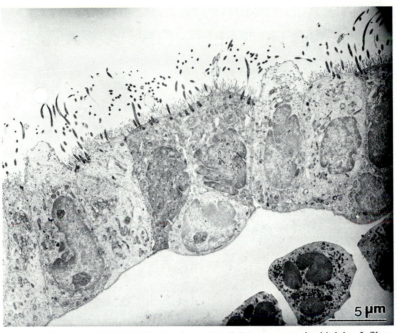

Figure 3 Electron micrograph showing the proximal site mucosa on the third day. Infiltration with polymorphonuclear leukocytes and cytoplasmic protuberances of epithelial cells are seen.

cilia in the eustachian tube and the middle ear close to the tube play an even more significant role in middle ear clearance.

REFERENCES

1. DeMaria TF, Briggs BR, Okazaki N, Lim DJ. Experimental otitis media with effusion following middle ear inoculation of nonviable *H. influenzae*. Ann Otol Rhinol Laryngol 1984; 93:52–56.

2. Ohashi Y, Nakai Y, Koshimo H, Esaki Y. Ciliary activity in the *in vitro* tubotympanum. Arch Otorhinolaryngol 1986; 243:317–319.

3. Ohashi Y, Nakai Y. Functional and morphological studies on chronic sinusitis mucous membrane. I. Decline of ciliary action in chronic sinusitis. Acta Otolaryngol (Stockh) 1983; Suppl 397:3–8.

4. Ohashi Y, Nakai Y, Kihara S. Ciliary activity of the middle ear lining in guinea pigs. Ann Otol Rhinol Laryngol 1985; 94:419–423.

5. Ohashi Y, Nakai Y, Ikeoka H, Koshimo H, Onoyama Y. Effects of irradiation on the ciliary activity of the eustachian tube and the middle ear mucosa. Arch Otorhinolaryngol 1985; 242:343–348.

6. Ohashi Y, Nakai Y, Esaki Y, Ikeoka H, Koshimo H, Onoyama Y. Acute effects of radiation on the middle ear mucosa. Ann Otol Rhinol Laryngol (in press).

7. Ohashi Y, Nakai Y, Esaki Y, Ikeoka H, Koshimo H, Onoyama Y. Mucosal pathology of the eustachian tube in experimental otitis media with effusion induced by x-ray irradiation. Am J Otolaryngol (in press).

8. Ohashi Y, Nakai Y, Esaki Y, Ikeoka H, Koshimo H, Onoyama Y. Mucociliary pathology of the eustachian tube in experimental otitis media with effusion induced by x-ray irradiation. Arch Otorhinolaryngol (in press).

9. Ohashi Y, Nakai Y, Kihara S, Ikeoka H. Effects of *Staphylococcus aureus* on the ciliary activity of the middle ear lining. Ann Otol Rhinol Laryngol 1987; 96:225–228.

10. Ohashi Y, Nakai Y, Esaki Y, Ikeoka H, Koshimo H. An experimental study on effects of bacterial endotoxin on the ciliary activity in the tubotympanum. Ann Otol Rhinol Laryngol (in press).

11. Ohashi Y, Nakai Y, Ikeoka H, Koshimo H, Esaki Y. Mucosal pathology of the eustachian tube after exposure to sulfur dioxide. Arch Otorhinolaryngol 1986; 243:274–279.

12. Ohashi Y, Nakai Y, Ikeoka H, Koshimo H, Esaki Y, Horiguchi S, Teramoto K, Nakaseko H. An experimental study on the acute effects of isopropyl alcohol on the middle ear mucosa. J Appl Toxicol 1987, 7:205–212.

IMMOTILE CILIA SYNDROME ASSOCIATED WITH OTITIS MEDIA WITH EFFUSION: A CASE REPORT

MARK J. SHIKOWITZ, M.D., CARL F. ILARDI, M.D., and MELANIE GERO, M.D.

In 1933 Kartagener described the syndrome that bears his name, consisting of a triad including chronic rhinosinusitis, chronic bronchitis with bronchiectasis, and situs inversus viscerum. Ciliated epithelium lines the upper and lower respiratory tract. These patients have a congenital abnormality of the cilia causing a defect in mucociliary transport.[1] This leads to stasis of secretions and is believed to be the cause of the chronic airway disease. Male patients with Kartagener's syndrome have shown a high incidence of sterility owing to the similar morphology in sperm tails and cilia.[2] It is now assumed that chance alone determines the final position of the viscera. In fact, situs inversus is found in only 50 percent of the individuals with ciliary defects.[3] It is the absence of dynein arms, defective radial spokes, or transposition of microtubules in both cilia and sperm tails that makes them immotile.[4,5]

Kartagener's syndrome is only one segment of the larger group of immotile cilia syndromes. The presence of otitis media in Kartagener's syndrome and the larger group of immotile cilia syndromes has been noted. It is only within the past 10 years that a few reports have specifically addressed the prominence of otitis media and the role played by immotile cilia in the middle ear space.[2,6,7] Here we report the case of a 5½ year old girl with chronic otitis media with effusion who was eventually diagnosed as having the immotile cilia syndrome.

CASE HISTORY

This was one of multiple admissions to the Schneider Children's Hospital for this 5½ year old white female who presented with recurrent pneumonia, productive cough, otitis media, and headaches. The patient was the product of a full term vaginal delivery, with a birth weight of 7 pounds and Apgar scores of 9 and 9.[1,5] At the age of 2 days she developed a "runny nose." Cultures of the nasal secretions revealed *Staphylococcus*, and she was treated intravenously with nafcillin sodium. A chest x-ray examination at this time revealed right upper lobe atelectasis. Following discharge the patient continued to suffer from recurrent pneumonia and was hospitalized seven times between birth and age 5½ years. During this period multiple sweat tests were performed, the results were normal, and cystic fibrosis was ruled out. A barium swallow and two bronchoscopies failed to reveal the presence of a tracheoesophageal fistula. Findings in an immunologic work-up were normal. At 5 years of age the patient underwent myringotomy by an outside physician with ventilation tube placement for chronic otitis media associated with a 30 db hearing loss.

Physical examination revealed a 5½ year old white thin female. The eyes were normal. The nose was congested with a thick yellow secretion. Examination of the ears showed bilateral myringotomy tubes in place with no discharge. Throat examination showed moderate tonsillar hypertrophy but no erythema. There were rales in both left and right lungs, with a mild end expiratory wheeze. The remainder of the findings in the physical examination were normal.

Laboratory values on admission were as follows: white cell count, 16.56×10^3 per cubic millimeter; hematocrit, 38.4 percent; hemoglobin level, 13.0 g per deciliter. The serum electrolytes, blood glucose, and BUN level were normal. A sputum culture revealed *Streptococcus mitis*. Chest x-ray examination revealed a right mediastinal density representing atelectasis or fibrosis and increased interstitial markings consistent with chronic airway disease. There was no situs inversus. A computed tomographic scan of the temporal bones and sinuses with contrast revealed diffuse soft tissue opacification of the maxillary and ethmoidal sinuses bilaterally. The sphenoidal and frontal sinuses were poorly developed. There was soft tissue opacification of the middle ear cavity and mastoid air cells bilaterally. No bone changes were identified (Fig. 1).

The patient was treated with intravenous doses of ceftazidime, theophylline anhydrous sustained action capsules, metaproterenol sulfate bronchodilator, and chest physiotherapy and postural drainage. The pneumonia resolved with antibiotic therapy, but the headaches persisted and were attributed to

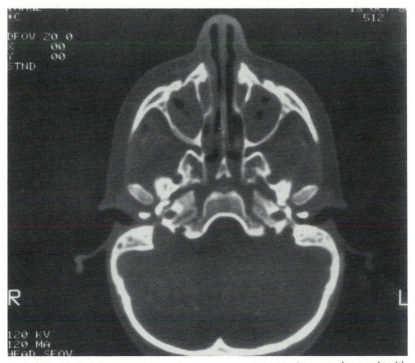

Figure 1 Computed tomographic scan of mastoids and sinuses demonstrating pansinusitis of the maxillary and ethmoidal sinuses bilaterally with soft tissue opacification of the middle ear cavity and mastoids bilaterally.

sinusitis. The patient was brought to the operating room and placed under general anesthesia.

Biopsy specimens were taken from the posterior two-thirds of the right inferior turbinate and sent for electron microscopy. At the same time brushings were taken from the left inferior turbinate for cilia immotility studies. Following this, bilateral maxillary antrostomies were performed through the inferior meatus with curettage and culture of the maxillary sinus contents. The ears were then examined with the operating microscope. The old myringotomy tubes were removed and the middle ear was examined through the myringotomy incision. No infection or fluid could be seen; however, the mucosa appeared somewhat thickened. Examination for possible ciliary movement was negative. Biopsy of the middle ear mucosa was performed through the myringotomy opening with microcupped forceps and specimens were placed directly in fixative for electron microscopy. A long lasting modified T tube was inserted bilaterally.

Pathologic examination revealed no cilia in any of the nasal biopsy specimens. The maxillary sinuses revealed mild chronic inflammation, and the biopsy examination of the middle ear mucosa revealed the presence of cilia (to be discussed). The sinus culture revealed *Streptococcus mitis*, as in the sputum.

The patient was discharged from the hospital on the twelfth day and has continued to do well.

MATERIALS AND METHODS

The middle ear biopsy specimens were placed in a modified Karnofsky's fixative, rinsed in 0.1 molar cacodylate buffer at a pH 7.4, and postfixed in cacodylate buffered 1 percent osmium tetroxide. The tissue was dehydrated and mounted in epoxy resin. Sections were cut at 1 μm and stained with methylene blue. Areas showing cross sections of cilia were thin sectioned and stained with uranyl acetate–lead citrate and examined with a Jeol Jem 100 MB electron microscope.

RESULTS

One hundred cilia were examined in cross section. Forty of these demonstrated normal ultrastructural features. The axoneme contained two central singlet microtubules and nine peripherally arranged doublet microtubules (Fig. 2A). The remaining 60 cilia examined demonstrated a variety of microtubular abnormalities, including extra central singlet

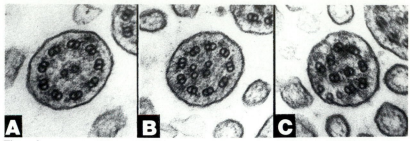

Figure 2 *A*, A normal cilium contains two central singlet microtubules surrounded by a ring of nine doublet microtubules. *B*, Note the presence of two extra central singlets. *C*, This cilium contains disordered doublets and singlets outside the central zone. (150,000×).

microtubules and extra doublets outside the peripheral ring (Fig. 2B, C). Total disorganization of microtubules was also noted. The cilia seen in perfect cross section had normal outer dynein arms.

DISCUSSION

The prevalence of Kartagener's syndrome has been estimated as being 1:40,000.[8] It has been shown that only 50 percent of the individuals affected by the immotile cilia syndrome have situs inversus, making the prevalence of the immotile cilia syndrome less rare, or approximately 1:20,000.[6,8,9]

Ciliated epithelium has been shown to line several sites in the human body, including the nasal passages, paranasal sinuses, eustachian tubes, middle ear mucosa, pharynx to the esophageal inlet, trachea, bronchioles, endometrial lining of the cervix, oviduct, ductuli efferentes, ependymal lining of the brain and ventricles, and the central canal of the spinal tract.[8] Any abnormality in the structure of the cilia can cause a change in their function, because it is ultimately the normal function of the cilia and not the structure that determines the effect on the individual patient. As in our case, the two prominent ultrastructural defects that could be identified are microtubular defects, yet the patient clearly appears to have demonstrated symptoms of deficient mucociliary transport since birth. It is believed that a change in the ultrastructure of the cilia may occur from childhood to adulthood with variable expression.[10]

Although many reports have noted the prevalence of otitis media in Kartagener's syndrome and the immotile cilia syndrome, only a few have stressed middle ear change as a significant part of the disease. Until recently most middle ear inflammatory disease was attributed to "eustachian tube dysfunction." Jahrsdoerfer et al[2] studied the mucosa of the middle ear in six patients with Kartagener's syndrome. Various abnormalities were noted in the cilia taken from the middle ear. Levinson et al[11] found that 100 percent of their 27 patients with the immotile cilia syndrome had associated recurrent otitis that often led to hearing loss.

Scanning electron microscopy has revealed three distinct ciliary drainage systems within the middle ear space. The presence or absence of beating cilia observed under the microscope during myringotomy and tube placement has been used as a sign in the management of problem cases of otitis media with effusion. Patients with actively beating cilia have a favorable course and rarely need a second set of ventilating tubes.[12] Any alteration in ciliary function leading to decreased mucociliary transport results in a diseased middle ear and mastoid.

Most physicians agree that the pulmonary disease seen in the immotile cilia syndrome must be treated aggressively with appropriate antibiotics and pulmonary physiotherapy. Bronchodilators have been used to increase mucociliary clearance. When patients develop localized bronchiectasis that is resistant to this therapy, a selective lobectomy may be indicated.

The management of the secretory otitis media is controversial as revealed in the literature. Some authors believe that repeated tympanometry and ventilation tube insertion should be avoided. They believe that these patients always have abnormal tympanograms and may develop a chronic purulent discharge from the ear after intubation.[13] Others believe that ear infections should be treated vigorously with antibiotics and ear drainage if necessary. They have found ventilating tubes to be useful in the management of chronic ear disease.[11] Our own patient has done well with antibiotic therapy in combination with ventilating tube insertion. The temporary use of hearing aids during an acute decrease in hearing may be indicated in these patients.[13]

The overall otolaryngologic prognosis in patients with the immotile cilia syndrome appears to be favorable.[12] Conservative therapy with minimal surgical procedures for ear and sinus complaints helps to minimize the long term sequela. The management of chronic pulmonary disease and male sterility may be of greater consequence to the patient and his physicians.

This study was supported in part by Captain L. Berger and the Otolaryngology Foundation, Incorporated.

REFERENCES

1. Mygind N, Pedersen M, Nielsen MH. Primary and secondary ciliary dyskinesia. Acta Otolaryngol 1983; 95:688–694.
2. Jahrsdoerfer R, Feldman PS, Rubel EW, et al. Otitis media and the immotile cilia syndrome. Laryngoscope 1979; 89:769–778.
3. Sturges JM, Chao J. A cause of human respiratory disease. N Engl J Med 1979; 300:53–56.
4. Sturges JM, Chao J, Turner JA. Transposition of ciliary microtubules. Another cause of impaired ciliary motility. N Engl J Med 1980; 303:318–322.
5. Afzelius BA. A human syndrome caused by immotile cilia. Science 1976; 193:317–319.
6. Ernstson S, Afzelius BA, Mossberg B. Otologic manifestations of the immotile cilia syndrome. Acta Otolaryngol 1984; 97:83–92.
7. Fischer TJ. Middle ear ciliary defects in Kartagener's syndrome. Pediatrics 1978; 62:443–445.
8. Jabourian Z, Lublin FD, Adler A, et al. Hydrocephalus in Kartagener's syndrome. Ear Nose Throat J 1986; 65:46–54.
9. Nadel HR, Stringer DA, Levinson H, et al. Immotile cilia syndrome: radiologic manifestations. Radiology 1985; 154:651–655.
10. Herzon FS, Murphy S. Normal ciliary ultrastructure in children with Kartagener's syndrome. Ann Otol 1980; 89:81–83.
11. Levinson H, Mindorff CM, Chao J, et al. Pathophysiology of the ciliary motility syndromes. Eur J Respir Dis 1983; 64:102–116.
12. Wacker DF, Howe ML. Middle ear cilia activity as a determinant of tympanostomy tube replacement. Otolaryngol Head Neck Surg 1986; 95:434–437.
13. Mygind N, Pedersen M. Nose-, sinus- and ear-symptoms in 27 patients with primary ciliary dyskinesia. Eur J Respir Dis 1983; 64:96–101.

ACUTE OTITIS MEDIA AND RESPIRATORY VIRUS INFECTION

OLLI RUUSKANEN, M.D., MIKKO AROLA, M.D., ANNE PUTTO-LAURILA, M.D., YUSSI MERTSOLA, M.D., OLLI MEURMAN, M.D., MATTI K. VILJANEN, M.D., and PEKKA HALONEN, M.D.

There is little information about the role of different viruses in the pathogenesis of acute otitis media.[1] This lack of knowledge might be ascribed to technical difficulties in virus isolation and insufficient sensitivity of conventional virus serologic tests in small children. We have extensively used rapid viral antigen detection of the nasopharyngeal mucus and report here the close association of acute otitis media and respiratory virus infections.

PATIENTS AND METHODS

From January 1980 to January 1986, 4,510 patients with acute otitis media were diagnosed in the Department of Pediatrics at Turku University Hospital. The diagnosis was based on the existence of fluid in the middle ear together with signs and symptoms of acute infection. In 3,332 ears the diagnosis was confirmed with positive tympanocentesis. Routine bacterial culture was carried out with all middle ear fluid samples. During the study period 5,092 nasopharyngeal mucus samples from children with respiratory tract symptoms or fever were collected. Samples were studied by immunofluorescence (the first 11 months) or by immunoassay for adenovirus, influenza A and B virus, parainfluenza virus types 1, 2, and 3, and respiratory syncytial virus antigens. The nasopharyngeal mucus was obtained by passing a polyethylene catheter into the nasopharynx through the nostrils and applying gentle suction. The details of immunoassay for viral antigens have been published earlier.[2] A total of 943 samples were positive (18.5 percent). Clinical data were obtained from 884 patients. Earlier we showed that the antigen detection method used detects true infection in respiratory syncytial virus and adenovirus diseases as well as in influenza A virus associated illnesses.

RESULTS

The relation between the monthly occurrence of acute otitis media and respiratory virus infections is shown in Figure 1. Epidemic peaks of respiratory syncytial virus infections in 1981–1982 and 1983–1984 were associated with peaks of acute otitis media. The elevated incidence of acute otitis media in the fall of 1984 and early 1985 possibly was associated with outbreaks of illness with adenovirus, parainfluenza virus, and influenza A vi-

rus. The otitis media peak in 1982–1983 was not clearly associated with any viral infection studied.

Middle ear fluid cultures were taken throughout the study period in the same proportion as the number of diagnosed cases of acute otitis media. The proportion of positive cultures (range, 33 to 80 percent; mean, 56 percent) did not follow the peaks of otitis media or respiratory virus infections. Neither was there any association of different pathogenic bacteria recovered from the middle ear fluid with peaks of otitis media or viral infections.

Thirty-four percent of the patients with verified viral infection had acute otitis media. Most commonly otitis media was recorded in patients with respiratory syncytial virus infections (53 percent). The occurrence of otitis media in other established viral infections was as follows: influenza A, 35 percent; parainfluenza type 3, 30 percent; adenovirus, 26 percent; influenza B, 21 percent; parainfluenza type 1, 19 percent; and parainfluenza type 2, 9 percent.

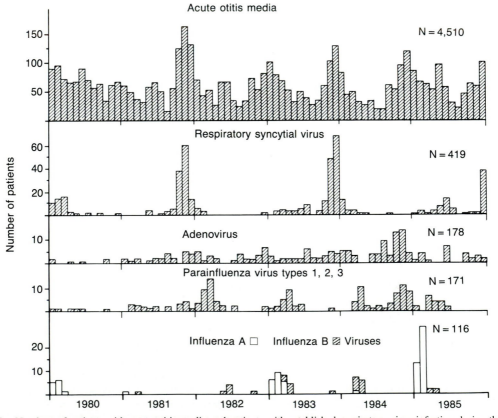

Figure 1 Numbers of patients with acute otitis media and patients with established respiratory virus infection during the 6 year study period.

DISCUSSION

Acute otitis media is one of the most common diseases in early childhood. Bacteria are generally considered to be the causative agents of acute otitis, but there are clinical observations suggesting an association with respiratory virus infections. Surprisingly few studies have been done to prove a viral etiology. This may be the result of minimal findings in studies carried out in the 1960s.[1] With modern virologic techniques three recent studies have demonstrated viruses or viral antigens in the middle ear fluid of 18 to 24 percent of the patients studied.[2-4]

Our study confirms the close association of acute otitis media with respiratory virus infections in a large number of patient specimens. Respiratory syncytial viruses most commonly induce acute otitis media. In this study 53 percent of the 419 patients with respiratory syncytial virus had acute otitis media. Earlier we showed that about half the patients with respiratory syncytial virus infection and otitis media also have the virus in the middle ear fluid.[2] In addition to respiratory syncytial virus, adenoviruses, and influenza A and B viruses have been shown to pose a risk of otitis media.[5]

A feature of this study is that in a large number of the patients with acute otitis media the diagnosis was confirmed by tympanocentesis. In addition the extensive use of the rapid virus antigen detection during the study period identified enough patients with definite viral infections to permit epidemiologic correlations.

Further studies are needed to define the exact role of different respiratory viruses in the etiology of acute and recurrent otitis media in children.[6] It is obvious that viral infections account for some cases of otitis media that do not respond to antibiotic therapy. In the future antiviral drugs may have some role in the prophylaxis of otitis in otitis prone children during epidemics of viral illness.

REFERENCES

1. Klein JO, Teele DW. Isolation of viruses and mycoplasmas from middle ear effusion: a review. Ann Otol Rhinol Laryngol 1976; (Suppl 25, Part 2) 85:140–144.
2. Sarkkinen H, Ruuskanen O, Meurman O, Puhakka H, Virolainen E, Eskola J. Identification of respiratory virus antigens in middle ear fluids of children with acute otitis media. J Infect Dis 1985; 151:444–448.
3. Klein BS, Dollete FR, Yolken RH. The role of respiratory syncytial virus and other viral pathogens in acute otitis media. J Pediatr 1982; 101:16–20.
4. Chonmaitree T, Howie VM, Truant AL. Presence of respiratory viruses in middle ear fluids and nasal wash specimens from children with acute otitis media. Pediatrics 1986; 77:698–702.
5. Henderson FW, Collier AM, Sanyal MA, Watkins JM, Fairclough DL, Clyde WA, Denny FW. A longitudinal study of respiratory viruses and bacteria in the etiology of acute otitis media with effusion. N Engl J Med 1982; 306:1377–1383.
6. Teele DW. Respiratory syncytial virus and otitis media with effusion. J Pediatr 1982; 101:62–63.

EUSTACHIAN TUBE RESPONSE TO PROVOCATIVE RHINOVIRUS CHALLENGE

TIMOTHY P. McBRIDE, M.D., WILLIAM J. DOYLE, Ph.D., FREDERICK G. HAYDEN, M.D., and JACK M. GWALTNEY Jr., M.D.

Because of its frequency and morbidity, otitis media is a serious public health problem. Research suggests that abnormal eustachian tube function plays a major role in the pathogenesis of this disease. Epidemiologic studies have revealed a relationship between upper respiratory infections and the development of otitis media.[1,2] Studies of patients with tympanostomy tubes reveal the presence of temporary eustachian tube dysfunction during upper respiratory illness of undefined etiology.[3]

We used the volunteer model of experimental rhinovirus infection to delineate the relationship between mild upper respiratory infection of defined viral etiology and tubal dysfunction.

MATERIALS AND METHODS

Twelve healthy college age subjects were enrolled in a study designed to document the effect of a nasal rhinovirus infection on function of the eustachian tube. Prior to entry all subjects were evaluated by routine physical and otolaryngologic examination and screened for serum antibody titer to the challenge rhinovirus. Subjects were included if the serum neutralizing antibody titer to the challenge rhinovirus was less than 1:4. No subjects had had otologic disease, allergic disorders, or sinusitis. The test used to detect tubal dysfunction was the nine step test; this test has been well described by both Bluestone and Williams.[3,4]

The study was performed at the University of Virginia in November 1986. Serotype 39 was the rhinovirus used for all subjects. Each subject was given two infecting doses of the virus on the morning of inoculation. Thirty-six hours later the subjects were confined to isolated hotel rooms for 5 days, after which they were released. Twenty-one days after challenge the subjects reported to study personnel for an exit visit.

Eustachian tube function tests and tympanometry were performed 24 hours before challenge, twice daily (9 AM and 4 PM) during the period of confinement, and then 21 days after challenge at an exit visit. During confinement daily symptom diaries were maintained and nasal virus cultures were performed.

RESULTS

Figure 1 summarizes the frequency of eustachian tube obstruction over the time of the study.

Nine subjects shed virus and symptomatically qualified for a cold according to the Jackson illness scale. Three subjects neither shed virus nor had an increase in the antibody titer; these three subjects did not feel symptomatically ill. There appeared to be a clear cut distinction between the two groups 72 hours after inoculation. The obstruction frequency in the infected group, 80 percent, was apparent by the third day and was maintained until the subjects left the hotel. When the subjects reported for exit studies on day 21 after inoculation, tubal function returned to the prechallenge baseline level. Subjects who were uninfected with the exception of one test session on the second day showed little change from the prechallenge baseline level.

The response of the two ears of an individual were relatively symmetrical with respect to observations of tubal function. When the number of observations of left sided obstruction were subtracted from the corresponding values for the right side, the majority of subjects showed a difference of two observations or less. For each of the ears the time of occurrence of a first observation of tubal obstruction was examined. Forty-eight hours after challenge and at the first test session eight ears showed obstruction. By the fourth day after challenge only one ear had a documented first observation of tubal obstruction, suggesting that the onset of obstruction is an early event.

The mean middle ear pressures for the infected and uninfected groups as a function of study day decreased to −90 mm H_2O by the fifth day. As in the tubal function results, the ears had recovered from these abnormal pressures by the exit visit on the twenty-first day. Ears showing early development of underpressure tended to develop more severe underpressures over the period of the study such that

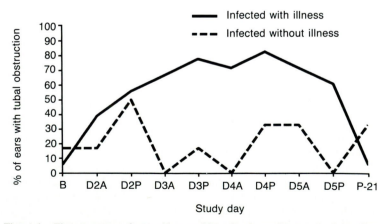

Figure 1 The percentage of ears with eustachian tube obstruction measured as a function of the study day.

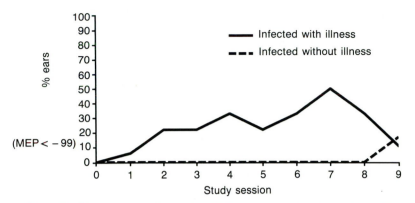

Figure 2   The percentage of ears with middle ear pressure less than −99 mm H_2O measured as a function of the study day.

by the fifth day five ears had underpressures less than −150 mm H_2O.

The percentage of ears with underpressures of less than −99 mm H_2O is shown as a function of the study day in Figure 2. Again there is a clear separation between the infected and uninfected group. Twenty-five percent of the infected group developed moderate underpressures of less than −99 mm H_2O within 60 hours after the viral challenge. This increased to a level of 50 percent by the fifth day, documenting the early development and secondary persistence of moderate underpressures.

DISCUSSION AND CONCLUSIONS

This study shows that a mild rhinovirus upper respiratory infection can be causally associated with the development of eustachian tube obstruction and abnormal middle ear underpressures. These changes occur early in the course of infection and resolve within 3 weeks. Persistent tubal obstruction appears to be a prerequisite to the development of significant middle ear pressures. These results suggest that nasal disease caused by infection with rhinovirus extends to anatomically contiguous structures, such as the eustachian tube. Although at present the mechanism responsible for the tubal dysfunction is unknown, one possibility is local tissue inflammation in or near the tubal orifice. In this regard previous work suggests that the nasopharynx is the site of greatest virus shedding following challenge.[5]

In regard to the role of tubal dysfunction in the pathogenesis of otitis media with effusion, these data suggest that the coincidence reported between upper respiratory infection and otitis media may be causally mediated by associated obstruction of the eustachian tube. Although no episodes of acute otitis media developed during this study, the observed changes in tubal function and middle ear pressure provide evidence that the milieu for overt disease was created. Moreover, in the pediatric population "at risk" for acute otitis media, tubal function is physiologically compromised.[2,4] Thus, the children's system may be less well buffered than that of adults, allowing for more complete expression of the disease.

REFERENCES

1. Henderson FW, Collier AM, Sanyal MA, Watkins JM, Fairclough DL, Clyde WA, Denny FW. A longitudinal study of respiratory virus and bacteria in the etiology of acute otitis media with effusion. N Engl J Med 1982; 306:1377–1383.
2. Tos M, Powlsen G, Borch J. Etiologic factors in secretory otitis. Arch Otolaryngol 1979; 105:582–588.
3. Bluestone CD, Cantekin EI, Beery QC. Effect of inflammation on ventilatory function of the eustachian tube. Laryngoscope 1977; 87:493–507.
4. Williams P. A tympanometric pressure swallow test for assessment of eustachian tube function. Ann Otol Rhinol Laryngol 1975; 84:339–343.
5. Winther B, Gwaltney J, Mygind N, Turner R, Hendley O. Sites of rhinovirus recovery after point inoculation of upper airway. JAMA 1987; 256:1763–1767.

OTITIS MEDIA WITH EFFUSION INDUCED BY HYPERBARIC OXYGEN TREATMENT

TETSUYA SHIMA, M.D., TAKEHIRO HANADA, M.D., FUMIO OHNO, M.D., and MASARU OHYAMA, M.D.

Hyperbaric oxygen treatment has been used in many diseases, such as carbon monoxide poisoning, caisson disease, cerebral infarction, and sudden deafness.[1] Since the advantages of hyperbaric oxygen treatment have been recognized, the number of patients in whom this treatment has been used has increased. However, there are many reports of disorders caused by hyperbaric oxygen treatment.[2] We have encountered otitis media with effusion during or after hyperbaric oxygen therapy. It is considered to result from middle ear barotrauma.

Middle ear barotrauma resulting from sea diving is well known, and several proposals for its classification have been proposed.[3] It has been reported that recovery takes 1 week. However, the barotrauma induced by hyperbaric oxygen treatment seems to be persistent and frequently advances to otitis media with effusion unless adequate treatment is provided. The prognosis in the middle ear barotrauma induced by hyperbaric oxygen treatment is different from that induced by diving. It has been suggested that the difference might be caused by daily exposure to high oxygen pressure. Moreover, it has been speculated that this middle ear disorder might be classified as otitis media with effusion rather than as barotrauma. We studied this type of otitis media induced by hyperbaric oxygen from the viewpoint of eustachian tube function.

MATERIALS AND METHODS

Eighty-five cases (165 ears) were investigated using hyperbaric oxygen treatment. Patients with perforated tympanic membranes were excluded from the study. The subjects consisted of 51 males and 34 females. Their ages varied from 27 to 88 years (mean, 66.5 years).

Of the 85 cases, 77 were patients with cerebral infarction, 5 had suffered sudden deafness, and 3 had facial palsy and other disorders. Hyperbaric oxygen therapy was administered for 5 days a week.

Prior to hyperbaric oxygen therapy, pure tone

audiometry and impedance audiometry were carried out in addition to routine otolaryngologic examinations. According to the type of tympanogram, the subjects were classified into three groups—A, C, and B. Nasopharyngeal examinations and eustachian tube catheterization were also performed in order to study the influence of the underlying diseases on the occurrence of otitis media with effusions. The effect of antithrombosis drugs was also investigated. When remarkable changes were noted in the eardrum after hyperbaric oxygen therapy, puncturing into the tympanic cavity was carried out. The levels of albumin, sodium, potassium and chloride in the effusion were determined biochemically.

The chamber pressure was changed in two different ways (Fig. 1). The subjects were divided into two groups, group A consisting of 55 patients (106 ears) and group B, 30 patients (59 ears). In group A the chamber pressure was increased gradually from 1.0 to 2.0 atmospheres absolute (ATA) for 12 minutes, maintained at 2.0 ATA for 33 minutes, and then decreased gradually to 1.0 ATA for 15 minutes. In group B the pressure was increased gradually from 1.0 to 2.0 ATA for 15 minutes including a 1 minute rest at 1.3 ATA, maintained at

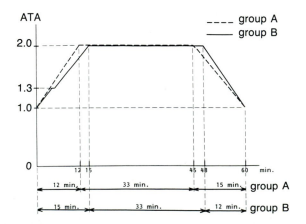

Figure 1 Patterns of chamber pressure in hyperbaric oxygen treatment.

2.0 ATA for 33 minutes, and decreased gradually to 1.0 ATA for 12 minutes.

RESULTS

The types of tympanograms obtained before hyperbaric oxygen treatment are summarized in Figure 2. In group A there were 95 ears with an A type of tympanogram, 8 with the C type, and 3 with the B type. In group B there were 57 ears of the A type and 2 of the C type. There was no case indicating the B type in group B.

The incidence of otitis media-like disorders induced by hyperbaric oxygen treatment is shown in Table 1 and Figure 3. The disorder was observed in 29 ears of the 165 (17.5 percent)—21 ears of the 106 (19.8 percent) in group A and 8 ears of the 59 (13.8 percent) in group B. According to types, the incidence was 14.7 percent (14 of 95) with the A type, 50.0 percent (4 of 8) with the C type, and 100.0 percent (3 of 3) with the B type in group A, and 14.0 percent (8 of 57) with the A type and 0 (0 of 2) with the C type in group B.

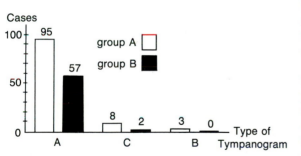

Figure 2 Distribution of ears before hyperbaric oxygen treatment classified by tympanogram types.

The levels of albumin, sodium, potassium, and chloride in the middle ear effusions and sera are shown in Figure 4. The sodium and chloride levels in the effusions were lower than those in the sera, whereas the albumin and potassium levels in the effusions were higher than those in the sera.

No close relationship was found between the incidence of otitis media with effusion and pure tone audiometric findings, nasopharyngeal disorders, or the administration of antithrombosis drugs.

DISCUSSION

Several theories regarding the pathogenesis of otitis media with effusion, have been proposed.[4-6] It has been suggested that the otitis media with effusion induced by hyperbaric oxygen therapy might be a type of otitic barotrauma at the onset. The incidence of middle ear barotrauma in sea diving has been reported to be as high as 25 to 36 percent in beginners and approximately 10 percent in experts.[7] In the present study most of the subjects were elderly patients with cerebral infarction. The incidence of otitis media with effusion was 17.6 percent, which was lower than the minimal incidence in beginner divers. It was thought that the slow change in the chamber pressure, such as 1.0 ATA for 12 to 15 minutes, might account for the low incidence.

The incidence was increased in correlation with the degree of impedance audiometric findings, especially in group A. It was suggested that eustachian tube function influenced the incidence of this kind of otitis media with effusion.[8] It was presumed that the middle ear effusion in this type of otitis media might be produced by a hydrops ex vacuo phenomenon. The middle ear effusion was suggested as being a transudation from vessels. The high potassium

TABLE 1 Incidence of Otitis Media with Effusion Induced by Hyperbaric Oxygen Treatment

Tympanogram (Before Hyperbaric Oxygen)	Incidence		
	Group A	Group B	Total
A	14.7% (14/95)	14.0% (8/57)	14.5% (22/152)
C	50.0% (4/8)	0.0% (0/2)	40.0% (4/10)
B	100.0% (3/3)	—	100.0% (3/3)
Total	19.8% (21/106)	13.8% (8/59)	17.5% (29/165)

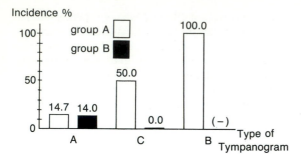

Figure 3 Incidence of otitis media with effusion induced by hyperbaric oxygen treatment classified by tympanogram types.

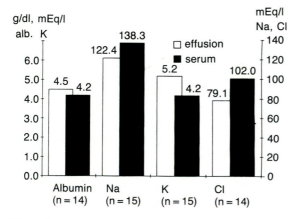

Figure 4 Levels of electrolytes and albumin in middle ear effusions and sera.

level in the effusion seems to support this theory.[9] The intermittent negative pressure might cause otitis media with effusion. Even if the patients could

equilibrate the middle ear pressure in the chamber, oxygen remained in the middle ear cavity at a high level after escaping from the chamber. Because of the absorption of oxygen, a negative pressure is induced in the tympanic cavity. It follows that the equilibration of the pressure might have been required even outside the chamber, which might have resulted in the occurrence of otitis media with effusion. It was speculated that daily exposure to a high oxygen pressure might cause barotrauma, advancing to this type of otitis media with effusion.

REFERENCES

1. Lamm H, Klimpel L. Hyperbare Sauerstofftherapie bei Innenohr- und Vestibularis-stoerungen. HNO 1971; 19:363–369.
2. Ledingham IM, Davidson JK. Hazard in hyperbaric medicine. Br Med J 1969; 3:324–327.
3. Teed RW. Factors producing obstruction of the auditory tube in submarine personnel. U.S. Nav Med Bull 1944; 44:293–306.
4. Senturia BH, Gessert DF, Carr DC, Barrman ES. Studies concerned with tubotympanitis. Ann Otol RhinolLaryngol 1958; 67:440–467.
5. Lim DJ, DeMaria TF. Pathogenesis of otitis media: bacteriology and immunology. Laryngoscope 1982; 92:278–286.
6. Palva T, Lehtinen T, Rinne J. Immune complex in middle ear fluid in chronic secretory otitis media. Ann Otol Rhinol Laryngol 1983; 92:42–44.
7. Bayliss GJA. Aural barotrauma in naval divers. Arch Otolaryngol 1968; 88:49–55.
8. Bluestone CD. Eustachian tube function: physiology, pathophysiology and role of allergy in pathogenesis of otitis media. J Allergy Clin Immunol 1983; 72:242–251.
9. Juhn SK, Huff SJ, Paparella MM. Biochemical analyses of middle ear effusions. Ann Otol Rhinol Laryngol 1971; 80:347–353.

CHRONIC SUPPURATIVE OTITIS MEDIA AS A COMPLICATION OF TYMPANOSTOMY TUBES

LOREN J. BARTELS, M.D., TIMOTHY B. MOLONY, M.D., and CARMELO SARACENO, M.D.

Tympanostomy tube insertion is the most common surgical procedure performed in children under general anesthesia in this country. It is estimated that over 2 million tubes are manufactured each year and placed in over 1 million patients.[1] The majority are children under the age of 8. Postoperative otorrhea develops in 5 to 20 percent. In 1 to 3 percent otorrhea is unresponsive to outpatient therapy.[2,3]

The concept of myringotomy with tympanic membrane intubation, credited to Politzer in the 1860s, was repopularized by Armstrong[4] in 1954. Since then numerous articles have described techniques, results, and complications. Now as in 1860 the most common complication is transient or chronic otorrhea. This article describes a management approach to chronic disease.

Reports of large series indicate that 1 to 3 percent of intubated ears develop chronic drainage emanating from a tympanostomy tube or post-tympanostomy perforation. The group of patients we are discussing is defined by a failure to respond to standard therapy of aural cleansing, ototopical therapy, and oral antibiotic therapy with and without tympanostomy tube removal. Although this problem is not rare, choices in management are not yet clearly defined.[5] As noted by Bluestone,[6] we believe that an initial trial of intensive medical therapy should precede surgical treatment. We present here our patient data, therapeutic results, and an empiric flow chart that we have used in managing these children over the past several years (Fig. 1).

MATERIALS AND METHODS

Subjects

We reviewed the charts of 25 children who developed chronic suppurative otitis media following tympanostomy insertion. The patient population was drawn from children treated by University of South Florida residents and faculty at Tampa General, University Community, and Saint Joseph's Hospitals and the University of South Florida Medical Center. Outpatient and inpatient records were reviewed.

Methods

When the complication of chronic otorrhea developed, each patient was seen and managed by University of South Florida faculty and residents. The ear was cleansed with the aid of a surgical microscope and ototopical medication was prescribed. If otorrhea persisted, culture and antibiotic sensitivity data were obtained. When organism sensitivity data permitted, orally administered antibiotics were prescribed. If pain, fever, postauricular swelling, cranial nerve palsies, or intracranial complications developed, a primary surgical procedure was carried out.

The ototopical medications we used included neomycin, polymyxin B, hydrocortisone drops, or gentamicin ophthalmic drops for sensitive gram negative organisms. The ear was inspected for cholesteatoma and granulation tissue was débrided. Patients were followed closely in the outpatient clinic with frequent visits and débridement as necessary. Many of the patients were evaluated for sinusitis, chronic adenoiditis, nasal airway obstruction, and immune deficiency disorders. If the otorrhea failed to clear in 2 to 4 weeks, the child was hospitalized for intravenous antibiotic therapy. Antibiotic combinations in most cases consisted of cefotaxime and clindamycin or tobramycin and ticarcillin. Depending on the age of the child, the availability of venous access, and the need for microscopic débridement, some children were examined under anesthesia. While the child was anesthetized, a central venous line was placed, tympanostomy tubes were removed, and when necessary granulation tissue was débrided. Material for culture and sensitivity was obtained from the middle ear during examination under anesthesia. Only aerobic cultures were done routinely.

Antibiotic therapy was adjusted on the basis of culture and sensitivity data. Thirty milliliters of 1 percent acetic acid in normal saline was used to irrigate the affected ears every 8 hours in most patients. In many, ototopical medication was continued.

Children whose otorrhea did not improve within 7 days were considered for complete mastoidectomy with myringoplasty. Findings at mastoidectomy determined how much longer intravenous antibiotic therapy was continued: soft bone suggestive of chronic osteitis and extensive granulation tissue was an indication for 6 weeks of intravenous antibiotic therapy. Comparatively minimal findings resulted in continued intravenous antibiotic therapy for another 7 to 10 days.

RESULTS

Twenty-five patients over the 3 years of study met the criteria of having suppurative otitis media following tympanostomy without other complications. A total of 32 ears were included in the study.

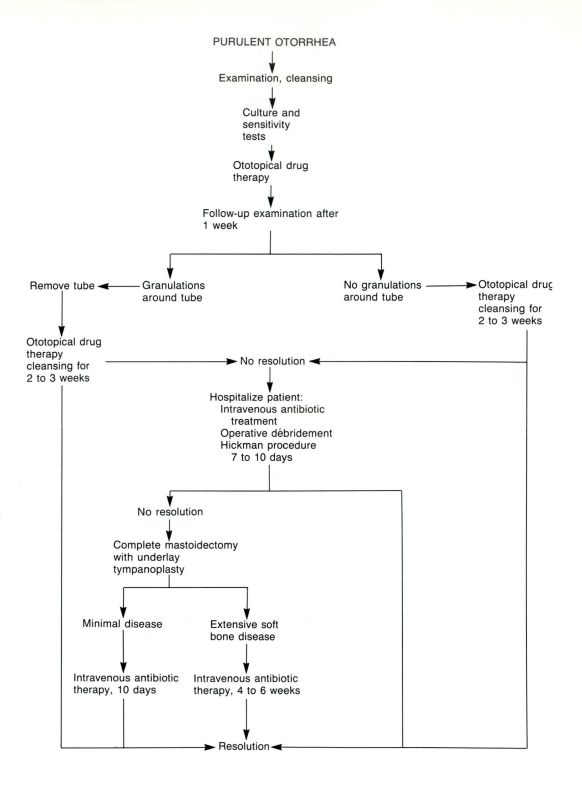

Figure 1   Management schema for patients with chronic post-tympanostomy tube otorrhea.

The 16 males and nine females ranged in age from 1 to 12 years; the average age was 3.7 years. Organisms cultured included gram negative bacilli, *Staphylococcus aureus*, and *Candida albicans* (Table 1). Anerobic cultures were not done routinely. Seventeen ears responded to initial medical therapy; 15 required surgical therapy. There were two relapses in the medical group and two in the surgical group (Table 2). The duration of follow-up varied from 2 months to 3 years; the average follow-up period was 17 months. The duration of hospital stay ranged from 4 days to 6 weeks. All ears treated eventually became dry.

Five of the 25 patients had documented immunologic disorders; these included agammaglobulinemia (1), hypogammaglobulinemia (2), serum IgA deficiency (1), and preleukemia (1). Four of these children underwent mastoidectomy. At surgery the principal author thought that patients in this group were more likely to have soft necrotic bone. Patients with polymicrobial infections appeared more likely to require surgery than those with single organism infections. These two findings will be addressed in another article.

TABLE 1   Organisms Isolated from Chronically Draining Ears

Pseudomonas aeruginosa
Proteus mirabilis, P. vulgaris
Providencia rettgeri
Klebsiella pneumoniae
S. aureus
Citrobacter
Beta streptococcus
Candida albicans

TABLE 2   Medical and Surgical Treatment and Results

	No. of Patients	Relapses
Medical treatment only	17	2
Surgical therapy	15	2
Totals	32	4

DISCUSSION

Chronic suppurative otitis media following tympanostomy is not an uncommon problem in modern otolaryngologic practice. A small but significant percentage of children develop this complication (1 to 3 percent). Previous studies have emphasized the long term risk to the middle and inner ear from chronic suppurative processes.[7] The incidence of cholesteatoma and intratemporal and intracranial complications is higher in these children.[8] Persistent infection may destroy conductive components and depress sensorineural hearing levels.[9]

The development of effective antimicrobial therapy for disease caused by gram negative organisms has changed the initial management from primarily surgical to primarily medical. With appropriate therapy over 50 percent of these patients can be managed without surgery. A small but significant incidence of relapse exists. These cases can be treated with either antibiotics or surgery. In essentially all these children middle ear and mastoid disease can be corrected with adequate therapy. Approximately 20 percent of our patients had significant immunologic disorders, prompting us to evaluate almost all these children for immune competence. Most of the children with immune system defects were under the age of 2 years when encountered.

REFERENCES

1. Bluestone CD. Surgical management of otitis media with effusion: state of the art. In: Lim DJ, Bluestone CD, Klein JO, Nelson JD, eds. Recent advances in otitis media with effusion. Proceedings of the Third International Symposium. Toronto: BC Decker, 1984:293.
2. Luxford WM, Sheehy JL. Myringotomy and ventilation tubes: a report of 1,568 ears. Laryngoscope 1982; 92:1293–1297.
3. McLelland CA. Incidence of complications from the use of tympanostomy tubes. Arch Otolaryngol 1980; 106:96–99.
4. Armstrong BW. A new treatment for chronic otitis media. Arch Otolaryngol 1984; 59:653–654.
5. Goodhill V. Ear disease: deafness and dizziness. New York: Harper & Row, 1979:348.
6. Bluestone CD. Chronic suppurative otitis media: antimicrobial therapy or surgery? Pediatr Ann 1984; 13:417–421.
7. Thomsen J, Jorgensen MD, Bretlau P, et al. Bone resection in chronic otitis media. A histological and ultrastructural study. I. Ossicular necrosis. J Laryngol Otol 1974; 88:975–981.
8. Browning GG. The unsafeness of "safe" ears. J Laryngol Otol 1984; 98:23–26.
9. Paparella MM, Brady DR, Hoel R. Sensorineural hearing loss in chronic otitis media and mastoiditis. Trans Amer Ophthal Otolaryng 1970; 74:108–115.

INCIDENCE OF OBSTETRICAL PATHOLOGY IN SEROUS OTITIS MEDIA BY FETAL LIQUID RETENTION

VINCENT M. BOUTON, M.D.

The etiopathogenesis of serous otitis media seems to involve multiple factors, such as immune mechanisms, the role of bacteria, enzyme activity, eustachian tube dysfunction, and obstetrical conditions at birth. The importance of obstetrical factors has been emphasized by van Cauwenberge[1] in regard to light birth weight and by Lisbonis et al[2] in regard to prematurity. More recently Wells[3] and Pestalozza[4] have raised the possibility of an obstetrical origin in cases of serous otitis media.

Study of obstetrical conditions at birth in cases of serous otitis media has helped in understanding the natural history of this affliction, partly explaining the results published by Giebink and Paparella[5] in regard to the high incidence of mucous effusion in newborn babies. "The highest frequency of mucous effusion had been observed in newborns and is decreasing with age," the authors noted, in addition to describing an immune insufficiency in newborn babies. Our own research has shown that up to 78 percent of the cases studied correspond to the end of a pregnancy or pathologic childbirth conditions.[6]

METHODS AND RESULTS

In 175 cases of serous otitis media with relapse and 75 cases of primary disease without or before relapse, we studied the effects of the end of pregnancy and those at birth up to the time of the newborn cry, without regard to sex and age. We found pathologic obstetrical conditions at birth in 75 percent of the cases (instead of 40 percent, the average incidence in France). The obstetrical disorders observed in 31 cases (18 percent) were divided as follows: prematurity (over 1 month), 6 cases (3.5 percent); fetal disease (e.g., cyanosis, bradycardia, dyspnea at birth), 17 cases (9.8 percent); and pathologic termination of pregnancy (e.g., maternal disease such as hypertension, infections, and nephropathy), 8 cases (4.6 percent). The study also included birth by cesarean section, 63 cases (36 percent); dystocia and forceps delivery, 34 cases (29.6 percent); and umbilical cord complications, 14 cases (8.0 percent). Birth weight is not considered in our statistics because sometimes light weight indicates prematurity and overweight may be a cause of dystocia, requiring forceps delivery, and is often associated with a large head circumference. The incidence exceeds 75 percent because of possible complications, such as cesarean section with fetal damage. Twenty-five percent of the cases did not involve obstetrical disorders.

These results suggest that the birth disorders might influence the development of serous otitis media. In order to have other means for comparison, we decided to conduct a second study of 75 cases of primary serous otitis media occurring without relapse or before relapse (regardless of sex and age). The results are presented in Table 1.

Thus we found practically the same incidence of obstetrical disorder (73 percent versus 75 percent) with and without relapse. This result, confirming the earlier findings, convinces us about the possibility of obstetrical disorder in the pathogenesis of serous otitis media. Looking more closely at both studies, we noted that the largest difference is in the incidence of cesarean section, which is higher in the first study pertaining to serous otitis with relapse than in the second study of serous otitis without or before relapse (Table 2).

The results clearly demonstrate that two con-

TABLE 1 Primary Serous Otitis Media Occurring Without Relapse or Before Relapse

Obstetrical Disorder	Percentage
Prematurity over 1 month (fetal disease, pathologic termination of pregnancy)	27
Birth by cesarean section	25.3
Dystocia of all types and forceps delivery	18.6
Umbilical cord complications	10.6
Normal birth	27

TABLE 2 Possibility of Obstetrical Disorder in the Pathogenesis of Serous Otitis Media

Possible Obstetrical Disorder	Relapse	No Relapse
Prematurity	3.4%	2.6%
Fetal disorder	9.7%	6.6%
Pathologic termination of pregnancy	4.5%	16 %
Cesarean section	36.0%	25.3%
Dystocia plus forceps delivery	19.4%	18.6%
Umbilical cord complications	8.0%	10.6%

ditions at birth are associated with an increased incidence of serous otitis media with and without relapse—birth by cesarean section and fetal disorders. The figures in dystocia and forceps deliveries are similar as well as are those in cases of umbilical complications and prematurity.

These findings lead us to think that we have a partial answer to the question of what criteria are needed to forecast the development of serous otitis media. It seems possible that birth by cesarean section and fetal disorders are among the criteria. A reasonable physiopathologic explanation could be insufficient middle ear ventilation at the time of the birth cry. The expiratory air flow is suddenly pushed through the nasopharynx by the high blood pressure in the head and neck and opening of the nasopharynx and the mouth, allowing the eustachian tube to open. Thus insufficient ventilation of the middle ear cavity may occur as a result of poor quality of the birth cry, which can be too short, to weak (even absent), or too late. The result is fetal mesenchymal retention, which creates a serous middle ear effusion.

Tympanometric measurements in 100 newborn babies (younger than 8 days) were performed without regard to the conditions of birth and confirm our etiopathogenic hypothesis. Under otoscopic control we used an automatic tympanograph. This procedure had been tested for 3 years in 1,000 cases with more than 85 percent reliability. Eleven of the recordings were difficult to interpret, 64 were normal, and 25 showed abnormalities. A normal recording includes a normal curve or twin peak graphs, normal amplitude, peak in the right position, and positive stapes reflexes at 80 and 100 db at three sound frequencies (500, 1,000, and 2,000 Hz). The anomalies included low amplitudes, flat graphs, a latent period before the peak, and absence of the stapes reflex. Two anomalies were necessary to label the response pathologic or abnormal. Among these 25 abnormal recordings we found 21 cases of obstetrical disease and 4 normal births. That is, in over 80 percent of the cases there was positive correlation between the birth conditions and the occurrence of fetal mesenchyme in the middle ear as checked by typanometry. Because of the reliability of the material (85 percent), we can say, in regard to abnormal graphs in newborns, that there is in 71.4 percent of the cases a possibility of serous otitis media occurring as a result of fetal liquid retention when delivery occurred under pathologic conditions. This figure needs to be compared with the normal graphs obtained in 48 normal births and in the 16 births under pathologic conditions. However, pathologic birth conditions do not always produce a flat graph or anomalies, probably because of efficient ventilation of the middle ear at the time of the cry. Presently we are beginning a study on newborn babies who die during the first year of life to study further the effect of liquid effusion in the middle ear cavities, comparing the conditions of birth and age. In some cases we have already found mucous effusions in the ear cavities in dead newborns. The results of this study will be published.

REFERENCES

1. van Cauwenberge P. Otitis media with effusion. Acta Otorhinolaryngol Belg 1982; 36:1.
2. Lisbonis JM, Block M, et al. Approche des facteurs perinataux de risque otitique. Soc ORL Litt Médit 1984.
3. Wells F. Symposium, Jerusalem, 1985. Personal communication.
4. Pestalozza G. Symposium, Jerusalem, 1985. Personal Communication.
5. Giebink S, Paparella M. Epidemiology of otitis media with effusion in children. Arch Otolaryngol 1982; 108:563-566.
6. Bouton VM. Pathologie de la naissance et otites séreuses. Soc Franc ORL, Congrès 1985:561-569.

QUANTITATIVE CYTOLOGIC AND HISTOLOGIC CHANGES IN THE MIDDLE EAR AFTER INJECTION OF NONTYPABLE *HAEMOPHILUS INFLUENZAE* ENDOTOXIN

THOMAS F. DeMARIA, Ph.D., TATSUJI YAMAGUCHI, M.D., and DAVID J. LIM, M.D.

Previous reports from this laboratory indicated that endotoxin derived from gram negative bacteria may play an important role in the pathogenesis of otitis media with effusion.[1] Nonviable *Haemophilus influenzae* or endotoxin purified from this organism has been shown to produce severe inflammatory changes in the middle ear,[2] and endotoxin has been found in a large percentage of sterile middle ear effusions.[3-6] The purpose of the present study was to investigate and quantitate the morphologic changes that occur in the middle ear after injection of *H. influenzae* endotoxin.

MATERIALS AND METHODS

Forty-eight healthy chinchillas (*Chinchilla laniger*, 350 to 670 g) were used.

Endotoxin Injection

The endotoxin used in this study was prepared from *H. influenzae* (nontypable biotype II) according to the method of Westphal and Jann.[7] The left superior bullae in six groups of chinchillas were injected with concentrations of endotoxin ranging from 0.001 to 100 µg per ear. All endotoxin solutions were prepared with sterile pyrogen free, phosphate buffered saline. The uninfected right ears served as controls. Two animals from each group were killed at days 1, 4, 7, and 14 after inoculation, and middle ear effusion specimens were collected at that time. When an effusion was not present, the bulla was washed by aspiration with 0.5 ml of RPMI 1640 culture medium (M.A. Bioproducts) containing 10 percent fetal calf serum.

Cytologic Analysis

Cellular analysis and culture of effusions or bulla washes were performed as described in an earlier report.[2] Briefly, 50 µl samples were centrifuged for 10 minutes in a Shandon Southern cytocentrifuge, air dried, and fixed in 95 percent methanol. Slides of each effusion and bulla wash were made for Gram staining and differential counts.

Morphologic Study

Eight chinchillas (two per sample time) were used in the morphologic investigation for each of the six concentrations of endotoxin. The chinchillas were anesthetized intraperitoneally by the use of sodium pentobarbital. After the effusions were collected, the temporal bones were fixed immediately with 2.5 percent glutaraldehyde buffered with 0.05 M sodium cacodylate (pH 7.2 to 7.4) for initial fixation (24 hours). They were then further dissected and decalcified with 0.1 M ethylenediaminetetraacetate (EDTA) in 2 percent glutaraldehyde (pH 7.2 to 7.3) for 3 to 6 weeks. EDTA solutions were changed every 1 to 3 days. The specimens were embedded in glycol methacrylate, and 5 µm sections were made with glass knives and stained with hematoxylin and eosin.

For quantitative analysis of histologic changes, the middle ear mucosa and the inferior bulla, including the tympanic orifice of the eustachian tube, were examined as described in a previous report.[2]

RESULTS

In most of the animals otoscopic findings were normal during the experiments. A few exhibited a slight translucency with a niveau line behind the tympanic membrane, but the tympanic membranes returned to normal within 1 week after inoculation.

In this experiment three middle ear effusions were obtained by tympanocentesis at days 1 and 4. The cells in these effusions were exclusively polymorphonuclear leukocytes and macrophages and exhibited a distinctly biphasic response, as previously reported by this laboratory.[1,2] A definite predominance of polymorphonuclear leukocytes was evident up to 4 days after injection. By 1 week after injection the numbers of polymorphonuclear leukocytes and macrophages were approximately equal. At 14 days after injection polymorphonuclear leukocytes were no longer evident. A slight increase in the number of lymphocytes occurred at days 4 through 7.

Although there were no marked otoscopic findings, histologic investigation of all specimens showed that there was some degree of inflammation of varying severity in the middle ear mucosa.

The thickness of the submucosal connective tissue increased (more in the experimental animals than in the controls) at day 1 and then gradually decreased during the experiment. The most thickened mucosa was induced by 100 μg of endotoxin at day 4. At all time periods the extent of thickening was not proportional to the dose of endotoxin.

The percentage of capillary area increased from day 1 through day 7 and then decreased. As observed in regard to the changes in thickness of the submucosal connective tissue, the increase in capillary area was not proportional to the dose of endotoxin. The greatest increase was observed with the 1.0 mg dose 4 days after injection.

The cellular density in the connective tissue was also examined. By 1 day after injection, a cellular infiltrate consisting of polymorphonuclear leukocytes, macrophages, and a few lymphocytes was observed at each dosage level (Fig. 1A). The degree of inflammation was the same, irrespective of dose. The capillaries were dilated, and bleeding and edema were found in the connective tissue.

The polymorphonuclear leukocyte response in the submucosa connective tissue was dramatically reduced by day 4 (Fig. 1B). Polymorphonuclear leukocytes were present only in the connective tissue from animals injected with 1.0 μg or more of endotoxin. Macrophages were the predominant cell type, and there was a significant increase in the number of lymphocytes at doses greater than 1.0 μg. Bleeding and capillary dilation were still predominant. Many osteoblasts could also be seen.

By 7 days after injection macrophages were the predominant type of cell in the connective tissue at all the doses of endotoxin. Lymphocytes were present by this time in the animals injected with doses of less than 1.0 μg of endotoxin (Fig. 1C). A very limited number of polymorphonuclear leukocytes were still present in the animals given 100 μg of endotoxin.

By 14 days after injection macrophages were still the predominant cell in the middle ear connective tissue (Fig. 1D). Polymorphonuclear leukocytes were evident, together with an increased number of lymphocytes at the lowest dose (0.001 μg).

At day 14 the connective tissue was thin compared with that at days 1 to 7. Bleeding and new bone formation were observed in over half the ears.

There was no increase in the number of secretory cells in the experimental ears as compared with those in the control ears. No pathologic changes were seen in the epithelial linings of the eustachian tubes in the experiments. However, macrophages and polymorphonuclear leukocytes were present in the tubal lumen. No increase in the number of osteoblasts was observed during the course of this experiment.

DISCUSSION

The histologic evidence from the present study indicates that as little as 1 ng of endotoxin purified from nontypable *H. influenzae* induces severe inflammatory changes in the middle ear, almost identical to those produced by the injection of nonviable *H. influenzae* reported previously from this laboratory.[2] The thickness of the submucosal connective tissue, cell density, and capillary permeability increased dramatically in all the experimental animals.

Capillary destruction and serum transudation are the probable major pathogenic factors in experimental endotoxin induced otitis media, as originally proposed by DeMaria et al.[1] In a recent study Nonomura et al[6] examined endotoxin induced otitis media in the guinea pig and stated that endotoxin induced transudation disturbed the mucociliary transport system, thereby promoting effusion formation.

Endotoxin is a potent and extremely biologically active material, capable of interaction with complement and components of the clotting system, and can effect the release of various vasoactive amines and other mediators of inflammation by direct interaction with macrophages, polymorphonuclear leukocytes, and other types of cells.[8] The exact mechanism responsible for the changes observed in the present study is not known.

It has been clearly established by numerous studies that endotoxin is present in middle ear effusions from patients with otitis media at concentrations in the range of those used in this study.

The single injection regimen used in this study

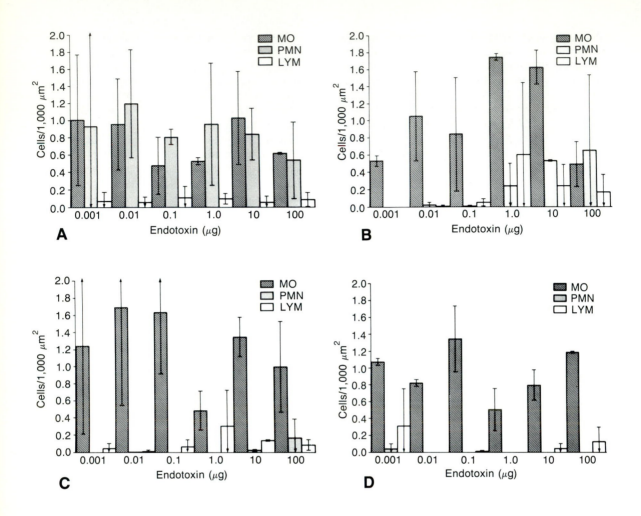

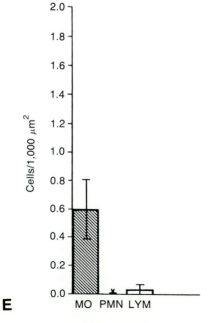

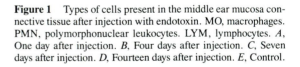

Figure 1 Types of cells present in the middle ear mucosa connective tissue after injection with endotoxin. MO, macrophages. PMN, polymorphonuclear leukocytes. LYM, lymphocytes. *A*, One day after injection. *B*, Four days after injection. *C*, Seven days after injection. *D*, Fourteen days after injection. *E*, Control.

produced a relatively short term serous type of otitis. One can speculate that with repetitive injections or concurrent tubal dysfunction, trapping endotoxin in the middle ear, inflammation could be sustained indefinitely.

This study was supported in part by grants from the NINCDS/NIH (NS08854) and the Deafness Research Foundation. Dr. Yamaguchi was on leave from Sapporo University Medical School.

REFERENCES

1. DeMaria TF, Briggs BR, Lim DJ, Okazaki N. Experimental otitis media with effusion following middle ear inoculation of nonviable *H. influenzae*. Ann Otol Rhinol Laryngol 1984; 93:52–56.
2. Okazaki N, DeMaria TF, Briggs BR, Lim DJ. Experimental otitis media with effusion induced by nonviable *Hemophilus influenzae*: cytologic and histologic study. Am J Otolaryngol 1984; 5:80–92.
3. Bernstein JM, Praino MD, Neter E. Detection of endotoxin in ear specimens from patients with chronic otitis media by means of limulus amebocyte lysate test. Can J Microbiol 1980; 26:546–548.
4. DeMaria TF, Prior RB, Briggs BR, Lim DJ, Birck HG. Endotoxin in middle ear effusions from patients with chronic otitis media effusion. J Clin Microbiol 1984; 20:15–17.
5. Iino Y, Kaneko Y, Takasaka T. Endotoxin in middle ear effusions tested with limulus assay. Acta Otolaryngol (Stockh) 1985; 100:42–50.
6. Nonomura N, Nakano Y, Satoh Y, Fujioka O, Niijima H, Fujita M. Otitis media with effusion following inoculation of *Haemophilus influenzae* type b endotoxin. Arch Otorhinolaryngol 1986; 243:31–35.
7. Westphal O, Jann K. Methods in carbohydrate chemistry. Vol 5. New York: Academic Press, 1965.
8. Morrison DC, Ulevitch RJ. The effects of bacterial endotoxin on host mediation systems. Am J Pathol 1978; 93:527–617.

MICROBIOLOGY

STANDARDIZED METHOD FOR QUANTITATIVE ESTIMATION OF BACTERIA IN MIDDLE EAR EFFUSION

LARS-ERIC STENFORS, M.D., Ph.D., SIMO RÄISÄNEN, M.D., Ph.D., and RIITTA YLITALO, M.D.

In most middle ear infections bacteria play a central role. The bacterium that occurs most frequently in acute otitis media, *Streptococcus pneumoniae*, can be isolated from 30 to 50 percent of middle ear effusions, followed in frequency by *Haemophilus influenzae* (15 to 20 percent).[1,2] *Branhamella catarrhalis* is found in about 10 percent.[3,4] Group A streptococci and *Staphylococcus aureus* are also said to cause acute otitis media.[5]

Secretory otitis media formerly was believed to be a noninfectious disease, with sterile effusion material filling the middle ear cleft.[6] However, most recent reports also describe positive bacteriologic findings in secretory otitis media, the microorganisms being among those just mentioned.[5]

In chronic suppurative otitis media with a continuously draining ear, the bacterial flora is quite different from that in acute and secretory otitis media. Here, *Streptococcus epidermidis*, *Pseudomonas aeruginosa*, *Proteus* species and gram negative rods are the predominating microorganisms.[7]

In treating otitis media early identification and quantification of the bacteria involved would seem to be self-evident. The isolation of large numbers of organisms is of greater clinical significance than the isolation of fewer bacteria of a certain species. However, bacteriologic examination of middle ear effusion material is a source of much controversy, mainly because of the lack of standardized techniques for sampling, handling, processing, and staining.

The purpose of the present work was to develop new ways to study middle ear effusions by microscopy in a standardized way. It also established a method for the rapid quantification of bacteria in effusion material.

MATERIAL AND METHODS

Patients suffering from acute otitis media, secretory otitis media, mucopurulent otitis media, and chronic suppurative otitis media composed the study material.

The external auditory canal was gently cleansed of wax and detritus and then washed with a 70 percent alcoholic solution for 2 minutes, after which myringotomy was performed in the anterior inferior quadrant. A cannula was inserted into the middle ear cavity without touching the canal walls, and effusion material was aspirated into a 1 ml syringe. The material was immediately transferred to the clinical laboratory for further processing.

The effusion material was homogenized by squeezing it through successively finer cannulas and then again aspirated into the syringe. A small sample (0.02 ml) of effusion material was flushed onto a clean glass slide, spread over it uniformly using another glass slide, and then allowed to dry. The smear was fixed in 70 percent ethanol for 1 minute, allowed to dry, and then stained with acridine orange for 2 minutes. The smears were examined by use of a fluorescence microscope (Leitz SM-Lux).

Theoretical Background for Quantifying Bacteria in Smears

As the dimensions of the microscope were known, the volume of the effusion cylinder corresponding to the circular field of the microscope could be calculated (Table 1). The volume of the effusion cylinder examined is $V_o = \pi r^2 h$, where r is the radius of the microscope field and h the thickness of the smear. At $h = 0.03$ mm all bacteria could

TABLE 1 Dimensions of the Microscope Used and Volumes of the Effusion Cylinders Examined

Magnification	Radius (mm)	Area (sq mm)	Thickness (mm)	Volume (ml)
250×	0.36	0.407	0.03 + 0.01	1.2×10^{-5}
400×	0.225	0.159	0.03 + 0.01	4.7×10^{-6}
1000×	0.09	0.0254	0.03 + 0.01	7.6×10^{-7}

be seen distinctly over the entire field without extra focusing.

The number of bacteria (n) per milliliter effusion material can be calculated as

$$n/\text{ml} = \frac{\text{number of bacteria in the microscopic field}}{\text{volume of the effusion cylinder in ml}}$$

With the same microscope and the same optics, r is constant. Provided the smears of the effusion materials are always processed in the same manner, the height (h) of the effusion cylinder also can be regarded as constant.

RESULTS

Figure 1 shows the correlation between the number of bacteria per microscopic field and the number of bacteria per milliliter of effusion material when the microscope is operated at 250 ×, 400 ×, and 1,000 × and the thickness of the smear is 0.03 ± 0.01 mm. If 10^5 bacteria per milliliter effusion material is considered as representing purulent otitis media, then one to two bacteria per 0.03 mm thick microscopic field should be seen in the sample when using 250 × magnification. At 400 × magnification the test is not so sensitive as when a 250 × magnification is used. On the other hand, if 10^7 bacteria per milliliter effusion material is considered to define purulent otitis media, three to five bacteria per microscopic field at 400 × magnification must be seen.

For draining ears with a perforation in the tympanic membrane, a bacterial content in the effusion material ranging from 10^8 to 10^{10} bacteria per milliliter was calculated. In contrast, sticky glue effusion material contained no or only very few bacteria (maximum, 10^5 bacteria per milliliter). In mucopurulent effusion material with an intact drum, the content was 10^6 to 10^8 bacteria per milliliter. In strictly serous effusion material we could not detect any bacteria at all.

DISCUSSION

The method for quantification of bacteria in middle ear effusion material just outlined has many advantages. As early as 15 to 20 minutes after sampling the aspirated material, the results are available. In a previous study it was demonstrated that staining with acridine orange was superior to Gram staining for detecting bacteria from middle ear material, while Giemsa stain gave more information about the inflammatory cells involved.[8] We fully agree with that opinion. Furthermore, the present technique is simple to carry out and does not require any expensive equipment. Today the fluorescence microscope is a standard item among the everyday equipment in most clinical laboratories.

It must be emphasized, however, that acridine orange staining provides only presumptive information about the presence and identification of microorganisms that may be present in the specimen. All smear results should be confirmed by culture.

Acridine orange does not distinguish between

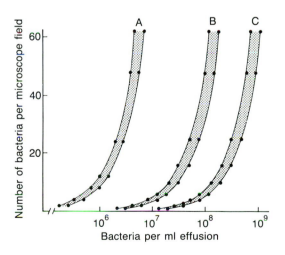

Figure 1 Estimation of quantity of bacteria in effusion fluid by microscopy. *A*, 250 × magnification; *B*, 400 ×; *C*, 1,000 ×.

gram positive and gram negative organisms. Approximately 10^4 to 10^5 bacteria per milliliter are required for detection by this method.

Sticky glue effusion material presented no or only a few bacteria per milliliter of effusion material. This means that secretory otitis media with a sticky glue effusion merely contained colony forming units for detection by this method. With the method outlined it is thus possible to accurately distinguish secretory otitis media from mucopurulent otitis media. This seems extremely important with respect to the treatment of these two conditions. The former, with no bacteria in the middle ear effusion, needs no antibiotic treatment, whereas in the latter case, with a bacterial content of 10^6 to 10^8 per milliliter, antibiotic treatment would seem to be self-evident.

REFERENCES

1. Howie VM, Ploussard JH, Lester RL Jr. Otitis media: a clinical and bacteriological correlation. Pediatrics 1970; 45:29–35.

2. Kamme C, Lundgren K, Mårdh P-A. The aetiology of acute otitis media in children. Occurrence of bacteria, L forms of bacteria and mycoplasma in the middle ear exudate, nasopharynx and throat. Scand J Infect Dis 1971; 3:217–223.

3. Klein JO. Microbiology of otitis media. Ann Otol Rhinol Laryngol 1980; (Suppl 68):98–101.

4. Coffey JD Jr, Booth HN, Martin AD. Otitis media in practice of pediatrics. Bacteriological and clinical observations. Pediatrics 1966; 38:25–32.

5. Qvarnberg Y. Acute otitis media. A prospective clinical study of myringotomy and antimicrobial treatment. Acta Otolaryngol (Stockh) 1981; Suppl 375.

6. van Cauwenberge P. Otitis media with effusion. Functional morphology and physiopathology of the structures involved. Acta Otorhinolaryngol Belg 1982; 36:5–240.

7. Jonsson L, Schwan A, Thomander L, Fabian P. Aerobic and anaerobic bacteria in chronic suppurative otitis media. A quantitative study. Acta Otolaryngol (Stockh) 1986; 102:410–414.

8. van Cauwenberge P, Rysselaere M, Waelkens B. Bacteriological and cytological findings according to the macroscopic characteristics of the middle ear effusions. Auris Nasus Larynx (Tokyo) 1985; 12(Suppl I):73–76.

SEMIQUANTIFICATION OF PATHOGENIC BACTERIA IN MIDDLE EAR EFFUSION AND IN NASOPHARYNX IN CHILDREN WITH SEROUS OTITIS MEDIA

ULF E.J. RENVALL, M.D., Ph.D., Per G.B. GRANSTRÖM, M.D., D.D.S., Ph.D., NILS G. KARLSSON, M.D., Ph.D., L. LIND, M.D., SVEN A.S. OLLING, M.D., and KRISTIAN P.L. ROOS, M.D., Ph.D.

The treatment of secretory otitis media is still a matter of controversy. Different kinds of treatment have been advocated over the years. An earlier generation of otolaryngologists used the Politzer maneuver, and the immediate hearing improvement that follows this procedure surely must have encouraged the doctor just as much as the patient. In the 1960s and 1970s oral decongestants seemed for a while to be the treatment of choice in secretory otitis media. Today these methods are used only infrequently. Since the early research of Sadé et al[1] we know that the middle ear effusion is not always sterile; during the past decade this has been confirmed repeatedly. Naturally this information has made otolaryngologists consider the use of antibiotics, and promising results have, in fact, been presented.[2-4] Therefore, the question whether antibiotic treatment should be recommended in secretory otitis media seems to be under serious discussion more often now than previously. The extent of microbial growth from middle ear effusions has been found to vary in different studies.[5-10]

MATERIAL AND METHODS

In the present study 70 children with secretory otitis media, ages 9 months to 8 years, were investigated. Only cases with a duration of secretory otitis media of more than 3 months were included. In all patients scheduled for grommet insertion, myringotomy was performed under general anesthesia. Before the myringotomy, cultures were taken from the tympanic membrane. After paracentesis the secretion was sucked into a 2 ml syringe without a piston with the syringe connected to an aspirator. After aspiration the piston was reintroduced and part of the fluid ejected was used for cytologic analysis. The remaining fluid was used for culture. The syringe with the remaining fluid was sealed and sent immediately for bacteriologic analysis.

Samples from the nasopharynx, the tympanic membrane, and the middle ear were cultivated aerobically on Colombia blood agar, on strepto agar containing human blood, on gentian violet with inhibitors of gram negative rods, and on chocolate agar. Anaerobically the samples were cultivated on Colombia blood agar and on chocolate agar with horse serum. Samples from the tympanic membrane and the middle ear were also inoculated in broth to detect small amounts of bacteria. The aerobic plates were incubated for 24 and 48 hours at 37° C and the anaerobic specimens for 96 hours. The broth was subcultivated after 24 hours in 37° C. The bacterial growths on the plates were counted and typed by conventional techniques.

RESULTS

Positive cultures were found in 25 percent of the middle ear fluid specimens. Tympanic membrane culture revealed no upper respiratory pathogenic bacteria, but in 47 of 117 ears diphtheroides or *Staphylococcus* was found, but these microbes were not regarded as upper respiratory pathogens. Cultures of the nasopharynx were positive in 81 percent of the cases. The microbes demonstrated in this location were *Haemophilus influenzae*, *Branhamella catarrhalis*, and *Streptococcus pneumoniae*. In the middle ear *Haemophilus influenzae*, was found in 76 percent, *Branhamella catarrhalis* in 14 percent, and *Streptococcus pneumoniae* in 10 percent (Table 1). Positive cultures exceeding 100 colony forming

units were found in 11 percent, and all these contained only one bacterium, *Haemophilus influenzae*. In the nasopharynx we found cultures with more than 100 colony forming units in 55 percent. In our study no beta lactamase producing *Haemophilus influenzae* were found. However, 15 *Branhamella catarrhalis* isolates produced beta lactamase, and two were isolated from the middle ear.

DISCUSSION

How should these results be interpreted? Do they supply any further knowledge about the indication for antibiotic treatment? Is there the same need for antibiotic treatment in the 25 percent group of patients as in the 11 percent group (scarce versus dense bacterial growth)?

It may be of some interest to relate this last problem to the prevailing attitudes concerning the treatment of tonsillitis. If only a few *Streptococcus* colonies are cultivated from the tonsils, this indicates a carrier state without infection, and treatment with antibiotics is not indicated.[11] Whether this way of looking at the problem can be applied when *Haemophilus influenzae*, *Branhamella catarrhalis*, and *Streptococcus pneumoniae* are found in the middle ear we cannot say as yet. However, we do not believe that our data justify the routine administration of antibiotics in secretory otitis media. Cultures from the middle ear are not normally available when the treatment decision has to be made. It is tempting of course to cultivate from the nasopharynx. However, some 80 percent of the patients have positive cultures, and 55 percent have more than 100 colony forming units in specimens from the nasopharynx, whereas only 25 percent have a positive culture from the middle ear and only 11 percent have more than 100 colony forming units. Consequently it is not easy to predict the ear in which antibiotic treatment might be more useful. If antibiotic treatment were to be recommended generally for secretory otitis media of more than 3 months' duration, considerable overtreatment, to our mind,

TABLE 1 Results from Cultures from 29 of 117 Middle Ears (25 Percent) and from the Nasopharynx in 58 of 70 Children (81 Percent) with Positive Cultures

	Middle Ear	Nasopharynx		Middle Ear	Nasopharynx
HI*	22/29 (76%)	25/58 (43%)	HI*	13/117 (11%)	21/25 (84%)
BC	4/29 (14%)	31/58 (53%)	BC	0	20/31 (65%)
SP	3/29 (10%)	36/58 (62%)	PN	0	10/36 (28%)

* HI, *Haemophilus influenzae*. BC, *Branhamella catarrhalis*. SP, *Streptococcus pneumoniae*.

would take place if one's aim were to combat the middle ear infection. Identification of the minority of patients with a solid growth of middle ear bacteria might be one way to identify patients in whom the indication for antibiotic treatment is clear.

REFERENCES

1. Sadé J, Carr C, Senturia B. Middle ear effusion produced experimentally in dogs. Ann Otol Rhinol Laryngol 1959; 68.
2. Sundberg L, Cederberg Å, Edén T, Ernstson S. Bacteriology in secretory otitis media. Acta Otolaryngol (Stockh) 1981; Suppl 384.
3. Healy GB. Antimicrobial therapy of chronic otitis media with effusion. In: Lim DJ, Bluestone CD, Klein JO, Nelson JD, eds. Recent advances in otitis media with effusion. Proceedings of the Third International Symposium. Toronto: BC Decker, 1984:285.
4. Ernstson S, Anari M. Cefaclor in the treatment of otitis media with effusion. Acta Otolaryngol (Stockh) 1985; Suppl 424.
5. Yea S, Lim D, Lang W, Birk G. Chronic middle ear effusion. Arch Otolaryngol 1975; 101.
6. Healy G, Teele D. The Microbiology of chronic middle ear effusion in children. Laryngoscope 1977; 87.
7. Giebink S, Mills E, Huff J, Edelman C, Weber M, Juhn S, Quie P. The microbiology of serous and mucoid otitis media. Pediatrics 1979; 63.
8. Sundberg L, Cederberg Å, Edén T, Ernstson S. Bacteriology in secretory otitis media. Acta Otolaryngol (Stockh) 1981; Suppl 384.
9. Giebink S, Carlson B, Juhn S, Heatherington S. Contributions of bacteria and polymorphonuclear leukocytes to middle ear inflammation in chronic otitis media with effusion. In: Lim DJ, Bluestone CD, Klein JO, Nelson JD, eds. Recent advances in otitis media with effusion. Proceedings of the Third International Symposium. Toronto: BC Decker, 1984:125.
10. van Cauwenberge P, Rysselaire M, Waelkens B. Bacteriological and cytological findings according to the macroscopic characteristics of the middle ear. Auris Nasus Larynx (Tokyo) 1985; 12 (Suppl 1):73–76.
11. Roos K. The diagnostic value of symptoms and signs in acute tonsillitis in children over the age of 10 and in adults. Scand J Infect Dis 1985; 17:259–267.

BIOTYPES OF *HAEMOPHILUS INFLUENZAE* ISOLATED FROM MIDDLE EAR FLUID OF CHILDREN WITH ACUTE OTITIS MEDIA WITH EFFUSION

WILLIAM A. HENDRICKSE, M.D., M.R.C.P., SHARON SHELTON, B.S., HELEN KUSMIESZ, R.N., and JOHN D. NELSON, M.D.

Haemophilus influenzae is second only to *Streptococcus pneumoniae* as a leading cause of acute otitis media. In our most recent study of acute otitis media conducted between the fall of 1985 and the fall of 1986, *H. influenzae* was isolated from 29 percent of 218 specimens of middle ear fluid obtained from 175 children; 24 percent were nontypable isolates and the remaining 5 percent were capsular serotype b.

Kilian[1] described a classification whereby species within the genus *Haemophilus* are subdivided into a number of biotypes on the basis of three biochemical reactions: indole production, urease activity, and ornithine decarboxylase activity.

The biotypes of *H. influenzae* have shown a relationship to the source of isolation, and there is also a correlation between biotype and capsular serotype. In the normal host invasive disease such as meningitis or epiglottitis is almost exclusively caused by serotype b organisms, the majority of which are biotype I, a much smaller number being either biotype II or III. In young children *H. influenzae* may be part of the constant bacterial flora of the healthy upper respiratory tract. The majority of such strains are serologically nontypable and of multiple biotypes with a predominance of biotypes II and III.

Previous reports of the biotypes of *H. influenzae* associated with otitis media have not described a consistent pattern of biotype distribution.

DeMaria et al[2] determined the biotypes of *H. influenzae* in the middle ear fluid and nasopharynx of 33 children undergoing myringotomy for chronic otitis media with effusion. They found that biotypes II and III were most frequent—53 and 23 percent, respectively. This finding is similar to the biotype distribution in the normal upper respiratory tract. Barenkamp et al[3] described similar findings in the middle ear fluid of 23 children with acute otitis media. However, the numbers in each biotype were small.

Kilian[1] biotyped 29 strains of *H. influenzae* associated with acute otitis media, 27 of which were nontypable. These 27 strains were almost equally distributed among biotypes I, II, and V. In another study by Oberhofer and Back[4] the majority of the 21 isolates were biotypes II and VI. This contrasted with data published by Long et al[5] in which 60 percent of the 14 isolates were biotype I. Almost every biotype except IV has been described as being predominant in acute otitis media.

One explanation proposed for the variation described in biotypes associated with acute otitis media has been that different biotypes may predominate in different geographic areas.[2] However, one factor is common to all these reports: the numbers are relatively small. This might account for the variation in results. Against this background we undertook biotype analysis of all our isolates of *H. influenzae* obtained from the middle ear fluid of children with acute otitis media. Our isolates had been obtained at various times between 1965 and 1986.

METHODS

Isolates obtained before 1975 had been lyophylized and stored at room temperature; those obtained since 1975 were stored at $-70°$ C in a solution of tryptose phosphate without dextrose and with 5 percent glycerol.

Identification of *H. influenzae* was undertaken by standard methods. The serotype was determined by direct slide agglutination with polyvalent and monovalent serum (Difco Laboratories). Biochemical characterization and determination of biotypes were done in batches using the Minitek kit commercially available from BBL Microbiology Systems.[6] Beta lactamase production was determined using a chromogenic cephalosporin spot test.[7]

RESULTS

There were 148 isolates of *H. influenzae*. Fifty-one percent were isolated between 1985 and 1986, 36 percent between 1982 and 1983, and the remaining 13 percent between 1965 and 1975. Twenty-three isolates, 15 percent of the total, were serotype b organisms; all but one of these were isolated after 1982. The remaining 125 isolates, 85 percent of the total, were serologically nontypable.

Fifty-two percent of the serotype b isolates were biotype I, with 35 percent biotype II and 13 percent biotype III.

These data contrast with the biotype distribution of our 125 isolates of nontypable strains of *H. influenzae* in which biotype II predominated, accounting for 41 percent of the total, and biotype III, 31 percent, with biotypes V, I, and VI accounting for 16, 10, and 2 percent, respectively (Fig. 1).

No beta-lactamase producing strains were isolated prior to 1975. Five of the 22 isolates (23 percent) of *H. influenzae* type b obtained between 1982 and 1986 were beta-lactamase positive, four were biotype I, and one was biotype III. Nine of the 107 nontypable strains isolated between 1982 and 1986 were beta-lactamase positive (8 percent of the total), and six of the nine were biotype III, despite the fact that biotype II was more common.

The distribution of biotypes of nontypable *H. influenzae* and *H. influenzae* type b in the four seasons was examined and the data analyzed as a percentage of the total of each species (*H. influenzae* type b or nontypable) in each season, for two 12 month periods in 1982–1983 and 1985–1986): nontypable *H. influenzae* biotypes II or III were the

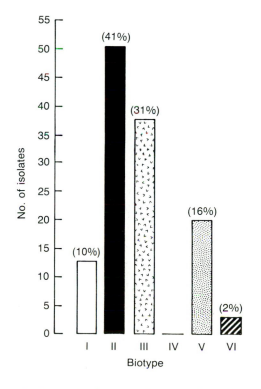

Figure 1   Biotype distribution of 125 isolates of *H. influenzae* from the middle ear fluid of children with acute otitis media with effusion (1965–1986).

most common in each season. In winter through spring, isolates were fairly evenly distributed between biotypes II (20 to 34 percent) and III (30 to 34 percent) and in smaller numbers between types V (25 to 29 percent) and I (20 to 26 percent). In the summer months biotype III accounted for 8 of 11 (73 percent) isolates and in the winter biotype II accounted for 11 of 23 (48 percent) of the total for that season.

There were only 15 isolates of *H. influenzae* type b during the two 12 month periods (seven biotype I, five biotype II, and three biotype III). None was isolated in the fall. Biotype I predominated in the winter and spring (four of six and three of five, respectively), but no biotype I isolates were obtained in the summer when biotype II accounted for three of four isolates.

We combined our data for nontypable isolates of *H. influenzae* with those of Long et al[5] and Barenkamp et al.[3] The combined data gives a total of 165 isolates, with biotype II accounting for just under 40 percent of the total, biotype III 28 percent, and biotypes I and V about 15 percent (Fig. 2).

DISCUSSION

The distribution of *H. influenzae* type b among biotypes I, II, and III, with a predominance of biotype I, is in keeping with the results of previous studies.

Nontypable strains of *H. influenzae* constitute part of the normal flora of the upper respiratory tract. These strains are most frequently biotypes II and III. It is postulated that they become pathogenic under certain conditions, such as during an acute viral upper respiratory tract infection. When such an infection causes abnormal eustachian tube function and inadequate drainage of the middle ear cavity, acute otitis media may result. The predominance of biotypes II and III in the middle ear fluid of children with acute otitis media in our study is in keeping with the results reported by Barenkamp et al.[3] We combined our data with those of two previous reports in which sufficient clinical information was given to ascertain that the isolates were from the middle ear fluid of children with acute otitis media. The combined data give a biotype profile similar to that observed in the healthy upper respiratory tract and in the middle ear fluid of children with chronic otitis media with effusion.[2]

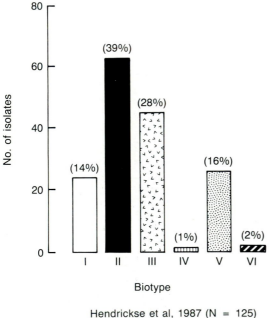

Figure 2 Biotypes of 165 isolates of *H. influenzae* (nontypable) in acute otitis media with effusion.

REFERENCES

1. Kilian M. A taxonomic study of the genus *Haemophilus*, with the proposal of a new species. J Gen Microbiol 1976; 93:9–69.
2. DeMaria TF, Lim DJ, Barnishan J, et al. Biotypes of serologically nontypable *Haemophilus influenzae* isolated from the middle ears and nasopharynges of patients with otitis media with effusion. J Clin Microbiol 1984; 20:1102–1104.
3. Barenkamp SJ, Munson RS, Granoff DM. Outer membrane protein and biotype analysis of pathogenic nontypable *Haemophilus influenzae*. Infect Immunol 1982; 36:535–540.
4. Oberhofer TR, Back AE. Biotypes of *Haemophilus* encountered in clinical laboratories. J Clin Microbiol 1979; 10:168–174.
5. Long SS, Teter MJ, Gilligan PH. Biotype of *Haemophilus influenzae*: correlation with virulence and ampicillin resistance. J Infect Dis 1983; 147:800–806.
6. Back AE, Oberhofer TR. Use of the Minitek system for biotyping *Haemophilus* species. J Clin Microbiol 1978; 7:312–313.
7. Montgomery K, Raymundo JR, Drew WL. Chromogenic cephalosporin spot test to detect beta-lactamase in clinically significant bacteria. J Clin Microbiol 1979; 9:205–207.

FREQUENCY OF FIMBRIATE ISOLATES OF NONTYPABLE *HAEMOPHILUS INFLUENZAE* FROM THE MIDDLE EARS AND NASOPHARYNGES OF PATIENTS WITH CHRONIC OTITIS MEDIA

LAUREN O. BAKALETZ, Ph.D., BARBARA TALLAN, M.S., TONI M. HOEPF, M.S., THOMAS F. DeMARIA, Ph.D., and DAVID J. LIM, M.D.

Bacterial fimbriae are defined as nonflagellar proteinaceous surface appendages that do not participate in the transfer of bacterial or viral nucleic acids. They are known to be critical to the successful adherence of many pathogens to host cells, which is considered to be the first step in the infectious process.[1] Although it has been shown by several investigators that nontypable *Haemophilus influenzae* is generally more adherent than type b strains,[2,3] to date the possession of fimbriae by nontypable isolates has been infrequently reported.[4,5]

Because of its importance as a causative agent in both acute and chronic otitis media, we investigated the frequency of fimbriation for minimally passaged middle ear and nasopharyngeal isolates of nontypable *H. influenzae*. In this study isolates from cases of chronic otitis media with effusion were assessed for the possession of fimbriae, both grossly by capacity to hemagglutinate and electron microscopically by a negative staining technique. In addition, we addressed the issue of whether the degree of fimbriation was influenced by biotype, site of isolation, type of effusion in the ear, or capacity to hemagglutinate and how fimbriation affected the capacity to adhere to chinchilla ciliated tracheal epithelium or to human oropharyngeal cells.

MATERIALS AND METHODS

Specimens

Middle ear effusions and nasopharyngeal samples were obtained from patients undergoing routine myringotomy and tube insertion for chronic otitis media with effusion at the Children's Hospital in Columbus, Ohio. All clinical specimens were held on ice until cultured for bacteria on blood and chocolate agars within 3 hours after surgery. Presumptive and definitive identification of nontyp-

able *H. influenzae* was made by conventional methods, as previously described.[6]

Negative Staining

Two percent ammonium molybdate–2 percent ammonium acetate in distilled water—was used to negatively stain bacteria. Organisms were taken from an 18 to 24 hour chocolate agar plate within one to four passages on artificial medium and suspended in a minimal amount of distilled water. Two drops of the bacterial suspension was mixed with an equal amount of stain, and a Formvar coated copper grid was floated on the surface for 5 minutes. Following staining, grids were blotted, allowed to air dry, and viewed immediately. One to 200 randomly chosen bacterial cells were scanned and rated for the presence or absence of fimbriae.

Hemagglutination

Fresh human erythrocytes were used to assess the capacity of these isolates to hemagglutinate. Erythrocytes were collected, washed twice in 0.15 M phosphate buffered saline (pH 7.4), and suspended to 5 percent (v/v) in phosphate buffered saline. The strength of hemagglutination was assessed within 2 days after blood collection by mixing 2 drops of erythrocytes with several colonies from an 18 to 24 hour chocolate agar plate and rocking for 5 minutes. The strength of the reaction was rated from 0 to 4+.

Adherence to Chinchilla Tracheal Epithelium

Adherence to tracheal epithelium was assessed as previously reported.[7] Briefly, chinchilla half-tracheas were embedded in a perfusion chamber modeled after the original design of Gabridge and Hoglund.[8] Colonies of nontypable *H. influenzae* from 18 to 24 hour chocolate agar plates were gently suspended to approximately 10^8 cfu per milliliter, and 2 ml was added to the perfusion chambers. The bacterial suspension was rocked back and forth through the tracheal lumen in a carbon dioxide incubator for 1 hour prior to homogenization of the tracheal tissue and determination of adherent cfu per average tracheal length.

Adherence to Human Oropharyngeal Cells

Oropharyngeal cells were harvested by gentle scraping of the soft palate in front of the uvula and suspension in cold phosphate buffered saline (0.01 M, pH 7.2). Cells were vortexed into separate clumps and collected over a 12 μm pore size polycarbonate membrane. Cells from several volunteers were pooled and adjusted to a density of 2 to 8 $\times$ 10^4 cells per milliliter of phosphate buffered saline. Bacterial suspensions were prepared as already described to a density of 10^8 to 10^9 cfu per milliliter as confirmed by plate count. Equal volumes of oropharyngeal cells and bacteria were mixed and incubated for 90 minutes at 37° C in a reciprocal shaking water bath. Controls consisted of oropharyngeal cells and sterile phosphate buffered saline. Cells with adherent bacteria were then collected over a 12 μm polycarbonate membrane and washed free of nonadherent bacteria with sterile phosphate buffered saline. Cells were harvested into a minimal amount of phosphate buffered saline, cytocentrifuged onto a glass slide, fixed with ETOH, and Gram stained. Determination of adherence was carried out by direct microscopic count of 25 nonoverlapping oropharyngeal cells per slide selected randomly and representing the four quadrants of the cytocentrifuged area of the slide. Only gram-negative bacilli resembling *H. influenzae* were counted. A total of 100 oropharyngeal cells were counted for each isolate per trial and a total of three replicates were studied. Only data collected from those trials in which control preparations rated less than three of 25 oropharyngeal cells with five or more adherent bacteria per cell were included.

Statistical Analysis

Determination of the correlation between a high degree of fimbriation and biotype, effusion type, site of isolation, or strength of hemagglutination was done by the chi square test. Comparison of adherence of nasopharyngeal cells and middle ear effusion statistic isolates to tracheal epithelium was carried out by individual Student t-tests. Differences in capacity to adhere to human oropharyngeal cells were determined by analysis of variance and the Student-Newman-Keuls multiple comparison procedure. A value of p $\leq$ 0.05 was chosen as the level of significance.

RESULTS

Examination of negatively stained preparations by transmission electron microscopy revealed that 100 percent of the isolates were capable of producing fimbriae. The percentage of cells bearing fimbriae within each isolate varied from less than 10 up to 100 percent. Fimbriae were either peritrichous or bipolar in distribution and were approximately 5.5 nm in width (range, 2.4 to 9.2 nm; Fig. 1).

When tested for the capacity to hemagglutinate erythrocytes, isolates varied in the strength of the hemagglutination reaction, and no correlation was found between a high degree of fimbriation and strength of the hemagglutination. In addition, a high degree of fimbriation did not correlate with either site of isolation, biotype, or effusion type.

When comparing the one isolate recovered that was both highly fimbriated and that gave a 4+ hemagglutination reaction with one that was minimally fimbriated and gave no or a weak hemagglutination, we found no significant difference in the capacity to adhere to chinchilla tracheal epithelium (Table 1).

The relative adherence of 10 isolates from five randomly selected nasopharynx–middle ear effusion pairs (isolated from the same patient) to chinchilla tracheal epithelium is illustrated in Table 2. An enhanced capacity to adhere did not consistently correlate with site of isolation, nor in the example of isolates 297 and 1714, in which the two were very different in terms of degree of fimbriation, was adherence related to the percentage of cells bearing fimbriae.

Adherence to human oropharyngeal cells by seven nontypable *H. influenzae* isolates, which varied in their fimbriate status and site of isolation, demonstrated no difference among six of the seven tested for either average number of adherent bacteria per 25 oropharyngeal cells or percentage of cells with five or more adherent bacteria (Fig. 2). One isolate (1128) adhered in numbers indistinguishable from background levels of normal flora resembling *H. influenzae*.

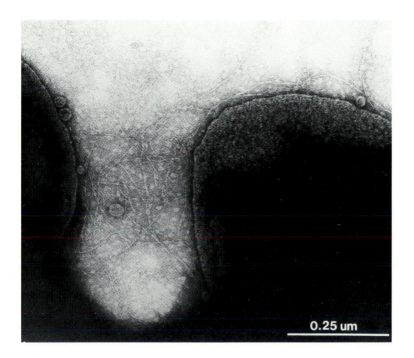

Figure 1 Transmission electron micrograph of a negatively stained fimbriated isolate of nontypable *H. influenzae*.

TABLE 1 Influence of Percentage of Fimbriation and Capacity to Hemagglutinate on Adherence

Isolate No.	Site of Isolation (Effusion Type)	Percentage of Cells Bearing Fimbriae	Capacity to Hemagglutinate	Average No. Adherent cfu/Half-trachea $\times$ 10^5 ($\pm$ SEM; n = 5)
1712	MEE (Se)	75%	+ + + +	5.3 $\pm$ 0.51
1657	MEE (Se)	< 10%	−/+	6.3 $\pm$ 0.50

TABLE 2 Relative Adherence of NP-MEE Pairs of Nontypable *H. Influenzae* Isolates to Chinchilla Tracheal Epithelium

Isolate No.	Site of Isolation*	Percentage of Cells Bearing Fimbriae	Average No. of Adherent cfu/Half-trachea $\times$ 10^6 ($\pm$ SEM; n = 5)
266	NP	25	1.9 $\pm$ 0.96
1590	MEE	< 10	1.2 $\pm$ 0.29
1848	NP	< 10	0.29 $\pm$ 0.05
1848	MEE	< 10	1.7 $\pm$ 0.59*
1885	NP	60–75	0.87 $\pm$ 0.25
1885	MEE	20	1.9 $\pm$ 1.1
214	NP	< 10	1.6 $\pm$ 0.28
1371	MEE	< 10	2.1 $\pm$ 1.3
297	NP	10	2.8 $\pm$ 0.62*
1714	MEE	90	1.1 $\pm$ 0.12

NP, nasopharynx. MEE, middle ear effusion.
* Significant difference.

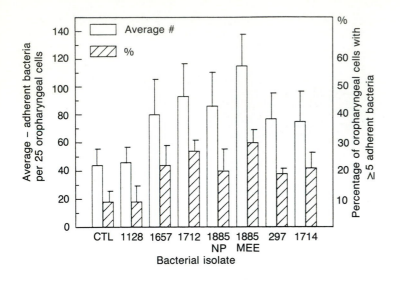

Figure 2 Adherence of various fimbriated clinical nontypable *H. influenzae* isolates to human oropharyngeal cells.

DISCUSSION

Our data have shown that all isolates of nontypable *H. influenzae* recovered from the nasopharynx and middle ear effusion of patients with chronic otitis media were fimbriated. The percentage of cells bearing fimbriae within each was highly variable but did not correlate with site of isolation, biotype, effusion type, or strength of hemagglutination.

Since several investigators have reported a strong correlation between the capacity to hemagglutinate and adherence for type b *H. influenzae*, we investigated this phenomenon for nontypable *H. influenzae* using the one isolate we had that was both highly fimbriated and that gave a 4+ hemagglutination reaction and another that was minimally fimbriated and gave no or a weak hemagglutination reaction. We found no difference in the capacity to adhere to chinchilla tracheal epithelium. Although this evidence is not conclusive, we had no indication on the basis of this pair that the capacity to hemagglutinate alone significantly affected adherence in this system. Since we were limited by the lack of additional highly fimbriated, strongly hemagglutinating isolates but had several nasopharynx–middle ear effusion pairs, we shifted our emphasis to an assessment of whether the site from which an organism was isolated had an influence on adherence. Using 10 isolates from five randomly selected pairs, we found no significant difference in adherence to tracheal organ culture based on site of isolation. The only significantly different values noted did not consistently relate to site.

In addition, we found no influence of site of isolation or degree of fimbriation on adherence to isolated human oropharyngeal cells with the seven isolates tested. One isolate, however, did show extreme variability in adherence, which may be due to its state of fimbriation upon retrieval from liquid nitrogen. Studies are under way to determine what effect, if any, this phenomenon has on adherence within any individual strain.

Although our data, to date, indicate that the degree of fimbriation does not significantly affect adherence per se, the possession of fimbriae appears to be important to this organism and may simply provide the mechanism by which the organism colonizes the nasopharynx, after which other pathogenic mechanisms or differences in immune status of the host determine whether otitis media will develop. Regardless of the exact mechanism of pathogenesis, the presence of these highly accessible appendages on most, if not all, isolates of nontypable *H. influenzae* makes them a highly likely antigen for use in the development of vaccines.

This study is supported in part by a grant from The Deafness Research Foundation.

REFERENCES

1. Beachey EH. Bacterial adherence: adhesin-receptor interactions mediating the attachment of bacteria to mucosal surfaces. J Infect Dis 1981; 143:325–345.
2. Lampe RM, Manson EO Jr, Kaplan SL, Umstead CL, Yow MD, Feigin RD. Adherence of *Haemophilus influenzae* to buccal epithelial cells. Infect Immunol 1982; 35:166–172.
3. Porras O, Svanborg-Eden C, Lagergard T, Hanson LA. Method for testing adherence of *Haemophilus influenzae* to human buccal epithelial cells. Eur J Clin Microbiol 1985; 4:310–315.
4. Apicella MA, Shero M, Dudas KC, Stack RR, Klohs W, La-

Scolea LJ, Murphy TF, Mylotte JM. Fimbriation of *Haemophilus* species isolated from the respiratory tract of adults. J Infect Dis 1984; 150:40–43.

5. Guerina NG, Langermann S, Schoolnik GK, Kessler TW, Goldmann DA. Purification and characterization of *Haemophilus influenzae* pili and their structural and serological relatedness to *Escherichia coli* P and mannose sensitive pili. J Exp Med 1985; 161:145–159.

6. DeMaria TF, Lim DJ, Barnishan J, Ayers LW, Birck HG. Bio-

types of serologically nontypable *Haemophilus influenzae* from the middle ears and nasopharynges of patients with otitis media with effusion. J Clin Microbiol 1984; 20:1102–1104.

7. Bakaletz LO, Rheins MS. A whole-organ perfusion model of *Bordetella pertussis* adherence to mouse tracheal epithelium. In Vitro Cell Devel Biol 1985; 21:314–320.

8. Gabridge MG, Hoglund LE. *Mycoplasma pneumoniae* infection of intact guinea pig tracheas cultured in a unique matrix-embed/perfusion system. In Vitro 1981; 17:847–858.

NASOPHARYNGEAL CARRIAGE OF PNEUMOCOCCI RESISTANT TO TRIMETHOPRIM-SULFA AND/OR BETA-LACTAM ANTIBIOTICS AMONG CHILDREN IN DAY CARE

FREDERICK W. HENDERSON, M.D. and PETER H. GILLIGAN, Ph.D.

Trimethoprim-sulfamethoxazole, erythromycin-sulfisoxazole, amoxicillin-clavulanate, and cefaclor have become frequently used alternatives to amoxicillin for the treatment of otitis media and sinusitis since strains of *Haemophilus influenzae* and *Branhamella catarrhalis* resistant to ampicillin have become prevalent. *Streptococcus pneumoniae*, however, remains the most common bacterial cause of infections of the paranasal sinuses and middle ear cleft. Although antibiotic sensitivity patterns of ampicillin susceptible and resistant strains of *H. influenzae* and *B. catarrhalis* have been examined in several studies, the susceptibility of pneumococci to trimethoprim-sulfamethoxazole, erythromycin-sulfisoxazole, amoxicillin-clavulanate, and cefaclor has not been monitored closely since the introduction of these antimicrobials for use in clinical practice. To address this problem, we studied antimicrobial susceptibility patterns of strains of *S. pneumoniae* cultured from the nasopharynx in children followed longitudinally in a research day care center between 1978 and 1985.

MATERIALS AND METHODS

The children studied attended the research day care program of the Frank Porter Graham Child De-

velopment Center in Chapel Hill, North Carolina. A cohort of 10 to 12 infants 2 to 3 months of age is admitted to the day care project each year; children are not admitted to the program after early infancy. Children attend the center 8 hours a day, 5 days a week, 50 weeks a year; they return home each evening and on weekends. Children recruited for participation are expected to remain in the program continuously until the age of kindergarten entry. For the present study we were interested in possible changes in patterns of antibiotic susceptibility in *S. pneumoniae* in relation to the introduction of trimethoprim-sulfamethoxazole for use in the treatment of otitis media in the day care population (introduced in 1979). Therefore, we identified all children enrolled in the day care center between July 1, 1978, and June 30, 1984, and studied pneumococci recovered from these children between July 1, 1978, and June 30, 1985.

Upper respiratory secretions were cultured for bacteria at the onset of all respiratory illnesses throughout the study period. Between July 1, 1978, and June 30, 1980, and between January 1, 1983, and June 30, 1985, surveillance cultures were taken each month independent of the occurrence of illness. Respiratory secretions were sampled by throat swab and saline nasal lavage. All pneumococcal isolates were serotyped by the quellung reaction using typing sera from Statens Seruminstitute, Copenhagen. Antibiotic susceptibility testing was performed with isolates that had been stored at $-70°$ C since their isolation.

Chronologic records were kept of nasopharyngeal cultures performed on each child. If the same serotype of *S. pneumoniae* was recovered from upper respiratory secretions in 2 of 3 consecutive months, the child was defined as having a period of "established" carriage of that organism. An episode of carriage was considered terminated after a 90 day interval with negative cultures for the serotype. We attempted to recover at least one isolate during each period of nasopharyngeal colonization occurring before a child's third birthday for antibiotic susceptibility testing.

All isolates were screened for susceptibility to trimethoprim-sulfamethoxazole and penicillin by the Kirby-Bauer technique using trimethoprim-sulfamethoxazole and oxacillin discs. Minimal inhibitory concentrations for penicillin G, amoxicillin-clavulanate, erythromycin, cefaclor, cefuroxime, trimethoprim, sulfamethoxazole, and trimethoprim-sulfamethoxazole (1:19 ratio) were determined by an agar dilution technique.

RESULTS

Seventy-two children entered the longitudinal day care program between July 1, 1978, and June 30, 1984. These children had 209 episodes of "established" nasopharyngeal colonization with *S. pneumoniae*. Antibiotic susceptibility testing was performed with at least one isolate from 189 episodes of carriage (90.4 percent). The average number of periods of carriage studied was 2.9 per child. Twenty-one additional random pneumococcal isolates that had been carried for shorter periods of time were also studied. Ten serotypes were represented in the episodes of carriage examined and serotypes 6, 14, 19, and 23 accounted for 85.7 percent of these.

Isolates from 63 episodes of carriage (30 percent) manifested reduced susceptibility to trimethoprim-sulfamethoxazole. Forty-one children carried the 63 strains of pneumococci with reduced susceptibility to trimethoprim-sulfamethoxazole. Reduced susceptibility to trimethoprim-sulfamethoxazole was common in serotypes 6 (52 percent), 14 (52 percent), and 23 (28 percent) but not in type 19 isolates (3 percent). There was a close correspondence between results obtained by disc diffusion screening and agar dilution minimal inhibitory concentration susceptibility testing. Isolates with zones of growth inhibition greater than 18 mm in diameter

around a trimethoprim-sulfamethoxazole disc (1.25/23.75; trimethoprim-sulfamethoxazole) were susceptible to the drug with a median minimal inhibitory concentration of 0.12/2.38 mcg per milliliter and a minimal inhibitory concentration-90 of 0.25/4.75 mcg per milliliter. Organisms with zones of growth inhibition between 9 and 17 mm had a median minimal inhibitory concentration of 1.0/19.0 mcg per milliliter and a minimal inhibitory concentration-90 of 4.0/76.0 mcg per milliliter. When there was no zone of growth inhibition around the trimethoprim-sulfamethoxazole disc, the median minimal inhibitory concentration was 4.0/76.0 mcg per milliliter and the minimal inhibitory concentration-90 was 8.0/152.0 mcg per milliliter. Isolates with 9 to 17 mm zones retained susceptibility to trimethoprim but were resistant to sulfamethoxazole (minimal inhibitory concentration greater than 152 mcg per milliliter). Organisms with no zone of growth inhibition in the Kirby-Bauer assay were resistant to both trimethoprim (median minimal inhibitory concentration, 4.0 mcg per milliliter) and sulfamethoxazole.

Trimethoprim-sulfamethoxazole was first used for the treatment of otitis media in the day care population in July 1979. It was administered to 57 percent of the study children at some time during the first 3 years of life. The first pneumococcal isolates with reduced susceptibility to trimethoprim-sulfamethoxazole were recovered in November 1980. Only 5.3 percent of the episodes of pneumococcal carriage studied before December 31, 1980 (N=57), included isolates with reduced susceptibility to trimethoprim-sulfamethoxazole, whereas 39.2 percent of the episodes of colonization studied between January 1, 1981, and June 30, 1985 (N=153), included trimethoprim-sulfamethoxazole resistant organisms.

Of the 106 pneumococcal isolates subjected to minimal inhibitory concentration testing to cefaclor, the median minimal inhibitory concentration was 1.0 mcg per milliliter and the minimal inhibitory concentration-90 was 2.0 mcg per milliliter. Organisms with penicillin G minimal inhibitory concentrations in this range would be categorized as being resistant to penicillin.

Twenty-five episodes of pneumococcal colonization (11.9 percent) included isolates with reduced susceptibility (minimal inhibitory concentration greater than or equal to 0.125 mcg per milliliter) to either penicillin G, amoxicillin, or cefuroxime; 15 of these isolates were relatively resistant to penicillin G or amoxicillin (7.1 percent), whereas all manifested reduced susceptibility to cefuroxime. Twenty-two children had carried the 25 strains with reduced susceptibility to beta lactam antibiotics.

DISCUSSION

Recent research has established day care attendance as an important factor influencing the epidemiology of many infectious diseases.[1-4] The data in this report suggest that day care attendance and patterns of antibiotic use in children in day care may influence the prevalence of antibiotic resistant microorganisms as well.

The prevalence of relative resistance to penicillin G and amoxicillin among isolates from the day care children was slightly higher (7.1 percent) than that usually observed in studies of isolates from hospitalized children in the general population.[5,6] Reduced susceptibility to cefuroxime was observed in 11.9 percent of the isolates, including all those with reduced susceptibility to penicillin G or amoxicillin. Cefaclor was much less active in vitro against all pneumococci studied (median minimal inhibitory concentration, 1.0 mcg per milliliter) than penicillin G, amoxicillin, or cefuroxime, and cefaclor minimal inhibitory concentrations were unrelated to oxacillin screening results. Oxacillin screening was effective in the identification of organisms with reduced susceptibility to cefuroxime.

Resistance to trimethoprim-sulfamethoxazole emerged soon after this drug was introduced for use as an alternative therapy for otitis media in the day care center. Within 2 years the prevalence of trimethoprim-sulfamethoxazole resistance among nasopharyngeal isolates of *S. pneumoniae* had increased from 5 percent to more than 30 percent; for certain serotypes the prevalence of trimethoprim-sulfamethoxazole resistance exceeded 50 percent. The prevalence of trimethoprim-sulfamethoxazole resistance in pneumococci is usually considered to be approximately 5 percent.[7,8] Organisms with 9 to 17 mm zones of growth inhibition by trimethoprim-sulfamethoxazole in the Kirby-Bauer assay (fully susceptible organisms had zones of growth inhibition greater than 18 mm) had developed resistance to sulfamethoxazole (minimal inhibitory concentration greater than 152 mcg per milliliter) but had retained susceptibility to trimethoprim. Organisms with no zone of growth inhibition by the trimethoprim-sulfamethoxazole disc were resistant to both sulfamethoxazole and trimethoprim.

For the clinician managing treatment resistant otitis media in the child with a history of day care attendance, these data suggest that infection with antibiotic resistant pneumococci must be considered in the etiologic differential diagnosis. From a public health perspective, the data suggest that the day care environment may be a focus where selection and spread of antibiotic resistant microorganisms could be a greater problem than has been perceived.

This chapter is part of an article originally published in the Journal of Infectious Diseases. Henderson FW, Gilligan PH, Wait K, Goff DA. Nasopharyngeal carriage of antibiotic-resistant pneumococci by children in group day care. J Infect Dis 1988; 157:256–263.

REFERENCES

1. Henderson FW, Giebink GS. Otitis media among children in day care: epidemiology and pathogenesis. Rev Infect Dis 1986; 8:533–538.
2. Daum RS, Granoff DM, Gilsdorf J, Murphy T, Osterholm MT. *Haemophilus influenzae* type b infections in day care attendees: implications for management. Rev Infect Dis 1986; 8:558–567.
3. Hadler SC, McFarland L. Hepatitis in day care centers: epidemiology and prevention. Rev Infect Dis 1986; 8:548–557.
4. Pickering LK, Bartlett AV, Woodward WE. Acute infectious diarrhea among children and day care: epidemiology and control. Rev Infect Dis 1986; 8:539–547.
5. Willett LD, Dillon HC, Gray BM. Penicillin-intermediate pneumococci in a children's hospital. Am J Dis Child 1985; 139:1054–1057.
6. Anderson KC, Maurer MJ, Dajani AS. Pneumococci relatively resistant to penicillin: a prevalence survey in children. J Pediatr 1980; 97:939–941.
7. Bach MC, Finland M, Gold O, Wilcox C. Susceptibility of recently isolated pathogenic bacteria to trimethoprim and sulfamethoxazole separately and combined. J Infect Dis 1973; 128:S508–S533.
8. Forsgren A, Walder M. Activity of common antibiotics against *Branhamella catarrhalis, Haemophilus influenzae,* pneumococci, group A streptococci, and *Staphylococcus aureus* in 1983. Acta Otolaryngol (Stockh) 1984; Suppl 407:43–49.

BACTERIOLOGY IN OTITIS MEDIA WITH EFFUSION: ARE *STAPHYLOCOCCUS AUREUS* AND *STAPHYLOCOCCUS EPIDERMIDIS* CAUSATIVE AGENTS?

YUICHI KURONO, M.D., KAZUHIRO TOMONAGA, M.D., and GORO MOGI, M.D.

Recent studies have demonstrated the presence of bacteria in high percentages of middle ear effusions. Although *Haemophilus influenzae, Streptococcus pneumoniae*, and *Branhamella catarrhalis* are commonly considered pathogens of otitis media with effusion, it is still controversial whether *Staphylococcus aureus* and *Staphylococcus epidermidis*, both frequently detected in middle ear effusions, are causative agents in otitis media with effusion. Riding et al[1] considered *S. aureus* and *S. epidermidis* as contaminants from the external ear canal, because these organisms were found frequently in both the external ear canal and the middle ear. On the other hand, Bernstein and Ogra[2] observed specific antibodies against *S. epidermidis* in the effusions in cases of otitis media with effusion and suggested that this organism may also be a pathogen. To clarify this problem, further study is needed in regard to the bacteriologic analysis of otitis media with effusion.

In the present study, further bacterial identification was attempted by determining the minimal inhibitory concentrations (MIC) of antibiotics. Bacterial isolates from the external ear canal, middle ear effusions, and the nasopharynx were compared. The possibility of *S. epidermidis* and *S. aureus* as causative agents of otitis media with effusion is discussed.

MATERIALS AND METHODS

The study group consisted of 282 children (ages 2 to 15 years) and 96 adults (ages 16 to 72 years) who underwent myringotomy or insertion of tympanostomy tubes between September 1984 and April 1987 at the Medical College of Oita, Japan. There were 345 mucoid, 157 serous, and 19 purulent effusions.

After removing most of the cerumen from the external auditory canal with a curet and irrigation with 1 percent povidone-iodine solution, iontophoretic anesthesia was induced. The external ear canal then was filled with 70 percent ethyl alcohol to which 0.05 percent Hibitane had been added, three times for 1 minute each. Then the alcohol was removed by suction. The external ear canal was swabbed with a sterile cotton tipped swab moistened with trypticase soy broth. Following myringotomy the middle ear effusion was collected by aspiration with a Juhn-Tym tap (Xomed) through the eardrum. Part of the specimen caught in the trap was removed with a sterile cotton tipped swab. A nasopharyngeal culture sample was obtained by swabbing the nasopharynx by way of the nose with a sterile cotton tipped swab. These samples were transported in a TCS porter (Clinical supply; TSB 2 ml, CO_2 20 percent) and were sent to the Tokyo Clinical Research Center.

Aerobic cultures were processed by inoculating specimens onto chocolate agar, bromthymol blue agar, and 5 percent sheep's blood agar. To isolate anaerobic organisms, phenylethyl alcohol blood agar and Gifu anaerobic medium agar were used. In parallel with those differential cultures, enrichment cultures were processed by inoculating to trypticase soy broth and Gifu anaerobic semisolid medium. Incubation was continued at 37° C for 7 days. Bacterial isolates were identified by standard procedures. Coagulase negative staphylococci were identified by use of API Staph-Ident strips. The minimal inhibitory concentrations of ampicillin, cefaclor, minocycline, and erythromycin were determined for each isolate by an agar dilution method. Beta lactamase production was determined by acidometry using benzylpenicillin for the substrate and by the chromogenic cephalosporin method.

RESULTS

Isolates of *S. epidermidis, S. aureus*, and other bacteria were found in the external ear canal in 159 (30.5 percent) of 521 ears in spite of sterilization with 70 percent alcohol. As shown in Table 1, 206 ears

(39.5 percent) yielded positive culture effusions. No effusion specimen contained anaerobic bacteria. In the positive cultures 35 with *S. epidermidis*, 12 with *S. aureus*, and 26 with other species were considered to be contaminants because these organisms had the same minimal inhibitory concentrations as those from the external ear canal. When those contaminants were excluded, the percentage of positive cultures was reduced to 25.7. The incidences of recovery of *H. influenzae* and *B. catarrhalis* were larger in the mucoid effusion group than in the serous effusion group; *S. aureus*, *S. epidermidis*, and *S. pneumoniae* were more common in the purulent effusion group.

The percentage of positive cultures from nasopharyngeal samples was 79.4. *S. aureus*, *S. pneumoniae*, *S. epidermidis*, and *H. influenzae* represented the bacterial flora of the nasopharynx. The finding of *H. influenzae*, *S. pneumoniae*, and *B. catarrhalis* in cultures of middle ear effusions agreed well with those findings from the nasopharynx, whereas there was less agreement between cultures for *S. aureus* and *S. epidermidis* (Table 2).

Thirty percent of the *H. influenzae* and 50 percent of the *B. catarrhalis* organisms cultured from effusions produced beta lactamase. The results were similar to those in the nasopharynx. Although the MIC_{50} for *H. influenzae* was smallest with ampicil-

lin, the MIC_{90} for the organism was largest with ampicillin and smallest with cefaclor.

DISCUSSION

The most common bacterial species we found in the middle ear effusions was *S. epidermidis*. This finding agrees with those of Senturia et al,[3] Riding et al,[1] and other investigators.[4,5] There are several possible explanations for the presence of *S. epidermidis* in middle ear effusions. One is that the organism is a contaminant from the external ear canal. In the present study we attempted to sterilize the external ear canal with povidone-iodine and alcohol. However, bacterial isolates were found in 30.5 percent of the samples from the external ear canal. This shows that sterilization using our method is not sufficient to avoid contamination from the external ear canal. Then to distinguish the contaminants, antibiotic minimal inhibitory concentrations were determined for each type of bacterial growth. Our analysis revealed that almost all the bacteria found both in effusions and in the external ear canal were contaminants. Another possibility in regard to recovery of *S. epidermidis* from middle ear effusions is that the organism may have ascended from the naso-

TABLE 1 Bacterial Isolates from Middle Ear Effusions in 521 Ears of Patients with Otitis Media with Effusion*

Species	Number of Organisms in Effusion	Found in Both Canal and Effusion Same MIC	Found in Both Canal and Effusion Different MIC	(1) − (2) (%)
S. epidermidis	76	35	3	41 (30.5)
S. aureus	46	12	2	34 (25.4)
H. influenzae	30	0	0	30 (22.4)
S. pneumoniae	18	0	0	18 (13.4)
B. catarrhalis	2	0	0	2 (1.5)
Others	40	26	0	14 (10.4)

* Positive cultures $= \dfrac{206\ (134)^{\dagger}\ \text{ears}}{521\ \text{ears}} = 39.5\ (25.7)\ \%.$

† Number of ears excluding contaminants.

TABLE 2 Bacterial Agreement Between Middle Ear Effusion and Nasopharynx

Species	Middle Ear Effusion	Agreed with Nasopharynx Culture (%)
S. epidermidis	41	2 (4.9)
S. aureus	34	7 (20.6)
H. influenzae	30	19 (63.3)
S. pneumoniae	18	11 (61.1)
B. catarrhalis	2	2 (100.0)
Others	14	0 (0.0)

pharynx to the middle ear. However, culture agreement in regard to *S. epidermidis* in the effusions and the nasopharynx was extremely uncommon in comparison with that of *H. influenzae* and *S. pneumoniae*, which are usually considered pathogens.

S. aureus was second in frequency in middle ear effusions and the most prevalent organism in purulent effusions. Moreover, the same antibiograms were found in *S. aureus* isolates from the effusions and the nasopharynx more frequently than was the case with *S. epidermidis*. These findings suggest that *S. aureus* in middle ear effusions is not always a contaminant but a causative agent in some cases of otitis media with effusion.

In our study the frequency of beta lactamase producing *H. influenzae* isolates was greater than that reported by Rohn et al.[6] Those strains are known to be resistant to ampicillin, which is commonly used for treating acute otitis media.

Our study suggests that *S. epidermidis* frequently isolated from middle ear effusions is not a pathogen in otitis media; rather it is a contaminant in many instances. There is a possibility that *S. aureus* is a causative agent in this disorder, although contamination from the external ear canal cannot be ruled out. The prevalence of antimicrobial resistant strains of *H. influenzae* resulting from beta lactamase production should be noted in the pathogenesis and treatment of otitis media with effusion.

REFERENCES

1. Riding KH et al. Microbiology of recurrent and chronic otitis media with effusion. J Pediatr 1978; 93:739–743.
2. Bernstein JM, Ogra PL. Mucosal immune system: implications in otitis media with effusion. Ann Otol Rhinol Laryngol 1980; 89(Suppl 68):326–332.
3. Senturia BH et al. Studies concerned with tubotympanitis. Ann Otol Rhinol Laryngol 1958; 67:440–467.
4. Healy BG, Teele DW. The microbiology of chronic middle ear effusions in children. Laryngoscope 1977; 87:1472–1478.
5. Geibink GS et al. The microbiology of serous and mucoid otitis media. Pediatrics 1979; 63:915–919.
6. Rohn DD, Vatman F, Cantekin EI. Incidence of organisms in otitis media. Ann Otol Rhinol Laryngol 1983; 92(Suppl 107):17.

ANTIBODY RESPONSE TO NONTYPABLE *HAEMOPHILUS INFLUENZAE*

HOWARD FADEN, M.D., JUNG J. HONG, B.S., DEBORAH A. KRYSTOFIK, R.N., JOEL M. BERNSTEIN, M.D., Ph.D., LINDA BRODSKY, M.D., JOHN STANIEVICH, M.D., and PEARAY L. OGRA, M.D.

In a longitudinal study of otitis media begun at the Children's Hospital of Buffalo in March 1986, children are enrolled from birth through age 5 years. They are examined four times each year at well visits and at each episode of an ear infection. Middle ear fluid and serum specimens are collected in order to identify the inciting organism and to determine the specific antibody response.

This discussion concentrates on the isotypic antibody response to nontypable *H. influenzae* in the general population and in children with otitis media. Previous studies have suggested that there are systemic and local immune responses to nontypable *H. influenzae* following otitis media.[1] Evaluation of isotypic antibody titers to nontypable *H. influenzae* in an earlier report indicated that IgG antibody was fairly common in the serum and middle ear fluid.[1] The present report confirms the presence of specific IgG, M, and A antibodies to nontypable *H. influenzae* in the serum and middle ear fluid. Furthermore, it suggests that recurrent middle ear disease is associated with larger concentrations of antibody in the middle ear fluid.

MATERIALS AND METHODS

Subjects

Seventy-eight children were enrolled in the study. Fifty-five were less than 1 year of age, 17 were between ages 1 and 2 years, and six were older than 2 years. Ninety tympanocenteses were performed; 62 yielded a pathogen and of these, 29 were nontypable *H. influenzae*.

Antibody Assay

An immunodot assay was developed. Nontypable *H. influenzae* was grown for 18 hours at 37° C in 5 percent carbon dioxide in brain-heart infusion broth with added nicotinamide-adenine dinucleotide and hemin. The organism was washed, suspended in Hanks' balanced salt solution, and sonicated. Five microliter aliquots of the preparation were applied to nitrocellulose paper and allowed to dry. A blocking buffer was added and rinsed. Appropriate dilutions of either serum or middle ear fluid were added next in 0.5 ml volumes and incubated at room temperature for 1 hour. Rabbit anti-human IgG, M, or A conjugated with peroxidase (0.5 ml) was added and incubated for 1 hour at room temperature. The preparation was rinsed before immersion in horseradish peroxidase color development solution for 45 minutes in the dark. The titer of antibody was the reciprocal of the last dilution that produced any detectable color. Controls in each test run included antibody negative and positive sera. Each specimen was tested on at least two occasions. Blocking experiments confirmed the specificity of the isotype of immunoglobulin. The antibody could be completely removed with nontypable *H. influenzae* but not *Staphylococcus aureus* or *Escherichia coli*. Homologous strains of bacteria were used whenever possible.

RESULTS

Serum Nontypable H. Influenzae Antibody Titers in the Normal Population

Sera were collected from 10 normal individuals in each of the different age groups: birth, 0.5, 1, 1.5, 2, 4, 6, 10 years, and adults. The sera in each age group were pooled for testing. Figure 1 shows the pattern of development for each of the type specific immunoglobulin classes. Newborn sera had the same IgG antibody titer as that in adults. At 0.5 year the IgG antibody titer fell to the lowest point. The titer gradually rose over the next 2 to 3 years and reached adult levels by age 4 years. Neither IgM or IgA was present at birth, but their concentrations rose rapidly in the first 2 years and approached adult concentrations at about 4 years.

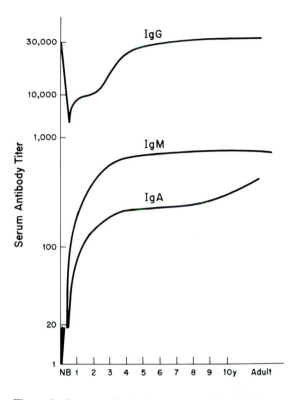

Figure 1 Serum antibody titer to nontypable *H. influenzae* according to age group. Sera from 10 normal individuals in each age group were pooled for the determination of antibody levels by an immunodot assay.

Acute and Convalescent Antibody Responses to Nontypable H. Influenzae in the Serum and Middle Ear Fluid in Children Treated with Antibiotics

Three children with acute otitis media caused by nontypable *H. influenzae* underwent tympanocentesis, were treated appropriately, and were then reevaluated 1 month later with repeat tympanocentesis because of persistent fluid. IgG specific antibody was present in the initial sera and middle ear fluid in each of the children (Table 1). Two of the subjects manifested a significant rise in antibody titer in the serum and only one in the middle ear fluid. The latter patient had a persistent infection with the same organism. None of the individuals had IgM specific antibody in the sera during the acute phase, but two developed it during convalescence. IgM was not present in the middle ear fluid in the acute phase; only the child with persistent nontypable *H. influenzae* in the middle ear fluid de-

TABLE 1   Acute and Convalescent Antibody Responses to Nontypable
H. Influenzae in Children Treated with Antibiotics

Case No.	Serum Antibodies			Middle Ear Fluid Antibodies		
	G (×10³)	M	A	G	M	A
1	1.6/25.6	< 25/100	< 25/<25	400/100	< 25/<25	<25/<25
2	6.4/ 6.4	<100/<100	<100/<100	100/100	<50/<50	<50/<50
3	1.6/12.8 *	<100/800	<100/800	100/3,200 *	<100/200	<100/400

* Persistently positive infection despite treatment.

veloped IgM specific antibody during the follow-up period; this infant was the only one to develop an IgA response in the serum or middle ear fluid.

Acute Antibody Titer to Nontypable H. Influenzae in Children with Otitis Media

Table 2 presents the serum and middle ear fluid titers in three representative children with otitis media due to nontypable *H. influenzae*. They differ in their history of otitis media; one child had had one episode, another child had had six episodes, and the third child had had more than 10 episodes. There was an apparent increase in antibody titer to nontypable *H. influenzae* in each of the immunoglobulin

subclasses as the number of episodes of otitis media increased. This progression was seen in the sera as well as in the middle ear fluids. The production of IgM and A lagged behind that of IgG. Although the serum concentrations of IgG and M in the second and third patients were similar, their titers in the middle ear fluid were markedly different. The titers were much higher in the child with a history of more ear infections, suggesting that local antibody production rather than passive transfer from the serum was the underlying cause of the increase.

Table 3 represents the geometric mean acute antibody titers to nontypable *H. influenzae* in the serum and middle ear fluid in children with different numbers of episodes of otitis media (i.e., 1 to 5, 6 to 10, and more than 10 episodes) at the time they

TABLE 2   Acute Antibody Titer to Nontypable H. Influenzae in Three
Children with Otitis Media

Case	Previous Episodes of Otitis Media	Serum			Middle Ear Fluid		
		G	M	A	G	M	A
1	1	1,600	200	<25	<25	<25	<25
2	6	6,400	400	50	200	<25	<25
3	>10	6,400	400	100	3,200	100	25

TABLE 3   Geometric Mean Acute Antibody Titer to Nontypable
H. Influenzae According to Number of Episodes of Otitis Media in Children
with at Least One Episode Due to Nontypable H. Influenzae

Episodes	Serum Antibodies			Middle Ear Fluid Antibodies		
	G	M	A	G	M	A
1–5	11.7 (7/7)*	7.9 (4/4)	5.9 (4/4)	7.8 (8/9)	0.1 (0/5)	0.1 (0/6)
6–10	12.9 (3/3)	5.8 (3/3)	5.6 (3/3)	8.3 (3/3)	4.4 (1/4)	0.1 (0/2)
>10	14.6 (3/3)	9.6 (3/3)	8.3 (3/3)	10.9 (3/3)	4.4 (2/3)	5.3 (3/3)
Persistent	13.1 (4/4)	9.6 (4/4)	5.5 (3/4)	10.5 (5/5)	4.1 (2/4)	6.9 (3/3)

* In parentheses, detectable antibody per number tested.

underwent tympanocentesis. As in Table 2, the serum and middle ear fluid titers of antibody increased as the number of episodes of otitis media increased. Although nontypable *H. influenzae* specific IgG, M, and A were present in the sera of all children in each group, the same was not true for the middle ear fluid. IgM and IgA specific antibodies were not detected in any of the six children with a history of one to five episodes of otitis media. IgA was absent in the group with six to ten episodes, but IgM was detected in one of the four children. In sharp contrast, IgM and A specific antibodies were found in the middle ear fluid in children with more than ten episodes of otitis media.

DISCUSSION

Otitis media is a recurrent problem for many children during early childhood. The role of humoral immunity in decreasing the frequency or severity of middle ear disease is currently under investigation. The data from the present study suggest that children of all ages possess IgG antibody to nontypable *H. influenzae* in the systemic circulation. However, the titer was lowest from 6 months to 2 years, a period when otitis media is most common. IgM and A specific antibodies were absent in early life but rapidly increased and reached adult concentrations at about 4 years of age. This pattern of immunoglobulin subclass evolution mirrors that for the total immunoglobulin subclasses in general.

The immune response to nontypable *H. influenzae* during acute otitis media was evident in the systemic circulation and locally in the middle ear. A fourfold rise in the IgG antibody titer was detected in the sera of two of three children during convalescence. The middle ear fluid did not reflect this rise except in one child with a persistent infection; the same child also manifested a significant rise in IgM and A antibody titers in the middle ear fluid. Sloyer et al [1] demonstrated a rise in the IgG or IgM antibody titer in the sera of one third of their subjects with otitis media due to nontypable *H. influenzae*. In addition they were able to detect IgG and A antibodies in the middle ear fluid in a large proportion of the children.

The relevance of specific antibody in the serum and middle ear fluid, as detected by a nonfunctional assay, i.e., immunodot, ELISA, and IFA, remains to be proved. The present study demonstrated a rela-

tionship of the antibody titer to the history of otitis media; many episodes were associated with increased titers of IgG antibody as well as the appearance of IgM and A antibodies. The appearance of local IgA specific antibody occurred only in individuals with a long history of recurrent disease or persistent infection.

Shurin et al [2] suggested that bactericidal antibodies to nontypable *H. influenzae* are generally absent in the serum at the start of otitis media and appear during convalescence. Animal studies have substantiated the protection afforded by serum antibodies through passive transfer experiments. [3] In certain situations the protection may not be completely effective, even with homologous strains of nontypable *H. influenzae*. [4]

The presence of IgG, M, and A classes of antibody to nontypable *H. influenzae* during the acute phase of the infection seen in our study suggests that the antibodies were not directed against protective antigenic epitopes. It is also possible that these early antibodies represented preexisting antibodies directed against heterologous strains of nontypable *H. influenzae*. [4] Further studies are needed to correlate isotypic antibody responses measured by immunodot assay with titers of bactericidal antibodies. Longitudinal studies are also needed to better understand the recurrent nature of nontypable *H. influenzae* disease. [5]

REFERENCES

1. Sloyer JL Jr, Cate CC, Howie VM, Ploussard JH, Johnston RB Jr. The immune response to acute otitis media in children. II. Serum and middle ear fluid antibody in otitis media due to *Haemophilus influenzae*. J Infect Dis 1975; 132:685–688.
2. Shurin PA, Pelton SI, Tager IB, Kasper DL. Bactericidal antibody and susceptibility to otitis media caused by nontypable strains of *Haemophilus influenzae*. J Pediatr 1980; 97:364–369.
3. Barenkamp SJ. Protection by serum antibodies in experimental nontypable *Haemophilus influenzae* otitis media. Infect Immun 1986; 52:572–578.
4. Pelton SI, Karasic RB. Serologic response in experimental otitis media due to nontypable *Haemophilus influenzae*. In: Lim DJ, Bluestone CD, Klein JO, Nelson JD, eds. Recent advances in otitis media with effusion. Proceedings of the Third International Symposium. Toronto: BC Decker, 1984:158.
5. Barenkamp SJ, Shurin PA, Marchant CD, Karasic RB, Pelton SI, Howie VM, Granoff DM. Do children with recurrent *Haemophilus influenzae* otitis media become infected with a new organism or reacquire the original strain? J Pediatr 1984; 105:533–537.

TUBERCULOUS OTITIS MEDIA—A SERIES OF 31 PATIENTS

EITAN YANIV, M.D.

The early diagnosis and treatment of tuberculous otitis media can prevent its becoming irreversible and prevent spread of the disease to other organs. Achieving an early diagnosis is difficult mainly because of the following factors:

1. Because only 0.04 percent of the cases of chronic suppurative otitis medias are of tuberculous origin,[1] the index of suspicion is often low.
2. The clinical signs of the disease have changed in recent years, making it more difficult to recognize.[2]
3. False negative results for culture often occur because of both the fastidious nature of the tubercle bacillus and other bacteria in the specimen interfering with its growth.[3]

A series of 31 patients with tuberculous otitis media is presented, and the clinical signs, diagnostic procedures, route of spread, and treatment of the disease are discussed.

MATERIALS

During the years 1984 to 1985, 31 patients were diagnosed as having tuberculous otitis media. All patients were evaluated carefully, and after the diagnosis was established, patients were transferred to a neighboring tuberculosis hospital for further treatment. Each patient was managed with 6 months of therapy with four antituberculous drugs. During the period all patients were regularly observed and managed by the staff of our clinic.

The ages of the patients ranged from 9 months to 67 years (mean, 18 years). Five patients were younger than 2 years and 7 were older than 20 years of age. There were 19 males and 12 females. The left side was affected in 16 cases and the right side in 14 cases; in one patient both ears were affected (total, 32 ears).

Signs and Symptoms

Otorrhea was present in all cases, the discharge varying from scanty to profuse (Table 1). Seven patients first presented to us with acute mastoiditis.

In 10 ears the handle of the malleus was stripped of soft tissue; we refer to this as a denuded malleus (Table 2). In one patient most of the bone in the tympanic cavity was bare of its mucosa, in addition to the denuded malleus. Three patients had bone sequestra in the middle ear. None of the patients had multiple perforations, including the seven patients

TABLE 1 Duration of Symptoms Prior to First Examination

Duration of Symptoms (Months)	No. Ears	Acute Mastoiditis
1	7	2
1–6	9	–
6–12	5	2
12–24	4	–
24	7	3
Total	32	7

TABLE 2 Condition of Ears When First Examined

	No. Ears	Granulation	Pale Granulation	Polyp	Denuded Malleus	Necrotic Bone	Facial Paralysis
Central perforation	11	5	5	1	2	–	–
Total perforation	15	4	10	1	8	3	2
Atelectatic eardrum	6	2	2	2	–	–	–
Total	32	11	17	4	10	3	2

who were seen within the first 10 days after onset of the disease.

Conductive hearing loss was a consistent finding in all patients and was often pronounced (Table 3).

The tuberculin skin test (Mantoux test) was positive in 29 patients and negative in two patients on admission. The latter two patients, had isolated tuberculous mastoiditis with symptoms for 1 week before admission. The Mantoux test became positive approximately 1 month after admission.

Radiographs of the mastoids showed sclerotic mastoids in 23 ears (74 percent) and 11 of these showed evidence of bone destruction. Poorly pneumatized mastoids with clouding of the cells were seen in six ears. Only two patients had well pneumatized mastoids. Chest radiographs showed tuberculous changes in 16 patients (52 percent).

In all patients the diagnosis was established by histologic examination of middle ear tissue. The diagnosis was made when a typical tubercle with central caseation, epithelioid cells, and Langhans giant cells was present. Only six cases were supported by positive culture of the bacillus. Other organisms cultured from aural swabs were *Proteus* (21 ears) and *Pseudomonas* (three ears). In two ears no growth was obtained.

Microscopic examinations for acid and alcohol fast bacilli were done in 28 patients; only four were positive, including two with negative cultures.

The Second Ear

Only 14 patients (47 percent) had a normal second ear. All the others had evidence of infection. Ten had chronic otitis media, four an atelectatic eardrum, and two secretory otitis media.

Treatment and Follow-Up

In the 18 patients undergoing surgery, 13 mastoidectomies (five cortical mastoidectomies and

TABLE 3   Hearing Status

Average Hearing Loss (db)	Conductive Hearing	Sensorineural Hearing
20	–	18
20–40	5	3
40–60	15	2
60	6	–
Not tested	6	9*

* Three patients had free field test only.

eight modified or radical mastoidectomies) were performed. The most common finding in the attic and antrum was pale, necrotic granulation tissue. Attic cholesteatomas were found in two patients, and in another three the cholesteatoma filled both the attic and the antrum. The ossicular chain was intact in only four patients and was missing in four patients. In the remaining 13 patients surgery consisted only of performing a biopsy.

All patients received four antituberculous drugs for 6 months. The drugs used were isonazid, ethambutol, rifampin (15 mg per kilogram per day each), and pyrazinamide (30 mg per kilogram per day). With this treatment significant improvement was noted within 3 weeks, and 80 percent of the ears stopped discharging within 2 months.

DISCUSSION

Excessive growth of granulation tissue and ears discharging for protracted periods were common findings, being noted in all the patients in our study. Granulations were either pale and necrotic or excessively large and occasionally polypoid. Of the 32 affected ears, none had multiple tympanic perforations.

Severe conductive hearing loss was evident in most of the ears tested and few patients had sensorineural hearing loss. Bone necrosis was seen in only four cases, one being associated with facial paralysis. In one third of the cases the handle of the malleus was denuded, without any soft tissue cover, and bare bone was present. We consider this a pathognomonic sign, as we could not find a similar feature in any other type of chronic otitis media. In regard to bacteriology, three quarters of the cases yielded positive cultures for organisms other than *Mycobacterium*. A positive culture for the tubercle bacillus or a positive microscopic examination for acid and alcohol fast bacilli was uncommon.

We believe that the majority of the tuberculous infections in our study were secondary to an existing chronic infection of the middle ear. We propose the following reasons in support of this:

1. Five of our patients were shown to have cholesteatoma. No evidence could be found to support tuberculosis as an etiologic factor for this.

2. Roentgenographic evidence of sclerosis of the mastoids was found in 74 percent of the patients in this study. This finding is common in ears in which otitis began in early childhood.[4]

3. Six patients had atelectatic eardrums, the

presence of which suggests long standing eustachian tube malfunction.

4. Fifty-three percent of the patients had disease of the second ear, not including tuberculosis. It is well known that chronic otitis media is bilateral in about 50 percent of the cases.

5. In 48 percent of our patients tuberculous otitis media was the primary infection. Of the 16 patients with underlying pulmonary tuberculosis, in only 11 (35 percent) could the pulmonary system have been a source of spread. The other five patients did not have open pulmonary tuberculosis—only hilar adenopathy.

We therefore assume that in most of our patients an air-borne bacillus was the source of the infection. Since the organism rarely invades through an intact mucosa, it would be logical to assume that previous infection allowed for penetration of the middle ear. This explanation would help to solve the old debate in the medical literature as to the route of spread of the tubercle bacillus to the middle ear.[5-7]

The clinical picture of tuberculous otitis media has changed during the past years. Although it is not a common cause of chronic otitis media, it is still an important cause to bear in mind—with or without mastoiditis—particularly in underdeveloped countries.

Since other organisms may cause infection secondary to the disease and, conversely, the disease may be secondary to other infections, bacteriologic findings are regarded as unreliable. It is our belief that a biopsy should be taken in all cases in which proliferation of granulation tissue is seen.

REFERENCES

1. Jeang MK, Fletcher EC. Tuberculous otitis media. JAMA 1983; 249:2231–2232.
2. Windle-Taylor PCW, Bailley CM. Tuberculous otitis media: a series of 22 patients. Laryngoscope 1980; 90:1039–1044.
3. Davis BD, Dulbecco R, Eisen HN, Gindber HS. Microbiology. 3rd ed. Hagerstown: Harper & Row, 1980:731–732.
4. Tos M, Stangerup S-E, Andreassen UK. Size of mastoid air cells and otitis media. Ann Otol Rhinol Laryngol 1985; 94:386–391.
5. American Thoracic Society: Diagnostic standards and classification of tuberculosis and other mycobacterial diseases. 14th ed. Am Rev Respir Dis 1981; 124:343–358.
6. Munzel MA: Tympanoplasty and tuberculosis of the middle ear. Clin Otolaryngol 1978; 3:311–313.
7. Banham TM, Runsame J. Tuberculosis mastoiditis treated with streptomycin. J Laryngol Otol 1951; 65:102–107.

DO ANAEROBIC BACTERIA PLAY A MAJOR ETIOLOGIC ROLE IN CHILDREN WITH CHRONIC OTITIS MEDIA WITH EFFUSION?

PHILLIP H. KALEIDA, M.D., MARGARET A. KENNA, M.D., JANET S. STEPHENSON, B.S., R.M., and GEORG KELETI, Ph.D.

The clinical importance and precise role of anaerobic bacteria in the pathogenesis of chronic otitis media with effusion have not been fully defined. Successful attempts to isolate anaerobic microorganisms from the middle ear fluid of such children have been reported by only relatively few investigators. In some studies contamination of the middle ear specimen with anaerobic bacteria from the external auditory canal could have occurred. In other studies the method of isolation of or examination for anaerobic bacteria, or both, may not have been optimal.

In this study we attempted to optimize conditions for the recovery of anaerobic bacteria from the middle ear fluid utilizing improved aseptic collection and planting techniques directly in the operating room. We studied the prevalence of anaerobic bacteria in the middle ear fluid of 41 children with chronic otitis media with effusion.

MATERIALS AND METHODS

Subjects with middle ear effusion of 2 to 3 months' duration or longer were selected from children scheduled for myringotomy with or without tympanostomy tube insertion at the Children's Hospital of Pittsburgh. The presence of a middle ear effusion had been documented by otoscopy, tympanometry, or both. Exclusion criteria were the presence of a nonintact tympanic membrane, otorrhea, or the initiation of antimicrobial therapy in the previous 2 weeks.

An attempt to meticulously sterilize the external auditory canal in all the subjects was performed with the patient under general anesthesia, as reported by Brook and colleagues.[1] After cerumen removal the external canal was filled with povidone-iodine solution for a timed 3 minutes. This solution was removed by irrigation with 50 ml of sterile saline. The external tympanic membrane surface was dried with sterile swabs, and then the culture swab was applied to the membrane for 20 seconds. The culture swab was placed immediately into enriched thioglycolate broth for the recovery of anaerobes. Only one ear was cultured per subject.

After myringotomy the effusion was aspirated into an Alden-Senturia trap with minimal exposure to air. Enriched thioglycolate broth was immediately added to the trap as a holding medium for anaerobes.

Each specimen of the external tympanic membrane and middle ear effusion pairs was planted on anaerobic and aerobic enrichment and isolation media. Planting was completed in the operating room within 10 minutes after collection. A slight modification of Brook's method[1] of facilitating the isolation and cultivation of anaerobic bacteria from the middle ear fluid was employed.

For anaerobic cultivation three prereduced anaerobic plates—anaerobic blood agar, kanamycin-vancomycin agar, and phenylethyl alcohol agar—were used. These plates were inoculated, streaked for isolation, and immediately placed into a GasPak jar. Thioglycolate broth was used as a secondary enrichment medium.

Standard cultivation methods for aerobic and facultative bacteria were also utilized.

Anaerobe jars were opened after 6 days of incubation. Aerobic plates were examined at 24 and 48 hours. Tubed media were examined daily until all isolates were identified or, if negative, until 10 days. Anaerobes, checked for aerobiosis, were identified using a rapid anaerobe panel (RapID ANA System, Innovative Diagnostic Systems, Atlanta, GA). Aerobes were identified conventionally. Beta lactamase production was assessed using a chromogenic cephalosporin test (Cefinase disk, BBL, Cockeysville, MD).

RESULTS

Forty-one subjects (41 ears) were entered into the study from February 21, 1985, to November 20, 1986. There were 23 males (56 percent) and 18 females (44 percent) enrolled, ranging in age from 1.1 to 11.2 years (median, 4.1 years). Most of the children (29; 71 percent) were white. All but one subject had received antimicrobial therapy for middle ear disease, but in only four subjects was antimicrobial therapy still being administered within the 2 weeks before surgery.

Twenty subjects (49 percent) had unilateral effusion and 21 subjects (51 percent) had bilateral otitis media with effusion. The duration of effusion was 2 to 2¾ months in 15 children (37 percent) and 3 months or more in 26 children (63 percent).

There were 21 different bacteria isolated from the chronic middle ear effusions in this study—4 anaerobes and 17 aerobes. Many middle ear fluid cultures grew multiple isolates. From 10 middle ear fluid specimens (24 percent) there was more than one isolate; 13 specimens (32 percent) had one isolate and 18 specimens (44 percent) had no bacterial growth.

Anaerobic bacteria were isolated from only the middle ear fluid specimen in four ears (10 percent) of four subjects (10 percent). They were *Peptococcus prevotii* only (one ear), *Peptostreptococcus micros* only (two ears), and *Peptostreptococcus micros*, *Bacteroides intermedius*, and *Bacteroides ureolyticus* in a single culture (one ear). In all four subjects the anaerobic bacteria were isolated from the middle ear fluid together with aerobic bacteria. Table 1 shows in detail the anaerobe positive culture results. Only one anaerobic isolate (*Bacteroides intermedius*) was documented as producing beta lactamase.

There were 39 isolates of aerobic bacteria in 23 subjects.

DISCUSSION

Fulghum and colleagues[2] isolated anaerobes in four of 10 patients with "chronic secretory otitis media." Brook and Finegold[3] found anaerobic bacteria

TABLE 1 Culture Results in Four Children with Anaerobic Bacteria Isolated from Four Chronic Middle Ear Effusions

Anaerobic Bacteria	Aerobic Bacteria
1. *Peptococcus prevotii*	*Streptococcus,* microaerophilic
2. *Peptostreptococcus micros*	*Staphylococcus,* coagulase negative
3. *Peptostreptococcus micros*	*Haemophilus influenzae,* type b *Streptococcus,* beta hemolytic, group C *Streptococcus,* alpha hemolytic *Eikenella corrodens* *Corynebacterium* species (diphtheroids)
4. *Peptostreptococcus micros* *Bacteroides intermedius* *Bacteroides ureolyticus*	*Streptococcus,* beta hemolytic, group F *Staphylococcus,* coagulase negative *Eikenella corrodens*

in 28 of 50 adult and pediatric subjects (56 percent) with chronic purulent middle ear fluid. From 110 middle ear fluid specimens (mucoid effusions) of 74 children with "secretory otitis media" Sipila and colleagues[4] recovered only one anaerobic bacterium (also present in the external auditory canal). In an earlier study of 60 subjects with "active chronic otitis media" Jokipii and co-workers[5] reported finding anaerobic bacteria in 23 of 70 middle ears (33 percent). However, in all these studies specific ear canal sterilization methods were not utilized.

After 1 minute of external auditory canal sterilization with 70 percent alcohol, Teele and colleagues[6] found no middle ear fluid anaerobes in 30 subjects (51 specimens) with "persistent effusions." Using the 3 minute povidone-iodine–sterile saline irrigation procedure for external auditory canal sterilization, Brook and co-workers[1] recovered anaerobes in 10 of 57 subjects (18 percent) who had had serous effusions for 6 months or longer. Lastly, with the use of a hydrogen peroxide–iodine–wash procedure to sterilize the external auditory canal, Edstrom and colleagues[7] found anaerobic bacteria in three of 30 children (45 specimens) with chronic (mucoid) effusion of 2 or more months' duration. In these three studies specimens were sent from the operating room to the laboratory for culture.

In the present study we not only used meticulous external auditory canal sterilization and bacterial cultivation methods but also attempted to enhance the recovery of anaerobic bacteria by inoculating specimens directly in the operating room within 10 minutes after collection. We found anaerobic bacteria in the middle ear fluid of only four of 41 (10 percent) children with chronic otitis media with effusion. Thus, anaerobic bacteria did not appear to play a major etiologic role in these subjects.

REFERENCES

1. Brook I, Yocum P, Shah K, Feldman B, Epstein S. Aerobic and anaerobic bacteriologic features of serous otitis media in children. Am J Otolaryngol 1983; 4:389–392.
2. Fulghum RS, Daniel HS, Yarborough JG. Anaerobic bacteria in otitis media. Ann Otol 1977; 86:196–203.
3. Brook I, Finegold SM. Bacteriology of chronic otitis media. JAMA 1979; 241:487–488.
4. Sipila P, Jokipii AM, Jokipii L, Karma P. Bacteria in the middle ear and ear canal of patients with secretory otitis media and with non-inflamed ears. Acta Otolaryngol 1981; 92:123–130.
5. Jokipii AM, Karma P, Ojala K, Jokipii L. Anaerobic bacteria in chronic otitis media. Arch Otolaryngol 1977; 103:278–279.
6. Teele DW, Healy GB, Tally FP. Persistent effusions of the middle ear: cultures for anaerobic bacteria. Ann Otol Rhinol Laryngol 1980; 89(Suppl 68):102–103.
7. Edstrom S, Ejnell H, Jorgenson F, Moller A. A microbiologicalstudy of secretory otitis media using an anaerobic technique. Otorhinolaryngol Relat Spec 1985; 47:32–36.

BIOCHEMISTRY

HYDROLASE ACTIVITY IN EXPERIMENTAL MIDDLE EAR EFFUSIONS: EFFECT OF ANTIBODY THERAPY

WARREN F. DIVEN, Ph.D., WILLIAM J. DOYLE, Ph.D., and BARBARA VIETMEIER, B.S.

Studies from several laboratories have documented the presence of significant activity levels for various hydrolytic enzymes in middle ear effusion from patients with acute, chronic, or recurrent otitis media.[1-4] It is conceivable that these enzymes could contribute to the pathogenesis of the disease.[5,6] Our own studies have focused in part on the comparison of microbiologic findings with enzyme activity.[4,7,8] Middle ear effusions removed from patients with chronic or acute otitis media have been cultured and analyzed for enzyme activity. The mean enzymatic activity was found to be higher in the culture positive effusions, but generally these differences were not statistically significant. These findings suggested that microorganisms could contribute to an increase in middle ear fluid enzyme activity perhaps by directly secreting enzyme into the middle ear or by promoting a host response. Either mechanism would result in enzyme activity that is increased relative to that resulting from a generalized host inflammatory response.

With the chinchilla animal model of acute otitis media, activities of several hydrolytic enzymes have been documented in experimentally induced middle ear effusion.[7] In that model one enzyme, neuraminidase, was shown to be capable of altering the middle ear mucosa with potentially detrimental results.[9] In the present study we investigated the effect of antibiotic therapy on the expression of hydrolytic enzyme activity in acute middle ear effusions induced by *Haemophilus influenzae* infections.

EXPERIMENTAL PROTOCOL

Thirty healthy adult chinchillas were entered into the study. The middle ears of the animals were bilaterally inoculated with $\simeq$ 150 cfu of *H. influenzae* (nontypable) via the transbullar approach. All ears were examined on day 2 to document middle ear inflammation and effusion using tympanometry and otomicroscopy. Beginning on day 3 and for the duration of the 10 day experiment, 15 of the animals received 100 mg of ampicillin intramuscularly every 12 hours. Four middle ear effusions from both treated and untreated groups of animals were recovered on days 4, 6, 8, and 10 by tympanocentesis. Sampled effusions were labeled, cultured, and submitted for enzyme analysis. The activities of α-mannosidase, β-glucuronidase, phosphatase, β-galactosidase, and hexosaminidase were determined at both an acid and neutral pH using previously published procedures.[4,7] The protein level was determined by the method of Lowry et al[10] using bovine serum albumin as the standard. Activities were then expressed as units per mg of protein. Median values of enzymatic activities in the effusions were calculated for the two groups of animals on each of the 4 sample days.

RESULTS

In the untreated animals, all recovered effusions were culture positive for *H. influenzae*. In contrast, effusions recovered from the ampicillin treated animals were sterile for aerobic bacteria. Activities measured for all enzymes were greater in the effusions of the untreated animals when compared to those of the ampicillin treated animals, and for the majority of the enzymes these differences were observed to increase with increasing time.

To define the pattern of change in enzymatic activity over time, the median values of the activities were plotted as a function of time for each of the enzymes in the effusions from the treated and untreated animals. Examples of these functions are shown in Figure 1. The graph of activity as a function of time for phosphatase assayed at pH 4.5 is shown in Figure 1A. The activity in the effusions from the untreated animals increased with time with a peak at 8 days, whereas those from the treated

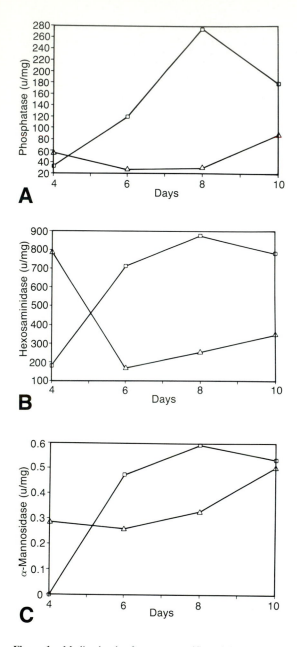

Figure 1   Median levels of enzyme specific activity in middle ear effusions obtained from control □-□-□ and △-△-△ animals treated with ampicillin as a function of time after infection with ≈ 150 cfu of *H. influenzae*. *A*, Phosphatase specific activity determined at pH 4.5. *B*, Hexosaminidase specific activity determined at pH 4.0. *C*, α-Mannosidase specific activity determined at pH 6.4.

animals were generally constant over the time course of the experiment. With the exception of day 4, the phosphatase activity in the effusions from the untreated animals was greater than that in the treated animals and this difference seemed to increase with

time. For hexosaminidase, the enzymatic activity measured at pH 4.0 increased with time in the effusions from the untreated animals with a peak at 8 days, whereas the median activity in the effusions from the treated animals decreased with time (Fig. 1*B*). Except for day 4, the activity in the untreated effusions is greater than that in the treated ones. For α-mannosidase measured at pH 6.4, the median activity in the effusions from the treated animals increased with time although the change was small (Fig. 1*C*). Except for day 4, the median activity in the untreated animals was greater than that in the effusions from the treated animals, but the difference was very small by the end of the experiment. The remaining enzymes were characterized by patterns of change similar to these.

DISCUSSION

These results show that the middle ear effusions of chinchillas inoculated with *H. influenzae* contain a number of hydrolytic enzymes also reported to be present in middle ear effusions from children that are culture positive for that organism. Moreover, the activities, and by implication concentrations, of these enzymes are characterized by well defined patterns of change over time. All the enzymes assayed in effusions from untreated animals showed an increase with increasing time after inoculation of the bacteria, with a peak at 8 days. The majority (6 of 10) of enzyme activities found in the treated effusions decreased with time over the course of the experiment. The unexpected finding was the behavior of α-mannosidase in the effusions from the treated animals. Both acidic and neutral α-mannosidase activities gradually increased over the course of the experiment, although the increase was less in the middle ear effusions from the treated animals. Perhaps this increase represents a different response to infection from that measured by the other enzymes.

Substrates for these hydrolases are found in the carbohydrate portions of membrane glycolipids and glycoproteins found in the middle ear. Removal of these sugar residues could enhance the pathogenesis of the disease by (1) exposing protease sensitive sites, which might allow bacterial protease to degrade membrane proteins and damage mucosal lining; by creating new terminal residues, which serve as adherence sites for bacterial colonization; or by exposing new sugar residues, which could provoke a local immune response. These observations and the results presented here suggest that sterilization of the middle ear cleft and the attendant decrease in activity of hydrolytic enzymes may be benefits of early antimicrobial activity and prerequisites to the healing of an inflamed mucosa.

This study was supported in part by grant NS-16337 from the National Institutes of Health.

REFERENCES

1. Juhn SK, Huff JS, Paparella MM. Certain oxidative and hydrolytic enzymes in the middle ear effusion in serous otitis media. Arch Otorhinolaryngol (NY) 1976; 212:119-125.
2. Juhn SK, Huff JS. Biochemical characteristics of middle ear effusions. Ann Otol Rhinol Laryngol 1976; 85:110-116.
3. Bernstein JM, Villari EM, Rattazi MC. The significance of lysosomal enzymes in middle ear effusions. Otolaryngol Head Neck Surg 1979; 87:845-851.
4. Diven WF, Glew RH, Bluestone CD. Lysosomal hydrolases in middle ear effusions. Ann Otol Rhinol Laryngol 1981; 90:148-153.
5. Lowell SH, Juhn SK. The role of bacterial enzymes in inducing inflammation in the middle ear cavity. Otolaryngol Head Neck Surg 1979; 87:859-870.
6. Giebink GS, Carlson BA, Hetherington SV, Hostetter MK, Le CT, Juhn SK. Bacterial and polymorphonuclear leukocyte contribution to middle ear inflammation in chronic otitis media with effusion. Ann Otol Rhinol Laryngol 1985; 94(4 pt.1):398-402.
7. LaMarco KL, Diven WF, Glew RH, Doyle WJ, Cantekin EI. Neuraminidase activity in middle ear effusions. Ann Otol Rhinol Laryngol 1984; 93:76-84.
8. Diven WF, Glew RH, LaMarco KL. Hydrolase activity in acute otitis media with effusion. Ann Otol Rhinol Laryngol 1985; 94:415-418.
9. LaMarco KL, Diven WF, Glew RH. Experimental alteration of chinchilla middle ear mucosae by bacterial neuraminidase. Ann Otol Rhinol Laryngol 1986; 95:304-308.
10. Lowry OH, Rosenbrough NJ, Farr AL, Randall RJ. Protein measurement with the Folin phenol reagent. J Biol Chem 1951; 193:265-267.
11. Bernstein JM, Boerst M, Hayes EM. Mucosubstances in otitis media with effusion. Ann Otol Rhinol Laryngol 1979; 88:334-338.
12. Kornfeld R, Kornfeld S. Comparative aspects of glycoprotein structure. Ann Rev Biochem 1976; 45:217-237.

HYDROLASE ACTIVITY IN EXPERIMENTAL MIDDLE EAR EFFUSIONS: CHARACTERISTIC ACTIVITY PROFILES

BARBARA VIETMEIER, B.S., WARREN F. DIVEN, Ph.D., and WILLIAM J. DOYLE, Ph.D.

One of the most common sequelae of a bacterial infection of the middle ear is the development and persistence of an effusion within the middle ear space. Such effusions are a potential source of information about the pathology of the disease. Effusions are routinely screened for aerobic bacteria, which if found are usually identified as the etiologic agent.[1,2]

Earlier work from our laboratory has demonstrated the presence of a variety of hydrolytic enzymes in middle ear effusions collected from children with both persistent and acute otitis media with effusion.[3-5] These data suggested that at least some of the enzymes (for example, neuraminidase) are produced by bacteria and are not of host cell origin. Furthermore, enzymatic expression appears to be somewhat specific for each bacterial species, suggesting the possibility that a pathogen induces or enhances a specific profile of enzymatic activity.

The purpose of this study was to investigate fur-ther these relationships in an animal model. We assayed a number of hydrolytic enzymes in middle ear effusions from chinchilla middle ears infected with *S. pneumoniae*, *H. influenzae*, *B. catarrhalis*, and *Pseudomonas*. To establish a baseline host response to local inflammation we performed similar assays on effusions collected from the chinchilla middle ear following pretreatment with *E. coli* endotoxin.

MATERIAL AND METHODS

Twenty healthy adult chinchillas were used in the study. For the endotoxin experiments, 12.5 μg per 100 microliters of lipopolysaccharide B from each of 4 strains of *E. coli* (0111:B4, 055:B5, 0127:B8, 0128:B12) was suspended in normal saline. With previously reported techniques, 100 μl of the suspension was inoculated bilaterally by the superior bullar approach into the middle ears of four chinchillas. Effusions were collected on day 4 after inoculation. All recovered effusions were cultured for aerobic bacteria and submitted for assay of enzymatic activity and total protein. Enzyme activity in these effusions served as a baseline for comparison with those induced by the bacterial infection models.

The 16 remaining animals were divided into four groups of four animals each. With the superior bullar approach, group I animals were inoculated bilaterally with ≃ 150 cfu of *S. pneumoniae* (type 3), group II with ≃ 150 cfu of nontypable *H. influenzae*, group III with 5,000 cfu of *B. catarrhalis*, and group IV with 50 cfu of *Pseudomonas*. All organisms utilized were recovered originally from the effusions of children with persistent (*B. catarrhalis, S. pneumoniae, H. influenzae*) or chronic (*Pseudomonas*) otitis media with effusion and previously had been shown to induce effusions at the inoculum dosage in the chinchilla animal model.[6] Effusions from all ears were recovered on day 4 by myringotomy and tympanocentesis. The collected effusions were labeled, cultured, and submitted for assay of enzymatic activity. The remaining effusion material for each bacterial pathogen was pooled, and the profile of activity as a function of pH for each of the six enzymes was determined.

The hydrolytic enzymes assayed were those previously shown to be present in middle ear effusions of children with persistent otitis media with effusion and included neuraminidase, hexosaminidase, α-mannosidase, phosphatase, β-galactosidase, and β-glucuronidase. Hydrolase activity was determined at acid (pH 4.0 to 5.5) and neutral (pH 6.4) pH levels using artificial substrates as previously described.[3,4] The total protein level was determined by the method of Lowry et al[7] using bovine albumin as the standard. Unless otherwise noted, all results are presented as activity per milliliter of effusion.

RESULTS

To establish a baseline enzymatic profile for noninfectious inflammatory processes, middle ear effusions were recovered on day 4 from a group of four animals bilaterally inoculated with endotoxin. The mean data for acidic and neutral enzyme activity for these effusions are reported in Table 1. For these effusions the activities assayed at the more acidic pH are greater than those assayed at neutral pH for all enzymes. This pattern would be observed if a single isoenzyme existed for each of the enzymes with a pH optima within the acidic range. This in-

terpretation is supported by the functions relating enzyme activity to pH for endotoxin induced effusions, presented in Figure 1.

TABLE 1 Hydrolase Activity in Endotoxin Induced Middle Ear Effusions

	Hydrolase Activity (U/ml): E. Coli Endotoxin
Neuraminidase	
Acid	210
Neutral	92
Hexosaminidase	
Acid	26,400
Neutral	4,290
α–Mannosidase	
Acid	4,410
Neutral	207
Phosphatase	
Acid	2,600
Neutral	1,460
β–Galactosidase	
Acid	632
Neutral	86
β–Glucuronidase	
Acid	256
Neutral	167

All middle ears inoculated with *S. pneumoniae, H. influenzae*, and *Pseudomonas* developed an effusion from which the inoculated organism could be recovered on culture. For *B. catarrhalis* inoculations, effusions developed in half the middle ears, but the organism was not recoverable from any effusion on culture. The ratios of the mean enzymatic activities in effusions collected at day 4 from animals infected with *S. pneumoniae, H. influenzae, B. catarrhalis*, and *Pseudomonas* sp. to the mean activities measured in the endotoxin induced effusions are shown in Table 2. These ratios serve as an index of relative activity and were designed to identify specific enzymatic activity not related to a general inflammatory response.

The enzyme ratios reported for *Pseudomonas* varied from 2.2 (α-mannosidase:acid) to 10.4 (phosphatase: neutral), indicating an increase in enzymatic activity across the spectrum of assayed hydrolases. No enzyme ratio documented a preferential elevation; this was supported by the similarity in the functions relating activity to pH for effusions induced by endotoxin and *Pseudomonas*. In all cases the

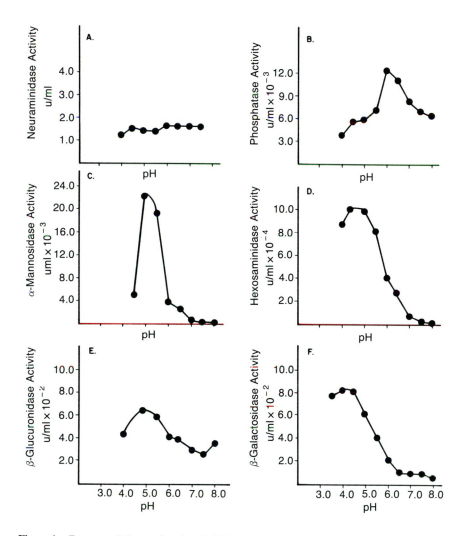

Figure 1   Enzyme activity as a function of pH for pooled *E. coli* endotoxin induced middle ear effusion. *A*, Neuraminidase. *B*, Phosphatase. *C*, α-Mannosidase. *D*, Hexosaminidase. *E*, β-Glucuronidase. *F*, β-Galactosidase.

**TABLE 2   Ratio of Enzyme Activity in Bacterial Induced Middle Ear Effusion
to that in Endotoxin Induced Middle Ear Effusion**

	Ratio of Bacterial Induced Activity to Endotoxin Induced Activity			
	H. Influenzae (nontypable)	*B. Catarrhalis*	*S. Pneumoniae*	*Pseudomonas*
Neuraminidase				
Acid	1.0	1.1	0.6	2.5
Neutral	1.4	0.9	29	5.2
Hexosaminidase				
Acid	2.5	1.1	1.2	6.7
Neutral	35	8.4	1.5	7.7
α–Mannosidase				
Acid	1.8	0.8	0.9	2.2
Neutral	2.8	1.2	1.7	4.6
Phosphatase				
Acid	7.6	1.7	3.4	7.3
Neutral	11	4.1	6.0	10.7
β–Galactosidase				
Acid	2.0	0.3	1.6	3.8
Neutral	7.9	1.8	2.4	4.7
β–Glucuronidase				
Acid	3.7	1.1	2.0	7.5
Neutral	1.3	1.2	1.2	4.6

overall activity was elevated for the *Pseudomonas* effusions, but the pH optima and forms of the curve were almost identical to those for endotoxin.

The ratios reported for enzyme activity in middle ear effusions resulting from *S. pneumoniae* infections were with two exceptions less than 2.5, indicating relatively little increase over baseline endotoxin levels. The two exceptions were neuraminidase (neutral) and phosphatase (neutral). Phosphatase activity was increased over the baseline level in effusions collected from all middle ears secondary to instillation of any viable organisms. Thus, this elevation probably reflects an active infection and is not specific to *S. pneumoniae*. However, the pH versus activity profile suggests the possibility of an additional species of phosphatase with a pH optima at approximately 7.5 (Fig. 2B). The 29-fold elevation relative to endotoxin for pH 6.4 neuraminidase activity does appear to be specific to *S. pneumoniae*, indicating a bacterial origin for this enzyme.

For *H. influenzae* infections the ratios of neutral hexosaminidase (35.0), acid phosphatase (7.6), and neutral β-galactosidase (7.9) in addition to the neutral phosphatase all suggest a significant increase in activity over the baseline level. However, the shape of the pH activity profiles are similar to those found for endotoxin, with the exception of phospha-

tase. For that enzyme there is an indication of an additional species with a pH optimum above pH 7.5.

The ratios reported for enzyme activity in middle ear effusions resulting from *B. catarrhalis* are with two exceptions less than 2.0, indicating no significant increase over baseline endotoxin activities. The two exceptions are hexosaminidase (neutral) and phosphatase (neutral). Phosphatase elevations seem to occur in every instance of instillation of viable organisms and as already mentioned, may be suggestive of an active infection. The elevations of hexosaminidase (neutral) also occurs in other microorganism induced effusions and also may be an indication of an active infection.

DISCUSSION

Middle ear effusions produced in response to either an acute bacterial infection or a sterile inflammatory response contain significant levels of hydrolytic enzyme activity. The elevated activities found relative to endotoxin seem to give a pattern that is characteristic of infection by a particular microorganism. Middle ear effusions resulting from *S. pneumoniae* infections are characterized by elevations in neutral neuraminidase and neutral phosphatase, whereas *H. influenzae* induced middle ear

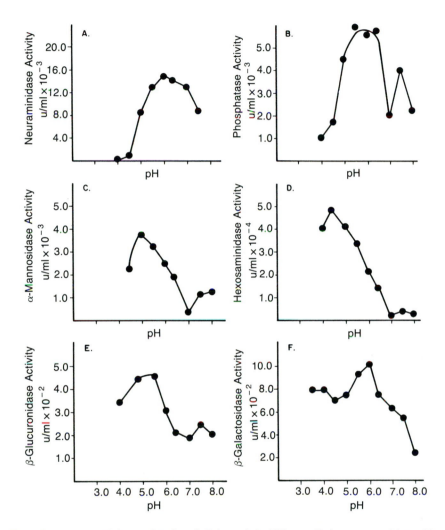

Figure 2 Enzyme activity as a function of pH for pooled middle ear effusions recovered from chinchillas infected with *S. pneumoniae*. *A*, Neuraminidase. *B*, Phosphatase. *C*, α-Mannosidase. *D*, Hexosaminidase. *E*, β-Glucuronidase. *F*, β-Galactosidase.

effusions are characterized by marked elevations in neutral hexosaminidase, neutral and acid phosphatase, and neutral β-galactosidase. *Pseudomonas* induced middle ear effusions show marked elevations in all the enzymes tested, whereas effusions resulting from instillation of *B. catarrhalis* showed elevations of only neutral hexosaminidase and neutral phosphatase activities. Elevation of the ratio for neutral phosphatase seems to occur in each case and thus may indicate the presence of an active microbial infection. It should be possible to use appropriate enzyme activity levels to predict the microorganism causing a particular effusion. Further studies are in progress to test these ideas.

This study was supported by grant NS 16337 from the National Institutes of Health/National Institute of Neurological and Communicative Disorders and Stroke.

REFERENCES

1. Lim DJ, Lewis DM, Schram JL, Birck HG. Otitis media with effusion: cytological and microbiological correlates. Arch Otolaryngol 1979; 105P:404–412.
2. Riding KH, Bluestone CD, Michaels RH, Cantekin EI, Doyle WJ, Pozivak CS. Microbiology of recurrent and chronic otitis media with effusion. J Pediatr 1978; 93:739–743.
3. Diven WF, Glew RH, Bluestone CD. Lysosomal hydrolases in middle ear effusions. Ann Otol Rhinol Laryngol 1981; 90:148–153.
4. LaMarco KL, Diven WF, Glew RH, Doyle WJ, Cantekin EI. Neuraminidase activity in middle ear effusions. Ann Otol Rhinol Laryngol 1984; 93:76–84.
5. Diven WF, Glew RH, LaMarco KL. Hydrolase activity in acute otitis media with effusion. Ann Otol Rhinol Laryngol 1985; 94:415–418.
6. Reilly JS, Doyle WJ, Cantekin EI, Supanze JS, Rohn DD. Actualized potential of pathogenetic microorganisms to cause acute otitis media with effusion in chinchillas. Ann Otol Rhinol Laryngol 1984; 92:107–128.
7. Lowry OH, Rosenbrough NJ, Farr AL, Randall RJ. Protein measurement with the Folin phenol reagent. J Biol Chem 1951; 193:265–267.

SECRETORY LEUKOCYTE PROTEASE INHIBITOR IN SEROUS OTITIS MEDIA

ULLA FRYKSMARK, M.D., Ph.D., BRITT CARLSSON-NORDLANDER, M.D., Ph.D., ÅKE REIMER, M.D., and KJELL OHLSSON, M.D., Ph.D.

Among the characteristics of inflammation found in middle ear secretions from patients with serous otitis media are granulocyte proteases.[1] These proteases are released in connection with phagocytosis and cell destruction.[2] If not inactivated, the proteases cause tissue damage. Sufficient amounts of protease inhibitors are therefore of importance for tissue protection.

The dominating protease inhibitors in middle ear secretions are α-1-proteinase inhibitor (α-1-PI), α-1-antichymotrypsin, α-2-macroglobulin, and antileukoprotease.[3] α-1-PI, α-1-antichymotrypsin, and α-2-macroglobulin are well known plasma protease inhibitors.[4]

Antileukoprotease, a low molecular weight inhibitor of granulocyte elastase, is present in respiratory tract secretions, including those of the middle ear.[3,5] It has recently been established that antileukoprotease is a degraded form of secretory leukocyte protease inhibitor (SLPI).[6] SLPI is a secretory protein found in goblet cells and in the serous parts of the seromucous glands of the mucosa. SLPI has been purified from parotid secretions, and the amino acid and nucleotide sequences have been determined. Like other secretory proteins, SLPI is found only in trace amounts in blood serum. The normal serum level of SLPI is about 40 μg per liter.

The purpose of this study was to see whether SLPI was present in middle ear secretions and to analyze its activity as an inhibitor of granulocyte elastase.

MATERIALS AND METHODS

Middle ear specimens were obtained from patients suffering from serous otitis media with a history of persistent middle ear effusion exceeding 2 months. The diagnosis was established by morphologic findings of a pale and retracted tympanic membrane and the serous fluid obtained in connection with myringotomy. Serous to seromucoid secretions were aspirated into a glass bottle and frozen at -20° C. Macroscopically blood contaminated secretions were excluded from the study. In all, 12 middle ear specimens from nine patients with serous otitis media were studied.

All specimens were analyzed for SLPI, α-1-PI, and protease activity. One specimen was subjected to gel filtration, and the fractions were analyzed for SLPI, α-1-PI, and granulocyte elastase.

Radioimmunoassays were used for the measurements of SLPI[7] and granulocyte elastase.[8] An electroimmunoassay was used for quantification of α-1-PI.[4] Gel filtration of serous secretions was performed on a Sephadex G-75 column. Protease activity was tested on fibrin agarose.

RESULTS

SLPI was found in every specimen, ranging from 0.2 to 4.6 mg per liter. α-1-PI was found in 10 of 12 specimens, ranging from 8 to 1,800 mg per liter. In two specimens the amounts of secretions were not large enough to allow analysis of α-1-PI (Fig. 1).

The amounts of SLPI and α-1-PI were compared in each specimen, and it was found that specimens with large amounts of SLPI also contained large amounts of α-1-PI (Fig. 2).

No free protease activity, tested on fibrin agarose, was detectable in the specimens.

Gel filtration of middle ear secretions is illustrated in Figure 3. The dominating part of SLPI was found in a free form, and a small part was found in the fractions corresponding to SLPI-granulocyte elastase complexes. Granulocyte elastase eluted in the fractions corresponding to granulocyte elastase-α-1-PI and granulocyte elastase-SLPI complexes.

DISCUSSION

In a previous study the degraded form of SLPI, antileukoprotease, was found in middle ear secretions from patients with serous otitis media.[3] In this investigation SLPI was found in every specimen. The levels of SLPI were very high, exceeding the levels found in normal blood serum. In addition, a majority of the specimens contained remarkably large amounts of α-1-PI. These results are in accordance with previous findings.[3]

Protease activity, tested on fibrin agarose, was not detected, indicating that the amounts of protease inhibitors were large enough to inhibit the proteases,

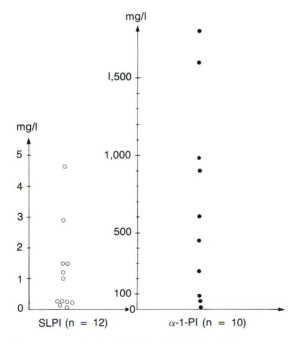

Figure 1 Distribution of SLPI and α-1-PI in middle ear secretions from patients with serous otitis media.

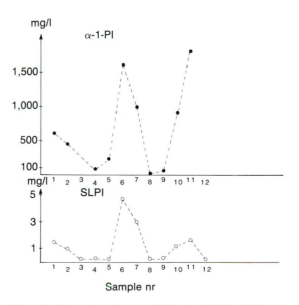

Figure 2 Comparison between SLPI and α-1-PI in middle ear secretions from patients with serous otitis media.

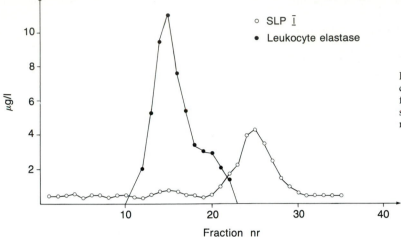

Figure 3 Partition of SLPI and leukocyte elastase in fractions obtained by gel filtration on Sephadex G-75 of middle ear secretions from patients with serous otitis media.

including granulocyte elastase. Gel filtration of the secretions and analysis of the fractions for SLPI, granulocyte elastase, and α-1-PI demonstrated that α-1-PI and SLPI were present in active forms, as they were found in complex forms with granulocyte elastase. The results suggest a potent inhibition of granulocyte elastase and a physiologic function of the inhibitors in the middle ear.

REFERENCES

1. Carlsson B, Lundberg C, Ohlsson K. Granulocyte proteases in middle ear effusions. Ann Otol Rhinol Laryngol 1982; 91:76–81.
2. Ohlsson K, Olsson I. The extracellular release of granulocyte collagenase and elastase during phagocytosis and inflammatory processes. Scand J Haematol 1977; 19:145–152.
3. Carlsson B, Lundberg C, Ohlsson K. Protease inhibitors in middle ear effusions. Ann Otol Rhinol Laryngol 1981; 90:38–41.
4. Laurell C-B. Electroimmunoassay. Scand J Clin Lab Invest 1972; 29(Suppl 124):21–37.
5. Fryksmark U, Prellner T, Tegner H, Ohlsson K. Studies on the role of antileukoprotease in respiratory tract diseases. Eur J Respir Dis 1984; 65:201–209.
6. Thompson RC, Ohlsson K. Isolation, properties, and complete amino acid sequence of human secretory leukocyte protease inhibitor, a potent inhibitor of leukocyte elastase. Proc Natl Acad Sci USA 1986; 83:6692–6696.
7. Fryksmark U, Ohlsson K, Rosengren M, Tegner H. A radioimmunoassay for measurement and characterization of human antileukoprotease in serum. Hoppe Seylers Z Physiol Chem 1981; 362:1273–1277.
8. Ohlsson K, Olsson A-S. Immunoreactive granulocyte elastase in human serum. Hoppe Seylers Z Physiol Chem 1978; 359:1531–1539.

ANTI-INFLAMMATORY EFFECTS OF A CORTICOSTEROID AND PROTEASE INHIBITOR AGENTS ON ANTIGEN INDUCED OTITIS MEDIA IN CHINCHILLAS

YUKIYOSHI HAMAGUCHI, M.D., STEVEN K. JUHN, M.D., and YASUO SAKAKURA, M.D.

It is well known that corticosteroid drugs exert inhibitory action against allergic inflammations, for example, suppression of the release of chemical mediators and lysosomal proteases from leukocytes, and inhibition of phospholipase A2, which, uninhibited, releases arachidonic acid from cell membranes.[1,2]

Aprotinin is one of the natural protease inhibitors and inhibits both plasma and glandular kallikrein activity to reduce the bradykinin level in the inflammatory locus.[3,4] Aprotinin has already been used clinically for the treatment of skin burns and endotoxin shock. Synthetic inhibitors with low molecular weights (e.g., leupeptin, antipain) have already been shown to reduce the release of chemical mediators and to suppress lysosomal protease activity.[5-7] However, in experimental otitis media models the effect of a protease inhibitor treatment has not yet been reported.

In the present study the anti-inflammatory effects of local treatment by a steroid and a protease inhibitor were studied to obtain baseline information for possible local treatment with these drugs in human otitis media with effusion.

MATERIALS

Normal chinchillas were systemically immunized by 0.1 ml of human serum albumin (HSA, 10 mg per milliliter) containing the same volume of complete Freund's adjuvant (Sigma Chemical Co., St. Louis). The emulsion was injected subcutaneously under the back skin of the animals, and then these animals were given booster doses twice, 3 days and 10 days after the first injection. When circulating antibody titers were elevated (2^4 to 2^6) enough to induce local inflammation, 1 ml of HSA (5 mg per milliliter) was instilled into the left middle ear bulla of 20 chinchillas (Arthus group), and 1 ml of HSA containing 12.5 mg per milliliter of triamcinolone diacetate (Aristocort, Lederle) or 5,000 kallikrein inhibitory units of aprotinin (Antagosan, Hoechst) was instilled into the right middle ear bulla

of 20 chinchillas (Arthus + steroid and Arthus + aprotinin groups). The bulla was exposed surgically, and the fluid retained in the bulla and blood samples were collected 24 hours after instillation. After cytologic analysis of the middle ear fluid, both fluid and blood samples were centrifuged at 2,000 rpm for 15 minutes at 4° C. The supernatants were stored at −70° C until use.

METHODS

Cellular Analysis of the Middle Ear Fluid

The middle ear fluid was diluted from 1 to 20 times with 0.1 M phosphate buffered saline (pH 7.4) immediately after sampling. Then the same amount of 0.1 M acetic acid was added. The number of leukocytes was counted using a Neubauer chamber. An aliquot of the middle ear fluid was placed on a slide glass and stained with May-Grünwald Giemsa stain. The leukocyte distribution was examined in two different areas and averaged.

Quantitation of Alpha-1-Antitrypsin (Alpha-1-AT) and Alpha-2-Macroglobulin (Alpha-2-M) Levels in the Recovered Middle Ear Fluid

The concentration of alpha-1-AT in the recovered middle ear fluid was measured by single radial immunodiffusion, and that of alpha-2-M was measured by electroimmunodiffusion, using specific rabbit antibodies against purified chinchilla alpha-1-AT and alpha-2-M.[8]

Bacteriologic Study of the Middle Ear Fluid

After collection of the middle ear fluid, an aliquot of each sample was plated directly onto sheep blood agar and chocolate agar plates for culture. The statistical significance between the groups was determined by either the Student's t test or the paired t test.

RESULTS

The bacterial cultures were negative for all the middle ear fluid samples.

Cellular Analyses

The total leukocytes were $2.17 \pm 1.54 \times 10^6$ per cubic centimeter in the Arthus group, $0.94 \pm 0.44 \times 10^6$ per cubic centimeter in the Arthus + aprotinin group, and $0.75 \pm 1.29 \times 10^6$ per cubic centimeter in the Arthus + steroid group. There were significant differences between the Arthus and Arthus + aprotinin groups and between the Arthus and Arthus + steroid groups ($p < 0.025$, 0.01; Fig. 1). The distribution of leukocytes was similar and no significant difference was observed among the three groups.

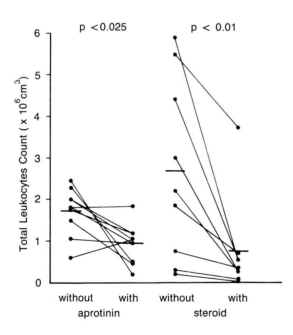

Figure 1 The number of leukocytes in the recovered middle ear fluid. Significant differences in the mean were observed with and without the treatments ($p < 0.025$ with aprotinin and $p < 0.01$ with a steroid).

Alpha-1-Antitrypsin (Alpha-1-AT) and Alpha-2-Macroglobulin (Alpha-2-M) Levels in the Middle Ear Fluid

The mean levels of alpha-1-AT in the middle ear fluid were 307.8 ± 118.6 mg per deciliter in the Ar-

thus group, 204.5 ± 146.1 mg per deciliter in the Arthus + aprotinin group, and 107.5 ± 100.0 mg per deciliter in the Arthus + steroid group. There were significant differences between the Arthus and Arthus + aprotinin groups and between the Arthus and Arthus + steroid groups ($p < 0.01$; Fig. 2A). The mean levels of alpha-2-M in the middle ear fluid were 163.8 ± 58.7 mg per deciliter in the Arthus group, 128.8 ± 60.6 mg per deciliter in the Arthus + aprotinin group, and 81.9 ± 48.7 mg per deciliter in the Arthus + steroid group. Similar trends in alpha-1-AT levels were observed among the three groups (Fig. 2B).

DISCUSSION

The anti-inflammatory effects of these two drugs depend on direct local action. For that reason they are very effective following topical application to ears. Triamcinolone diacetate (molecular weight 478.5) is one of the synthetic corticosteroids, and its suspension form (Aristocort) is usually used for the local treatment of joint disease, such as bursitis, synovitis, and arthritis.[1]

In the present study we measured the levels of protease inhibitors, alpha-1-antitrypsin and alpha-2-macroglobulin, in the recovered middle ear fluid. Alpha-1-AT and alpha-2-M are protease inhibitors derived mainly from the blood, and their levels are found to be very low in the normal middle ear.[8] Therefore the levels of both inhibitors in the middle ear fluid may be useful in determining the degree of vascular leakage from the middle ear mucosa in Arthus otitis media. The significant decreases of both alpha-1-AT and alpha-2-M levels in the middle ear fluid by steroid treatment suggest that a steroid drug (triamcinolone) reduces vascular leakage in the early stage of Arthus otitis media. A steroid drug also reduced the number of leukocytes in the middle ear fluid, suggesting that leukocyte infiltration into the middle ear bulla is suppressed by steroid treatment. This may be the result of suppression of the production of chemotactic factors, namely, active complement fragments (C3a, C5a) and prostaglandins.[1,9]

Aprotinin, (molecular weight 6,500) is one of the natural polyvalent protease inhibitors and has strong inhibitory function against the serine type of proteases, such as trypsin, kallikrein, plasmin, and elastase.[3–5] Its significance in clinical usage is to inhibit both the kallikrein-kinin and the fibrinolytic systems. Bradykinin released from high molecular weight kininogen by plasma kallikrein is one of the

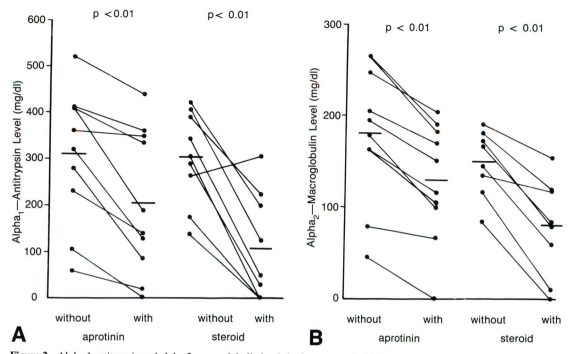

Figure 2   Alpha-1-antitrypsin and alpha-2-macroglobulin levels in the recovered middle ear fluid. *A*, Alpha-1-antitrypsin. Significant differences in the mean were observed with and without the treatments (p < 0.01 in both treatments). *B*, Alpha-2-macroglobulin. A trend similar to that of the alpha-1-antitrypsin level was observed (p < 0.01 in both treatments).

strong vascular permeability enhancing and pain inducing factors.[3,4] The significant decreases in the levels of alpha-1-AT and alpha-2-M in the middle ear fluid by aprotinin treatment indicate that aprotinin remarkably reduces the leakage of the middle ear fluid and that bradykinin is related to the enhanced vascular leakage in the early stage of Arthus otitis media.

It is concluded that both steroid and aprotinin are very effective in reducing the vascular leakage and leukocyte infiltration associated with Arthus otitis media. The kallikrein-kinin system seems to be related to the inflammatory process in the early stage of Arthus otitis media.

This research was supported by NINCDS grant NS-14538 for the Otitis Media Pathogenesis Research Program.

REFERENCES

1. Haynes RC Jr, Murad F. Adrenocortical steroids. In: Gilman AG, Goodman LS, Gilman A, eds. The pharmacological basis of therapeutics. 6th ed. New York: Macmillan, 1975:1966.

2. Lewis GO, Piper PJ. Inhibition of release of prostaglandins as an explanation of some of the actions of anti-inflammatory corticosteroids. Nature (London) 1975; 254:308–311.

3. Werle E. Über einen Hemmkörper für Kallikrein und Trypsin in der Rinderlunge. Hoppe-Seyler Z Physiol Chem 1964; 338:228–230.

4. Schachter M. Kallikrein and kinins. Physiol Rev 1969; 40:510–540.

5. Suda H, Aoyagi T, Hamada M, Takeuchi T, Umezawa H. Antipain, a new protease inhibitor isolated from actinomycetes. J Antibiot 1972; 25:263–266.

6. Takahashi K, Tamoto K, Koyama J. Effects of protease inhibitors of actinomycetes on the first component of human complement. J Antibiot 1976; 29:983–985.

7. Schiessler H, Ohlsson K, Ohlsson I, Arnhold M, Birk Y, Fritz H. Elastase from human and canine granulocytes. II. Interaction with protease inhibitors of animal, plant and microbial origin. Hoppe-Seyler Z Physiol Chem 1977; 358:53–58.

8. Hamaguchi Y, Edlin J, Juhn SK. Protease inhibitors in middle ear effusions from experimental otitis media. Otolaryngol Head Neck Surg 1986; 8:28(abstract).

9. Willoughby DA, DiRosa M. Vasoactive chemical mediators. In: Forscher BK, Houck JC, eds. Immunopathology of inflammation. Amsterdam: Excerpta Medica, 1971:28.

ACTIVATION OF THE COMPLEMENT AND COAGULATION-FIBRINOLYTIC PATHWAYS IN SECRETORY OTITIS MEDIA

JAMES R. CARLSON, M.D., K. JOZAKI, M.D., ALAN DESPINS, B.S.,
MARTHA MERROW, B.S., KATHLEEN FLAHERTY, B.S., GERALD LEONARD, M.D.,
ABRAHAM TZADIK, M.D., THOMAS L. KENNEDY, M.D.,
and DONALD L. KREUTZER, Ph.D.

Activation of the complement and coagulation-fibrinolytic pathways has long been recognized as a hallmark of inflammation. The metabolic products of these activations have been shown to control a wide variety of inflammatory reactions, including vasopermeability as well as leukocyte accumulation in a variety of tissues. However, virtually nothing is known about the existence or significance of these activation products in chronic otitis media with effusion. In the present study we characterized the level of the major activation products of the complement (i.e., C3a and C4a) and coagulation-fibrinolysis (i.e., Bb1–42 and Bb15–42) in middle ear effusion specimens obtained from patients with chronic otitis media with effusion. General inflammatory markers (C3 and total protein levels) were also determined in the samples for correlation with the various activation products. We compared the levels of fibrinogen derived factors and complement products to provide insight into the interaction of these two inflammation systems in middle ear effusions.

METHODS

In this study 66 middle ear effusion specimens were collected from 43 patients—20 females and 23 males with ages ranging from 11 months to 73 years. Thirty-four patients were children less than 16 years of age and nine patients were adults. Their medical problems included cleft palate (one), Down Syndrome (one), premature birth (two), asthma (one), laryngeal cleft (one), and squamous cell carcinoma of the tonsil (one). We classified the effusions on the basis of clinical and laboratory observation as serous (n=22) or mucoid (n=44).

The effusion specimens were collected from patients by use of Juhn Tymtaps at the time of myringotomy. The effusion samples were suspended in 1 mm of Hanks' balanced salt solution, sonicated, centrifuged, the supernatant decanted, and the

volume measured. Aliquots of the resulting effusion specimens were frozen at $-70°$ C and assayed at a later date. Activated C components (C3a, C4a, C5a) were assayed with commercially available radioimmunoassay kits (Upjohn Diagnostics, Kalamazoo, Michigan). Whole C components were determined by enzyme linked immunospecific antibody assay (ELISA).[1] The total protein levels were measured by the Bradford assay.[2] Both normal and complement activated (zymogen) serum levels were measured in all RIA, ELISA, and protein assays and used as a reference standard.[3] The products of plasmin and thrombin cleavage of fibrin, Bb1–42 and Bb15–42, were assayed in commercially available kits (New York Blood Center peptide assay, New York, New York). All data are expressed as total amounts of products in individual effusion specimens. Data were analyzed after logarithmic transformation using the Mann-Whitney and Pearson product correlation tests.

RESULTS

We characterized the antigenic levels of complement and fibrinogenic products of 66 effusion specimens from patients with chronic otitis media. The range of Bb1–42 values was 4 to 28 picomoles and that of Bb15–42 was 3.5 to 90 picomoles. Complement levels ranged from 83 to 9,504 ng for C3a, 545 to 5,721 ng for C4a, and 1 to 292 mg for C3. Total protein levels ranged from 0.16 to 4.15 mg. Serous mucoid and effusion specimens were compared for each of the components, and no significant difference was seen ($p < 0.01$) for complement or fibrinogen products. However, there was a significant difference ($p=0.0085$) for the ratio of Bb1–42 to Bb15–42, such that the serous effusions averaged 1.22 and the mucoid, 0.80 (Table 1). There was a significant and predictable positive relationship ($p < 0.001$) for all complement products except C4a for both serous and mucoid effusions (Table 2).

TABLE 1 Comparison of Serous and Mucoid Middle Ear Effusions for Complement and Fibrinolytic Markers

	Serous	Mucoid
C3a	NS	NS
C4a	NS	NS
C3	NS	NS
Total protein	NS	NS
Bb1–42	NS	NS
Bb15–42	NS	NS
Bb1–42/Bb15–42	1.22 p<0.001	0.80

TABLE 2 Complement Correlation in Serous and Mucoid Middle Ear Effusions

		Serous	Mucoid
Total protein with	C3a	+*	+
	C3	+	+
	C4a	0	0
C3a with	C3	+	+
	C4a	+	+
C3 with	C4a	+	+

* p <0.001

However, there was no correlation between Bb1–42 and Bb15–42 in either serous or mucoid middle ear effusions. Also there was no correlation with levels of Bb1–42 and Bb15–42 and complement product or total protein levels for serous effusions. In mucoid effusions no correlation existed for C3, C3a, C4a, total protein, and Bb1–42 or for total protein, C4a, and Bb15–42. However, C3a and C3 levels correlated significantly with Bb15–42 levels (p=0.004 and p=0.002; Table 3).

TABLE 3 Complement Correlation with Coagulation in Serous and Mucoid Middle Ear Effusions

		Serous	Mucoid
Bb1–42 with	total protein	0	0
	C3a	0	0
	C3	0	0
	C4a	0	0
Bb15–42 with	total protein	0	0
	C3a	0	+
	C3	0	+*
	C4a	0	0

* p<0.005

DISCUSSION

The presence of inflammatory reactions in otitis media with effusion is well established, with various researchers measuring components of the complement, kinin, coagulation, and fibrinolytic systems.[4-8] Compartmentalization of these systems is necessary initially to begin understanding their roles in the pathogenesis of this disease. However, it is well established that these systems interact in the blood and their interaction can alter the outcome of inflammation. Studies have shown that in blood both fibrinolytic and complement system enzymes—serum proteases—can activate and amplify the reaction of their substrates.[9] Experiments have shown that plasmin can activate complement components C2, C3, and C5, that thrombin can cleave C3 and C5, and that complement activation promotes fibrinolysis.

An examination of the interaction of these two systems in middle ear effusions begins with a comparison of the levels of activated products and metabolites of individual effusions. In serous effusions there was no correlation between fibrinolytic products and whole C3, total protein or activated C3, C4. One can infer that despite evidence of the presence of enzymes from both systems, there is no synergism between the complement enzymes and fibrinolytic activation. However, in mucoid effusions a significant correlation existed for plasmin metabolites of fibrinogen products (Bb15–42) and levels of activated C3. One can only infer that plasmin, thrombin, and C3a interactivity promoted generation of their metabolic products in proportion to their presence. The lack of this interactivity in serous effusions may be secondary to the elevated fibrolytic activity on perhaps some other unknown factor. At the very least there appears to be a difference between the two types of effusions in a measurement that excludes differences in collection, dilution, or handling by comparing levels of components within individual effusions.

Other studies have shown differences between serous and mucoid effusions in other immunologic parameters. Lim et al[10] found greater IgA, G, and M activity and functional enzyme levels in mucoid effusions. However, the mucoid effusions in that study were sonicated with glass beads, which perhaps released or altered the immunoglobulins not normally exposed in middle ear effusions and may have increased the concentrations of these products. In fact, in measuring another parameter tested before sonication, the presence of bacteria, there were no differences between serous and mucoid effusions. Another study showed no differences between serous and mucoid effusions in the number of immunologic cell types, both types having T cells.

With similar total levels of complement and fibrinolytic products, it becomes difficult to envision different mechanisms for the generation of serous and mucoid effusions. However, differences were evident when the ratio of fibrinolytic to fibrinogenic products was examined. Serous effusions had a 50 percent greater amount of fibrolytic activity than mucoid effusions. We speculate that this increase in fibrinolysis may prevent the formation of clots within the middle ear space and that in mucoid effusions this lowering of fibrinolytic activity (or raising of fibrinogenic activity) may allow the formation of a "clot," i.e., the mucoid plug. Biochemical examination of this "clot" is necessary to support this theory.

CONCLUSION

The middle ear effusion of otitis media is a complex collection of enzymes, substrates, and products of the various inflammatory systems. C3, C3a, and C4a, as well as total protein levels, were detectable in both serous and mucoid effusions. These levels were positively correlated with each other in all samples, with a $p < 0.01$. Values of the fibrinogen Bb1–42 levels in serous effusions ranged from 4 to 34 picomoles per sample and Bb15–42 levels from 4 to 28 picomoles per sample range. No correlation between levels of Bb15–42 and Bb1–42 were seen in either the serous or mucoid samples. A positive correlation ($p < 0.1$) occurred in mucoid effusions between Bb15–42 and C3–C3a. Finally, when activation product levels in serous and mucoid effusions were compared, only the ratio Bb1–42 to Bb15–42 showed a significant difference between the serous and mucoid samples. The ratio of Bb1–42 to Bb15–42 reflects the relative activities of both plasmin and thrombin in middle ear effusions. Significant differences in the ratios between the serous and mucoid effusions suggest that alterations in these important proteases occur during secretory otitis media. The mechanism responsible for this alteration may involve changes in either protease or antiprotease activity in the middle ear effusions. The impact of these alterations on potent proteases such as plasmin may cause a change in structure, function, and repair of the middle ear and may affect the course or outcome of chronic otitis media with effusion. Currently we are investigating these possibilities, but further studies are necessary to help define these interactions and their possible effects on the pathogenesis of this disorder.

Study partially supported by a grant from the Deafness Research Foundation.

REFERENCES

1. Bullock SL, et al. Evaluation of some parameters of the enzyme linked immunospecific assay. J Infect Dis 1977; 136:5279–5285.
2. Bradford MM. A rapid sensitive method for quantitation of microgram quantities of protein utilizing the principle of protein die binding. Anal Biochem 1976; 72:248–254.
3. Kreutzer DL. Personal communication.
4. Bernstein JM, et al. Complement activity in middle ear effusion. Quinn Exp Immunol 1978; 33:340–346.
5. Prellner K, et al. Complement and CIQ binding substances in otitis media. Ann Otol Rhinol Laryngol 1980; 89(Suppl 68):129–132.
6. Carlson JR, et al. Characterization of complement activation products in SOM. Proceedings, International Conference on Acute and Secretory Otitis Media. Part I, 1986. (In press.)
7. Bernstein JM, et al. The fibrinolysis system in otitis media with effusion. Am J Otolaryngol 1979; 1:28–32.
8. Hamaguchi U, et al. Activities of antiplasmin and antiplasminogen activator in serous middle ear effusions. Ann Otolaryngol 1985; 94:293–298.
9. Sunsmo JS, et al. Relationships among the complement, kinin, coagulation and fibrinolytic systems in the inflammatory reaction. Chn Physiol Biochem 1983; 1:225–284.
10. Lim DJ, et al. Ultrastructural pathology of the middle ear mucosa of secretory otitis media. Ann Otol Rhinol Laryngol 1971; 80:838–855.

IMPORTANCE OF FIBRINOLYTIC ENZYMES ON SECRETORY OTITIS MEDIA PATHOGENESIS

DESIDERIO PASSALI, M.D., LUISA BELLUSSI, M.D.Ch., and MARIA LAURIELLO, M.D.

We would like to discuss in detail the presence of proteases and their physiologic inhibitors in middle ear effusions. In the present study we assessed modifications in the protease-protease inhibitor system in various phases of otitis media with effusion.

Other researchers have pointed out variations in the rate of protease production in various forms of secretory otitis media, i.e., an increase in protease production in the serous as compared to the mucous form.[1]

The behavior of alpha$_1$ antitrypsin also has been assessed in studies of secretory otitis media showing that this inhibitor was present in greater quantities in effusions than in the plasma.[1,2] High levels of unsaturated alpha$_1$ antitrypsin were demonstrated in chronic effusions, which showed a good capacity for neutralizing trypsin.[3] There was also a lower proportion of unsaturated alpha$_2$ macroglobulin available for the inhibition of papain, which may lead to mucosal damage. Collagenolytic activity also has been noted in effusions.[4]

On the basis of these considerations, we provoked secretory otitis media in adult rabbits in order to accurately assess the role played by imbalance of the protease inhibitor system.

MATERIAL AND METHODS

We closed the eustachian tube in 18 adult rabbits (12 males and 6 females) chosen on the basis of normal tympanographic findings. All the animals were anesthetized with pentothal by means of an intraperitoneal injection. In 10 rabbits ligature of the tubes was undertaken after pharyngotomy across the neck, following the technique adopted earlier in cats by Tos et al.[5] In six rabbits we used the method involving the coagulation of the tubes used by Kuijpers and Van der Beek[6] in mice. Finally, in the last two rabbits we used cotton wool and fibrin glue to close one nostril. Thereafter, at 12 hour intervals, each animal was subjected to bilateral tympanometric examination.

In this way it was possible in all cases except one to demonstrate flattening of the tympanometric curve.

With a fine needle and an insulin syringe, the middle ear effusions were removed in varying quantities and subjected to laboratory tests. In 20 samples used for biochemical examination—16 "first samples" and 4 "second samples" (carried out 10 days after flattening of the curve)—fibrinolytic activity was measured.

In order to make the material more fluid, each sample of effusion (0.25 ml) was diluted with saline solution up to 1 ml and mixed with mercaptoethanol to a concentration of 10^{-3} M and kept at $-4°$ C for one night. Then the sample, freed from excess mercaptoethanol by dialyzing with a saline solution, was kept in a freezer at $-20°$ C. Each 0.05 ml of the sample thus treated was placed on a standard fibrin plate (Boehringer Mannheim). After incubation at $37°$ C for 12 hours, on the basis of the transparent halo of lysis forming around each sample, it was possible to assess the lytic activity of the effusion (the square of the diameter of the lysis halo gives the extent of the lytic area in square millimeters). The amounts of alpha$_2$ macroglobulin and alpha$_1$ antitrypsin were measured by spectrophotometry; bacterial cultures were done with 12 samples.

Finally, by inserting a cotton pad into each nostril alternately and leaving it in situ for 20 minutes, 26 nasal samples were obtained.

RESULTS

All the samples sent for culture examination were found to be sterile, and 2 to 7 days after closing of the tubes, flattening of the tympanogram occurred.

The samples taken immediately after these procedures showed lower levels of protease inhibitors than those obtained 10 days later (Tables 1, 2). Proteolytic activity of the effusions compared to that of nasal secretions was greater in the "first samples," whereas in "second samples" this activity was similar to that of the nasal secretions; that is to say, it was practically negligible.

TABLE 1 Fibrinolysis Area and Levels of Alpha₁ Antitrypsin and Alpha₂ Macroglobulin in Middle Ear Effusions Immediately After Flattening of Tympanogram

	Mean and S.D.
Fibrinolysis area (sq mm) on standard fibrin plate	23.25 ± 12.19
α_1 AT (mg %)	250.47 ± 56.88
α_2 MG (mg %)	47.37 ± 19.35

TABLE 2 Fibrinolysis Area and Levels of Alpha₁ Antitrypsin and Alpha₂ Macroglobulin in Middle Ear Effusions 10 Days After Flattening of Tympanogram

	Mean and S.D.
Fibrinolysis area (sq mm) on standard fibrin plate	
α_1 AT (mg %)	330.47 ± 30.92
α_2 MG (mg %)	77.55 ± 11

DISCUSSION

The results of our study are in accordance with a modification over time of the characteristics of the effusion in relation to the protease to antiprotease ratio. In fact, as the effusion induced experimentally by closing of the eustachian tube became chronic, a shifting of the balance of the system was observed in favor of the inhibitors. Thus, we hypothesize that mechanical occlusion of the tube causes modifications in the middle ear, resulting in excessive activation of trypsin and papain released by the neutrophilic granulocytes. The excess of proteolytic activity is responsible for metaplasia of the mucosa toward a pseudostratified epithelium of the respiratory type, with a high level of production of mucus and enzymes,[5] as well as damage to the cell component.

In the absence of prompt recovery of physiologic tubal ventilation, there is an excess of antifibrinolytic enzymes, such as alpha₁ antitrypsin and alpha₂ macroglobulin, which firmly oppose the lytic action of trypsin and papain, inevitably leading the process to become a chronic one.

It should be mentioned also that in the rabbits subjected to the closing of one nasal fossa, an effusion formed in the ear homolateral to the occluded nostril. The significance of this observation requires further study.

REFERENCES

1. Diven WF, Glen RH, Bluestone CD. Lysozyme hydrolases in middle ear effusion. Ann Otol Laryngol 1981; 14:990–995.
2. Carlsson B, Lundberg C, Ohlsson K. Protease inhibitors in middle ear effusion. Ann Otol Rhinol Laryngol 1981; 90:38–41.
3. Hamaguchi Y, Majima Y, Ukai K, Sakakura Y, Miyoschi Y. The significance of protease inhibitors in the pathogenesis of otitis media with effusion. Abstracts, International symposium on recent advances in otitis media with effusion. Kyoto, 1985:75.
4. Granström G, Holmquist J, Jarlstedt J, Renvale V. Collagenase activity in middle ear effusion. Abstracts, International symposium on recent advances in otitis media with effusion. Kyoto, 1985:74.
5. Tos M, Wiederhold M, Larsen P. Experimental long term tubal occlusion in cats. A quantitative histopathological study. Acta Otolaryngol (Stockh) 1984; 97:580–592.
6. Kuijpers W, Van der Beek JMH. Experimental occlusion of the eustachian tube: the role of short- and long-term infection and its sequelae. In: Lim DJ, Bluestone CD, Klein JO, Nelson JD, eds. Recent advances in otitis media with effusion. Proceedings of the Third International Symposium. Toronto: BC Decker, 1984:204–207.

GLYCOCONJUGATES IN EUSTACHIAN TUBE OF THE JAPANESE MONKEY

YUTAKA HANAMURE, M.D., HIROSHI TSURUMARU, M.D., and MASARU OHYAMA, M.D.

Glycoconjugates are integral components of mucosal epithelium and play important roles not only as mucin participating in the mucociliary transport system but also as tissue matrix and specific receptor sites for a variety of substances, resulting in the modulation of cell metabolism.[1] It has been suggested that middle ear effusions contain large amounts of acid glycoconjugates and sugars, especially mucoid effusions.[2,3] Our study was performed to elucidate the cellular and regional differences in the glycoconjugates in the eustachian tube in Japanese monkeys, using lectins that bind to specific saccharide residues or residue sequences of glycoconjugates.

MATERIALS AND METHODS

Tissue Processing

Four adult healthy Japanese monkeys *Macaca fuscata* were used for this study. Under general anesthesia they were subjected to cardiac perfusion with 10 percent neutral buffered formalin. The temporal bones were removed and kept in the same fixative for 3 days. After dissection, the eustachian tube tissues were dehydrated with graded ethanols and embedded in paraffin.

Histochemical Staining

Consecutive 4-μm sections were deparaffinized and stained with alcian blue (pH 2.5), periodic acid–Schiff (AB-PAS) stain, and seven lectins in conjunction with the avidin-biotin-peroxidase complex: *Ulex europeus* agglutinin (UEA-1), peanut agglutinin (PNA), *Dolichos biflorus* agglutinin (DBA), soy bean agglutinin (SBA), *Ricinus communis* agglutinin (RCA), concanavalin A (Con A), and wheat germ agglutinin (WGA; Vector Laboratories, Burlingame, CA). For each lectin staining, deparaffinized and rehydrated sections were immersed into 0.3 percent hydrogen peroxide with methanol at room temperature to block endogenous peroxidase activity and incubated in the following sequence of reagents at room temperature: (1) 1 percent bovine serum albumin in 0.01 M phosphate buffered saline for 5 minutes; (2) 10 μg per ml biotinylated lectin for 30 minutes; and (3) avidin-biotin-peroxidase complex for 30 minutes. All these steps were alternated with three rinses in phosphate buffered saline. The sections were next incubated in freshly prepared 0.05 percent 3,3′-diaminobenzidine tetrahydrochloride, 0.01 percent hydrogen peroxide, and 0.05 M-trishydrochloride buffer (pH 7.2) for 5 minutes. After rinsing with distilled water to stop the peroxidase reaction, the slides were counterstained with hematoxylin. As a negative control we used a lectin absorbed with each inhibitory sugar in place of lectin.

RESULTS

Periodic Acid–Schiff Staining

Goblet cells in the luminal epithelium and subepithelial glands stained an intense purple with AB-PAS, evidence of abundant acid glycoconjugates. Serous cells and mucous cells were distinguishable in the glands; the former possessed well defined small granules and the latter, poorly defined secretory granules (Fig. 1*A*).

Lectin Staining

As shown in Table 1, each cell and its component in the eustachian tube mucosa revealed a striking and selective affinity for each lectin. Mucus in the lumen showed affinities for UEA-1, RCA, Con A, and WGA (Fig. 1*B*, *D*, *E*, *F*). Secretory cells in the luminal epithelium and subepithelial glands showed lectin specific affinities resembling those observed in mucus in the lumen. However, major sugar components of the secretory granules of the secretory cells differed from each other, as demonstrated by the staining intensity for each lectin. For example, in the mucous cells of the glands the secretory granules contained large amounts of fucose, whereas in the serous cells the secretory granules had large amounts of mannose or glucose. In addition, the supranuclear region probably the Golgi complex of the secretory cells disclosed lectin affinities. The supranuclear region of the mucous cells was stained with PNA and SBA and that of serous cells was stained with WGA in the glands, whereas goblet cells showed no affinity for lectin in the supranuclear region (Fig. 1*C*, *F*).

Cilia and the luminal surface of the epithelium stained intensely with RCA and WGA (Fig. 1*D*, *F*), demonstrating the glycocalyx of the cell membrane. Ciliated cells showed diffuse staining for Con A (Fig. 1*E*). Furthermore, the supranuclear region, presumably the Golgi complex, was stained with PNA, SBA, and WGA (Fig. 1*C*, *F*).

DISCUSSION

One of the functions of the eustachian tube is to protect the tympanum by preventing or eliminating invading organisms that enter through the eustachian tube by means of the secretory products and the mucociliary transport system. Glycoconjugates participate in the formation of such secretory products and the mucociliary transport system.

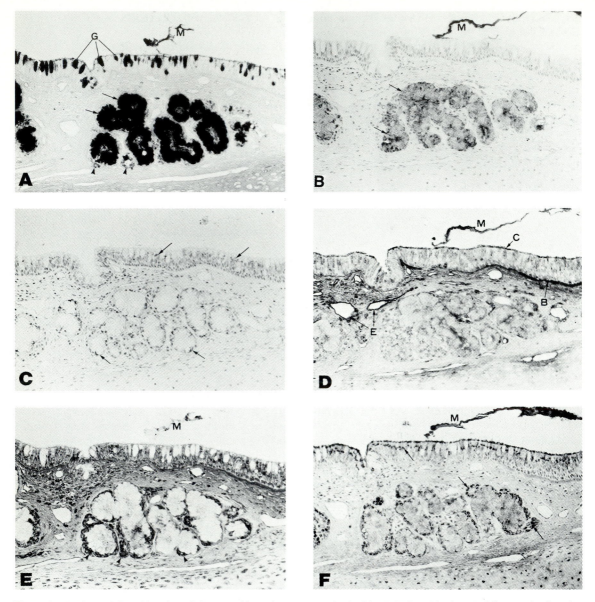

Figure 1 Sections of the midportion of the eustachian tube mucosa stained with AB-PAS and lectins. *A*, Micrograph of section stained with AB-PAS, showing mucus (M) in the lumen, luminal goblet cells (G), and mucous (arrows) and serous (arrow heads) cells of the glands. *B*, Section stained with UEA-1 lectin, showing mucus (M) in the lumen and mucous cells (arrows) of the glands. *C*, Section stained with PNA lectin showing supranuclear regions (arrows) of the ciliated cells and mucous cells of the glands. *D*, Section stained with RCA lectin, showing mucus (M) in the lumen, cilia (C), basement membrane (B), and endothelium of blood vessels (E). *E*, Section stained with Con A lectin, showing mucus (M) in the lumen and serous cells (arrow heads) of the glands. *F*, Section stained with WGA lectin, showing mucus (M) in the lumen and supranuclear region (arrows) of the ciliated cells and serous cells of the glands.

TABLE 1 Lectin Affinities of Glycoconjugates in Eustachian Tubes of Japanese Monkeys

Eustachian Tube	UEA-1*	PNA[†]	DBA[‡]	SBA[§]	RCA[#]	Con A**	WGA[††]
Mucus	3[‡‡]	0	0	0	3	1	3
Cilia	0–1	0	0	0	3	1	3
Ciliated cell (cell body,	0	0	0	0	0–1	2	1
supranuclear region)	0	2–3	0–1	2–3	0	0	3
Goblet cell	0–2	0	0	0	1–2	0–1	1
Basal cell	0	0	0	0	0	3	0
Basement membrane	0	0	0	0	3	3	1
Mucous cell (granule,	3	0	0	0	1–2	0–1	1–2
supranuclear region)	0	3	0	3	0	0	0
Serous cell (granule,	0–1	0	0	0	1–2	3	1
supranuclear region)	0	0	0	0	0	0	3
Endothelium of blood vessel	0	0	0	0	3	1–2	0

* Sugar component: Fucose
[†] Sugar components: Galactose B(1→3) N-acetylgalactosamine
[‡] Sugar component: N-acetylgalactosamine
[§] Sugar components: Galactose, N-acetylglucosamine
[#] Sugar component: Galactose
** Sugar components: Mannose, Glucose
[††] Sugar components: N-acetylglucosamine, Sialic Acid
[‡‡] Numbers indicate staining intensity.

Recent studies with middle ear effusions have shown that the biochemistry of the constituents of mucous glycoconjugates may be an important factor in determining rheologic properties and in insuring effective clearance by the mucociliary transport system.[4] Three kinds of secretory cells—luminal goblet cells and serous and mucous cells of the glands—secrete different kinds of substances composed of glycoconjugates.[5] However, information about the saccharide residues of the glycoconjugates in the secretory cells of the eustachian tube is insufficient.

The present study clarified the nature of saccharide residues in the eustachian tube and demonstrated the main sugar constituent of the three kinds of secretory cells. In our study the major components of the mucus in the lumen of the eustachian tube were fucose, galactose, N-acetylglucosamine, and sialic acid, which are also the main saccharide residues in the secretory granules of the mucous cells of the glands.

It is suggested that the mucous cells of the glands are the major supplier of the mucus involved in the mucociliary transport system in the eustachian tube of normal Japanese monkeys. Tos[6] has reported in autopsy series of adults with secretory otitis media that the mucosa of the eustachian tube was thickened to varying degrees and that there was an increase in goblet cell and gland density. In the pathologic eustachian tube there is an alteration of the constituents and the volume of the glycoconjugates, influencing effective clearance of mucus by ciliary function.

We also discovered that the supranuclear regions, probably the Golgi complex, of the ciliated cells and secretory cells of the glands have affinities for some lectins. It is conceivable that the saccharide residues are transferred by each glycosyltransferase at the Golgi complex and that the affinities of lectins may reflect the biosynthesis of glycoconjugates in the Golgi complex.

REFERENCES

1. Sharon N. Complex carbohydrates. Their chemistry, biosynthesis and function. Boston: Addison-Wesley, 1975.
2. Palva T, Raunio V, Nousiainen R. Middle ear specific proteins in glue ears. Acta Otolaryngol 1975; 79:160–165.
3. Kobayashi K, et al. Sugar components of glycoprotein fractions in middle ear effusions. Arch Otorhinolaryngol 1985; 242:177–182.
4. Brown DT, Litt M, Potsic WP. A study of mucous glycoproteins in secretory otitis media. Arch Otolaryngol 1985; 111:688–695.
5. Hanamure Y, Lim DJ. Normal distribution of lysozyme and lactoferrin-secreting cells in the chinchilla tubotympanum. Am J Otolaryngol 1986; 4:410425.
6. Tos M. Production of mucus in the middle ear and eustachian tube. Ann Otol Rhinol Laryngol 1974; 83:4458.

HYALURONIC ACID IN THE HEALTHY AND DISEASED MIDDLE EAR: A MARKER FOR CONNECTIVE TISSUE INVOLVEMENT?

CLAUDE LAURENT, M.D., STEN O.M. HELLSTRÖM, M.D., Ph.D,
ANDERS TENGBLAD, Ph.D., and KARIN LILJA

In recent years increasing interest has been focused on the importance of the subepithelial connective tissue layer in the middle ear in its normal state and in disease. Paparella et al[1] reported that the subepithelial connective tissue layer exhibited typical structural differences in the various forms of otitis media.

Hyaluronic acid, a high molecular weight polysaccharide, is a major component of all soft connective tissue.[2] It is important in the structural organization of the extracellular matrix and has been considered a marker substance for involvement of the connective tissue in inflammatory disorders.[3] It is tempting to speculate that it also could play a role in modulation of the inflammatory process in the middle ear. In the present study the hyaluronic acid content was determined in various tissue sites in healthy rat middle ears and in middle ears with experimentally provoked serous and purulent otitis media. The hyaluronic acid content also was analyzed in middle ear effusions from rats with experimentally induced serous and purulent otitis media.

MATERIALS AND METHODS

Healthy adult male Sprague-Dawley rats weighing 250 to 350 g were used for the study. Normal middle ears from 25 rats were included. In 31 rats serous otitis media was induced unilaterally by blocking the tympanic orifices of the eustachian tubes with gutta-percha plugs. In 14 rats purulent otitis was provoked bilaterally by splitting the soft palates along the midline.

Tissue specimens were collected from four well defined areas of the middle ear (the pars tensa and pars flaccida of the tympanic membrane and the mucosa of the nasal fossa and the occipital sulcus of the medial wall) and analyzed to determine hyaluronic acid concentration by sensitive and specific radioassay.[4]

Middle ear effusion specimens were obtained after the time periods shown in Tables 1 and 2. The hyaluronic acid concentrations in the serous and purulent effusions were determined by use of the same specific radioassay.[4]

RESULTS

The hyaluronic acid concentrations in pooled tissue samples from the four areas of normal middle ears are shown in Figure 1. The pars flaccida of the tympanic membrane exhibited a level of hyaluronic acid 20 to 30 times higher than that of

TABLE 1 Hyaluronic Acid Concentrations in Effusion Material from Rats with Experimentally Provoked Serous Otitis Media

Duration of Serous Otitis Media (Days)	Hyaluronic Acid Concentration (μ/ml)	
	Mean	Range
3	70.6 (n=6)	43.7 – 95.0
6	86.0 (n=4)	53.7 – 129.3
9	75.4 (n=11)	20.0 – 120.3
14	83.9 (n=4)	26.2 – 116.5
28	94.8 (n=6)	25.3 – 190.0

TABLE 2 Hyaluronic Acid Concentrations in Effusion Material from Rats with Experimentally Induced Purulent Otitis Media

Duration of Purulent Otitis Media (Days)	Hyaluronic Acid Concentration (μ/ml), Left and Right Ears	
	Mean	Range
9	18.4 (n=9)	8.0 – 42.2
24	18.4 (n=9)	3.0 – 29.8
32	9.7 (n=7)	2.4 – 21.8

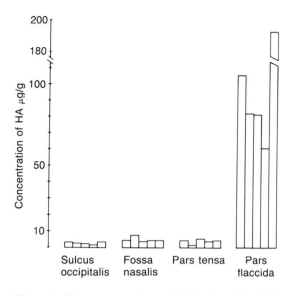

Figure 1 Tissue concentrations of hyaluronic acid in healthy middle ears. Each bar represents a pooled sample (n=5).

the pars tensa and the two mucosal areas of the medial wall.

The hyaluronic acid concentrations in pooled tissue samples from the middle ears with otitis media are shown in Figure 2. The major alteration was that in purulent otitis media the pars flaccida contained considerably less hyaluronic acid than in serous otitis media and normal middle ears (Fig. 1.) The other tissue sites showed variable but slightly increased hyaluronic acid concentrations as compared with the range observed in normal middle ears (see Fig. 1.)

The concentrations of hyaluronic acid in the effusions from the ears with serous otitis media are shown in Table 1. Hyaluronic acid was present in the effusion material after 3 days and remained at approximately the same level throughout the study. The hyaluronic acid concentrations in the effusion material in purulent otitis media are shown in Table 2. The purulent effusion material had a considerably lower concentration of hyaluronic acid than the serous effusion material Table 1, and in purulent otitis media the concentration had a tendency to decrease with time.

DISCUSSION

The present study shows that hyaluronic acid occurs in middle ear tissues at all sites analyzed but with regional differences. In the tympanic membrane the concentration is considerably higher)20 to 30 times) in the pars flaccida than in the pars tensa.

This is an interesting observation, because these two portions of the tympanic membrane are also structurally different in regard to fiber composition, occurrence of mast cells, and innervation.[5-7]

Large amounts of hyaluronic acid appeared early in the serous and purulent effusion materials in both serous and purulent otitis media. The concentration in the effusion material in serous otitis was higher than in purulent otitis media. In serous otitis the hyaluronic acid remained at almost the same level throughout the study, whereas in the purulent form it had a tendency to decrease with time. The lower concentration in the pars flaccida and in the effusion material in purulent otitis may depend on the degradation of hyaluronic acid by invading inflammatory cells or bacteria, producing hyaluronidase and other slow acting enzymes.[8] The concentrations of hyaluronic acid in both serous and purulent effusion materials were 1,000 times higher than in the circulating blood and were comparable to those previously determined for lymph.[9]

That middle ear effusions contain significant amounts of hyaluronic acid indicates involvement of the connective tissue in otitis media. It is possible that hyaluronic acid in the diseased middle ear may play a role in modulating the inflammatory process, for it has been reported that hyaluronic acid can interact with and regulate the function of granulocytes, macrophages, and immune competent cells.[10] Because hyaluronic acid occurs in significant concentrations in healthy and diseased middle ears, the substance must be considered when we attempt to understand the function of the middle ear under normal circumstances and in various inflammatory disorders.

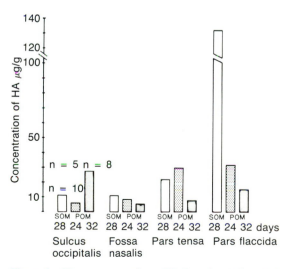

Figure 2 Tissue concentrations of hyaluronic acid in middle ears with serous (SOM) and purulent (POM) otitis media.

REFERENCES

1. Paparella MM, Sipilä P, Juhn SK, Jung TTK. Subepithelial space in otitis media. Laryngoscope 1985; 95:414–420.
2. Laurent TC. Chemistry, structure and metabolism of hyaluronic acid. In: Balazs EA, ed. Chemistry and molecular biology of the intercellular matrix. New York: Academic Press, 1970:703–732.
3. Hällgren R, Eklund A, Engström-Laurent A, Schmekel B. Hyaluronate in bronchoalveolar lavage fluid: a new marker in sarcoidosis reflecting pulmonary disease. Br Med J 1985; 290:1778–1781.
4. Laurent UBG, Tengblad A. Determination of hyaluronate in biological samples by a specific radioassay technique. Anal Biochem 1980; 109:386–394.
5. Lim DJ. Human tympanic membrane. An ultrastructural observation. Acta Otolaryngol Stockh 1970; 70:176–186.
6. Alm PE, Bloom GD, Hellström S, Stenfors LE, Widemar L. Mast cells in the pars flaccida of the tympanic membrane. A quantitative morphological and biochemical study in the rat. Experentia 1983; 39:287–289.
7. Widemar L, Hellström S, Schultzberg M, Stenfors LE. Autonomic innervation of the tympanic membrane. An immunocytochemical and histofluorescence study. Acta Otolaryngol Stockh 1985; 100:58–65.
8. Lowell SH, Juhn SK. The role of bacterial enzymes in inducing inflammation in the middle ear cavity. Otolaryngol Head Neck Surg 1979; 87:859–870.
9. Tengblad A, Laurent UBG, Lilja K, Cahill RNP, EngströmLaurent A, Fraser JRE, Hansson HE, Laurent TC. Concentration and relative molecular mass of hyaluronate in lymph and blood. Biochem J 1986; 236:521–525.
10. Laurent TC. Biochemistry of hyaluronan. Acta Otolaryngol Stockh 104(Suppl 442):7–29.

SEQUELAE

SPECIAL LECTURE: OTITIS MEDIA WITH EFFUSION AND THE DEVELOPMENT OF LANGUAGE

JEAN B. GLEASON, Ph.D.

Delayed language development is one of the most troubling of the many possible negative sequelae of otitis media with effusion in young children. Numerous researchers have attempted to document that such effects do indeed occur; less effort has been directed toward providing a theoretical rationale. In the light of contemporary interactional theory, language delay does not appear to be ineluctable, and recent research on language development in normal populations provides some insight into how possible language problems might be mitigated through careful attention to the at-risk child's language environment.

THE NORMAL COURSE OF LANGUAGE DEVELOPMENT

One of the reasons for the theoretical weakness in typical studies of otitis media with effusion is that although researchers on language are agreed about the nature of the general course of development, we disagree about how to account for development theoretically. We agree, for instance, that there are nearly universal stages in prelinguistic development during the first year of life: infants produce mostly vegetative sounds and reflexive crying during the first couple of months. In the next stage the baby begins to coo and laugh. Then, at about the age of 6 months the infant begins to babble, to play with speech sounds and syllables. By the age of 1 year, infants in all language communities babble reduplicated syllables such as "mama." In the last of these prelinguistic stages a kind of babbling, called jargon, which has the intonational pattern of adult sentences, is produced by many infants even after they have begun to say some real words.[1]

Even during the first year, infants have sophisticated auditory and cognitive capacities: They are capable of making fine phonetic discriminations; they pay attention to the intonation of what is said to them; and they understand individual words like "no" and "blanket" long before they can produce them. During the early months, babies also learn many principles of conversation, such as turn taking, as part of their interactions with adults; this occurs in "conversations" in which the babies' burbles, coughs, and sneezes are given the status of conversational turns by adults.[2]

After infants begin to speak, they go through some other typical stages as well; for some time most are at a one word stage. Once they have about 50 words, there is often a sudden spurt in vocabulary size, and at about this time (frequently late in the second year) children begin to make rudimentary "telegraphic" sentences consisting of two or three words, without any grammatical markers such as articles, plural markers, or verb endings. "There Daddy" and "Kitty eat lunch" are typical utterances at this stage.

In the next stage of development, English speaking children acquire some simple grammatical forms, such as the plurals, past tenses, and articles that previously were absent from their speech, and they learn to make a number of different types of sentences, such as questions and negatives. Thus, by the age of 3 or 4 they have acquired the basic system; more complex forms, such as passives, come later, but by the time children enter school, the major tasks of language development have been accomplished.[3] If otitis media with effusion affects language acquisition, it must do so during the child's first 3 or 4 years.

THEORETICAL PERSPECTIVES

Just how to account for language development is a matter of historical disagreement in the field of developmental psycholinguistics. In order to evaluate the claim and the evidence that during the first 3 years of life the fluctuating hearing loss characteristic of otitis media with effusion may adversely affect language development, it is necessary to consider some current theoretical perspectives: behaviorist, innatist, cognitive, and interactionist.[4]

Behaviorism

Behaviorists and others who emphasize the role of learning contend that language, like other behavior patterns, is learned according to the general laws of learning. They assume that, for instance, the progression from babbling to speech that has been outlined here is a result of selective reinforcement by adults, who reward the child for making sounds that resemble the target language. This Skinnerian view holds that language is not a special capacity, and it is one that often offends scholars in linguistics, yet until recent times it was the theoretical perspective of most language intervention or remediation programs. A behaviorist explanation for why children with otitis media could have language problems might be that parents of such children are unaware of the associated hearing loss and fail to adjust their teaching methods to account for the child's lessened acuity. Alternatively a child with ear pain might associate the pain with listening, and thus find language unrewarding.

Innatism

A contrasting theoretical perspective is provided by adherents of a linguistic-innatist position. This Chomskyan view holds that adults have little to do with language development in children, except insofar as they provide samples of the target language for the child to analyze. Innatists believe that children are born preprogrammed for language, equipped with a conceptual language acquisition device, ready to abstract the rules of language from the language they are exposed to. The innatist position assumes that the child has built in language processing and filtering capacities. This theory appears to be implicit in many of the studies of otitis media that have been reported,[5] and it provides the most commonly stated rationale for possible language problems. Researchers assume that the mild fluctuating hearing loss caused by otitis media interferes with the child's ability to process the incoming acoustic signal; as a consequence the child is not able to make the correct hypotheses about how the language system works. The child's task is made especially difficult, according to this view, because the signal is variable and inconsistent.

The Cognitive View

This basically Piagetian view sees language development as secondary to cognitive development. According to this theory, children first learn about the world (for instance, what a dog is and what dogs are like); then they learn the word "dog." Piagetians believe that general cognitive ability underlies language acquisition and development. From this perspective we would expect that if otitis media has negative effects, they would therefore not be limited to language but rather would be more pervasive and affect all types of cognitive functioning.

Social Interactionist

Supporters of this theory agree with behaviorists that some parts of language are explicitly taught to children. For instance, our own work has shown that contrary to what was previously believed, babies' first conventionalized communicative expression in the United States is "bye bye," which parents train even prelinguistic infants to say.[6] Unlike behaviorists, however, social interactionists agree with innatists that humans come into the world with neural mechanisms that subserve language and with a predisposition to acquire language. We agree also that there are some cognitive prerequisites to acquiring language.

However, social interactionists put a great deal of emphasis on the child's social and communicative motivations for acquiring language and on special adjustments in their own speech that adults make when speaking to young children that may facilitate language development. During the prelinguistic period, for instance, infants use their vocal abilities to get and hold the attention of adults. Adults interact with infants in a way that fosters language development. They assume that babies have something to say, and they hold conversations with them: even a burp or sneeze counts as a turn.[2]

As children approach the end of the first year, recent research has shown that adults speaking to them modify their speech to make the phonology (sounds) of the language clearer and cleaner; for instance, they distinguish between words that are often pronounced alike, such as "kiddie" and "kitty." As children begin to acquire the language, adults' speech to them is simpler, slower, more redundant, child centered, clearly articulated, and better formed grammatically than speech to other adults. It appears to be fine tuned to the child's current linguistic state.[7]

A social interactionist rationale for language problems as a result of otitis media would assume that the disease contributes in some way to a disruption of the communicative matrix that exists between parent and child such that the child does not receive the optimal linguistic input.

Research on Otitis Media and Language: Possible Models

The literature relating to the effects of otitis media on language development presents conflicting results. Some studies have shown no adverse long term effects, whereas others have reported, variously, reduced auditory acuity as measured by the auditory brainstem response, lower IQ, worse performance on a variety of expressive measures, and poorer narrative and discourse skills. It is not surprising that the studies have such disparate results, since most of them were retrospective rather than prospective, and they have used different methods and measures and widely varying populations. It is now important to develop models relating to possible effects and to design research that is theory driven and related to those models.

The work of Feagans et al[7] for instance, attempts to do this, citing three possible models for developmental effects: First, the problem might occur simply because the child has been ill, rather than because of anything specific to otitis media; children with the common cold, for instance, also have more difficulty than well children. A second model, which has been alluded to here already, postulates that a fluctuating hearing loss during the language formative years may cause problems directly by degrading the incoming auditory signal and making it more difficult for the child to categorize language. This model predicts a delay in basic lower order language acquisition.

The third model that Feagans et al propose is an attentional one: Because the auditory signal is unclear or unstable during bouts of otitis media for young children, they may develop the habit of paying less attention to language than normal hearing children. This would have long term effects on higher order processes, such as discourse and narrative, which require sustained attention, but not on basic lower order processes. Feagans reports experimental results that uphold this model: A group of children who had a history of otitis media were compared with controls on attention measures, basic linguistic measures, and narrative tasks. As predicted, the children with a history of otitis media showed more attentional deficits and poorer narrative skills but were equivalent in basic syntactic development.

The social interactionist theoretical position offers a model that is more inclusive than what has just been described. First, we must recognize that there are individual differences in children—different cognitive styles and motivations. Thus, the same environmental factors might have differential effects on different children. Some children, even with otitis media and reduced hearing, may be strongly motivated to communicate and willing to work very hard to overcome any processing problems; others might be inclined to tune out.

More important, subtle changes may take place in parent-child interaction when the child has otitis media that may cause the parent to provide a less than optimal linguistic environment. If the child is not hearing well, she may also not provide the kind of feedback that the parent needs to adjust his speech. Even such behavior as the child's smiling has a strong effect on parental behavior: We know that children who smile less receive less speech from their parents. We need to conduct research on otitis media that deals with the entire communicative environment of children with the disease. We do not presently know, for instance, whether children with otitis media are talked to less or differently than other children because of these subtle but pervasive interactive effects.

CONCLUSION

We are not certain that otitis media with effusion has long term effects on language development but there are many theoretical reasons why it might. Language is, however, a robust and well buffered system and it is likely that there are many ways to offset the kinds of problems posed by otitis media with effusion. Until we have definitive research results, there is a conservative stance to adopt in terms of intervention, and that is to make sure that parents understand that the child with otitis media with effusion will have temporarily diminished hearing, and to encourage parents of children with otitis media with effusion to provide them with varied and full linguistic experiences in an environment that assures that the child can hear what is being said and is responsive. This linguistic enrichment is, of course, appropriate for all children, but it might serve a protective function for children who are prone to frequent bouts of otitis media with effusion.

REFERENCES

1. Sachs J. Prelinguistic development. In: Gleason JB, ed. The development of language. Columbus: CE Merrill, 1985:37.
2. Snow CE. The development of conversations between mothers

and babies. J Child Lang 1977; 4:1–22.
3. Brown R. A first language. Cambridge: Harvard University Press, 1973.
4. Bohannon JN, Warren-Leubecker A. Theoretical approaches to language acquisition. In: Gleason JB, ed. The development of language. Columbus: CE Merrill, 1985:173.
5. Menyuk P. Predicting speech and language problems with persistent otitis media. In: Kavanagh JF, ed. Otitis media and child development. Parkton, MD: York, 1986:83.
6. Gleason JB, Perlmann RY, Greif EB. What's the magic word: learning language through routines. Discourse Processes 1984; 6:493–502.
7. Feagans L, Sanyal M, Henderson F, Collier A, Appelbaum M. The relationship of middle ear disease in early childhood to later narrative and attention skills. J Pediatr Psychol (in press).

AUDITORY DEFICIT IN INFANTS WITH OTITIS MEDIA WITH EFFUSION: MORE THAN A "MILD" HEARING LOSS

ROBERT J. NOZZA, Ph.D.

The notion that delays in language and speech development can occur as a result of chronic middle ear effusion in early childhood relies, in part, on theories of auditory deprivation and critical periods. Proponents of that position believe that the hearing loss associated with middle ear effusion during language learning years is sufficient to disrupt the processing of speech and results in the failure to properly acquire the phonology, syntax, and semantics of language.

Skeptics argue that the hearing loss that accompanies middle ear effusion is only a "mild" one and is insufficient to cause major disruptions of auditory input. The average hearing thresholds of older children with otitis media with effusion are typically about 20 to 25 dB hearing level (HL),[1] a mild impairment according to traditional criteria for judging the severity of hearing loss. On the other hand, it has been suggested that the criteria for categorizing degrees of impairment should be different for younger children and infants from those for subjects who are older because of the extraordinary need for high quality auditory input during language acquisition.[2] That is, a 25 dB hearing loss may be more than a mild impairment in the infant or young child.

The latter proposition assumes that the hearing loss associated with otitis media with effusion in infants and the very young is the same as that in older children and adults. There is no reason to suspect that an effusion in the infant's ear causes a greater threshold shift than it does in the older child's ear. Therefore, it is reasoned, the need for a lower "fence" for impairment in the infant must be due to processes that are beyond the sensory system and that are related to the organization of speech input into a meaningful language system.

The purpose in this article is to suggest that there is more than one reason infants with otitis media with effusion might have a greater impairment than older children with the disease. As noted, the complexity of the auditory-linguistic challenge faced by infants during the first year of life makes it reasonable to hypothesize that infants are more impaired with a given amount of hearing loss than are older children. What has not been recognized, however, is that infants with otitis media with effusion do not respond to sound until it is presented at higher intensity levels than are required by older children with otitis media with effusion. With respect to our standards for normal hearing, the minimal response levels of infants with otitis media with effusion suggest a greater hearing loss than do the thresholds obtained in older children. In addition, recent research suggests that the relationship between the intensity level required to detect speech and the intensity level required to perform more complex tasks, such as discrimination or recognition of speech, is different for infants than for older groups. In the following section three lines of evidence are discussed to support the position that, in addition to requiring a different criterion for impairment, infants as a group have a greater reduction in auditory capability than is commonly thought during episodes of otitis media with effusion.

MEASURES OF HEARING IN INFANTS AND CHILDREN

Infant Minimal Response Levels Are Elevated Relative to Those in Older Children and Adults

Behavioral measures of infant hearing have improved greatly in recent years. Use of new techniques, such as visual reinforcement audiometry, and the introduction of strict psychophysical procedures have produced reliable estimates of infant hearing. In fact, several experimental studies have been done with infants using earphone presentation of test sounds to better compare with data from older groups.

Data from two studies using the head-turn procedure with normal hearing 6 month olds reveal that infant minimal response level for pure tone signals presented monaurally under earphones are elevated relative to audiometric standards and thresholds of older children.[3,4] In addition, infant minimal response levels have a different variation with frequency, with relatively poorer hearing in the low to middle frequencies. For example, the mean minimal response levels at 500 and 1,000 Hz in infants with normal middle ear function are 25 and 15 dB HL, respectively. These are similar to the mean thresholds (about 25 dB HL for both frequencies) in older children with otitis media with effusion.[1] The shift in hearing associated with effusion (about 15 to 20 dB), if added to the normal infant minimal response level, would place infant minimal response levels well above (i.e., much poorer than) thresholds typically found in older children with otitis media with effusion.

In a recent study of masking and binaural hearing, a monaural minimal response level for a speech sound presented in quiet was estimated for adults, preschool children, and infants, all with normal middle ear function.[5] A computer based visual reinforcement audiometry procedure was used to establish this speech awareness threshold for infants under earphones, and play audiometry was used for the preschool children. The speech awareness threshold for infants was about 17 dB poorer than that for the adults and about 9 dB poorer than that for the preschoolers, again demonstrating an age related difference in normal ability to respond to auditory stimuli.

The Speech Recognition Threshold and the Speech Awareness Threshold Do Not Measure the Same Feature of Auditory Function

At this point one might ask why data from our clinical studies do not reflect this apparent age related difference in hearing. The reason is that the measure typically used with older children is the speech recognition threshold and the measure used with infants for comparison is the speech awareness threshold. For example, in a recent article on hearing and otitis media with effusion, infant speech awareness threshold data were presented side by side with speech recognition threshold data from older children.[1] There was a great similarity between both the means and the distributions of the two measures (speech recognition threshold: mean = 22.7 dB, SD = 10.9; speech awareness threshold: mean = 24.6 dB, SD = 11.3). A fact that is sometimes ignored or misunderstood, however, is that the speech awareness threshold and the speech recognition threshold do not measure the same dimension of auditory function. For one, the speech awareness threshold is usually measured in the sound field with infants, whereas the speech recognition threshold is determined monaurally with older children. Moreover, the speech awareness threshold is an estimate of the lowest hearing level at which a listener can detect the presence of speech, whereas the speech recognition threshold is an estimate of the lowest hearing level at which simple words can be identified with about 50 percent accuracy.[6] Among those who can provide both measures, there is typically about a 10 dB difference between the speech awareness threshold and the speech recognition threshold.

As mentioned, the speech awareness threshold in normal hearing infants is poorer than that in older children and adults. Clinical measures of hearing in older children are also consistent with the 10 dB difference between the two thresholds found in adults. If we extrapolate, the ability of the infant to recognize speech must be at least 10 dB poorer than the speech awareness threshold. In that case the "speech recognition threshold" (estimated) of the normally developing infants would be about 20 dB HL, a level that is near the point of impairment (20 to 25 dB HL) according to our traditional definitions.

At the same time that the group of normal hearing infants was providing minimal response levels for the speech sound, already discussed, a group of infants who met tympanometric criteria for effusion were also being tested under the same protocol.[5] In this group the speech awareness threshold was about 18 dB poorer than that of the normal group. This 18 dB difference between ears with effusion and ears without effusion in infants is consistent with data from older children. The monaural speech awareness threshold in infants with otitis media with effusion is about 30 dB HL. If we adjust the speech awareness threshold in infants with otitis media with effusion by 10 dB to predict their speech recognition threshold, as done already for the normal hearing infants, it is apparent that the infants with otitis media with effusion are operating at a level (40 dB HL) that is in a region of greater impairment than that suggested by the speech awareness threshold data commonly reported.

Performance Versus Intensity in Speech Discrimination

The relationship between the speech awareness and speech recognition thresholds in infants, of course, is only speculative, because we have no way to measure the speech recognition threshold in infants. Besides, one might argue that the difference between the speech awareness threshold and the speech recognition threshold in the older groups is only 10 dB and does not provide sufficient evidence that the infant is experiencing the auditory world at a greater handicap. Investigations in our laboratory of the ability of infants to discriminate among various speech sounds as a function of the intensity level of the stimuli apply directly to the question of hearing loss and higher level processing of speech. Data collected so far relating to speech-sound discrimination in infants lend support to the notion that infants have at least as great, and probably a greater, difference between their speech awareness threshold and their ability to discriminate among speech sounds than do adults. Through a modification of the head-turn procedure, infants are taught to respond with a head turn to a change in a repeating background speech sound. The ability to discriminate one speech sound from another then can be assessed. We have determined that normal hearing infants do not reach their maximal level of performance in such a task until speech is at least 40 or 45 dB HL. This is 25 dB or more above their speech awareness threshold. Adults in the same task reach nearly maximal performance levels within 10 dB of their speech awareness threshold.

Performance versus intensity for discrimination of /ba/ from /da/ in normal hearing infants and adults is illustrated in Figure 1.[7] Note that the infants' performance does not reach a maximum until intensity levels are well above their speech awareness threshold (10 dB HL) and well above those at which adults achieve their maximum. Although this measure is not the same as the speech recognition threshold, it reflects complex discrimination processes that underlie recognition. Note that for infants the difference between the speech awareness threshold and optimal performance on a simple

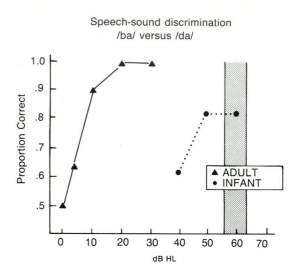

Figure 1 Performance versus intensity in a speech-sound discrimination task (/ba/ versus /da/) for infants and adults. The infant performance function is adapted from data reported in reference 7 and converted to approximate decibel hearing level values. The discrimination functions were measured in a sound field. The shaded bar approximates the long-term average intensity level of conversational speech.

speech discrimination task is much greater than the 10 dB difference between the speech awareness and speech recognition thresholds in older children.

It should also be noted that the intensity level at which infants reach maximal performance is not very far below levels generally considered to be the levels at which conversational speech is heard. If we assume a level of 60 dB HL for conversational speech, normal hearing infants will be at their maximal performance (proportion correct [P(C)] = 0.80 to 0.85) for this procedure. However, if the presentation level is reduced to about 40 dB HL, simulating a reduction in hearing of only 20 dB, infant performance is degraded considerably, down to P(C) = 0.62, which is only slightly above chance performance of P(C) = 0.50 in this procedure. This is not the case for the adults who continue to perform near maximum with presentation levels down to 20 dB HL and below.

DISCUSSION

It is clear from recent data relating to infant auditory function that infants with middle ear effusion encounter their auditory environment with more than a mild hearing loss. This occurs because the threshold shift accompanying the effusion overlays a developmental requirement for greater stimulus intensity before an infant can either respond to or discriminate speech. This places them nearer the margin of impairment than previously thought. This situation may be obscured in clinical data because the methods for testing the hearing of infants (e.g., the speech awareness threshold) are not directly comparable to those used with older children (e.g., the speech recognition threshold), but often produce similar values and are reported in a similar context. The data reveal that, besides a need to redefine categories of severity for hearing loss in the very young, continued efforts must be directed toward defining the nature of the auditory deficit of infants with middle ear effusion. Such data must be paired with a better understanding of speech acoustics and the phonologic, syntactic, and semantic problems the infant attempts to solve at various stages of language and speech development. Until these things are done, it will be difficult to generate testable hypotheses regarding the long term consequences of otitis media.

Study funded by NIH grant NS 163337, the Deafness Research Foundation, and the Pennsylvania Lions Hearing Research Foundation.

REFERENCES

1. Fria TJ, Cantekin EI, Eichler JA. Hearing acuity of children with otitis media with effusion. Arch Otolaryngol 1985; 111:10–16.
2. Northern JL, Downs MP. Hearing in children. 3rd ed. Baltimore: Williams & Wilkins, 1984:1.
3. Nozza RJ, Wilson WR. Masked and unmasked puretone thresholds of infants and adults: developmental change in frequency selectivity and sensitivity. J Speech Hear Res 1984; 27:613–622.
4. Hesketh LJ, Wilson WR. Pure-tone thresholds and ear-canal pressure levels in infants and adults. Paper presented at the annual convention of the American Speech-Language-Hearing Association, November 1984, Detroit, MI.
5. Nozza RJ, Wagner EF, Crandell MA. Binaural release from masking for a speech sound in infants, preschoolers and adults. J Speech Hear Res (in press).
6. Hirsh IJ, Davis H, Silverman SR, Reynolds EG, Eldert E, Benson RW. Development of materials for speech audiometry. J Speech Hear Disord 1952; 17:321–337.
7. Nozza RJ. Infant speech-sound discrimination testing: effects of stimulus intensity and procedural model on measures of performance. J Acoust Soc Am 1987; 81:1706–1718.

BRAINSTEM AUDITORY EVOKED POTENTIALS IN CHILDREN WITH TYMPANOSTOMY TUBES

MARY JEAN OWEN, M.D., KARYL NORCROSS, M.D., Ph.D., VIRGIL M. HOWIE, M.D., LAWRENCE DUSSACK, B.S., and BARRY D. BOONE, B.A.

Owing to its widespread prevalence, otitis media is the leading cause of hearing loss in childhood. The placement of tympanostomy tubes to treat chronic otitis media with effusion or recurrent acute otitis media is one of the most common surgical procedures performed during early childhood. The peak incidence of otitis media occurs during the first 3 years of life, a time when reliable use of standard audiometric techniques is difficult or impossible. Information regarding the hearing status of young children with otitis media with effusion is needed to make clinical treatment decisions, to test the safety

and efficacy of treatment interventions, and to perform studies addressing the potential long term sequelae of this common condition. Two techniques are currently available to evaluate hearing in these young children: behavioral audiometry using operant conditioning techniques and brainstem auditory evoked potential (BAEP) testing.

BAEPs were first described in the early 1970s.[1] They can be used to assess peripheral and brainstem auditory function in very young children. The BAEP consists of electrical activity recorded from scalp electrodes in response to the presentation of a sound stimulus to one ear. Computer averaging of the responses to repeated clicks cancels the background electroencephalographic activity and allows detection of the series of five reproducible waves that appear in the first 10 milliseconds after the stimulus. Wave I, and possibly wave II, arise from the auditory nerve.[2] Waves III through V are generated in the ascending brainstem auditory pathways. Waves after wave V are probably due to activity rostral to the brainstem. A conductive hearing loss delays transmission of sound through the middle ear or decreases the intensity of sound presented to the cochlea. Both these effects result in a delay in the appearance of wave I, or a prolongation of the wave I latency. If brainstem function is intact, subsequent waves are displaced by an equal amount of time.

Although BAEPs are widely used clinically, few reports have been published regarding the use of this technique in young children with otitis media with effusion.[3-6] This observational study reports our results using BAEPs in the clinical assessment of hearing loss due to otitis media with effusion and of the effect of tympanostomy tube placement on the hearing function in young children.

METHODS

Study Population

BAEP testing was performed on 63 children who presented to the pediatric clinic between June 1986 and March 1987 with a history of chronic otitis media with effusion. Forty-nine children were tested immediately before and after myringotomy and placement of tympanostomy tubes. Nineteen were tested at a follow-up visit for tubes placed 3 weeks to 18 months previously (mean duration of tube presence, 7 months). Five were studied both at the time of tube insertion and at follow-up. The children ranged in age from 3 months to 6 years (mean age, 21 months). Eighty-four percent of the subjects were less than 3 years of age. Thirty-five subjects were males; 28 were females. Fifty-four of the subjects were Caucasians and nine were blacks.

Tympanostomy Tube Placement Procedure

The clinical decision to place tympanostomy tubes was based upon a documented history of persistent otitis media with effusion lasting for 6 weeks or more. After obtaining parental informed consent, bilateral myringotomy with placement of tympanostomy tubes was performed under chloral hydrate sedation after the administration of a Xylocaine and epinephrine local anesthetic via iontophoresis. General anesthesia was not used. Chloral hydrate is the standard sedative used for BAEP testing and is known to have no effect upon BAEP results. To determine whether the local anesthetic affected any BAEP parameters, several subjects were tested immediately before and after its administration, prior to tube placement. No differences were found, and this variable was excluded from further consideration.

BAEP Technique

BAEPs were recorded using a 200 microsecond duration, mixed frequency, rarefaction click sound stimulus presented monaurally via earphones at a rate of 31.1 clicks per second. The nonstimulated ear was masked with white noise 30 db below stimulus intensity. Recording electrodes were applied via a standard technique to the vertex and over each mastoid area. A midfrontal electrode was used as a ground. A Pathfinder II evoked potential machine (Nicolet Biomedical, Inc.) was used to amplify, filter (150 Hz to 3 kHz), and average the electrical activity in the first 15 milliseconds following presentation of 2,000 clicks for each trial. Movement artifact was automatically rejected by the averaging computer. Each trial was repeated at least once to ensure reproducibility of responses.

For each ear the initial BAEP tracing was recorded using a 75 db intensity stimulus. Stimulation was then performed at 30, 20, and 10 db, and additional intensities as indicated, until a minimum of three BAEPs with an identifiable wave V were recorded at different stimulus intensities. The type of hearing loss was characterized and the degree of hearing deficit measured by generation of a wave V latency versus click intensity curve, as described by Galambos and Hecox.[7] Thus, hearing losses reported represent a deviation from a laboratory established normal range for age and cannot be considered directly equivalent to an audiometric threshold value or air-bone gap.

RESULTS

The 137 ears in 63 subjects tested were divided into four clinical categories: ears with effusion tested before and after tube placement (effusion present), ears without effusion tested before and after tube placement (effusion absent), ears with dry functional tubes (dry tubes), and ears with tubes that had otorrhea present at the time of testing (draining tubes). The effusion absent ears had had otitis media in the

TABLE 1   Mean (SD) Peak Latencies Using 75 db Stimulus in the Four Clinical Categories of Ears Tested*

		Wave I	WaveV
Effusion present (56 ears)	Before tubes	2.51 (0.68)	6.64 (0.54)
	After tubes	2.07 (0.37)†	6.28 (0.40)†
Effusion absent (24 ears)	Before tubes	1.99 (0.39)	6.26 (0.39)
	After tubes	2.01 (0.30)	6.29 (0.34)
Dry tubes (28 ears)		1.88 (0.27)	6.01 (0.22)
Draining tubes (9 ears)		2.58 (0.81)	6.85 (0.93)
Upper limit of normal range for children ≥ 6 months (laboratory mean + 2SD)		2.00	6.12

* All values expressed in milliseconds.
† After tube mean peak latency significantly different from tube mean peak latency (p < 0.001 via Wilcoxon signed ranks test).

past that had cleared at the time of tube placement, but cannot be considered normal ears.

Table 1 presents the mean peak I and V latencies for the four clinical categories of ears in subjects 6 months of age and older. In the 56 effusion present ears, mean wave I and V peak latencies were prolonged beyond the laboratory established normal range (mean + 2 SD). Immediately after tube placement, the mean peak latencies in these ears improved significantly (p < 0.001 via Wilcoxon signed ranks test). In the 24 effusion absent ears, the mean wave I and V peak latencies were at the upper limit of the normal range, and did not change significantly after tube placement. In the 28 dry tube ears, the mean peak latencies were normal. The nine draining tube ears had markedly prolonged mean I and V peak latencies compared to normal.

Because there is a normal maturational decrease in BAEP peak latencies during the first 6 months of life, results for the subjects less than 6 months of age were analyzed separately and were similar to those of the older children. Values for the subjects less than 6 months of age were included in the mean hearing loss calculations for the four clinical categories, because the method of calculating hearing loss incorporates a correction for age.

The 63 effusion present ears had a mean hearing loss of 22 db. Immediately after tube placement, the hearing loss in the same ears was significantly improved (p < 0.001 via Wilcoxon signed ranks test) to 11 db. Table 2 shows that before tube placement, 65 percent of the effusion present ears had clinically significant hearing loss of 15 db or more. Hearing losses before and after tube placement in these ears differed significantly (p < 0.001 by chi square testing).

The 35 effusion absent ears had a mean hearing loss of 8 db before tube placement, and there was no significant change after tube placement. The 28 ears with dry tubes had a mean hearing loss of only 3 db. The 11 ears with draining tubes had a mean hearing loss of 31 db. Five of the 11 ears with otorrhea had mild hearing losses (0 to 20 db range), but the other six ears had moderately severe hearing losses (40 to 60 db range). The reason for this dichotomy was not clinically apparent in this small sample.

DISCUSSION

Our data show the presence of clinically significant conductive hearing loss in the majority of young children with otitis media with effusion. The placement of tympanostomy tubes resulted in an immediate and significant improvement in mean hearing loss. In the presence of dry functional tympanostomy tubes, hearing was normal for age. The presence of otorrhea was associated with significant hearing loss. This result suggests that the presence

TABLE 2   Comparison of Hearing Losses in the 63 Effusion-Present Ears Immediately Before and After Tube Placement*

	Before Tubes	After Tubes
0–14 db	22 ears	45 ears
15–24 db	14 ears	10 ears
25–39 db	13 ears	6 ears
40–60 db	14 ears	2 ears

* Before tube and after tube distributions significantly different by chi square test (p < 0.001).

of tympanostomy tubes alone does not insure normal hearing, and that otorrhea must be actively detected and treated. Longitudinal studies to determine the long term effects of otitis media with effusion and tympanostomy tubes upon auditory function are in progress.

The hearing losses measured in these young children using BAEP techniques are similar in magnitude and range to those reported in older children with otitis media with effusion using audiometry[8] and in young children with otitis media with effusion using behavioral audiometry.[9] Studies are under way in our laboratory and others to compare the hearing losses in young children as estimated by BAEP and behavioral audiometry. BAEP testing does have limitations as the sole measure of hearing function. It does not provide frequency specific information, does not detect selective low frequency hearing losses, and provides no information about cortical level auditory processes. BAEP testing does, however, provide a reliable method to evaluate auditory function in the hard to test subject and is a valuable tool in the auditory evaluation of young children with otitis media with effusion.

REFERENCES

1. Jewett DL, Romano MN, Williston JS. Human auditory evoked potentials: possible brain stem components detected on the scalp. Science 1970; 167:1517–1518.
2. Moller AR, Jannetta P, Bennet M, Moller MB. Intracranially recorded responses from human auditory nerve: new insights into the origin of brainstem evoked potentials. Electroenchephalogr Clin Neurophysiol 1981; 52:18–27.
3. Mendelson T, Salamy A, Lenoir M, McKean C. Brainstem evoked potential findings in children with otitis media. Arch Otolaryngol 1979; 105:17–20.
4. Fria TJ, Sabo DL. Auditory brainstem responses in children with otitis media with effusion. Ann Otol Rhinol Laryngol 1980; 89(Suppl 68):200–206.
5. Friel-Patti S, Finitzo-Hieber T, Conti G, Brown KC. Language delay in infants associated with middle ear disease and mild, fluctuating hearing impairment. Pediatr Infect Dis 1982; 1:104–109.
6. Chisin R, Gapany-Gapanavicius B, Gafni M, Sohmer H. Auditory nerve and brainstem evoked responses before and after middle ear corrective surgery. Arch Otorhinolaryngol 1983; 238:27–31.
7. Galambos R, Hecox KE. Clinical applications of the auditory brainstem response. Otolaryngol Clin North Am 1978; 11:709–722.
8. Kokko E. Chronic secretory otitis media in children: a clinical study. Acta Otolaryngol 1974; Suppl 327:6–44.
9. Fria TJ, Cantekin EI, Eichler JA. Hearing acuity of children with otitis media with effusion. Arch Otolaryngol 1985; 111:10–16.
10. Sohmer H, Kinarti R. Survey of attempts to use auditory evoked potentials to obtain an audiogram: review article. Br J Audiol 1984; 18:237–244.

IDENTIFICATION OF CHILDREN WITH LANGUAGE DELAYS DUE TO RECURRENT OTITIS MEDIA

MARION P. DOWNS, M.A., D.H.S., DEWEY D. WALKER, M.D.,
JERRY L. NORTHERN, Ph.D., and SUSAN GUGENHEIM, M.S., CCP-Sp.

Middle ear effusion has become a disease of early childhood and is often associated with language problems. However, early childhood is a time when language delays have traditionally been difficult to identify. A 4-year study in Denver attempted to answer the question whether early language delays that might be related to recurrent episodes of otitis media with middle ear effusion could be identified. The first phase of this study evaluated the status of medical practice in regard to language and hearing problems by analyzing a random sample of 1,200 case files in 24 primary care physicians' offices, clinics, and a neighborhood health center of children between birth and 3 years of age. The chart review showed that referrals for speech-language disorder evaluations were made for less than 0.4 percent of this population, yet later studies in this project revealed that 8 percent of this age group failed a language screening test. These discrepant results strongly suggest that primary care physicians need a language screening tool in order to detect language disorders that may arise early in life, whether from recurrent middle ear effusions or from other causes.

An additional finding in the random chart audits showed that 50 percent of all the children had had a first attack of otitis media by 10 months of age, confirming the early nature of the disease. Inasmuch as many reports have noted a relationship between early otitis media and later language deficiencies,[1-4] we applied a new language screening test to a large childhood population to determine whether such a tool might be useful in the management of children with recurrent middle ear effusions.

SUBJECTS AND METHOD

Six hundred and fifty-seven children from birth to 3 years of age were given language and hearing screening tests in the 24 physicians' offices and clinics that constituted the project test sites. The children of this age who were entered into the study were those who appeared in the physicians' offices for well baby or sick baby visits during a planned 2 week period. The screening tests included the early language milestone scale (ELM), a tympanometric test, and a behavioral hearing screening test using selected noisemakers.[5,6] Each parent received a basic data questionnaire while in the physician's office, recording the number of episodes of otitis media among other factors.

All children who failed the ELM tests, in addition to a random sample of those who passed the tests, were given an in-depth language evaluation utilizing the sequenced inventory of communication development. Children who were found to have significant language delays on this inventory were referred by their physicians for therapy; those who had borderline problems were given a home language enrichment program that could be managed through the physicians' offices.[7]

FINDINGS

Results of the Screening

The ELM screen was found to be a satisfactory tool to identify language delays in children ages 12 to 36 months. Its validity for different age groups was determined by sensitivity-specificity measures derived by comparing children who passed and children who failed on the ELM with the results of the sequenced inventory of communication development language evaluation. The sensitivity represents the agreement between the rating of a child as positive (abnormal) on the screening test and his rating of positive on the diagnostic evaluation. The specificity refers to the agreement between the screening test's classification of a child as negative (normal) and the diagnostic test's designation of him as normal. Two ELM tests were applied, an initial screen and a rescreen, at the time of the sequenced inventory of communication development test. The results are presented in Table 1.

The data shown in Table 1 indicate that in children under 12 months of age the ELM test is unacceptable, as it does not accurately identify infants with language delay. In the overall age range of 13 to 36 months, a satisfactory application was found in the rescreen ELM test, with a sensitivity of 88 percent and a specificity of 83 percent. With the initial ELM's specificity of 68 percent, too many children without language delays would be referred for unnecessary testing. Therefore despite the 100 percent sensitivity, one initial ELM screen alone cannot be recommended. However, in the 25 to 36 month age group a sensitivity of 100 percent and a specificity of 91 percent were obtained, indicating that ELM screening in this age range produces the most effective results.

An overall 8 percent of the population failed the ELM screening test. The age related failure incidence is shown in Table 2; the figures of Table 2 represent the increased number of language delays

TABLE 1 Sensitivity-Specificity Incidences for the Early Language Milestone Screening Test as a Function of Age

Age (in months)	Initial ELM (Percentage)		Rescreen ELM (Percentage)	
	Sensitivity	Specificity	Sensitivity	Specificity
0–12	0	86		
13–18	100	58	100	67
19–24	100	63	67	100
25–30	100	91	92	100
31–36	100	58	100	66
Overall: 13–36	100	68	88	83

TABLE 2   Age Related Failure Incidence for the Early Language Milestone Screening Test

Age (in months)	Percentage
0–12	3.9
13–18	9
19–24	8
25–30	12
31–36	14

that appear as the child matures.

Relationship of Results to Otitis Media

The number of episodes of otitis media were related to the number of ELM screening failures as shown in Table 3. A chi square significance of 0.098 was found in the overall relationship of ELM screen failures to otitis media episodes.

Of particular interest was the statistical analysis of failure on the ELM expressive language and the ELM receptive language sections of the screening test when compared to more than six bouts of otitis media. The results showed that the ELM expressive language failure plus six bouts of otitis media produced a significant chi square value of 0.046. However, the ELM receptive language failure with six bouts of otitis media was statistically nonsignificant. These findings suggest that expressive language skills as measured by the ELM are more sensitive to recurrent otitis media episodes than the recessive language aspects. Why expressive language should be the most fragile part of language skills on this test, in relation to otitis, is not known. It may be noted that expressive language is the last function to appear in the hierarchy of language development.

Relationship of Hearing Test Results and Early Language Milestone Scale Results

The behavioral hearing screening tests (local-

TABLE 3   Otitis Media Episodes Versus ELM Screening Failures*

29% had 0 episodes; of these, 2.5% failed the ELM

43% had 1 to 5 episodes; of these, 12% failed the ELM

28% had 6+ episodes; of these, 8% failed the ELM

* Chi square = 0.098 significance.

ization to soft noisemakers) showed a significant chi square relationship of 0.013 with the sequenced inventory of communication development (SICD) evaluation, indicating that gross behavioral hearing screening tests are more sensitive to language status than had been thought. These results point to the need for a determination of how the various degrees of hearing loss from otitis media are related to language delays. When possible, future studies should utilize definitive audiologic threshold tests with such young children to determine what degree of loss may contribute to later language problems.

CONCLUSIONS

1. The early language milestone scale is an adequate tool for primary care physicians to screen for language delays in children 12 to 36 months of age.
2. More than six episodes of otitis media are significantly related to expressive language failure on the ELM test.

We strongly urge primary care physicians to utilize a standardized screening test to identify language delays in children from birth to 3 years, particularly in the population having recurrent episodes of otitis media or middle ear effusion. The ability to identify language delays enables the physician to refer the otitis prone child more appropriately for the requisite evaluation and treatment.

REFERENCES

1. Teele D, Klein J, Rosner B. Otitis media with effusion during the first three years of life and development of speech and language. Pediatrics 1984; 74:282–287.
2. Sak R, Ruben R. Effects of middle ear effusion in preschool years on language and learning. Dev Behav Pediatr 1982; 3:7–11.
3. Zinkus P. Psychoeducational sequellae of chronic otitis media. Sem Speech Lang Hear 1982; 3:305–312.
4. Feagans L. Otitis media: a model for long term effects with implications of intervention. In: Kavanagh J, ed. Otitis media and child development. Parkton, MD: York Press, 1986:192.
5. Coplan J, Gleason J, Ryan R, et al. Validation of an early language milestone scale in a high risk population. Pediatrics 1982; 70:677–683.
6. Coscarelli-Buchanan JE. Finding ears that do not hear. Tenn Med Assoc J 1986; 79(1):39.
7. Sparling J, Lewis I. Learning games for the first three years. New York: Walker Educational Book Co., 1981.

This study was entirely supported by a grant from the Robert Wood Johnson Foundation, Princeton, New Jersey.

OTITIS MEDIA IN EARLY CHILDHOOD AND ITS RELATIONSHIP TO LATER SPEECH AND LANGUAGE

JOANNE E. ROBERTS, Ph.D., MARGARET R. BURCHINAL, Ph.D.,
MATTHEW A. KOCH, M.D., ALBERT M. COLLIER, M.D.,
and FREDERICK W. HENDERSON, M.D.

The relationship between the occurrence of otitis media with effusion during the first 3 years of life, and later speech and language development was examined in a group of socioeconomically disadvantaged children who attended a research day care program. Study children were part of a longitudinal multidisciplinary program in which the number of episodes of otitis media with effusion, the duration of each episode, and the psychoeducational development of each child were charted prospectively from infancy.

MATERIALS AND METHODS

Study Population

The children studied attended the Frank Porter Graham Child Development Center, a multidisciplinary research day care program. Study children were identified at birth as biologically normal and classified as being at risk for poor school performance because of socioeconomic and cultural factors. Children entered the day care program of the center between the ages of 6 weeks and 3 months. They attended the center for 5 full days a week, 50 weeks a year until entry into kindergarten. While in the day care program, children received complete medical care provided by two pediatricians and two nurse practitioners. Each weekday nurses reviewed the children's health status. Physical examinations, including ear examinations, were performed when parents, day care teachers, or medical staff observed signs or symptoms of illness in a study child.

Otitis Media Experience

During the study period 1975 to 1986 the diagnosis of otitis media with effusion was based on the findings of pneumatic otoscopy. It was diagnosed when middle ear fluid was seen or when the mobility of the tympanic membrane was markedly reduced or absent. Between 1978 and 1986 tympanometry using the tympanogram classification of Jerger[1] was used to corroborate the diagnosis. During symptom free periods the middle ear status of the children was monitored once a month by otoscopy and tympanometry. Throughout the study, ears with persistent effusion were examined every 2 weeks until the effusion resolved. A total otitis media with effusion score (total OME, 0 to 3) for each child was calculated by summing the total number of days with episodes of unilateral and bilateral otitis media with effusion over the first 3 years of life.*

Speech Measures

Between 1982 and 1986 the speech and language of all high risk children between the ages of 2½ and 8 years were assessed. Children were tested in the fall of each year in a sound treated room. Testing occurred if a child had passed a hearing screening and had a type A or C tympanogram according to Jerger's tympanogram classifications.[1] First, speech was assessed using the Goldman-Fristoe Test of Articulation, and then language was examined during a 15 minute conversational speech sample. Responses on the articulation tests were coded live using narrow transcription, and both speech and language outcomes were recorded on audiotape. Interexaminer agreement based on 10 percent of the test sessions was 87.2 percent for narrow transcription of consonant sounds.

Each consonant on the articulation test was coded for phonological processes according to Ingram's classification.[3] Phonological processes are systematic simplifications of adult words or error patterns in sound usage. Dialect features were coded but were excluded from the analysis. A total phonological process TPP score for each child was computed by summing the frequency of the following

---

* See article by Roberts et al[2] for additional details.

phonological processes that are common in the developing speech of normal children: deletion of final consonant, consonant cluster reduction, fronting, stopping, liquid gliding, reduplication, assimilation, and unstressed syllable deletion. The total phonological process score was selected as the primary speech variable in the analyses, because individual phonological processes were observed infrequently after age 4.

Language Measures

To compute language measures, 15 minutes of the conversational speech sample were transcribed and segmented on the basis of the communication unit. Each child's transcribed language sample was processed by the Systematic Analysis of Language Transcripts (SALT)[4] program, a computer program for language analysis. The language measures were the mean number of words per communication unit, the mean number of dependent clauses (adjectival, adverbial, and noun clauses) per communication unit, the ratio of the total number of different words to the total number of communication units, the ratio of the total number of different conjunction words excluding "and" to the total number of communication units, and the mean number of utterances per turn.

RESULTS

Otitis Media with Effusion and Speech Measures

Fifty-five high risk children participated in the speech study. Fifty-one were black and four were white; 37 were boys and 18 were girls. The mean and median number of days of total otitis media with effusion (0 to 3) were 242.6 and 196.0, respectively; these ranged from 8 to 931 days. Table 1 shows that although there is a marked decrease in children's use of phonologic processes between the ages of 3

and 4 years, the number of processes becomes relatively stable, with only a gradual decline after the age of 4 years. Since children between the ages of 2½ and 8 years were tested annually, each child contributed one to five observations to these data.

In our first analysis we used Spearman correlations to determine whether a linear relationship existed between ranks on total otitis media with effusion (0 to 3) and TPP at any given age. No significant correlations ($p > 0.05$) between total otitis media with effusion (0 to 3) and TPP were found (Table 1). However, though not significant, all rank order correlations observed in the 4 through 8 year olds were in the hypothesized direction.

Second, a growth curve approach was used to determine whether otitis media with effusion was related to indices of speech development during the period in which the phonological processes were exhibiting their greatest change. The TPP was transformed by computing natural logarithms after recording each zero as 0.1. Individual linear polynomial growth curves were fitted to the transformed data of 18 children who had at least three observations of otitis media with effusion over time and whose first articulation test was given when they were between 2½ and 3½ years of age. Two indices of development were estimated: the intercept (i.e., the predicted log of TPP at age 3) and the linear slope associated with age in months. No significant relationships between otitis media with effusion and these indices were found; the Spearman correlation of total otitis media with effusion (0 to 3) with the intercept was $r = 0.07$ ($p = 0.79$) and with the rate of change (the slope) was $r = 0.01$ ($p = 0.97$).

In a third analysis we examined the age period during which phonological processes exhibited little change, that is, the TPP observed when children were 4½ years or older. Forty-five children were tested one to three times after the age of 4½. The median of these one to three scores was selected as a robust measure of central tendency of TPP during these years.

TABLE 1 Means and Medians for Total Number of Phonologic Processes and Correlations with Otitis Media with Effusion Across Age

	Age (Years)					
	3 (N = 27)	4 (N = 25)	5 (N = 24)	6 (N = 30)	7 (N = 29)	8 (N = 19)
Mean	22.5	6.2	2.9	3.1	0.9	1.4
SD	13.6	6.0	2.1	4.2	1.5	1.9
Median	20.0	4.0	3.0	2.0	0.0	1.0
Spearman coefficient	−0.04	0.29	0.31	0.29	0.18	0.10
P Value	0.85	0.16	0.15	0.13	0.34	0.69

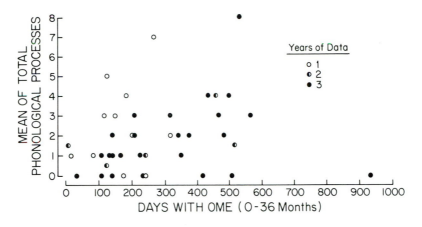

Figure 1 Plot of medians of total common phonologic processes by number of days with otitis media with effusion during the first 3 years of life (total OME, 0 to 3).

Figure 1 shows the plot of the relationship between the median number of TPP and total otitis media with effusion (0 to 3). The plotting symbol indicates the number of times each child was tested after the age of 4½ years. Spearman rank-order correlations were used to test the association between otitis media with effusion and the median of TPP, weighted by the number of times TPP was assessed after 4½ years of age. A small but significant rankorder correlation (r=0.35, p=0.017) was observed. Even after partialing out median age of testing, the parameter reflecting the observed association was still significant (t(42)=0.22, p=0.035). Median age was a nonsignificant predictor (t(42)= −1.3, p=0.21), suggesting that the observed association is probably not explained by age.

Otitis Media with Effusion and Language Measures

Thirty-four high risk 5 year olds participated in the language study. Thirty-two were black and two were white; 24 were boys and 10 were girls. The language sample for each child taken closest to 60 months of age was used in the language analysis. Table 2 shows the means and medians on each language measure. To determine whether a relationship existed between ranks on total otitis media with effusion (0 to 3) and the language measures, Spearman rank-order correlations were conducted. As shown in Table 2, no significant correlations p>0.05 were found.

DISCUSSION

The results of this exploratory study did not show a relationship between the number of days of otitis media with effusion in the first 3 years of life and either the total number of common phonological processes observed during the preschool years or language measures at age 5. Early otitis media with effusion was associated with the total number of phonological processes used by children between the ages of 4½ and 8 years. However, this finding

TABLE 2   Means and Medians for Language Measures and Correlations with Otitis Media with Effusion

	Mean No. of Words per Communication Unit	Mean No. of Dependent Clauses per Communication Unit	No. of Different Words per Communication Unit	No. of Different Conjunctions per Communication Unit	No. of Different Pronouns per Communication Unit
Mean	3.80	0.13	1.26	0.06	0.11
SD	0.60	0.05	0.21	0.04	0.06
Median	3.75	0.11	1.24	0.04	0.10
Spearman coefficient	−0.04	0.17	−0.03	0.20	0.09
P value	0.83	0.33	0.89	0.26	0.62

should be interpreted carefully, since the final speech analysis was conducted because of trends observed in the first analysis and not on a priori basis. Moreover, these data were subjected to multiple analyses.

Whether early otitis media with effusion has detrimental effects on later speech and language has been debated. Early disease has been shown to be related to delay in speech and language development in preschool and school aged children.[5-6] However, the results of these studies are not conclusive.[9,10] In the present study the otitis media with effusion history and speech and language development were documented prospectively, and the otitis media with effusion history was documented more intensively than in previous studies.

For socioeconomically disadvantaged children attending day care, the magnitude of any adverse speech or language outcome associated with early childhood otitis media with effusion is small and is more likely when children are school age.

This study was supported in part by grants from the Office of Special Education Programs (Department of Education G008400664) and the Deafness Research Foundation.

REFERENCES

1. Jerger J. Clinical experience with impedance audiometry. Arch Otolaryngol 1970; 92:311–324.
2. Roberts JE, Sanyal MA, Burchinal MR, Collier AM, Ramey CT, Henderson FW. Otitis media in early childhood and its relationship to later verbal and academic performance. Pediatrics 1986; 78:423–430.
3. Ingram D. Phonological disability in children. New York: Elsevier, 1976.
4. Miller JF, Chapman RS. Salt—systematic analysis of language transcripts. Users manual, Apple version. 1983.
5. Teele DW, Klein JO, Rosner BA, et al. Otitis media with effusion during the first three years of life and development of speech and language. Pediatrics 1984; 74:282–287.
6. Shriberg LD, Smith AJ. Phonological correlates of middle-ear involvement in speech-delayed children: a methodological note. J Speech Hear Res 1983; 26:293–297.
7. Lehmann KD, Charron K, Kummer A, Keith RW. The effects of chronic middle ear effusion on speech and language development—a descriptive study. Int J Pediatr Otorhinolaryngol 1979; 1:137–144.
8. Holm VA, Kunze LH. Effect of chronic otitis media on language and speech development. Pediatrics 1969; 833–838.
9. Paradise JL, Rogers KD. On otitis media, child development, and tympanostomy tubes: new answers or old questions? Pediatrics 1986; 77:88–92.
10. Paradise JL. Long-term effects of short-term hearing loss—menace or myth? In: Bluestone CD, Klein JO, Paradise JL, et al. Workshop on effects of otitis media on the child. Pediatrics 1983; 71:639–652.

OTITIS MEDIA AND ITS EFFECT ON LANGUAGE IN INFANCY

INA F. WALLACE, Ph.D., JUDITH S. GRAVEL, Ph.D., CECELIA M. McCARTON, M.D., DAVID R. STAPELLS, Ph.D., RICHARD S. BERNSTEIN, Ph.D., and ROBERT J. RUBEN, M.D.

Otitis media with effusion is a common illness in young children, by some estimates affecting two-thirds of infants in their first years of life.[1] Research has indicated that the disease may result in mild to moderate hearing losses as well as language and learning difficulties.[2-4] At our Clinical Research Center for Communicative Disorders in Children we serve a population who, as a result of environmental conditions and perinatal complications, are at risk for both otitis media and language disabilities. We are currently following a large cohort of these children in order to examine the development of their communicative competence. The present report is based on several studies designed to examine the sequelae of otitis media with effusion in this population.[5,6]

MATERIALS AND METHODS

The cohort from whom our study babies were drawn included 53 high risk infants (i.e., very low birth weight, perinatally asphyxiated, or mechanically ventilated) and 21 healthy full term babies, all of whom had reached 1 year post term. All the children (high risk and full term) receive medical, neurologic, audiologic, and developmental assessments through the LIFE Program of the Rose F. Kennedy Center. The babies in this study were born to families of low socioeconomic background; all but three infants were black (34) or Hispanic (37). There were 39 girls and 35 boys in the sample.

Infants were first scheduled for medical evaluations at 40 weeks postconceptional age; thereafter they were scheduled monthly from 1 to 6 months of age and every 2 months through 1 year of age. A pediatric nurse practitioner, who was trained and supervised by our pediatric otolaryngologist (R.J.R.), determined the otologic status via pneumatic otoscopy during each medical examination. At every visit the nurse practitioner completed a nine item checklist, which queried tympanic membrane characteristics such as position, color, and mobility. Each ear was then judged as "clear," "suspicious," or "positive" for otitis media with effusion.

Two groups of infants were selected from the larger cohort of 74 babies on the basis of these otoscopy records. The 15 babies (8 high risk and 7 full term) who had normal ratings in both ears in 80 percent or more of their visits to the LIFE Program were designated as "otitis free." Another 13 babies (10 high risk and 3 full term) judged to have bilateral otitis media in 30 percent or more of their first year visits were designated as "otitis positive."

Infants were also regularly scheduled for behavioral hearing evaluations and electrophysiologic assessments (i.e., auditory brainstem responses and cortical auditory evoked potentials). Electrophysiologic and behavioral hearing assessments revealed that the infants in the study did not have sensorineural hearing loss. At 1 year of age the children were administered the Bayley Scales of Infant Development, which measures global cognitive and motor development. Children with subnormal cognitive ability (i.e., Bayley Mental Development Index less than 80) were eliminated. No significant differences between the groups were detected in either perinatal or demographic characteristics.

RESULTS

Study 1

Our first study was designed to examine cognitive and language outcomes at 1 year of age as a function of otitis media.[5] Using only the children designated as otitis positive and otitis free, we compared the groups on the Bayley Mental Development Index and the receptive and expressive scales of the Sequenced Inventory of Communication Development (SICD). To correct for slight variations in ages at which infants were tested, the age scores from the SICD were divided by the child's chronologic age (corrected if premature) and multiplied by 100.

The results indicated that the two groups differed very little on either the Bayley or the receptive scale of the SICD. In contrast, the mean expressive language score of the otitis positive group of 79.2 differed significantly from the score of 106.6 achieved by the otitis free group (t [24] = 2.97; p < 0.01). The results were identical when we examined outcome as a function of both risk status and middle ear disease and controlled for cognitive ability.

Study 2

Our next study[6] was designed to examine the impact of otitis media with effusion on auditory sensitivity as measured by the auditory brainstem response (ABR). ABRs were scheduled at term, 3 months, 6 months, 9 months, and 1 year of age after term. ABR thresholds for clicks were obtained when possible from both ears of each infant, in natural or sedated sleep (seven infants were able to be assessed in only one ear at one of their visits). The click-ABR threshold values used in the following analyses are the lowest stimulus intensity level evoking a replicable response on a given day.

In most cases infants' ears were otoscopically examined on the same days they received an ABR. For a few children these data are not available, but for some of these children we have tympanometric data collected on those days. Data on the ear status at the time of ABRs represent both ears unless indicated, except for the seven children for whom ABRs were assessed on only one ear; for these children data concerning effusion are given for the same ear as the ABR. For children in the otitis free group,

24 ABR assessments were made, collapsing over all visits. In this group 20 of the 24 children were considered normal by either otoscopy or tympanometry on the day of testing; two were considered suspicious or positive; and data on two were not available. There were 28 ABR assessments for infants in the otitis positive group. In this group 10 were considered normal by otoscopy or tympanometry on the day of testing; 16 were considered suspicious or positive; and data on 2 were not available.

In order to examine the differences in ABR threshold as a function of otitis media status, distributions of threshold values were made at three time intervals (i.e., 3 to 5 months, 6 to 8 months, and 9 to 12 months) for each ear for both the otitis positive and the otitis free groups. We considered a threshold of 30 dB nHL or higher to be elevated. An inspection of the distributions revealed that at each window sampled, the majority of otitis free children did not have elevated thresholds. In contrast, the majority of otitis positive children had elevated threshold values. Threshold values ranged from 30 to 80 dB nHL, even though none of these infants has sensorineural hearing loss.

The ABR threshold estimates for each child were then summarized in two ways. First, we considered whether an infant's thresholds were never elevated (that is, always less than 30 dB nHL) or were elevated at least some of the time. Five of the 13 otitis free children never had an elevated ABR in contrast to only one of the 12 otitis positive children. Second, we pooled the ABR thresholds over both ears at all available visits and obtained a mean threshold. The difference in mean ABR threshold values between the otitis free (M=22 dB nHL; SD=7.3) and otitis positive groups (M=33 dB nHL; SD=10.8) was significant (t [23]=3.1; p < 0.01) and clinically meaningful.

The association of ABR status and otitis media on the developmental outcome was then examined. Using ABR threshold categories (i.e., elevated or not elevated) and otitis media groups, we found that the otitis positive group performed significantly poorer on the expressive language measure than the otitis free children. Neither the Bayley nor the receptive language measures differed across the groups. Because of the great variability in auditory sensitivity that was masked by grouping children as elevated or not, correlations were computed to examine the relationships between otitis media, auditory sensitivity, and language outcome. For these analyses we used mean ABR thresholds, the percentage of time the ears were clear, the percentage of time that children had bilateral episodes of otitis media with effusion, and the three outcome meas-

ures. We found that lower scores on the expressive scale of the SICD were associated with both increases in episodes of otitis media (r=0.55, p < 0.05) and elevations in ABR thresholds (r=0.55; p < 0.05), although no significant relationships were obtained with either the Bayley cognitive scores or the SICD receptive language scores.

Study 3

Now that many of the children are 2 years old, we have the opportunity to examine whether group differences in language development remain. Because not all the children have been seen for their 2 year visit, the data are only preliminary. In addition to receiving the Sequenced Inventory of Communication Development, the children also were videotaped with their parent (usually the mother) in both a free play and a structured teaching task. Many of the videotapes have been transcribed and from the language samples we have calculated the children's mean length of utterance (MLU).

The data from the SICD show that children in the otitis positive group were more likely than the otitis free group to have expressive language scores 8 or more months below their chronologic ages. Specifically, four of the 10 otitis positive children had such delays in contrast to only one of the nine otitis free children. Likewise, analysis of the spontaneous language data indicates that the average MLU of the otitis positive children was 1.2 words, whereas it was 1.5 words for the otitis free children. In contrast, there were no differences between the groups on the receptive scale of the SICD as five in each group had receptive language scores 8 or more months below their chronologic age.

DISCUSSION

These findings suggest that infants with recurrent otitis media during the first year of life display expressive language deficits and reduced auditory sensitivity when compared to a group of infants considered otitis free. Although we included both high risk and healthy full term babies, no differences were associated with risk status. Although our results are consistent with reports by Friel-Patti et al[3] and Klein et al,[4] we have demonstrated language deficits at 1 year of age, which is earlier than that reported by these other investigators. Moreover, our results indicate that there is a modest dose-response relationship between bilateral episodes of otitis media, elevated ABR thresholds, and expressive language development. Furthermore, it appears that as a group, the children who were identified as otitis positive in their first year of life continue to display less well developed expressive language at 2 years of age.

The failure to find differences between the groups in global ability is not surprising given that infants with severe abnormalities were excluded. In contrast, it was surprising that receptive language was not associated with either the otitis media or ABR measures, since previous investigators have reported deficits in receptive as well as expressive language. However, it may be that the SICD, which includes many nonspeech items at 1 year of age, is not sensitive to the kinds of deficits these children may eventually display. At age 2 years our lack of group differences in receptive language seemed to be a result of the fact that a majority of children in both groups faired poorly on the SICD receptive scale.

We did not obtain ABR results each time the children's ears were otoscopically examined, which limits the statements that can be made about otitis media, auditory sensitivity, and language development. In addition, because pure tone audiograms for each child were not available, we are unable to examine functional hearing loss as it relates to these other measures. However, newly recruited subjects will undergo an expanded protocol, which will offer us the opportunity to validate and elaborate upon associations found in this investigation.

Although we do not as yet know the long term outcome, at the end of the first year infants with repeated episodes of middle ear disease appear to be at risk for developmental language disorders. Given these findings, it may be appropriate to consider early language stimulation programs for such infants.

REFERENCES

1. Howie VM. Acute and recurrent otitis media. In: Jaffee BF, ed. Hearing loss in children. Baltimore: University Park Press, 1977:421.
2. Bess F. Hearing loss associated with middle ear effusion. In: Workshop on effects of otitis media on the child (special issue). Pediatrics 1983; 71:640–641.
3. Friel-Patti S, et al. Language delay in infants associated with middle ear disease and mild, fluctuating hearing impairment. Pediatr Infect Dis 1982; 1:104–109.
4. Klein JO, et al. Otitis media with effusion during the three years of life and development of speech and language. In: Lim DJ, Bluestone CD, Klein JO, Nelson JD, eds. Recent advances in otitis media with effusion. Proceedings of the Third International Symposium. Toronto: BC Decker, 1984:332.
   dia and language development at 1 year of age. J Speech Hear Disord (in press).
6. Wallace IF, Gravel JS, McCarton CM, Stapells DR, Bernstein RS, Ruben RJ. Otitis media, auditory sensitivity and language outcome at 1 year. Laryngoscope 1988; 98:64–70.

EFFECT OF OTITIS MEDIA WITH EFFUSION ON LANGUAGE DEVELOPMENT OF PRESCHOOL CHILDREN: PRELIMINARY RESULTS OF A CONTROLLED RANDOMIZED LONGITUDINAL STUDY

GEROLD H. RACH, M.D., GERHARD A. ZIELHUIS, M.Sc., Ph.D., and PAUL VAN DEN BROEK, M.D., Ph.D.

Otitis media with effusion is a widespread silent disease among young children.[1] It is suggested that the fluctuating conductive hearing loss experienced in otitis media with effusion may lead to psychologic, educational, and behavioral problems. Language and speech development can be negatively influenced.[2] Because the research design of most studies involves many methodologic problems, most reviewers have been highly critical of the results,[3,4] and suggestions have been given to improve research in this area. This study of the effect of otitis media with effusion on language development in young children was designed to be prospective, longitudinal, and randomized to control for all the pitfalls mentioned in the literature.

MATERIALS AND METHODS

Subjects for the study were recruited from an apparently healthy birth cohort in Nijmegen—1439 2 year old children—on the basis of tympanometric measurement every 3 months until the fourth birthday. The measurements were done at the children's homes by three qualified audiometric assistants. The Grason-Steadler impedance meter (GSI-27) was used to obtain the tympanograms. To classify the tympanograms, the classification proposed by Jerger[5] was used. The visits also included the filling out of a questionnaire relating to the ear, nose, and throat history and risk factors related to otitis media with effusion.

Children with a bilateral B type tympanogram at two consecutive measurements were referred to the otolaryngologic surgeon for further evaluation, where they underwent a standardized otolaryngologic examination, including otoscopy and tympanometry.

These children were eligible for a randomized trial in which half the group was treated with ventilating tubes in both ears and the other group was not (after informed consent of the parents). (When this was done, randomization in the two groups was effected after balancing the variables.) Also a reference group of healthy children (ears with type A tympanograms) was recruited from the cohort. In both groups (the otitis media and reference groups) two language development tests were performed successively—one at the beginning of the trial (and before treatment) and one 6 months later. The Reynell Developmental Language Scale (Revised) was used by a speech therapist, who was unaware of the child's history or study group. Scores were measured for language comprehension and language expression according to the age in months.

The groups were balanced on the basis of age, sex, educational level of the mother, language comprehension, and language expression score. Excluded from the study were children with chronic ear discharge, perceptive hearing loss, emotional disturbances, hospitalization for more than 6 weeks, congenital malformations, visual disorders, or other neurologic problems.

RESULTS

Here we present the results obtained in the first 62 children who entered the trial and who underwent the first language development test. The total population with otitis media with effusion consisted of 49 children with bilateral disease and a reference group of 13 healthy children.

The language comprehension score of the otitis media population (N=49) had a mean value of −0.17, which is in accordance with the standard (p=0.16). By contrast, the language expression score (N=48) was depressed and had a mean value of −0.70; this is statistically significant (p<0.0001).

The healthy group (N=13) scores are in accord with the standard for both language comprehension (N=13) and language expression (N=13) (mean values, 0.23 and 0.14, respectively; p=0.11 and p=0.43).

To study the effect of short and longstanding persistent bilateral otitis, a distinction was made between children with otitis media for more than 6 months and a group with otitis for 3 to 6 months and a normal tympanogram before the onset of disease.

Again the language comprehension score in both groups was not lowered significantly, in contrast to the language expression level. The mean value for the longstanding disease (N=31) was −0.71 (p< 0.0001). The 3 to 6 month group (N=14) had a mean value on the language expression score of 0.49 (p=0.05).

STATISTICAL ANALYSIS

All scores were converted to Z scores with a mean of 0 and a standard deviation of 1. This was done to allow for direct comparison of all measures. If the mean value of the Z score compared to the standard is not statistically significant, the procedure tests the null hypothesis that there are no differences between the values. The Student t test was used.

DISCUSSION

As already noted by many authors, it is extremely difficult to link chronic persistent otitis media with effusion to language and developmental problems. No study has yet been published in regard to children in the age group 2 to 4 years on a randomized and longitudinal basis. We controlled for many items, although we admit that during the test procedure these children had hearing loss (except the healthy group) that could have influenced the scores, according to Paradise.[4] However, this is only a theoretical possibility because the hearing loss due to otitis media with effusion is a moderate one of 10 to 35 db; thus the children are able to understand the instructions of an experienced speech therapist.

Our preliminary results lead to the following conclusions:

1. The group with a history of chronic persistent bilateral otitis media with effusion has a statistically significant depressed language expression level compared to the standard. The language comprehension level meets the standard.

2. The effect on the language expression level for the subgroup with a long history of otitis is greater than that in the group with a shorter history of bilateral otitis.

3. The reference group, consisting of healthy children, meets the standard in regard to both comprehension and expression levels.

Thus there is now a clear-cut link between chronic persistent bilateral middle ear effusion and language development in preschool children. The longer the otitis media persists, the more the language expression level is affected. Middle ear disease in preschool children should not be regarded as a harmless condition. It is a potentially dangerous disability that deserves the close attention of doctors and educators.

REFERENCES

1. Paradise JL. Pediatrician's view of middle ear effusions: more questions than answers. Ann Otol Rhinol Laryngol 1976; 85(Suppl 25):20–24.
2. Sak RJ, Ruben RJ. Recurred middle ear effusion in childhood: implications of temporary auditory deprivations for language and learning. Ann Otol Rhinol Laryngol 1981; 90:546–551.
3. Ventry IM. Effects of conductive hearing loss fact or fiction. Speech Hear Disord 1980; 45:143–156.
4. Paradise JL. Otitis media during early life: how hazardous to development? A critical review of the evidence. Pediatrics 1981; 68:869–873.
5. Jerger J. Clinical experience with impedance audiometry. Arch Otolaryngol 1970; 92:311–324.

SECRETORY OTITIS MEDIA AND VERBAL INTELLIGENCE: A SIX-YEAR PROSPECTIVE CASE CONTROL STUDY

JØRGEN LOUS, M.D., MOGENS FIELLAU-NIKOLAJSEN, M.D., and ANNA LISE JEPPESEN, M.A.

A prospective case control study was undertaken to elucidate the relationship between early long-lasting tubal dysfunction and secretory otitis media, and language development and reading achievement. The study was a part of the second Hjørring cohort study.

METHODS

All 463 of the 3 year old children in Hjørring, Denmark, were invited for middle ear screening (Fig. 1). About 94 percent were fully examined four times from August 1978 to January 1979.[1] Because of capacity problems, some of the normal subjects only had three tests. All the children underwent a general otolaryngologic examination, including pneumatic otoscopy and impedance and pure tone audiometry at each test session.

The 40 children (9 percent of the cohort) with continuing secretory otitis media or a negative middle ear pressure of at least 200 decapascal (daPa) in one or both ears were regarded as "case" pupils for this study.

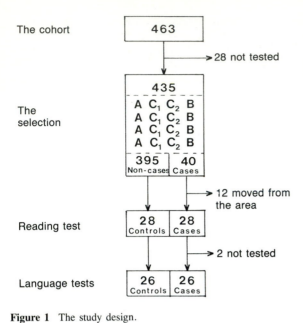

Figure 1 The study design.

In the second grade all the children were given a silent reading test (OS-400). In this reading test, performed with a whole class at a time, each pupil identifies as many as possible of 400 written test words with four illustrations, only one of which is correct for each word.

After another year all the case and control pupils took two language tests—a Danish translation of the Peabody Picture Vocabulary Test (revised version) and the verbal part of the WISC test. One of the boys in the case group had moved from the community during the year and the parents of another case pupil would not give the permission for their daughter's participation in the two language tests, leaving 26 pairs for language testing (see Fig. 1).

RESULTS

Reading

In the case-control pupil analysis of the reading test results, a correction was made for an important classroom factor[2] in the 10 cases in which the case and control pupils were from different classrooms. In these 10 control pupils the reading score was corrected with the difference between the mean values of the reading score in the two classrooms:

Corrected control pupil's reading score = control pupil's reading score + (case pupil's classroom mean reading score − control pupil's classroom mean reading score).

The correction was positive in 5 control pupils and negative in the other 5. The range was from −86 to +87 points, and the mean correction for the 10 control pupils was −4 points.

The analysis showed no difference in reading achievement between the case pupils and the control pupils (Wilcoxon signed ranks test, p=0.25).

The reading scores of the case pupils also were

About 5 years later, at the second grade level, 12 of the case pupils had moved from the community, leaving 28 case pupils, 19 boys and 9 girls. The case pupils were subdivided into two groups, 12 with continuing bilateral ear disease and 16 with continuing unilateral ear disease.

Each case pupil was matched with a "control" pupil who had joined the cohort testing at the age of 3 and who had had no ear disease during that period, i.e., type A (or C1 tympanogram; Table 1). Each control pupil was of the same sex, from the same school and grade level, and as far as possible from the same classroom (18 of 28) and with parents from the same socioeconomic level as the case pupil. In 10 cases it was impossible to find a suitable control pupil among the classmates. In these cases the control pupil was found in one of the other classrooms in the same school at the same grade level.

TABLE 1   Number of Different Tympanogram Types in the 28 Case Children, the 12 Dropout Children, and the 28 Control Children at the Age of 3

	Cases (N = 28)	Dropouts (N = 12)	Controls (N = 28)
Type A	20 (9%)	5 (6%)	184 (89%)
Type C1	21 (9%)	7 (8%)	22 (11%)
Type C2	44 (20%)	38 (43%)	0
Type B	139 (62%)	38 (43%)	0
Number of tympanograms	224 (100%)	88 (100%)*	206 (100%)†

* Two of the dropout children had only two tests. Chi square (case children) = 18; df = 3; p <0.0005.
† Nine of the control children had only three tests. Chi square (case children) = 318; df = 3; p <0.0001.

compared with their own classroom mean reading scores, without finding any difference (Wilcoxon, p = 0.50).

Separate analysis of the 12 pairs in which the case pupil had had bilateral middle ear disease also revealed no difference (Wilcoxon, p = 0.27).

Peabody Picture Vocabulary Test (Revised)

The analysis of the Peabody Picture Vocabulary Test (revised version) standard scores showed no difference between the 26 case pupils and the 26 control pupils (Wilcoxon, p = 0.61).

Verbal Part of the WISC Test

The analysis of the five verbal subtests of the WISC test also failed to show any significant difference between the case and control pupils (Fig. 2; Wilcoxon, p = 0.35 on standardized WISC scores and 0.27 on nonstandardized WISC scores).

DISCUSSION

The study design used, a case control study in a prospective cohort study, eliminated some of the possible flaws in comparing diseased with non-diseased children. On the other hand, the possibility of overmatching may be considered. In our study none of the matched variables (i.e., sex, socioeconomic status of the parents, classroom) interfered significantly with the frequencies of serous otitis media.

In an earlier similar study from the first Hjørring cohort study we also found no significant difference between case pupils who had had continuing serous otitis media or high negative middle ear pressure for 6 months at the age of 3 and control pupils without any ear problems at that age.[3]

With the silent reading test (OS-400) the results in the case pupils did not differ from those for the other pupils in the classroom or from those in individual control pupils matched by sex and socioeconomic status and controlled for classroom.

In the two language tests, the Peabody Picture Vocabulary Test (revised version) and the verbal part of the WISC test, we found no significant difference between the case and control pupils.

Considering the high frequency of secretory otitis media during childhood and the divergent views of its influence on learning,[4] more controlled studies in this field are needed before the importance of screening[5] and treating long-lasting asymptomatic secretory otitis media can be established.

WISC - Verbal

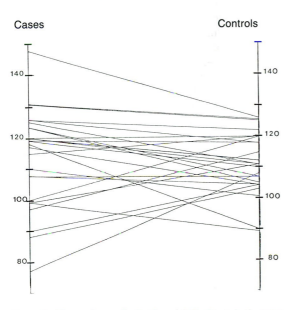

Figure 2 The total score in the five verbal subtests in the WISC test in 26 case pupils and 26 control pupils.

This study was supported by grants H 11/57-82 and H 11/61-86 from the Sygekassernes Helse-fond.

We thank the Education Committee in Hjørring for permission to use the results of the reading tests and the School Psychological Service for their kindness in taking part in the investigation.

REFERENCES

1. Fiellau-Nikolajsen M. Tympanometry and secretory otitis media. Acta Otolaryngol 1983; Suppl 394:1–73.
2. Lous J. Secretory otitis media and reading achievement in Hjørring and Hirtshals municipality: some preliminary results. In: Tronhjem K, ed. Aspects of reading processes: with special regard to the hearing-impaired students. København; 12th Danavox Symposium, 1986:227–240.
3. Lous J, Fiellau-Nikolajsen M. A 5-year prospective case-control study of the influence of early otitis media with effusion on reading achievement. Int J Pediatr Otorhinolaryngol 1984; 8:19–30.
4. Lous J. Linguistic and cognitive sequelae to secretory otitis media in children. Scand Audiol 1986; Suppl 26:71–75.
5. Lous J. Screening for secretory otitis media: evaluation of some impedance screening programs for longlasting secretory otitis media in 7-year-old children. Int J Pediatr Otorhinolaryngol 1987; 13:85–97.

OTITIS MEDIA AND THE DEVELOPMENT OF SPEECH, LANGUAGE, AND COGNITIVE ABILITIES AT SEVEN YEARS OF AGE

JEROME O. KLEIN, M.D., CYNTHIA CHASE, Ph.D., DAVID W. TEELE, M.D.,
PAULA MENYUK, Ph.D., BERNARD A. ROSNER, Ph.D., and the GREATER BOSTON
OTITIS MEDIA STUDY GROUP: CAROLE ALLEN, M.D., LORNA BRATTON, M.B., Ch.B.,
GILBERT FISCH, M.D., MIRJANA KOSTICH, M.D., LILLIAN McMAHON, M.D.,
SIDNEY STAROBIN, M.D., PETER STRINGHAM, M.D., and LLOYD TARLIN, M.D.

Otitis media and effusion of the middle ear are most prevalent in early infancy, a time that coincides with rapid cognitive and linguistic development. To determine whether disease of the middle ear in infancy is associated with problems in development, we assessed cognitive abilities, speech, and language in 7 year old children who had been observed for ear disease prospectively since birth.

METHODS

Beginning in 1975, pediatricians working in private practices in Holliston and Framingham, Massachusetts, and in an urban health center in East Boston began to follow a cohort of consecutively enrolled children. This cohort comprised every child aged less than 3 months seeking care at these two sites. Enrollment was continuous for 2 years (N = 1068). Diagnoses of middle ear disease were made by pediatricians, using pneumatic otoscopy until age 3 and both pneumatic otoscopy and tympanometry in years 4 through 7.

The criterion for the diagnosis of acute otitis media was middle ear effusion in addition to signs of acute illness. Children with effusion who were well were considered to have asymptomatic middle ear effusion.

Our criteria for effusion consisted of otorrhea, gas-liquid levels visible on otoscopy, or marked reduction of mobility using both positive and negative pressure. Our tympanometric criterion for effusion was a "type B curve," essentially a flat tracing.

To calculate the time spent with effusion, we assigned a "window" of 23 days to each observation of effusion, whether accompanied by signs of illness or not. Time with effusion could be shortened or extended by multiple examinations.

From this original cohort of 1,068 children, we tested a randomly selected subset of children still active in the practices. Selection occurred several months before the oldest child's seventh birthday. The 642 then active children were ranked by time with middle ear effusion during the first 2 years of life. Testing was offered for every third child; if testing was declined, testing was offered for the next child on the list. The tested sample included 196 children, 30.2 percent of the then active children.

Reasons for exclusion included parental refusal, nonwhite race, a child in whose home English was not the primary language, seizures, mental retardation, cerebral palsy, and bilateral hearing loss greater than 20 db at the time of testing. Children in the last group were deferred until they could pass the hearing screen.

Tests administered at the seventh birthday (± 3 months) included the Wechsler Intelligence Scale for Children—Revised (WISC-R) for cognitive ability, the Goldman-Fristoe-Woodcock test, the WUG test, the Peabody Picture Vocabulary Test, the Boston Naming Test, a recorded language sample (all for assessment of speech and language), and the Metropolitan Achievement Test (reading and mathematics) for school achievement.

RESULTS

We found that the time spent with middle ear effusion during the first 3 years of life and especially during the first year was associated with significantly lower scores in many aspects of cognitive ability, speech, and language. Multivariate analysis was used to control for confounding variables such as socioeconomic status and sex. Results on the full scale WISC-R are shown in Table 1. Similar results were found in both the performance and ver-

TABLE 1 Cognitive Abilities and Otitis Media During the First 3 Years of Life: Mean Scores on WISC-R*

	Full Scale WISC-R	
Effusion Group[†]	LS Mean	S.E. LS Mean
1. <32 days	113.4	1.41
2. 33–108 days	107.5	1.49
3. >108 days	105.6	1.34

Group 1 versus group 2, p = 0.005
Group 1 versus group 3, p < 0.0001
Group 2 versus group 3, p = NS

* General linear models procedure–least squares (LS) means controlling for socioeconomic status and sex.
† Time with effusion during the first 3 years of life.

bal scores. Speech and language measures significantly associated with otitis media during the first 3 years of life included aspects of speech production, speech perception, morphologic production, morphologic comprehension, lexical production, and syntactic production. Results of the Metropolitan Achievement Test indicated that after controlling for socioeconomic status and sex, the time spent with middle ear effusion during the first 3 years of life was associated with significantly low-er scores in mathematics (p < 0.009) and in reading (p = 0.045).

After controlling for disease during the first 3 years of life, middle ear disease occurring during years 4 to 7 showed no significant association with lower scores on these tests.

Similar results were found after substituting the number of episodes of acute otitis media for the variable of time spent with middle ear effusion.

PNEUMATIZATION IN SECRETORY OTITIS IN DIFFERENT TREATMENT GROUPS

SVEN-ERIC STANGERUP, M.D. and MIRKO TOS, M.D.

For several years it has been debated whether hypocellularity of the mastoid air cell system is a predisposing factor in the development of secretory otitis media, as claimed by advocates of the hereditary theory,[1] or whether the pneumatization process is hampered by reduced middle ear ventilation and an abnormal middle ear mucosa, as claimed by advocates of the environmental theory.[2]

In our previous studies, in which children were followed closely from birth to the age of 10 years, a close correlation was found between the severity and duration of secretory otitis media and the size of the mastoid air cell system.[3,4] The children with the longest and most severe episodes had the smallest air cell area, whereas children with normal middle ear ventilation had the largest air cell system. These results strongly support the environmental theory.[3,4]

Another finding was that in children with different degrees of tubal dysfunction on the right and left sides, the largest cell system was found in the less affected ear.[4,5] Furthermore, we found that girls generally had a larger cell system than boys, which is consistent with the fact that the girls had fewer episodes of secretory otitis media than the boys.[5]

In experimental animal studies van der Beek et

al[6] showed that artifical tubal occlusion had an inhibitory effect on the pneumatization process. Hug and Pfaltz[7] found an increase of 18.8 percent in the size of the mastoid air cell system in children treated with adenoidectomy, compared with an increase of 52 percent in children treated with adenoidectomy and the insertion of grommets. These findings indicate that it is possible to increase the area of the air cell system by improving the middle ear ventilation. A roentgenographic examination of children with bilateral secretory otitis media 7 years after intubation on the right side and paracentesis on the left showed a larger cell area on the grommet side, i.e., on the better ventilated side, which in our opinion is a strong point in favor of the environmental theory.[8]

PATIENTS AND METHODS

From 1977 to 1978, 224 consecutive children with bilateral secretory otitis media were treated with adenotomy, insertion of a grommet on the right side, and paracentesis on the left. During the first postoperative year the children were reexamined every third month. Follow-up examinations conducted in 1980 and 1984 were attended by 193 and 150 children, respectively. Tympanometry, audiometry, and otoscopy were performed at each examination; the follow-up examinations also included otomicroscopy.

At the last follow-up examination some of the children were selected for roentgenography on the basis of the following criteria: a type B tympanogram (flat curve) on both sides preoperatively, and middle ear effusion on both sides perioperatively. Of the 150 children, 83 fulfilled both these criteria. Of these, 47 children had received no additional treatment since the initial insertion of a grommet on the right side and paracentesis on the left (Table 1). In 1984 these children were invited to undergo roentgenography of the mastoid cell system using Runström's lateral projection. This examination was attended by 33 children and the results have been published previously.[8] The remaining 36 children, who in addition to the initial procedure in 1977–1978 had been treated with grommet insertion either unilaterally or bilaterally (see Table 1), were invited for a similar x-ray examination in April 1987. Of these 36 children, 25 attended the examination. Thus, a total of 58 children were subjected to roentgenography and form the basis of this investigation. The roentgenograms were given code numbers and the air cell area was measured by planimetry.

TABLE 1 Total Treatment at Time of X-ray Examination in 83 Children

	Invited	Attended
Grommet inserted in right ear only	47	33
Grommet inserted in both ears once	24	16
Grommet inserted in both ears twice	12	9
Total	83	58

RESULTS

The median age of the children was 4 years at the initial procedure in 1977–1978, 11 years at the x-ray examination in 1984, and 14 years at the examination in 1987. The study comprised 33 boys (57 percent) and 25 girls (43 percent). At the last follow-up examination the ratio of boys to girls was 61 to 39, which corresponds well with that found in our cohort studies of children with secretory otitis media and thus supports the judgment that more boys than girls have the disease.

Only two children had identical areas of the air cell system on the two sides, whereas the remaining showed varying degrees of asymmetry. Right-left asymmetry was either in agreement with the hypothesis that the better ventilated ear has the larger air cell area, or in disagreement with the hypothesis, so that the larger cell system was found on the side with poorer ventilation. Of the 33 children who underwent insertion of a grommet on the right side alone, the results in 19 showed agreement with the hypothesis and in 14 showed disagreement (Tables 2 and 3). Results in children who underwent more than one grommet insertion on both sides showed agreement in 16 cases, disagreement in seven, and symmetrical areas in two (Table 4).

TABLE 2 Mean Size of Mastoid Air Cell Area in Grommet Ear and Paracentesis Ear in 33 Children

	Grommet Ear (sq cm)	Paracentesis Ear (sq cm)
Agreement (n=19)		
Mean area	15.00	11.53
SD	4.94	4.59
SEM	1.13	0.98
	$p < 0.05$	
Disagreement (n=14)		
Mean area	9.47	11.51
SD	3.89	5.17
SEM	1.04	1.38
	n.s.	

TABLE 3   Difference in Mastoid Air Cell Area Between Grommet and Paracentesis Ear in 33 Children

Difference Groups (sq cm)	Agreement (n=19), %	Disagreement (n=14), %
0.25–1.25	11	36
1.50–2.50	32	36
2.75–3.75	5	14
4.00–5.00	26	7
5.25+	26	7
	p<0.05	

The median cell area in the children showing agreement with the hypothesis was 15.00 sq cm on the grommet side and 11.53 sq cm on the side with paracentesis (see Table 2). This difference is statistically significant (Student's t test, $p < 0.05$). In children with disagreement, the median cell area was 9.47 sq cm on the grommet ear and 11.51 sq cm on the ear with paracentesis—a difference that is nonsignificant.

Because of the differences in age at the time of roentgenography, the exact size of the cell system is not as important as the difference in size between the better and poorer ventilated ear of the individual child, who thus acts as his own control. The significantly largest differences occurred among children with agreement with the hypothesis, whereas almost all the minor differences were found in the group with disagreement (see Table 3). Also among children who underwent more than one grommet insertion on both sides the largest difference in cell area between the short and long term ventilated ear was found in the group with agreement.

The median difference in the period of ventilation in the three treatment groups was 10 months for children with one grommet insertion, 3 months

TABLE 4   Mean Difference in Air Cell Area Between Ear with Longest Ventilation Time and Ear with Shortest Ventilation Time

	Agreement (n=35)		Disagreement (n=21)	
	sq cm	n	sq cm	n
Grommet inserted in right ear only	3.6	19	2.0	14
Grommet inserted in both ears once	3.1	10*	2.0	4
Grommet inserted in both ears twice	1.9	6	1.2	3

* In this group two children had symmetry of the air cell size.

for those with grommet insertion on both sides, and 4 months for children in whom grommet insertion was performed twice or more on both sides.

DISCUSSION

The advantage of this study is that each patient acts as his own control, thus eliminating uncertainties regarding history, the x-ray examination, and determination of the size of the cell area, just as the genetically determined growth rate of the mastoid cell system must be considered to be similar on the two sides.

One of the cornerstones in the hereditary theory of pneumatization is the demonstration of a gaussian distribution of the size of the air cell area in a group of children who had "healthy" ears at the time of examination.[1] In this as well as in our previous reports,[3,4] a gaussian distribution of the size of the cell system was found, and the children had "healthy" ears at the time of roentgenography. It was evident, however, that the children with the smallest cell systems were those with a history of secretory otitis media, whereas the largest cell systems were found among children who had never had the disease.

In this as well as in our previous studies,[3,4,8] we have attempted to show that improvement of middle ear ventilation in childhood increases the size of the mastoid cell system. The significance of having a large cell system, however, remains uncertain. Some otosurgeons claim that a large air reservoir is of importance for the functional results of intact wall mastoidectomy,[9] and similar arguments have been brought forward to support the use of mastoidectomy in myringoplasty.[10] This argument is based on the assumption that a small cell system is the direct cause of chronic otitis. So far the underlying mechanisms remain obscure, but the discussion about pneumatization is undoubtedly of clinical relevance.

REFERENCES

1. Diamant M. Otitis and pneumatisation of the mastoid bone. Lund, Sweden: Hakon Olsons Boktryckeri, 1940:1.
2. Wittmaack K. Über die normale und pathologische Pneumatisation des Schlafenbeins. Jena, East Germany: Fischer, 1918:1.
3. Tos M, Stangerup S-E, Hvid G. Mastoid pneumatisation. Evidence of the environmental theory. Arch Otolaryngol 1984; 110:502–508.
4. Tos M, Stangerup S-E. The causes of asymmetry of the

mastoid air cell system. Acta Otolaryngol (Stockh) 1985; 99:564–570.

5. Tos M, Stangerup S-E. Secretory otitis and pneumatisation of the mastoid process: sexual differences in the size of the mastoid cell system. Am J Otolaryngol 1985; 6:199–205.

6. van der Beek JMH, van den Broek P, Kuijpers W. Effect of tubal occlusion on bone formation in the middle ear of the rat. ORL 1983; 45:87–95.

7. Hug JE, Pfaltz CR. Temporal bone pneumatisation. A planimetric study. Arch Otolaryngol 1985; 233:145–156.

8. Stangerup S-E, Tos M. Treatment of secretory otitis and pneumatisation. Laryngoscope 1986; 96:680–684.

9. Holmquist J, Bergstrom B. The mastoid air cell system in ear surgery. Arch Otolaryngol 1978; 104:127–129.

10. Proud CO, Duff WE. Mastoidectomy and epitympanotomy. Ann Otol Rhinol Laryngol 1976; 85(Suppl 25):289–292.

OCCURRENCE OF POSTINFECTIOUS AND SILENT MUCOID SECRETORY OTITIS MEDIA: A PROSPECTIVE LONG TERM STUDY

PEKKA H. KARMA, M.D. and MARKKU M. SIPILÄ, M.D.

Secretory otitis media has been intensively studied during recent years. However, the data and opinions of the disease differ widely: even the definition secretory otitis media is different among different authors.[1] Its incidence figures, although often reported to be high, are very variable.[2,3] Opinions about its etiopathogenesis vary from infection to related to mechanical.[4–6] The real need for active treatment is unknown. To clarify these questions we determined the incidence of mucoid secretory otitis media necessitating tympanostomy treatment in a large and unselected childhood population. We also tried to clarify the characteristics and etiologic background in these cases.

MATERIAL AND METHODS

The study material was composed of 1,679 unselected children (51.9 percent boys) born between December 1978 and March 1980 in the city of Tampere, Finland (74 percent of the whole age group). They were followed for ear morbidity up to the age of 6¾ to 8 years (median, 7 5/12 years) in the Department of Otolaryngology at the Tampere University Central Hospital, where the ear related surgery, including tympanostomies, was also performed. Among those who were subjected to tympanostomy because of secretory otitis media with verified mucoid effusion, all the data concerned with ear related and other morbidity were recorded. The data were collected from the medical records; in order to include information regarding possible visits outside the study clinic, questionnaires were sent to the parents when the children were 5 years old. To study the role of middle ear infections in the etiopathogenesis of mucoid secretory otitis media, we paid special attention to recording all the episodes of acute otitis media before the first tympanostomy for secretory otitis media. An episode was clinically diagnosed as acute otitis if the child had acute ear related symptoms and otoscopic signs suggesting middle ear effusion. Acute attacks were treated with myringotomy (and aspiration) and antimicrobial drugs, primarily penicillin-V, 25 to 35 mg per kg twice daily orally. The ear was regularly reexamined at 2 to 3 week intervals until it was completely healed. Statistical analyses were done with the Student's t test or the X^2 test.

RESULTS

Altogether 142 (8.5 percent) of the children, 85 boys (59.9 percent) and 57 girls (40.1 percent), developed mucoid secretory otitis media, necessitating tympanostomy in 218 ears during the follow-up. Of the ears, 154 (70.6 percent) were subjected to tympanostomy only once, 40 (18.3 percent) twice, and 24 (11.1 percent) three or more times. The median age of the children at the time of the first tympanostomy was 18 months.

Only three (2.1 percent) of the children with secretory otitis media had never contracted acute otitis media, and 20 (14.1 percent) had experienced it three or fewer times during their lifetime before tympanostomy (Table 1). Within 1 year preceding the first tympanostomy for secretory otitis media, 105 (73.9 percent) of the children had had at least four attacks of acute otitis media. If the children were grouped into those with recurring acute otitis media during the last year (four or more attacks) and those having acute otitis media only occasionally (0 to 3 attacks during the last year), there were distinct differences in the age and sex profiles in the two groups (Table 2). Mucoid secretory otitis media preceded by recurrent acute otitis media was seen at a median age of 16 months, 62.9 percent of the patients being boys, whereas the cases with occasional otitis attacks were found at a median age of 42 months and with the same frequency among boys and girls. Both these differences are statistically highly significant (p < 0.001).

Of all the children with secretory otitis media, 76 (53.5 percent) had bilateral disease. In the infectious group this proportion was 58.1 percent and in the noninfectious group, 40.5 percent; this difference, however, was not statistically significant. The age or sex distribution of bilateral cases did not differ from that of the unilateral cases in either group. On the other hand, tubes had to be reinserted into 33.7 percent of the ears in the infectious group, but only into 15.4 percent of the noninfectious ears with secretory otitis (p < 0.025).

At the time of tympanostomy, the adenoids usually were also removed, if not done earlier (11 children). Large adenoids, as defined according to age by the surgeon, were found in 67.6 percent of the noninfectious children but in only 36.2 percent

TABLE 1 Occurrence of Acute Otitis Media Before Mucoid Secretory Otitis Media

	During Last Year				*Since Birth*				
	0	*1–3*	*4–6*	*>6*	*0*	*1–3*	*4–6*	*7–10*	*>10*
Boys									
Number	4	15	58	8	2	9	53	15	6
Age*	54	40	17	14	54	40	14	20	50
Girls									
Number	3	15	28	11	1	8	24	22	2
Age	87	26	18	15	35	12	17	37	43
All									
Number	7	30	86	19	3	17	77	37	8
Age	56	31	17	15	51	21	15	20	44

*Median age in months.

TABLE 2 Mucoid Secretory Otitis Media and Otitis: History

	Attacks of Acute Otitis Media Within Preceding Year		
	0–3	*≥ 4*	*All*
Boys			
Number	19	66	85
Age*	44	16	18
Girls			
Number	18	39	57
Age	33	16	20
All			
Number	37	105	142
Age	42	16	18

*Median age in months.

of the infectious group (p < 0.001); (Table 3). The size distribution was not different in the two sexes.

DISCUSSION

Our practice was to carry out tympanostomy if the middle ear effusion persisted without acute symptoms for longer than 1 month and was mucoid in character at myringotomy. Only 7 percent of the effusions in the present series had persisted for longer than 3½ months. Thus, as in acute otitis, we were rather active in surgical treatment in secretory otitis media too.

With the foregoing criteria our study showed that in the Finnish urban child population every twelfth child will develop mucoid secretory otitis media necessitating tympanostomy during the first 7 years of life. As far as we know there are no other studies of the occurrence of mucoid secretory otitis media using the same kind of criteria. In most studies, with very much higher incidence figures, the diagnosis of secretory otitis media has been made tympanometrically[2,3] or otoscopically.[7] Thus our figures reflect the clinical importance of the problem in terms of the need for active treatment. On the other hand, because we were very active in doing tympanostomy, our figures, although low, are probably overestimated rather than underestimated.

Our study showed that there are two clinically different groups of cases of mucoid secretory otitis media. Three-quarters of the cases are preceded by the otitis prone condition with frequent attacks of acute otitis. In these cases secretory otitis media developed, as with recurrent acute otitis in general,[8] more often in boys than in girls. One-quarter of the cases, with a "normal" otitis history, were seen at

TABLE 3   Adenoid Size in Children with Mucoid Secretory Otitis Media

| Size | Attacks of Acute Otitis Media Within Preceding Year | | | |
| | 0–3 | | ≥ 4 | |
	Girls	Boys	Girls	Boys
Small	1	2	13	15
Medium	6	2	13	25
Large	10	15	13	25
Unknown	1	0	0	1
All	18	19	39	66

a somewhat older age and with the same frequency in both sexes. These differences suggest that there is a different etiopathogenetic background in the two groups. It is probable that in a majority of the cases, middle ear infections play a major role,[5] while a smaller number of the cases are more silent, without an apparent infectious background, but more directly caused by mechanical tubal factors. However, these basic etiologic factors do not exclude each other, but both contribute, with a different importance in different cases, to the process resulting in inflammation and finally in the increase in secretory elements in the middle ear mucosa.

REFERENCES

1. Paparella MM, Bluestone CD, Arnold W, Bradley WH, Hussl B, Munker G, Naunton RF, Sadé J, Tos M, van Cauwenberge P. Panel report 1A. Definition and classification. In: Lim DJ, ed. Recent advances in otitis media with effusion. Report of research conference. Ann Otol Rhinol Laryngol 1985; 94(Suppl 116):8–9.
2. Tos M, Stangerup S-E, Andreassen UK, Hvid G, Thomsen J, Holm-Jensen S. Natural history of secretory otitis media. In: Lim DJ, Bluestone CD, Klein JO, Nelson JD, eds. Recent advances in otitis media with effusion. Proceedings of the Third International Symposium. Toronto: BC Decker, 1984:36–40.
3. Casselbrant M, Brostoff LM, Cantekin EI, Flaherty MR, Doyle WJ, Bluestone CD, Fria TJ. Otitis media with effusion in preschool children. Laryngoscope 1985; 95:428–436.
4. Senturia BH, Gessert DF, Carr CD, Baumann ES. Studies concerned with tubotympanitis. Ann Otol Rhinol Laryngol 1958; 67:440–467.
5. Karma PH, Sipilä PT, Luotonen JP, Grönroos PW. Bacteriological aspects of acute otitis media in secretory otitis media. In: Sadé J, ed. Acute and secretory otitis media. Amsterdam: Kugler Publications, 1986:181–188.
7. Virolainen E, Puhakka H, Aantaa E, Tuohimaa P, Ruuskanen O, Meurman OH. Prevalence of secretory otitis media in seven to eight year old school children. Ann Otol Rhinol Laryngol 1980; 89(Suppl 68):7–10.
8. Pukander J, Karma P, Sipilä M. Occurrence and recurrence of acute otitis media among children. Acta Otolaryngol (Stockh) 1982; 94:479–486.

IMMUNOHISTOCHEMICAL ANALYSIS OF CONNECTIVE TISSUE COMPONENTS IN TYMPANOSCLEROSIS

BURKHARD HUSSL, M.D., RUPERT TIMPL, Ph.D., DAVID J. LIM, M.D., MONIKA GINZEL, B.S., and GEORG G. WICK, M.D.

Tympanosclerosis is a frequent sequel of otitis media. Whereas its histology and ultrastructural morphology are well established,[1-3] its pathogenesis remains to be clarified. Recent animal experiments by Poliquin and co-workers[4] and by Yoo et al[5] suggest that immunologic hypersensitivity to tympanic membrane connective tissue, e.g., an autoimmune response against type II collagen, may play a pathogenetic role. In this study we attempted to identify the main connective tissue components in normal and tympanosclerotic tympanic membranes by immunohistochemical methods, in order to elucidate the pathogenesis.

MATERIALS AND METHODS

Seventeen normal tympanic membranes were obtained from autopsies, and 21 specimens from tympanosclerotic tympanic membranes were obtained during middle ear surgery for chronic otitis media. All normal tympanic membranes and five of the tympanosclerotic specimens were immediately immersed into N-ethyl maleimide buffer (pH 7.0), transported to the laboratory, washed and snap frozen in liquid nitrogen. The other tympanosclerotic specimens were embedded in glycol methacrylate (JB-4) following EDTA decalcification. Frozen unfixed sections 4 μm thick were either stained with hematoxylin and eosin or processed for indirect immunofluorescence using specific polyclonal cross absorbed and affinity chromatography purified antibodies against the following collagenous and noncollagenous connective tissue components: collagen type I, procollagen type I, collagen type II, collagen type III, procollagen type III, collagen type IV, collagen type V, fibronectin, and laminin. In addition, sections of the tympanosclerotic specimens were treated with 0.1 percent trypsin for 15 minutes and with 0.1 percent hyaluronidase for 30 minutes, respectively, before being stained for indirect immunofluorescence. Preparation of antibodies and performance of the immunofluorescence tests were done according to established procedures.[6-8]

RESULTS

The distribution of the different connective tissue components in normal tympanic membranes is summarized in Table 1. The predominant collagens of the collagenous (radial and circular) fiber layer were types III and II (Fig. 1) and to a lesser extent also type I. Type II collagen was also present in the center of the tympanic anulus. Procollagens I and III showed a preponderance in the subepidermal and submucosal connective tissue layers, but in addition procollagen III was found throughout the collagenous fiber layer. Collagen type IV and laminin were present only in epithelial and vascular basement membranes. Antifibronectin gave strong reactions with all basement membranes and the subepithelial connective tissue layers and also stained the collagenous fiber layer, albeit less intensively. Collagen type V could be demonstrated only in vascular walls.

The results of the immunohistochemical analysis of the connective tissue components in tympanosclerotic tympanic membranes are summarized in Table 2. In native frozen sections the center of the plaques could not be stained with any of the antibodies employed. However, after hyaluronidase treatment a reaction with anticollagen type III could be observed in these areas. Trypsin treatment, on the other hand, had no effect on the staining pattern of the plaques. However, in areas of the sections unaffected by tympanosclerosis the intensity of staining with antiprocollagen I, antiprocollagen III, anticollagen IV, antilaminin, and antifibronectin was reduced or even abolished, because the molecules in question carry nonhelical trypsin sensitive portions.

TABLE 1 Immunohistochemical Analysis of Connective Tissue Components in Normal Human Tympanic Membranes

	a-pI	a-I	a-II	a-pIII	a-III	a-IV	a-V	a-FN	a-lam
Epidermis	-	-	-		-	-	-		-
Basement membrane	-	-	-	-	-	+++	-	++	+++
Subepidermal layer	+++	+	+	++	+	-	-	++	-
Collagenous fiber layer	-	+	++	++	++	-	-	+	-
Submucosal layer	++	+	-	++	+	-	-	++	-
Basement membrane	-	-	-	-	-	+++	-	++	+++
Mucosal epithelium	-	-	-	-	-	-	-	-	-
Vascular basement membrane	-	-	-	-	-	+++	+	++	+++

- , no reaction. + , weak reaction. ++ , strong reaction. +++ , very strong reaction.

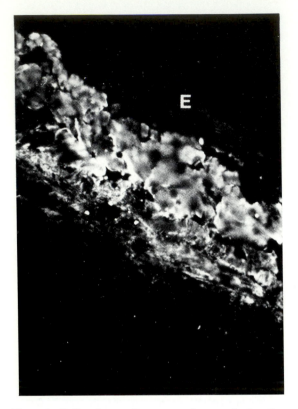

Figure 1 Indirect immunofluorescence, frozen unfixed section of normal human tympanic membrane. Rabbit anticollagen type II antibodies strongly stain the outer strata of the collagenous fiber layer. E, epidermal epithelium. (Original magnification 250x.)

The connective tissue around the plaques was rich in collagen type I (Fig. 2) and procollagen type III (Fig. 3), but collagen types II and III as well as procollagen I and fibronectin could be demonstrated there. The plaques seemed to displace and compress the preexisting connective tissue layers. In peripheral areas of the plaques some reactivity with anticollagen I, antiprocollagen III, and anticollagen

III could be observed. Anticollagen IV and antilaminin impressively revealed the increased vascularization of the connective tissue adjacent to the plaques and the extreme paucity of the vessels within the plaques proper (Fig. 4). Collagen type V again was present only in vascular walls.

DISCUSSION

Collagens are the most important structural components of connective tissue. They form a family of proteins with a largely triple helical structure. Several genetic variants of collagen exist, which differ in their molecular chain composition, distribution, and biologic function. Whereas collagen types I, II, and III are so-called interstitial collagens, types IV and V are basement membrane specific. In addition type V was found around smooth muscle fibers of the vascular walls. Collagen type II has been demonstrated in hyalin cartilage, the vitreous body of the eye, and the nucleus pulposus of the intervertebral disk. Procollagens are precursor forms of collagens that possess nonhelical N terminal and C terminal domains. In addition to collagens and procollagens, the connective tissue contains noncollagenous glycoproteins, the most prominent being laminin and fibronectin demonstrated in basement membranes. The latter is found in codistribution with types I, III, and IV collagen and is functional in various biologic processes, such as cell attachment.[9]

Information concerning the distribution of connective tissue components in normal and tympanosclerotic tympanic membranes has been scanty. In guinea pigs, collagen types I and III were identified in normal tympanic membranes by biochemical methods.[10] In primates, collagen type II has been demonstrated in the lamina propria and in the tympanic anulus of normal tympanic membranes.[11]

TABLE 2   **Immunohistochemical Analysis of Connective Tissue Components in Human Tympanosclerosis**

	a-pI	a-I	a-II	a-pIII	a-III	a-IV	a-V	a-FN	a-lam
Connective tissue around plaque	+	+ +	+	+ + +	+	-	-	+	-
Vascular basement membrane	-	-	-	-	-	+ +	+	+ + +	+ + +
Peripheral areas of plaque	-	+	-	+	+	-	-	-	-
Center of plaque									
without hyaluronidase	-	-	-	-	-	-	-	-	-
with hyaluronidase	-	-	-	-	+	-	-	-	-

- , no reaction. +, weak reaction. + + , strong reaction. + + + , very strong reaction.

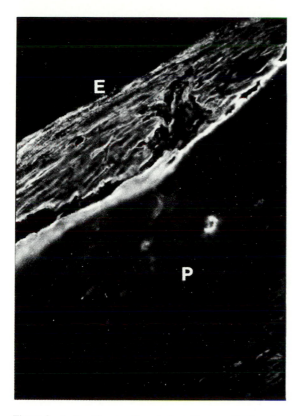

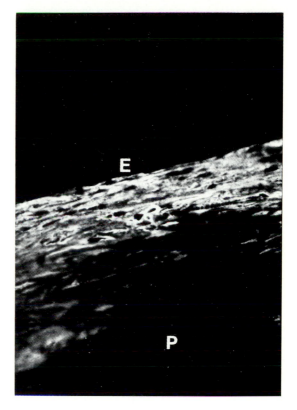

Figure 2 Indirect immunofluorescence, frozen unfixed section of tympanosclerotic tympanic membrane. Rabbit anticollagen type I antibodies produce strong staining in the connective tissue adjacent to the plaque but not in the center of plaque. E, epidermal epithelium. P, plaque. (Original magnification 250x.)

Figure 3 Indirect immunofluorescence, frozen unfixed section of tympanosclerotic tympanic membrane. Rabbit antiprocollagen type III antibodies stain the connective tissue surrounding the plaque and peripheral areas of the plaque but not its center. E, epidermal epithelium. P, plaque. (Original magnification 250x.)

In humans Birchall et al[10] found collagen type I as the predominant constituent in normal tympanic membranes, whereas Yoo et al[12] demonstrated the presence of collagen type II in the tympanic anulus of normal tympanic membranes.

Our study shows that collagen types III and II and—to a lesser extent—type I are the major constituents of the normal human tympanic membrane. The demonstration of collagen type II is of particular interest in view of the hypothesis that an autoimmune response against type II collagen may play a role in the pathogenesis of tympanosclerosis. The subepithelial connective tissue layers of the normal tympanic membrane seem to be main sites of collagen I and III turnover, similar to that in skin. The distribution of collagen types IV and V, laminin, and fibronectin corresponds to the pattern of reactivity found in other areas of connective tissue in the body.

In tympanosclerotic specimens taken from human tympanic membranes at surgery, Birchall et al[10] detected collagen type I employing biochemical methods. Ishibe et al[13] using indirect immuno-

fluorescence, demonstrated the presence of collagen type II in lamellar dense connective tissue in tympanosclerotic foci in surgical specimens from patients with tympanosclerosis.

In the present study this observation could not be confirmed. In tympanosclerotic tympanic membranes the center of the plaques could not be stained with the antibodies employed, with the exception of anticollagen III after hyaluronidase treatment. This indicates that antigenic determinants were made accessible after cleavage of hyaluronic acid. The question remains whether the plaques are composed of yet other constituents with masked antigenic determinants that prevent reactivity of the respective antibodies or whether they contain a still different material, e.g., another type of collagen, which was not recognized by the antibodies used in this investigation.

In peripheral areas of the plaques, and especially in some areas of the surrounding connective tissue, an increased turnover of collagen type III was noted. This points to a continuing fibrotic process,

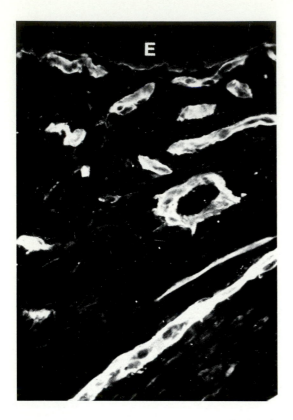

Figure 4 Indirect immunofluorescence, frozen unfixed section of tympanosclerotic tympanic membrane. Rabbit antilaminin antibodies brilliantly stain the vascular basement membranes, outlining the increased vascularity of the connective tissue adjacent to the plaque. E, epidermal epithelium. (Original magnification 500x.)

since fibrosis in any tissue studied, such as liver, skin, lung, and cornea, always starts with an increased production of type III collagen; only later, in chronic stages, does type I collagen production prevail.[14] The latter phenomenon was also noted in some areas of the connective tissue adjacent to the plaques, where a strong reactivity with anticollagen type I was present, indicating that the disease process might have reached an irreversible state. The increased vascularity of the connective tissue adjacent to the tympanosclerotic lesions outlined with anticollagen IV and antilaminin is consistent with the postulated increased metabolic activity in these areas.

The specific reagents used in the present immunohistochemical study allowed the exact typing of the collagenous and noncollagenous connective tissue components in normal and tympanosclerotic human tympanic membranes. The predominant collagens are types III and II and—to a lesser extent— type I in normal tympanic membranes. In tympanosclerotic plaques only collagen type III

could be demonstrated. Although we cannot determine whether autoimmunity to type II collagen is the basis for the development of tympanosclerosis, the absence of type II collagen in the plaque is noteworthy.

This study was supported by the Austrian National Research Council project S–41/05 and by grant NS 08854 from NINCDS-NIH.

REFERENCES

1. Hussl B, Lim DJ. Fine morphology of tympanosclerosis. In: Lim DJ, Bluestone CD, Klein JO, Nelson JD, eds. Recent advances in otitis media with effusion. Proceedings of the Third International Symposium. Toronto: BC Decker, 1984:348–353.
2. Friedmann J, Galey FR, Odnert S. The ultrastructure of tympanosclerosis. The source of matrix vesicles and the pattern of calcospherules. Am J Otol 1981; 3:144–149.
3. Moeller P. Tympanosclerosis of the eardrum. A scanning electron microscopic study. Acta Otolaryngol 1981; 91:215–221.
4. Poliquin JF, Catanzaro A, Robb J, Schiff M. Adaptive immunity of the tympanic membrane. Am J Otol 1981; 2:94–98.
5. Yoo TJ, Sudo N, Tomoda K, Yazawa Y, Ishibe T, Takeda T, Floyd R. Type II collagen mediated autoimmune middle ear disease: eustachian tube disease, otitis media with effusion and tympanosclerosis. Auris Nasus Larynx Japan 1985; 12:91–93.
6. Timpl R. Antibodies to collagens and procollagens. Methods Enzymol 1982; 82A:472–498.
7. Wick G, Traill KN, Schauenstein K, eds. Immunofluorescence technology. Selected theoretical and clinical aspects. Amsterdam: Elsevier Biomedical Press, 1982.
8. Timpl R, Wick G, Gay S. Antibodies to distinct types of collagens and procollagens and their application in immunohistology. J Immunol Methods 1977; 18:165–182.
9. Wick G, Ginzel M, Timpl R. Immunohistochemical analysis of connective tissue components. Fresenius Z Anal Chem 1984; 317:648–649.
10. Birchall JP, Pearman K, Dawes JDK. The collagens of middle ear structures and tympanosclerotic plaques. J Laryngol Otol 1982; 96:797–800.
11. Ishibe T, Yoo TJ. Type II collagen distribution in the monkey ear. In: Lim DJ, ed. Abstracts of the eighth midwinter research meeting, Association for Research in Otolaryngology, 1985:91–92.
12. Yoo TJ, Tomoda K. Type II collagen distribution in the external and middle ears. In: Lim DJ, ed. Abstracts of the sixth midwinter research meeting, Association for Research in Otolaryngology, 1983:111.
13. Ishibe T, Yoo TJ, Shea JJ, Tomoda K. Immunohistochemical studies in Meniere's disease, otosclerosis and tympanosclerosis. In: Lim DJ, ed. Abstracts of the eighth midwinter research meeting, Association for Research in Otolaryngology, 1985:92.
14. Wick G, Brunner H, Penner E, Timpl R. The diagnostic application of specific antiprocollagen sera. II. Analysis of liver biopsies. Int Arch Allergy Appl Immunol 1978; 56:316–324.

WHY DO TYMPANOSTOMY TUBES BLOCK?

ANDREW P. REID, F.R.C.S. (Edin), LESLEY SMALLMAN, F.R.C.Path., and DAVID PROOPS, F.R.C.S.

The modern otologist devotes a large part of his practice to treating childhood otitis media with effusion. The surgical treatment involves insertion of a tympanostomy tube, which was introduced into present practice by Armstrong[1] in 1954. The problem with these tubes is the finite period for which they function. They cease to function as a result of blockage or eventual extrusion from the tympanic membrane. The incidences of extrusion of different types of tubes have been studied,[2-4] and possible mechanisms for the extrusion have been postulated consequent upon studies of the migratory pattern of the outer layer of the tympanic membrane.[5,6] A review of the literature shows no studies related specifically to the problem of blockage of tympanostomy tubes. It was the intention in this study to identify the material and associated factors causing tympanostomy tube blockage.

METHOD

One hundred extruded tympanostomy tubes were retrieved from the ear canals of children under continuing review following surgical treatment of otitis media with effusion. These tubes were examined macroscopically to record the presence of blockage and to determine the pattern of material around the outer aspect of the tube. Each tube was then sliced longitudinally and reinspected with specific reference to whether the blockage lay within the lumen or across the opening at the base of the tube.

The luminal material and the outer debris were then examined microscopically in 20 of the specimens using hematoxylin and eosin staining.

These findings were correlated with surgical details recorded at the time of tube insertion. These related to the appearance of the tympanic membrane, the state of the middle ear mucosa, and the type of middle ear effusion present. The occurrence of middle ear infections after tube insertion was recorded together with the time of tube extrusion.

FINDINGS

Macroscopic examination revealed the lumen of the tubes to be blocked by an amorphous material and the outer surface to be covered with a cast or crust of lamellar material. This outer material was shown to consist of layers of desquamated squamous epithelium identical to the casts and crusts described by Weinberger et al.[7] This was situated mainly across the base of the tube and was found in 70 percent of the specimens. The luminal material was entirely different. Light microscopy revealed a largely eosinophilic collection with polymorphonuclear leukocytes, some clumps of gram positive organisms, and occasional red blood cells. Initial examination showed that 77 percent of the tubes had blocked lumens but reinspection after slicing reduced this figure to 56 percent as in some cases the lumen was "blocked" simply by a cast across the base, which can appear only after extrusion.

There is no relationship between the occurrence of tube blockage and the appearance of the tympanic membrane or middle ear mucosa at the time of tube insertion. There is a definite association between the presence of thick fluid and subsequent lumen blockage ($p < 0.02$). This is not seen in association with thin fluid. This association is still found even in the reduced numbers of blocked tubes after slicing. It was also noted that the presence of tube blockage did not influence the time the tube remained in situ.

DISCUSSION

We demonstrated the material present in the lumen of a blocked tympanostomy tube. The appearances would suggest that it is derived from the middle ear effusion found in these patients. It has been clearly demonstrated that it is the thick middle ear effusion that is associated with subsequent tube blockage. The presence of organisms in some specimens raises the possibility that episodes of suppurative otitis media after tube insertion may be responsible for this blockage. Our long term follow-up in all these cases fails to demonstrate any association between blockage and infective episodes.

The mechanisms relating to the extrusion of tympanostomy tubes might lead one to believe that a blocked tube would be extruded more easily than an unblocked tube. This study has shown that there is no difference in extrusion times between blocked and unblocked tubes. This fact together with the clearly demonstrated layers of squames on the outer aspect of the tubes supports the role of this unique migrating surface epithelium in the extrusion of a tympanostomy tube.

REFERENCES

1. Armstrong BW. A new treatment for chronic secretory otitis media. Arch Otolaryngol 1954; 59:653–654.
2. Gibb AG. Long term assessment of ventilation tubes. J Laryngol Otol 1980; 94:39–51.
3. Mackenzie IJ. Factors affecting the extrusion rates of ventilation tubes. J R Soc Med 1984; 77:751–753.
4. Gibb AG, Mackenzie IJ. The extrusion rate of grommets. Otolaryngol Head Neck Surg 1985; 93:695–699.
5. O'Donoghue GM. Epithelial migration on the guinea pig tympanic membrane; the influence of perforation and ventilating tube insertion. Clin Otolaryngol 1983; 8:297–303.
6. O'Donoghue GM. The kinetics of epithelial cells in relation to ventilation tubes. Acta Otolaryngol (Stockh) 1984; 98:105–109.
7. Weinberger J, Proops DW, Hawke M. Casts and crusts of the tympanic membrane. Acta Otolaryngol (Stockh) 1986; 102:44–51.

LABYRINTHINE INVOLVEMENT IN OTITIS MEDIA—CURRENT STATUS

MICHAEL M. PAPARELLA, M.D., PATRICIA A. SCHACHERN, B.S., MARCOS V. GOYCOOLEA, M.D., M.S., Ph.D., and TAE-HYUN YOON, M.D.

Otitis media can lead to complications or sequelae in the middle ear cleft, intracranial space, or labyrinth. We report here current information about labyrinthine problems resulting from or associated with otitis media.

CLASSIFICATION AND CONTINUUM

Because some sequelae and complications result from some forms of otitis and not from others, it is important to define the type under study. As agreed upon by the 1983 Task Force on Terminology, each author defines the type(s) considered in his study.[1] Figure 1 shows our classification and continuum (interrelationships of various types of otitis media). Our classification modifies that recommended at the 1983 symposium:

1. Suppurative otitis media
   a. Acute
   b. Chronic
2. Nonsuppurative otitis media (secretory otitis media or otitis media with effusion)
   a. Serous
   b. Mucoid

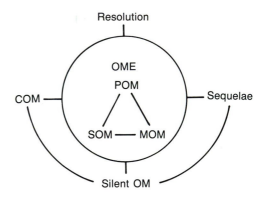

Figure 1 Classification and continuum of otitis media.

Chronic otitis media was defined in that report, and in many textbooks, as being associated with otorrhea and perforation of the tympanic membrane, but in an earlier study 81 percent of 92 cases studied in human temporal bones showed intractable disease with no perforation or otorrhea.[2] Labyrinthine sequelae are more likely to occur with acute purulent or chronic suppurative otitis media, regardless of whether the tympanic membrane is intact or not (silent otitis). The 1,383 temporal bones (474 with otitis media) studied in our laboratory were classified as shown in Table 1.[2]

CLASSIC COMPLICATIONS

Labyrinthine complications can be distinguished more easily than the subtle labyrinthine sequelae accompanying otitis media. Established classic complications include cholesteatoma, fistula, and tympanogenic suppurative labyrinthitis.

Cholesteatoma and Fistula

Chronic otitis media is defined as intractable disease including cholesteatoma, granulation tissue, or cholesterin granuloma. Cholesteatoma can result in fistulas of the labyrinth (usually the horizontal semicircular canal) and rarely the promontory or windows. Vertigo and deafness are cardinal symptoms. The pathophysiologic effects include the direct effects of the lesion and secondary effects from serous labyrinthitis (which can produce temporary threshold shifts) or purulent labyrinthitis (permanent threshold shifts).

Tympanogenic Suppurative Labyrinthitis

Tympanogenic suppurative labyrinthitis can result from purulent or chronic suppurative otitis media. The usual portal of entry is the round window. The other major form of labyrinthitis is the meningogenic form (most often bilateral); tympanogenic suppurative labyrinthitis can be unilateral. The classic findings documented in Europe about 1900 can result in three stages—purulent, fibrous, and ossificans.[3]

COEXISTING PATHOLOGIC FINDINGS

Pathologic study is important in diagnosing and treating otologic disease. In a recent study multiple pathologic correlates were documented in the middle ear cleft or inner ear.[4] Of 1,383 human temporal bones, 152 had more than one pathologic lesion. In those 152 otitis media was found most commonly, followed by otosclerosis, endolymphatic hydrops, labyrinthitis, and cancer (Table 2).

Probable Coincidental Relationship

Table 3 lists the disorders, otosclerosis and ear cancer (mostly metastatic), occurring with various types of otitis media. Although cancer may help initiate some of the changes of otitis media, the coexistence of otosclerosis and otitis media is probably coincidental.

Possible Causative Relationship

Earlier studies associated Meniere's disease with or resulting from otitis media, especially the chronic suppurative form.[5] One of two temporal bones from patients with Meniere's disease in a 1938 study by Hallpike and Cairns[6] exhibited changes of the chronic suppurative form; the possible causative relationship was discussed. This classic report established endolymphatic hydrops as the most important pathologic correlate of Meniere's disease. Table 4 lists the types of otitis media (especially the chronic suppurative form) associated with hydrops.

Tympanogenic suppurative labyrinthitis can result from otitis media. Table 5 lists the types associated with or resulting from otitis media. Some temporal bones were acquired from very sick

TABLE 1 Temporal Bones with Otitis Media (474)

Type of Otitis Media	SOM	SPOM	POM	MPOM	MOM	COM
No. of bones	30	113	110	9	9	203
% of bones	6.3	23.8	23.2	1.9	1.9	48.5

SOM = Serous otitis media
SPOM = Serous purulent otitis media
POM = Purulent otitis media
MPOM = Mucopurulent otitis media
MOM = Mucoid otitis media
COM = Chronic suppurative otitis media

TABLE 2   Bones with Multiple Diseases (152 of 1,383 Temporal Bones)

Category of Disease	Number of Ears	Percentage of Ears
Otitis media	108	71.9
Otosclerosis	66	43.4
Endolymphatic hydrops	59	38.8
Labyrinthitis	39	25.0
Metastatic ear cancer	37	24.3
Acoustic neuroma	7	4.6
Hemorrhage in inner ear	5	3.3
Mondini's disorder	4	2.6
Arteritis of middle ear	4	2.6
Fungus in inner ear	3	2.0
Bulging round window membrane	2	1.3
Fracture of temporal bone	1	0.7

patients who may have developed pneumonia, acute otitis media, and labyrinthitis with the terminal illness. However, chronic labyrinthine changes were seen most frequently with chronic otitis media and probably were not part of the terminal illness.

SENSORINEURAL HEARING LOSS

Since 1970 our clinics and laboratories have studied sensorineural hearing loss resulting from otitis media and have published several reports, 27 of them recently documented. Another 41 investigators before and since have observed and described sensorineural hearing loss and otitis media. Some have reported a relationship of sensorineural hearing loss to otitis media with effusion (secretory otitis) in children.[7] The pathologic correlate may be serous labyrinthitis localized in the perilymph at the basal turn, which can result in a temporary threshold shift. With continued exposure to otitis media, a permanent threshold shift or permanent sensorineural loss can result with subsequent apical involvement of lower frequencies.

Studies in animals have included tracer studies to assess the permeability of the round window membrane in otitis media and electrophysiologic evidence of cochlear loss in the basal turn in experimentally induced acute otitis media.[7,8] Other findings include the passage of inflammatory elements (polymorphonuclear leukocytes) across the round window membrane to the scala tympani. Walby et al[9] have confirmed sensorineural hearing loss as a sequela of chronic suppurative otitis media and hypothesized that the pathogenesis may involve stiffening or collagenation of the basilar membrane.

Morphology

Assessing the role of the round window membrane in the pathogenesis requires a detailed understanding of its normal cytoarchitecture. In ultrastructural studies in animals (monkeys, guinea pigs, chinchillas) and more recently in man we evaluated the thickness and morphologic characteristics of normal round window membranes and those from cases of serous, purulent, and chronic otitis

TABLE 3   Otitis Media and Other Diseases

	SOM	SPOM	POM	MPOM	MOM	COM
Otosclerosis	1	2	7	1	0	24
Ear cancer (metastatic)	2	5	2	0	0	15

TABLE 4 Temporal Bones with Otitis Media and Endolymphatic Hydrops

Type of Otitis Media	SOM	SPOM	POM	MPOM	MOM	COM
Number of bones with hydrops	4	5	4	0	0	16

media.[7] Bones in chronologic order in six age ranges were studied to determine the possibility of age related differences. No significant difference appeared by age group in the mean thickness of the round window membrane in normal temporal bones or bones with otitis media, but a difference was observed in the mean thickness of the membrane in various forms of otitis media, as compared to the thickness in the normal membrane, in all age groups (Table 6). The membrane was thickest in cases of chronic suppurative otitis media when compared to the normal round window membrane or that in patients with serous or purulent otitis media.

To determine the layer in which the change in mean thickness occurred, the epithelial layer (including the subepithelial space) and fibrous layer were measured individually. Measurements showed involvement of all layers of the round window membrane in groups with otitis media; maximal involvement occurred in the combined epithelial layer and subepithelial space (see Table 6).[10] A thickening of the round window membrane may help provide protection to the inner ear in cases of chronic suppurative otitis media.

Permeability

Because the toxins and cellular components of otitis media and the pharmacologic agents used in its treatment may cross the round window membrane and pass into the inner ear, it is important to study the permeability of the membrane during otitis media. In an electron microscopic evaluation the round window membranes of 25 cats were studied to follow the passage of a tracer substance (horseradish peroxidase) through the normal membrane as well as through the membrane 3 days, 1 week, and 2 weeks after eustachian tube obstruction. Passage at 3 days following obstruction was like that through the normal membrane, but after 1 to 2 weeks the membrane's permeability was greatly reduced (Fig. 2). The reduction was probably due to residual effusion overlying the round window membrane, granulation tissue within the niche, and thickening of the membrane.

Grafting Studies

Grafting of the round window may be used in the treatment of perilymphatic fistulas and sudden deafness. Uncommonly perilymphatic fistulas have been reported with otitis media.[7] The permeability of the round window membrane may be decreased in chronic otitis media, and a thickened membrane may afford protection to the labyrinth in cases of chronic disease. We have not found reports of experimental (animal) studies of round window membrane grafting, which might interest patients with perilymphatic fistulas or sensorineural hearing loss and otitis media. Grafting the round window membrane as a procedural step during tympanoplasty can afford protection to the inner ear.

In our animal study grafts were packed against intact round window membranes (part I, completed)

TABLE 5 Temporal Bones with Otitis Media and Labyrinthitis (23)

Type of Otitis Media	SOM	SPOM	POM	MPOM	MOM	COM
Purulent labyrinthitis	0	1	10	0	0	6
Fibrous labyrinthitis						1
Labyrinthitis ossificans						5

TABLE 6 Thickness of Round Window Membrane

	Normal	SOM	POM	COM
Number of temporal bones	37	23	34	55
Mean thickness, mm	0.0694	0.0889	0.0956	0.1141
Standard deviation, mm	0.0043	0.007	0.0223	0.0183

and grafts were also packed against perforated membranes (part II, to be completed). In 15 cats Gelfoam grafts packed tightly into the round window niche were compared to grafts of collagen-adipose tissue.

Although Gelfoam grafts over an open oval window result in a thin membrane, a different result is seen when Gelfoam is grafted against an intact membrane. The round window uniformly and consistently thickens as a result of fibroblastic proliferation in the subepithelial space and the middle layer. Tracers did not permeate these thickened membranes as well as they permeated nongrafted membranes. Collagen-adipose grafts resulted in nonuniform grafting, secondary membranes of granulation tissue, and adhesions and air pockets; healing characteristics and tracers were inconsistently seen when this material was used.

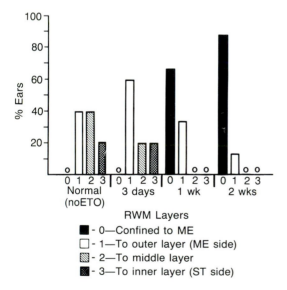

Figure 2 Passage of horseradish peroxidase (2 minutes) through the round window membrane.

DISCUSSION

Otitis media is classifiable by type along a continuum. Most labyrinthine complications and sequelae result from suppurative forms of otitis media (purulent and chronic suppurative). Classic complications include chronic suppurative otitis, cholesteatoma resulting in a fistula (usually of the horizontal semicircular canal), and tympanogenic suppurative labyrinthitis resulting from invasion of inflammatory elements and toxins through the round window membrane.

Multiple disorders can be seen in a given temporal bone; of 1,383 bones, 11 percent revealed more than one disorder—most commonly otitis media, especially the chronic suppurative form. The relationship of otitis media to cancer or otosclerosis may be coincidental, but a causative relationship may exist in the types (especially chronic suppurative disease) occurring with hydrops in Meniere's disease and labyrinthitis.

Many reports (68) have cited sensorineural hearing loss with various forms of otitis media. Studies have included electron microscopy of the round window membrane in animals and humans. Although the morphology of the round window membrane does not appear to change between infancy and old age, thickening of the membrane occurred in cases of chronic suppurative otitis media, affording probable protection to the inner ear. Animal studies using tracers showed decreased permeability in chronic experimentally induced otitis media; the changes were like those in humans—thickening of the round window membrane. Studies of experimental grafting of the round window comparing packed Gelfoam to grafts to collagen-adipose tissue showed Gelfoam to afford more consistent and more uniform thickening of the round window membrane.

Evidence of labyrinthine involvement resulting from otitis media continues to accumulate in regard to both subtle (sensorineural hearing loss) and classic complications. The hypothesis that otitis media (especially the suppurative forms) can insidiously lead to labyrinthine problems requires further clinical and basic research to better understand the implications for its diagnosis and treatment in patients.

This research was supported in part by National Institute of Neurological and Communicative Disorders and Stroke grant NS 14538 and by a grant from the National Temporal Bone Banks Program.

REFERENCES

1. Lim DJ, et al. Recent advances in otitis media with effusion. Ann Otol Rhinol Laryngol 1985; 94 (Suppl):116.
2. Meyerhoff WL, Kim CS, Paparella MM. Pathology of chronic otitis media. Ann Otol Rhinol Laryngol 1978; 87:749–760.
3. Paparella MM, Sugiura S. The pathology of suppurative labyrinthitis. Ann Otol Rhinol Laryngol 1976; 76:554–586.
4. Paparella MM, Schachern PA, Goycoolea MV. Multiple otological pathology. Ann Otol Rhinol Laryngol 1988; 97(1):14–18.
5. Pararella MM, deSousa LC, Mancini F. Meniere's syndrome and otitis media. Laryngoscope 1983; 93:1408–1415.
6. Hallpike CS, Cairns H. Observations on the pathology of Meniere's syndrome. J Laryngol Otol 1938; 53:625–654.
7. Paparella MM, Goycoolea MV, Schachern PA, Sajjadi H. Current clinical and pathological features of round window diseases. Laryngoscope 1987; 97(10):1151–1160.
8. Morizono T, Giebink GS, Paparella MM, Sikora MH, Shea DH. Sensorineural hearing loss in experimental purulent otitis media due to *Streptococcus pneumoniae*. Arch Otolaryngol 1985; 111:794–798.
9. Walby PA, Barrera A, Schuknecht HF. Cochlear pathology in chronic suppurative otitis media. Ann Otol Rhinol Laryngol 1983; 92 (Suppl. 103):3–19.
10. Sahni RS, Paparella MM, Schachern PA, Goycoolea MV, Le CT. Thickness of the human round window membrane in different forms of otitis media. Arch Otolaryngol 1987; 113:630–634.
11. Schachern PA, Paparella MM, Goycoolea MV, Duvall AJ, Choo YB. The permeability of the round window membrane during otitis media. Arch Otolaryngol 1987; 113:625–629.

EFFECTS OF TOPICAL ANESTHESIA ON EARDRUM AND INNER EAR

STEN-HERMANN SCHMIDT, M.D., STEN O.M. HELLSTRÖM, M.D., Ph.D., and MATTI ANNIKO, M.D., Ph.D.

Myringotomy plays an important role in otologic therapy. This procedure requires efficient anesthesia, which can be provided without general anesthesia. However, the use of local anesthetics on the tympanic membrane has been abandoned in many places because general anesthesia has been readily available. Local anesthetics are still used, but we know little about their effects on the tympanic membrane and what they might do accidentally to the inner ear. In the present evaluation the effects of some commonly used topical anesthetics on tympanic membrane structure and inner ear function were studied in an animal model.

MATERIALS AND METHODS

Four anesthetic compounds were used for the study (Table 1). The drugs were applied to the tympanic membrane in the animals (rats and guinea pigs), which were sacrificed at different intervals, ranging from 10 minutes to 5 months after application. At sacrifice the tissue was fixed and the tympanic membrane was analyzed by light microscopy and transmission electron microscopy. In some

TABLE 1 Anesthetics Tested

Xylocaine spray	Lidocaine, 10 mg
	Cetylpyridinium chloride
	Ethanol, Macrogol, Aroma
Emla	Lidocaine, 25 mg
	Prilocaine, 25 mg
	Polyoxyethylene
	Carboxypolyethylene
	Sodium hydroxide
Bonain's liquid	Phenol
	Menthol
	Cocaine hydrochloride
Phenol, 96 percent	

animals phenol, Xylocaine spray, or Emla was applied into the round window niche, and auditory brainstem response recordings were made 24 hours to 6 months after exposing the round window area to the various compounds. After the final auditory brainstem response evaluation the animals were killed and the cochleas were prepared for microscopy.

RESULTS

Phenol and Bonain's liquid caused instant destruction of the epidermis of the tympanic membrane[2] followed by long lasting hyperplasia of the epithelium and connective tissue. Even more pronounced hyperplasia of these two layers was noted with the Xylocaine spray group—but without immediate destruction of the epidermis. The extent of structural change differed in relation to the extent of spread with each drug. Emla caused few if any signs of epithelial reaction and had no effect on the connective tissue. Quantitative changes in tympanic membrane thickness are shown in Figure 1.

Emla, Xylocaine spray, and phenol induced a significant loss of hearing, as determined by auditory brainstem response thresholds (Fig. 2). It affected mainly the higher frequencies. However, the change in the auditory brainstem response threshold was reversible, and at the end of the experiment there was no significant loss of hearing compared with control data (Fig. 3). All the drugs induced damage to the hair cells in the basal part of the cochlea as shown by cytocochleography and scanning electron microscopic analysis.

DISCUSSION

The drugs studied caused profound connective tissue reactions. The manner of application, depending on the physical properties of the drug, determined the extent of structural change. For example, a slight touch of a slender cotton applicator moistened with 96 percent phenol anesthetizes the tympanic membrane and causes the area to take on a grayish appearance. In accord with observations by other authors,[3,4] instant destruction of the epithelium seems to be necessary for an instant anesthetic effect. The changes in the connective tissue occurred mainly in the submucosal layer, which seems to be the area for reconstruction of the damaged tympanic membrane, as evidenced by the multitude of fibroblasts appearing there.[5]

All the drugs tested caused morphologic and functional inner ear changes.[6] Despite the structur-

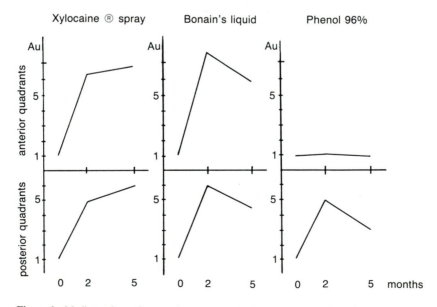

Figure 1 Median values of tympanic membrane thickness in the anterior and the posterior quadrants after application of anesthetic drugs to the posterior quadrants.

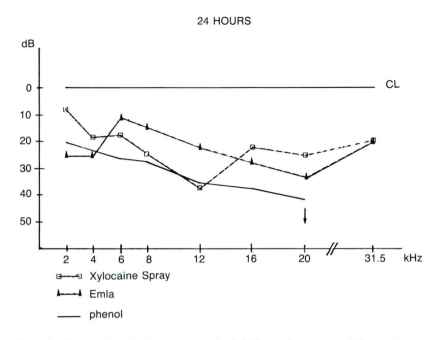

Figure 2 Mean auditory brainstem response levels 24 hours after exposure of the round window area to the anesthetics. Each point represents the mean in three animals (rats). CL, level before application of the anesthetic.

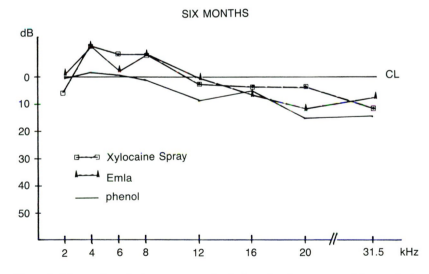

Figure 3 Mean auditory brainstem response levels 6 months after exposure of the round window area to the anesthetics. Each point represents the mean in three animals (rats). CL, mean level before application of the anesthetic.

al alteration of the hair cells, the functional changes were reversible. However, it is reasonable to assume that with auditory brainstem response evaluation exceeding 31.5 kHz, the region of the permanently damaged hair cells would be accessible for electrophysiologic testing.

It seems obvious that in regard to the extent of the tympanic membrane damage and inner ear changes, the skill and experience of the physician who handles these drugs are as important as their properties.

REFERENCES

1. Bonain A. Note au sujet de l'anesthésique local employé en oto-rhinolaryngologie sous la dénomination "liquide de Bonain." Ann Mal Oreil Laryngol 1907; 33:216–217.
2. Schmidt S-H, Hellström S, Carlsöö B. Short term effects of local anesthetic agents on the structure of the rat tympanic membrane. Arch Otolaryngol 1984; 240:153–166.
3. Freystadtl B. Studien der Oberflächenanasthesie. Acta Otolaryngol (Stockh) 1934; 20:235–251.
4. Storrs LA. Topical anesthesia for myringotomy. Laryngoscope 1968; 78:834–839.
5. Schmidt S-H, Hellström S, Carlsöö B. Fine structure of the rat tympanic membrane after treatment with local anesthetics. Acta Otolaryngol (Stockh) 1986; 101:88–95,
6. Schmidt SH, Hellström S, Anniko M. Effects on the inner ear of the clinically used local anesthetics Xylocaine, Emla and phenol. (Submitted for publication.)

VESTIBULAR FUNCTION IN OTITIS MEDIA WITH EFFUSION

IWAO HONJO, M.D., YASUSHI NAITO, M.D., JUICHI ITO, M.D., and NOBUYA YAGI, M.D.

Patients with otitis media with effusion sometimes complain of slight dizziness, and it is suggested that the disease influences human vestibular function. Fukuda[1] reported that stepping deviation of a patient with unilateral otitis media with effusion disappeared immediately after air was inflated into the affected middle ear.

In our study the head movements of patients with otitis media with effusion were observed to evaluate the influence of the disease on human equilibrium. Since the eardrums of such patients are retracted and the middle ear pressures are generally negative,[2] the effects of eardrum retraction and negative middle ear pressure were also investigated. The influence of changes in middle ear pressure on vestibular function was studied electrophysiologically in cats.

MATERIALS AND METHODS

Study A

Twenty-five patients with unilateral otitis media with effusion were examined. The head movement of a subject standing upright was measured from above using an infrared position sensor system. Measurement was carried out for 60 seconds with the subject's eyes open and then for another 60 seconds with the eyes closed. The data obtained were digitalized at a sampling frequency of 20 Hz and analyzed by use of a microcomputer (PC9801, NEC, Japan). The center of the head movement was calculated by averaging the X-Y coordinates of 1,200 points obtained during a 1-minute period. Movement along the X axis (the movement from side to side) was analyzed in this study.

The center of the head movement deviates when the eyes are closed. The deviation ratio was calculated from the degree of this deviation divided by the standard deviation of the distribution of X coordinates obtained with eyes closed for 1 minute (Fig. 1). This ratio reflects the inclination of human posture.

In experiments on the effects of middle ear pressure on vestibular nerve activity in cats, the orifice of the eustachian tube was blocked, and a small perforation was made in the tympanic membrane (Fig. 2). Middle ear pressure was measured with a transducer. The cats were mounted in a

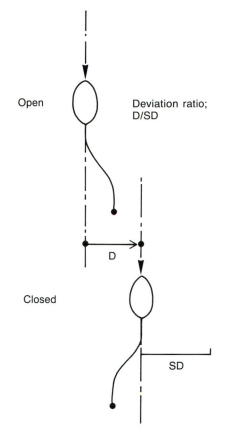

Figure 1 Calculation of deviation ratio. D, the degree of deviation of the movement center. SD, the standard deviation of the distribution of X coordinates obtained with eyes closed for 1 minute.

stereotaxic apparatus on a turntable that could be rotated in three dimensions. Intra-axonal vestibular nerve action potentials were recorded using a glass microelectrode filled with 3M potassium chloride.

RESULTS

Figure 3 shows the deviation ratio before and immediately after myringotomy in patients with unilateral otitis media with effusion. On the average the center of head movement deviated to the affected side before treatment. This deviation was observed on the opposite side immediately after myringotomy. This shift in the direction of deviation was significant (Student's t test, $p < 0.01$).

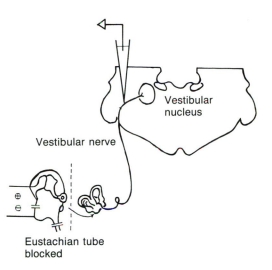

Figure 2 Deviation ratio in patients with otitis media with effusion before and immediately following myringotomy.

Next we examined 15 normal volunteers. The external auditory canal chosen at random was made airtight, and a pressure of 300 mm H_2O above or below atmospheric pressure was applied to cause retraction or protrusion of the eardrum. Compared to the state before the pressure was applied, the head tended to deviate significantly to the side to which positive pressure was applied (Fig. 4). The eardrum is thought to be retracted in this condition.

Then patients with a middle ear ventilation tube were examined in the same way. Pressure was applied directly to the middle ear through the tube. This time the head tended to deviate to the side to which negative middle ear pressure was applied. This tendency was also significant (Fig. 5).

In the animal experiments the vestibular nerve axons were classified into three groups according to their regularities of spontaneous firing, that is, regular type, irregular type, and intermediate type.

The vestibular nerves originating in the horizontal semicircular canal were investigated first. In five of six regular type fibers, the firing rates increased when positive pressure was applied to the middle ear and decreased with negative pressure (Fig. 6). Most of the intermediate and irregular type fibers examined did not respond to the middle ear pressure changes. Of the 26 fibers originating in the vertical canal, only one responded to the changes in the middle ear pressure.

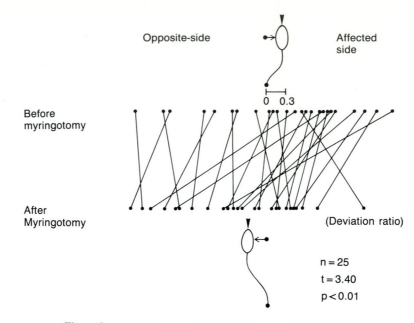

Figure 3   Effects of external ear canal pressure in normal subjects.

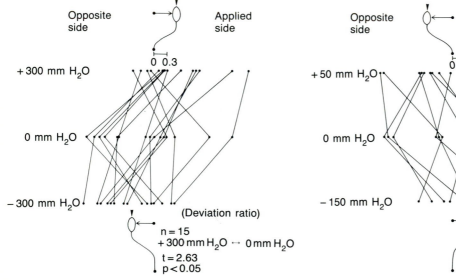

Figure 4   Effects of middle ear pressure in subjects with middle ear ventilation tubes.

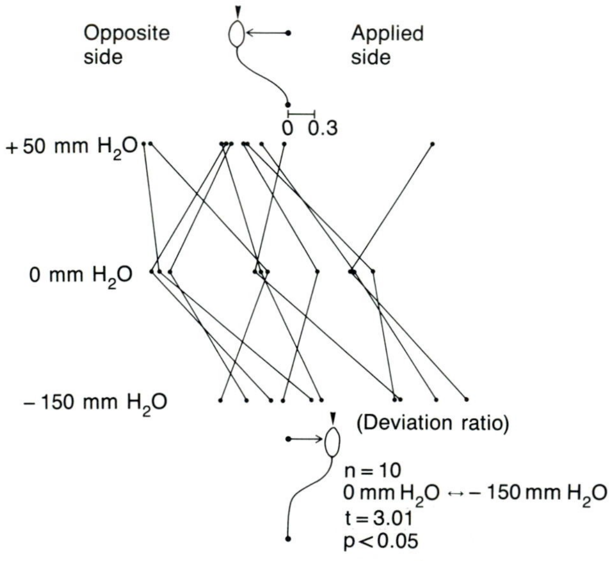

Figure 5   Effects of middle ear pressure on vestibular nerve activity.

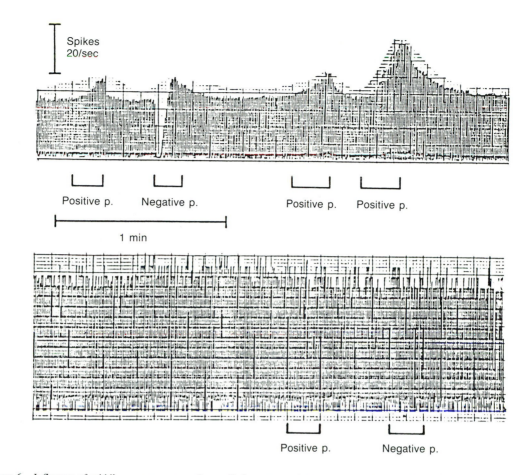

Figure 6   Influence of middle ear pressure on the vestibular nerves originating in the horizontal semicircular canal. 1, regular type of fiber. 2, intermediate type of fiber.

DISCUSSION

The results of our clinical study suggested that patients with otitis media with effusion have a slight tendency to incline to the affected side; this tendency could be caused by either eardrum retraction or negative middle ear pressure. Inputs from the various portions around the middle ear could cause such head deviations. However, from the results of animal experiment B, we conclude that there is a pathway, including the inner ear vestibular system, that responds to changes in middle ear pressure and alters the firing rates of the vestibular fibers. These findings support the idea that the head deviation found in our clinical study could be derived from changes in vestibular function caused by abnormal middle ear pressure. Studies of the effects of abnormal position of the eardrum on the inner ear vestibular system are in progress.

REFERENCES

1. Fukuda T. Statokinetic reflexes in equilibrium and movement. Tokyo: University of Tokyo Press, 1984:119.
2. Takahashi H, Hayashi M, Honjo I. Direct measurement of middle ear pressure through the eustachian tube. Arch Otorhinolaryngol 1987; 243:378–381.

TINNITUS IN CHILDREN WITH CHRONIC SECRETORY OTITIS MEDIA

ROBERT P. MILLS, M. Phil., F.R.C.S., DAVID M. ALBERT, F.R.C.S., and CAROLINE E. BRAIN, M.R.C.P.

Adult patients with middle ear effusions sometimes report tinnitus dating from other symptoms referable to the effusion. Children seldom mention tinnitus spontaneously, but often admit to it when questioned about noises in the ears.[1,2] Nodar[1] studied children undergoing routine audiometric screening. There was a higher incidence of tinnitus in children who failed the screening test than in those who passed. Graham[2] studied children with sensorineural hearing loss. According to Leonard et al,[3] tinnitus occurs in children with chronic secretory otitis media, particularly when they are taking aspirin. In the present study the incidence of tinnitus, reported on direct questioning and spontaneously, was studied in children with secretory otitis media and in those without evidence of ear disease.

MATERIALS AND METHODS

A group of children with the typical clinical picture of chronic secretory otitis media were questioned about noises in their ears. Only children who were able to describe the noise were considered to have tinnitus. Similar questions were put to a group of children with no evidence of ear disease. They were interviewed during routine school and community medical examinations, had normal tympanic membranes on pneumatic otoscopy, and had passed an age appropriate screening test for hearing (distraction, Kendal toy test, Stycar test, or sweep audiometry). The incidence of tinnitus in the two groups was compared using the chi square test.

Details in children attending pediatric otolaryngology clinics in the King's College Hospital group were recorded over a 6-month period. Spontaneous reports were recorded, and the condition of the child's ears at the time of interview was noted. A comparison was made using the chi square test between the incidence of tinnitus in children without evidence of ear disease and that in those with middle ear effusions at the time of interview or with ventilation tubes in situ for the treatment of secretory otitis media.

RESULTS

Sixty-six children with secretory otitis media were questioned about tinnitus (ages 5 to 15 years; mean, 8.4 years). Of these, 29 (43.9 percent) reported tinnitus. Of the 93 children with healthy ears who were questioned (ages 5 to 17 years; mean, 8.7 years), 27 (29 percent) described noises in their ears. This difference is not statistically significant (chi square = 3.756; p = >0.05; 1 d.f.). During the 6-month study period 105 children with evidence of middle ear effusion(s) at the time of their outpatient visits were seen. Five of these children described tinnitus. During the same period 116 children with ventilation tube(s) in situ were also seen, and 5 of these described tinnitus. The overall incidence of tinnitus in children with secretory otitis media (ages 5 to 13 years; mean, 6.8 years) was therefore 10 percent. None of the 136 children without evidence of ear disease (ages 5 to 15 years; mean, 6.8 years) who were seen during the study described noises in their ears. This difference is statistically significant (chi square = 6.35; p = <0.02; 1 d.f.). Table 1 lists the spontaneous descriptions given by children with secretory otitis media during the second half of the study.

TABLE 1 Spontaneous Descriptions of Tinnitus Given by Children with Secretory Otitis Media

Description	Number of Reports
Ringing	2
Beeping	1
Bubbling	1
Rattling	1
"Like water rushing"	1
"Like shouting"	1
"Like hearing test noises"	1
"Like drums"	1
"Like marching"	1
"Like a heartbeat"	1
"Angel noise"	1
"Monster noise"	1
"Clowns laughing"	1
Total	14

DISCUSSION

If tinnitus is a symptom of middle ear effusion in childhood, one might have expected a significantly higher incidence of the symptom in a group of children with secretory otitis media as opposed to a group of normal children. In the first part of the study no such difference was demonstrated, although the incidence in the group with secretory otitis media was higher. However, direct questioning of children is likely to produce misleading results. Although every effort has been made to avoid suggesting answers to the children, it would be naive to believe that all the reports obtained are genuine. In the second part of the study, this difficulty has been eliminated. However, in view of the reticence of children to report tinnitus, which has been reported by previous authors,[3,4] it is likely that the number of descriptions of noises recorded in the second part of the study represents an underestimate of the true incidence of tinnitus in this group. However, the significantly higher incidence of tinnitus in the children with secretory otitis media in this part of the study supports the view that tinnitus is a symptom of this disease.

Leonard et al[3] and Goodhill et al[5] have suggested that conductive hearing loss unmasks physiologic tinnitus, while Adams et al[6] believe that tinnitus may be caused by the movement of fluid within the middle ear. In either case tinnitus is just as likely to occur in children with middle ear effusions as it is in adults. Parents are sometimes worried by their children's reports of noises in the ears. They can be reassured that tinnitus is a common symptom of secretory otitis media with no more sinister significance.

REFERENCES

1. Nodar R. Tinnitus aurium in school age children: a survey. Audit Res 1972; 12:133–135.
2. Graham J. Paediatric tinnitus. J Laryngol Otol (Suppl) 1981; 4:117–120.
3. Leonard G, Black FO, Schramm VL. Tinnitus in children. In: Bluestone C, Stool S, eds. Pediatric otolaryngology. Philadelphia: WB Saunders, 1983:24.
4. Fowler EP, Fowler EP Jr. Somatopsychic and psychosomatic factors in tinnitus, deafness and vertigo. Ann Otol Rhinol Laryngol 1955; 64:29–37.
5. Goodhill V, Brockman SJ. Secretory otitis media. In: Goodhill V, ed. Diseases, deafness and dizziness. Hagerstown, MD: Harper & Row, 1972:307.
6. Adams GL, Boies LR, Paparella MM. Secretory otitis media. In: Boies' fundamentals of otolaryngology. 5th ed. Philadelphia: WB Saunders, 1978:201.

ROUND WINDOW MEMBRANE PERMEABILITY: AN IN VITRO MODEL

LARS LUNDMAN, M.D., DAN BAGGER-SJÖBÄCK, M.D.,Ph.D., LEIF HOLMQUIST, Ph.D., and STEVEN K. JUHN, M.D.

The round window membrane is regarded as the main route for passage of potentially ototoxic substances from the middle ear cavity into the inner ear. This is of clinical importance in acute and chronic otitis media in which sensorineural hearing impairment sometimes develops.[1] Little is known about the ototoxicity of substances that develop in the middle ear during these disorders. Most bacteria present in the middle ear in these infections have the capacity to produce several different toxins. These toxins have been held responsible for sensorineural hearing impairment in patients suffering from these ailments (chronic otitis media in particular). In the treatment of chronic otitis media, ear drops containing antimicrobial drugs are often used for long periods, and there is a risk that these drugs may have ototoxic effects.[2]

Previous reports have shown that the round window membrane seems to be impermeable to macromolecules like ferritin with a molecular weight of 415 kd,[2] but the normal round window membrane is permeable to albumin, with a molecular weight of only 68 kd, when it is applied in the middle ear for 12 hours.[3] Substances with low molecular weights such as antibiotics and corticosteroids pass into the inner ear within minutes when applied in the middle ear cavity.[2,4] Substances known to be ototoxic have been shown to cause damage to the organ of Corti with hearing loss when applied in the middle ear.[5] In previous in vivo permeability studies of the round window membrane, it has been difficult to isolate the membrane from other possible transport routes, such as lymphatic pathways and bone communications, and it has also been difficult to estimate the exact rate of passage of different substances through the round window membrane.

The aim of this study was to describe an in vitro method to study the permeability of the round window membrane. With this experimental design it may be possible to study the rate of passage of different potentially ototoxic substances under controlled conditions.[6]

MATERIAL AND METHODS

The round window membrane together with its bony niche was dissected out from healthy mongolian gerbils (*Meriones unguiculatis*). The preparation was mounted over a 1 mm hole in a thin glass plate and attached with epoxy resin (Fig. 1). The glass disc was inserted between two glass chambers representing the middle ear cavity and the inner ear, respectively. The entire dissection and mounting procedure was performed in tissue culture medium at room temperature. Both chambers were filled with tissue culture medium. The reliability and accuracy of the system were tested in the following experiments:

1. High molecular weight substances were introduced into the middle ear side of the model. Low density lipoprotein, a spherical molecule with a diameter of 20 nm and a molecular weight of 2,300 kd, was introduced into the middle ear chamber in seven trials. Low density lipoprotein was estimated as apolipoprotein B, the major protein component of the low density lipoprotein molecule. The concentrations of the apolipoprotein B in the middle ear side of the chamber ranged from 0.9 to 1.8 g per liter. High density lipoprotein with a diameter of 9 nm and a molecular weight of 115 to 300 kd was also introduced into the middle ear side of the model in six trials. High density lipoprotein was estimated as apolipoprotein A-I, which is the major protein component of this molecule. The concentrations of apolipoprotein A-I in the middle ear side ranged from 2.8 to 14.3 g per liter. Samples from the inner ear chamber were collected after 1 and 3 hours.

2. Horseradish peroxidase, which is known to penetrate the round window membrane, was introduced into the middle ear side of the model in 10 trials. The purpose of this experiment was to determine the rate of passage of this substance (molecular weight 48 kd). Horseradish peroxidase concentrations were estimated using enzymatic and spectrophotometric methods. Samples from the inner ear chamber were collected at regular intervals from 30 minutes to 5 hours.

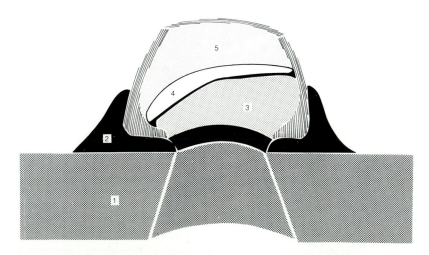

Figure 1 Diagram of technique for preparation of round window membrane and fixation to glass plate of the in vitro model. 1, Glass plate. 2, Epoxy resin. 3, Bony niche. 4, Round window membrane. 5, Inner ear side of model.

3. In order to demonstrate the reliability of the epoxy resin seal, the round window membrane preparation was exchanged for a piece of bone from the bulla. Horseradish peroxidase and toluidine blue, a low molecular weight dye, were introduced into the middle ear chamber in concentrations of 10 and 1 g per liter, respectively. The toluidine blue content was estimated spectrophotometrically. Samples were collected after 10 hours.

RESULTS

Low density lipoprotein did not penetrate the round window membrane in six of the seven trials after 3 hours. In one of the trials slight passage through the membrane was seen (Table 1). High density lipoprotein did not penetrate the round window membrane at all in two of six trials, but slight passage occurred in four trials after 3 hours (see Table 1).

The mean passage rate of horseradish peroxidase was estimated to be 6 µg per hour (Fig. 2). There was a spread of the values, but the mean and median values demonstrated a clear linear relationship. Neither horseradish peroxidase nor toluidine blue passed the epoxy resin seal.

DISCUSSION

Previous permeability studies of the round window membrane have indicated that the critical molecular weight for passage is between 70 and 400 kd.

The round window membrane in vitro model was impermeable to low density lipoprotein within 3 hours in all but one trial. The spherical low density lipoprotein has a molecular weight of 2,300 kd and a diameter of about 20 nm. In order to pass through the round window membrane, pores of this size are needed. We concluded that no such pores developed in the in vitro model within 3 hours.

The also spherical high density lipoprotein particles have molecular weights of 115 to 350 kd and diameters of about 9 nm. Theoretically they should not pass through the tight junctions of the round window membrane, since previous studies have failed to demonstrate passage of other high molecular weight compounds, such as ferritin, through the intercellular junctions of the epithelial cells in the normal round window membrane.[2] No passage of high density lipoprotein was demonstrated in trials 11 and 13. High density lipoprotein, however, was found to pass through the round window membrane to a minor degree in trials 8, 9, and 10. In addition to molecular weight and size, the configuration of a protein presumably also affects its penetration properties. Thus the globular high density lipoprotein particles are expected to be less retarded by the round window membrane than nonglobular protein molecules of the same molecular weight. The concentrations obtained were close to the detection limit and probably reflect an extremely low passage rate.

TABLE 1 Concentrations of Low and High Density Lipoproteins in the Inner Ear*

Trial No.	30 Minutes[†]	1 Hour[†]	3 Hours[†]
1	—	0	0
2	—	0	0
3	—	0	0
4	0	—	0
5	0	—	7
6	0	—	0
7	0	—	0
8	—	1	1
9	—	2	3
10	—	0	1
11	0	—	0
12	3	—	22
13	0	—	0
14	2	—	>100

* The concentrations (mg per liter) of low density lipoprotein were estimated as apolipoprotein B (trials 1 to 7), and high density lipoprotein concentrations were estimated as apolipoprotein A-1 (trials 8 to 14) as a function of time in the inner ear chamber in 14 trials.
† 0, Detection limit of methods used for measuring apolipoprotein B and apolipoprotein A-1 concentration was 0.5 mg per liter.
A-1 concentration was 0.5 mg per liter.
—, Measurement not performed.

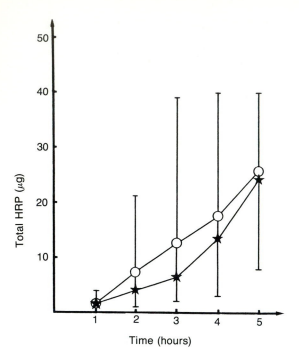

Figure 2 Passage of horseradish peroxidase through the round window membrane in the in vitro model as a function of time. Concentration of horseradish peroxidase on the middle ear side = 10 g per liter. ○ = Means and maximal spread. ★ = Median value.

The present in vitro model demonstrates that the round window membrane is permeable to horseradish peroxidase. The mean passage rate in 10 trials was calculated to be 6 μg per hour. No quantitative analyses of this type have been performed previously, but it has been found that horseradish peroxidase penetrates the round window membrane of guinea pigs within minutes.[7] The spread of the values between the individual trials may be due to biologic variations.

Morphologically the round window membrane consists of three layers. The outer epithelial cell layer is continuous with the epithelial layer of the tympanic cavity. The cells are flat and nonciliated, with microvilli covering the surface. No secretory cells are found. The cells are interconnected by tight junctions classified as intermediate to tight. This cell layer is believed to be the main barrier against penetration of substances from the middle ear to the perilymphatic space through the round window membrane.[2] The lamina propria consists of numerous elastic and collagen fibers, and the inner endothelial cell layer consists of flat cells interconnected by tight junctions classified as loose.

The present study demonstrates the possibility of removing the intact round window membrane from an animal and using it in a two compartment permeability model. The sealing of the preparation to prevent leakage artifacts is accomplished by using a rapid setting epoxy resin. No major functional disturbances seem to develop under these experimental conditions. In using the in vitro model to test the permeability to low molecular weight substances, it is necessary to include a high molecular weight substance in the experiment in order to detect possible artifactual leakage. Conclusions regarding the passage rate so far have been drawn only from short term experiments, owing to the risk of subsequent autolytic changes in the round window membrane that can alter the permeability properties.

Study supported by grants from Foundation Tysta Skolan, the Swedish Medical Research Council (00720), and Foundation Nachmansson.

REFERENCES

1. Paparella MM, Hiraide F, Oda M, Brady D. Pathology of sensorineural hearing loss in otitis media. Ann Otol Rhinol Laryngol 1972; 81:632–647.
2. Nomura Y. Otological significance of the round window. Basel: Karger, 1984.
3. Hamaguchi Y, Morizono T, Juhn SK. The round window membrane permeability to human serum albumin in Chinchilla. Am J Otolaryngol, in press.
4. Smith BM, Myers MG. The penetration of gentamicin and neomycin into perilymph across the round window membrane. Otolaryngol Head Neck Surg 1979; 87:888–891.
5. Brummett RE, Harris RF, Lindgren JA. Detection of ototoxicity from drugs applied topically to the middle ear space. Laryngoscope 1976; 86:1177–1187.
6. Lundman LA, Holmquist L, Bagger-Sjöbäck D. Round window membrane permeability. An in vitro model. Acta Otolaryngol (Stockh) 1988; 103:1–9.
7. Tanaka K. Motomura S. Permeability of the labyrinthine windows in guinea pigs. Arch Otorhinolaryngol 1981; 233:67–75.

RELATIONSHIP BETWEEN MIDDLE EAR INFLAMMATION AND ROUND WINDOW MEMBRANE PERMEABILITY IN ANTIGEN INDUCED OTITIS MEDIA

STEVEN K. JUHN, M.D., YUKIYOSHI HAMAGUCHI, M.D., and TETSUO MORIZONO, M.D., D.M.S., M.S.

The round window has been recognized for many years as one of the routes through which middle ear inflammation spreads to the inner ear. Permeability of the round window membrane is an important aspect in understanding the mechanism of inner ear disease, such as sensorineural hearing loss associated with otitis media and that following ototopical administration of drugs.

Studies of round window membrane permeability to various substances and drugs have been carried out in animals. The passage through the round window membrane of macromolecular proteins, such as exotoxin (12 K),[1] horseradish peroxidase (45 K),[2] human serum albumin (67 K),[3,4] and ferritin (445 K),[5] seems to depend on the time after instillation, the molecular weight, and the state of the round window membrane. With an antigen induced otitis media model in chinchillas sensitized with human serum albumin, antigen levels in both the middle ear fluid and the perilymph were measured after local instillation of human serum albumin. The purpose in this study was to explore the effects of antigen induced otitis media on the rate of transport of human serum albumin from the middle ear cavity into the perilymph through the round window membrane. The effect of a corticosteroid drug on membrane permeability to human serum albumin was also investigated.

MATERIALS

The experimental procedures are summarized in Figure 1.

Control Group

Normal chinchillas weighing 400 to 600 g were used throughout this study. Seven animals were anesthetized with ketamine hydrochloride (20 mg per kilogram intramuscularly). One milliliter of human serum albumin (5 mg per milliliter, Sigma Chemical Co.) dissolved in sterile saline was instilled into the middle ear bulla of the chinchillas. The middle ear bulla was exposed surgically, and middle ear fluid retained therein was recovered 24 hours after instillation. After the middle ear bulla was washed several times with sterile saline, the perilymph was collected with a capillary glass tube through the round window membrane.

Sensitized Groups

Twenty-two normal chinchillas were systemically immunized with 0.1 ml of human serum albumin (10 mg per milliliter) containing the same volume of complete Freund's adjuvant (Sigma). The emulsion was injected subcutaneously under the back skin of the animals, and then the animals were given booster doses twice—3 and 10 days after the first injection. When circulating antibody titers were elevated high enough to induce local inflammation (2^4 to 2^6), 1 ml of human serum albumin (5 mg per milliliter) was instilled into the left middle ear bulla of 22 chinchillas (Arthus group), and 1 ml of human serum albumin containing 25 mg per milliliter

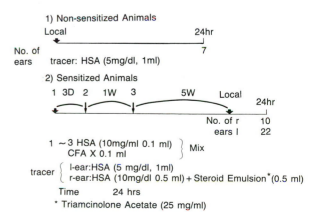

Figure 1 Experimental procedures in this study.

of triamcinolone diacetate (Aristocort, Lederle Parenterals Co.) was instilled into the right middle ear bulla of 12 chinchillas (Arthus plus steroid group). The middle ear fluid and perilymph samples were collected by the procedures already described. After cytologic analysis the middle ear fluid samples were centrifuged at 2,000 rpm for 10 minutes at 4° C. Blood samples were collected by cardiac puncture and centrifuged. The serum and middle ear fluid samples were stored at −70° C until use. The perilymph was analyzed immediately following sampling.

METHODS

Quantitation of Human Serum Albumin Levels in Middle Ear Fluid and Perilymph

The concentration of human serum albumin was measured by electroimmuno diffusion[6] using a commercial goat antihuman serum albumin antibody (Cooper Biomedical). Its detection limit was 10 mcg per milliliter. In order to avoid the cross reaction of chinchilla albumin against antihuman serum albumin antibody, the commercial antibody was preincubated with the same volume of normal chinchilla serum for 1 hour at 37° C. The middle ear fluid sample was diluted 10:1 prior to this assay.

Bacteriologic Study of Middle Ear Fluid

After collection of the middle ear fluid, an aliquot of each sample was plated directly onto both sheep blood agar and chocolate agar plates for culture.

The statistical significance among the different groups was determined by either Student's t test or the paired t test. Human serum albumin levels in the perilymph were transformed to a logarithmic scale.

RESULTS

The bacterial cultures were negative for all the middle ear fluid samples.

Human Serum Albumin Levels in Middle Ear Fluid

The mean levels of human serum albumin in the middle ear fluid samples were 2.77 ± 0.61 mg per milliliter in the control, 1.29 ± 0.87 in the Arthus, and 1.63 ± 0.73 in the Arthus plus steroid groups. The values in the Arthus plus steroid group were significantly higher than that of the Arthus group and significantly lower than in the control group (p < 0.01; Fig. 2).

Human Serum Albumin Levels in Perilymph

Human serum albumin levels in the perilymph were 3.31 ± 2.71 mg per deciliter in the control, 2.71 ± 4.42 in the Arthus, and 3.23 ± 6.75 in the Arthus plus steroid groups. There was no significant difference in levels in the perilymph between the groups. The incidences of animals with human serum albumin positive perilymph were 6/7 (85.7 percent) in the control, 5/22 (22.7 percent) in the Arthus, and 4/12 (33 percent) in the Arthus plus steroid groups (Tables 1, 2). The percentage of human serum albumin positive perilymph samples in

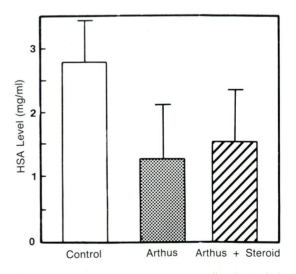

Figure 2 Mean values of human serum albumin levels in middle ear fluid in control, Arthus, and Arthus plus steroid groups. Mean ± S.D. Human serum albumin levels were significantly lower in both the Arthus and Arthus plus steroid groups as compared to the control group (p <0.01).

TABLE 1   Results of Cytologic and Biochemical Analyses of Recovered Middle Ear Fluid

Parameters	Control	Arthus	Arthus + Steroid
Total leukocytes			
(x10⁶)	0.51± 0.15	2.17± 1.54	0.75± 1.09
1–Antitrypsin (mg/dl)	19.7 ±13.2	307.8 ±118.6	107.5 ±100.0
2-Macroglobulin (mg/dl)	2.2 ± 1.76	163.8 ± 58.7	81.9 ± 48.7
Human serum albumin (mg/ml)	2.77± 0.61	1.29± 0.87	1.63± 0.87

the control group was significantly higher than that of the Arthus group (chi square test, p < 0.01).

Relationship Between Human Serum Albumin Levels in Perilymph and Middle Ear Fluid

In both the Arthus and the Arthus plus steroid groups, perilymph samples were divided into two groups: human serum albumin positive and human serum albumin negative perilymph samples. Levels in the middle ear fluid were 2.27 ± 0.31 mg per milliliter in the Arthus human serum albumin positive perilymph group and were significantly higher than that in the Arthus human serum albumin negative perilymph group (0.94 ± 0.73 mg per milliliter; p < 0.01). In the Arthus plus steroid group, human serum albumin levels in the middle ear fluid were 2.25 ± 0.06 mg per milliliter in the human serum albumin positive perilymph group and were significantly higher than that in the human serum albumin negative perilymph group (1.21 ± 0.78 mg per milliliter; p < 0.01; Fig. 3).

DISCUSSION

In the Arthus group, human serum albumin (antigen) levels in the middle ear fluid decreased significantly after human serum albumin instillation, compared to the control group. This may be due to the formation of immune complexes with specific antihuman serum albumin antibodies, masking the antigenicity of human serum albumin. A dilutional effect by enhanced vascular leakage may also contribute to the decrease in human serum albumin lev-

els in the middle ear fluid. In the control group, human serum albumin in the perilymph was more frequently detected than in the Arthus group. In both the Arthus and the Arthus plus steroid groups, human serum albumin levels in the middle ear fluid were significantly higher in animals with human serum albumin positive perilymph than in those with human serum albumin negative perilymph (Fig. 3). These results suggest that human serum albumin levels in the perilymph seem to be closely related levels in the middle ear fluid in these groups.

The round window membrane permeability to macromolecular antigenic proteins such as human serum albumin seems to decrease with the development of Arthus otitis media because of the decrease in human serum albumin (antigen) levels in the middle ear due to elimination from the middle ear bulla through the eustachian tube, a dilution effect of antigenic proteins by enhanced vascular leakage, and elimination from the middle ear bulla via immunologic protective reactions (immune complex formation and phagocytosis). The pathologic

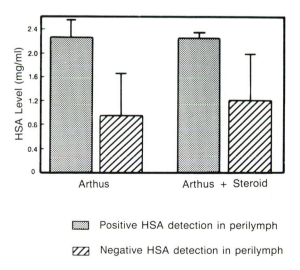

Positive HSA detection in perilymph

Negative HSA detection in perilymph

Figure 3   Human serum albumin levels in recovered middle ear fluid in Arthus and Arthus plus steroid groups. Mean ± S.D. In both groups, human serum albumin levels were significantly different between the perilymph positive and perilymph negative subgroups (p <0.01).

TABLE 2   Incidence in Animals with Human Serum Albumin Positive Perilymph

Control Group	Arthus Group	Arthus + Steroid Group
85.7%	22.7% *	33.3%
(6/7)	(5/22)	(4/12)

* Significantly lower than control group (chi square test; p<0.01).

changes in the round window membrane, such as deposition of inflammatory products on the middle ear surface of the membrane may also reduce the passage of human serum albumin.[7] Although a corticosteroid was found to reduce the decrease in human serum albumin levels in the middle ear fluid, there was no significant difference in human serum albumin levels in the perilymph between the Arthus and Arthus plus steroid groups.

It is well known that many pathologic conditions in the middle ear contribute to the mechanism of sensorineural hearing loss and that inflammatory products in otitis media can spread through the round window membrane to cause labyrinthitis.[8] However, our present study has shown that a passage of antigenic proteins through the round window membrane depends on the level of the protein in the middle ear fluid and the stage of middle ear inflammation.

One interesting concept that can be derived from this study may be the existence of minimum threshold concentrations for potentially toxic substances in both the middle ear fluid and the perilymph. Since the passage of human serum albumin from the middle ear into the inner ear appears to depend on the middle ear fluid level, if the concentration of inflammatory products in the middle ear cavity is not high enough to reach threshold levels and thus cross the round window membrane, they may not cause any inner ear damage or dysfunction. It is also conceivable that certain factors can either enhance or reduce the rate of transport of substances through the round window membrane by direct effects on the round window membrane. The existence of these multifactorial events may explain the variable levels of incidence of sensorineural hearing loss as a sequela of otitis media.

The round window membrane is permeable to various substances, including inflammatory products. The rate of transport of substances from the middle ear cavity through the round window membrane into the inner ear depends on the molecular weight of the substances, the state of the round window membrane, and the concentrations of the substances in the middle ear cavity. The present study with human serum albumin suggests the existence of threshold concentrations of toxic substances in both the middle ear and the inner ear fluids. In addition to direct toxic effects of substances transported into the inner ear, local biochemical and immunochemical reactions may be responsible for inner ear dysfunction.

This research was supported by grant 5P50—NS—14538 from the National Institute of Neurological and Communicative Disorders and Stroke.

REFERENCES

1. Goycoolea MV, Paparella MM, Goldberg B, Schlievert P, Carpenter AM. Permeability of the middle ear to staphylococcal pyogenic exotoxin in otitis media. Int J Pediatr Otorhinolaryngol 1980; 1:301–308.
2. Saijo S, Kimura RS. Distribution of horseradish peroxidase in the inner ear after injection into the middle ear cavity. Acta Otolaryngol (Stockh) 1984; 97:593–610.
3. Goldberg B, Goycoolea MV, Schlievert P, Shea D, Schachern PA, Paparella MM, Carpenter AM. Passage of albumin from the middle ear to the inner ear in otitis media in chinchillas. Am J Otolaryngol 1981; 2:210–214.
4. Hamaguchi Y, Morizono T, Juhn SK. Round window membrane permeability to human serum albumin in chinchilla (in preparation).
5. Nakai Y, Kaneko M. Round window membrane. Submicroscopic structure and permeability. Pract Otol Kyoto 1975; 90:38–41.
6. Laurell CB. Quantitative estimation of proteins by electrophoresis in agarose gel containing antibodies. Anal Biochem 1966; 15:45–52.
7. Meyerhoff WL, Kim CS, Paparella MM. Pathology of chronic otitis media. Ann Otol Rhinol Laryngol 1978; 87:749–760.
8. Paparella MM, Goycoolea MV, Schachern PA, Sajjadi H. Current clinical and pathological features of round window diseases. Laryngoscope (in press).

PATHOLOGY

ULTRASTRUCTURE OF MUCOUS BLANKET OF OTITIS MEDIA WITH EFFUSION

YASUO SAKAKURA, M.D., MASASHI INAGAKI, M.D., KAZUHIKO TAKEUCHI, M.D.,
KENJI SAKAKURA, M.D., YUICHI MAJIMA, M.D., and KOTARO UKAI, M.D.

Two mechanisms are involved in the elimination of middle ear effusion through the eustachian tube—muscular and mucociliary. Both mechanisms of clearance may be mutually complementary in the normal situation. However, these different systems of evacuation essentially cannot compensate for each other. With ciliary dyskinesia in Kartagener's syndrome, otitis media with effusion develops in spite of normal muscular clearance, and with muscular dysfunction in cleft palate otitis media with effusion develops in spite of normal mucociliary clearance. Although muscular clearance can expel more fluid than mucociliary clearance, muscular drainage is unlikely to occur in the presence of negative middle ear pressure. Therefore, mucociliary transport may play a major role in the clearance of middle ear effusion under negative pressure.

The purpose in the present study was to determine the mucociliary function of the middle ear cleft and to clarify the ultrastructure of the mucous blanket of the promontory in pediatric patients with otitis media with effusion.

MATERIALS AND METHODS

Determination of Mucociliary Transport

An aliquot of 0.01 ml of human serum albumin tagged with technetium-99m was used as a tracer material. The tracer material was instilled into the middle ear cavity through a myringotomy incision. Transport of the tracer was monitored by gamma-camera in 40 ears of pediatric patients with otitis media with effusion.

Transmission Electron Microscopic Study of the Mucous Blanket

Biopsy samples of the promontory were ob-

tained from eight children aged 5 to 9 with otitis media with mucoid effusion. To insure good preservation of the mucous blanket in situ with a conventional glutaraldehyde-osmium fixative, we used small samples of tissue, avoided trauma to the samples, and tried to keep the samples from moving during fixation.

Plastic embedded thin sections were stained with uranyl acetate and lead citrate and studied by use of a JEM 100B electron microscope.

RESULTS

Mucociliary Function of the Middle Ear Cleft in Otitis Media with Effusion

The 40 ears were classified into two groups depending on the presence or absence of middle ear effusions. All those in group 1 without middle ear effusions (n=13) had mucociliary function, whereas 66.7 percent of the group 2 ears with effusions (n=27) failed to clear in 15 minutes. The average mucociliary transport rate was $2.41 + 1.63$ mm per minute in group 1 and $0.63 + 1.26$ mm per minute in group 2. The difference between the two groups was statistically significant ($p < 0.01$, Wilcoxon test).

Ultrastructure of the Mucous Blanket

The mucous blanket consisted of two layers. The mucous layer was located at the tips of the cilia. The periciliary fluid layer (5 to 6 μ) was the electron lucent layer between the lower edge of mucous layer and the luminal surface of the epithelium. There was an electron lucent zone over the nonciliated surface of the epithelium. The majority of the surface cells were secretory; ciliated cells were scarce.

Two other layers were identified in the mucous layer—luminal and inner layers. Numerous specks floated in the luminal layer. Fragments of the cell organelles often were seen between fibrous strands of varying size. The inner layer contained cells that had migrated, mainly macrophages and neutrophils, desquamated epithelial cells, and various secretory vesicles. In loci where secretory activity was marked in goblet cells, ciliated cells crowded by the adjacent goblet cells, which were densely packed with secretory vesicles. In these areas the mucous layer penetrated deeply into the periciliary space, leaving 0.5 to 0.75 μ. This finding suggests that there was a lack of normal interaction between the cilia and the mucus.

DISCUSSION

It has been reported that there is mucociliary dysfunction in otitis media.[1,2] We found that mucociliary transport was absent in 70 percent of the middle ear clefts in children with otitis media with mucoid effusion. Mucociliary transport is governed by three factors—cilia, mucus, and the interaction of cilia and mucus. Abnormality of any one or any combination of these factors causes mucociliary dysfunction.[3] The depth of the periciliary fluid layer is crucial to the interaction of the cilia and mucus. Normally its depth is shorter than that of a cilium. If it is too shallow, the cilia beat in the sticky mucous layer. If it is too deep, the energy of ciliary beating is not transmitted to the mucous layer.

To clarify the cause of the mucociliary dysfunction in the middle ear cleft in otitis media with mucoid effusion, we endeavored to study the ultrastructure of the mucous blanket with special reference to the depth of the periciliary fluid layer, which represents morphologically the interaction of cilia and mucus.

In the large portion of the ciliated surface the mucous layer was located at the tips of the cilia, and the layer between the lower edge of the mucous layer and the luminal surface of the epithelium was electron lucent where the ciliary shafts were immersed. In this part of the promontory the mucociliary transport system was functioning.

On the rest of the ciliated surface the mucous layer deeply penetrated into the periciliary space. It is obvious that the frequency and amplitude of the ciliary beat are depressed. Mucociliary transport cannot take place in this situation. This finding is the same as that observed in the promontory mucosa in patients with otitis media with effusion[6] and in

otitis media with effusion induced experimentally in animals.[7]

This effect could be caused by an increase in the amount or a change in the biochemical composition of the mucus. Mucosubstances in the mucus may prevent it from settling into the periciliary space under normal circumstances.[8] On the contrary, the affect may be due to a decrease in the periciliary fluid by an unknown cause or a combination of both.

Although the present study was not quantitative, intensive goblet cell hyperperplasia was also observed.[8,9] The majority of the epithelial surface was secretory and the rest was ciliated. The intense hyperplasia of goblet cells caused the relative decrease in the number of ciliated cells. Ciliated cells were too scarce for abundant mucus to be transported.

Moreover, the lowered mucous layer disturbs ciliary activity. The ciliary beat would decrease or cease, and the amplitude would not be sufficient in sticky mucus.

These results indicate that there is mucociliary dysfunction in the middle ear in otitis media with effusion caused by a lack of cilia and abnormal interaction of the cilia and mucus. This dysfunction could be a cause of mucus accumulation in the middle ear cavity in this disease.

REFERENCES

1. Kärja J, Nuutinen J, Karjalainen P. Mucociliary function in children with secretory otitis media. Acta Otolaryngol 1983; 95:544–546.
2. Nuutinen J, Kärja J, Karjalainen P. Measurement of mucociliary function of the eustachian tube. Arch Otolaryngol 1983; 109:669–672.
3. Sakakura Y. Pathogenesis of mucociliary dysfunction in the upper respiratory tract. Pract Otol (Kyoto) 1987; 80:1–18.
4. Majima Y, et al. Mucociliary clearance in chronic sinusitis; related human nasal clearance and in vitro bullfrog palate clearance. Biorheology 1983; 20:251–262.
5. Lucas AM, Douglas LC. Principles underlaying ciliary activity in the respiratory tract. II. A comparison of nasal clearance in man, monkey and other mammals. Arch Otolaryngol 1934; 20:518–541.
6. Shibuya M, et al. Ultrastructure of the middle ear mucosa and effusion in otitis media. Ear Res Jpn 1985; 16:352–357.
7. Takasaka T, Kawamoto K. Mucociliary dysfunction in experimental otitis media with effusion. Am J Otolaryngol 1985; 6:232–236.
8. Thacte LG, Spicer SS, Spock A. Histology, ultrastructure, and carbohydrate cytochemistry of surface and glandular epithelium of human nasal mucosa. Am J Anat 1981; 162:243–263.
9. Tos M. Anatomy and histology of the middle ear. Clin Rev Allergy 1984; 2:267–284.
10. Móller P, Dalen H. Ultrastructure of the middle ear mucosa in secretory otitis media. Acta Otolaryngol 1981; 91:95–110.

LONGITUDINAL STUDY OF THE HISTOPATHOLOGY OF EXPERIMENTAL OTITIS MEDIA DUE TO NONTYPABLE *HAEMOPHILUS INFLUENZAE*

TREVOR J. McGILL, M.D., MIREILLE LEMAY, M.D., DENISE PAGE, M.D., and STEPHEN I. PELTON, M.D.

Chronic otitis media with effusion is a common sequela of acute otitis media, which is associated with conductive hearing loss and continued chronic middle ear disease. Animal models of otitis media have been used extensively to investigate the pathogenesis of chronic otitis media with effusion.[1,2]

The chinchilla is an ideal animal model because of its easily accessible middle ear and the thin bullar wall, which can be penetrated easily to inoculate the middle ear.

The purpose of this article is to document the results of a longitudinal study of the histopathology of experimental otitis media due to nontypable *Haemophilus influenzae* over an extended period.

MATERIAL AND METHODS

Sixteen healthy chinchillas free of middle ear infection were used in this experiment. The left bulla in these animals was inoculated with 10 CFU of nontypable *Haemophilus influenzae*. The right bulla was inoculated with sterile saline to serve as a control.

Animals were sacrificed at days 1, 3, 7, 14, 28 and 42. The chinchillas were perfused at the time they were sacrificed, and the heads were removed, decalcified, and embedded in paraffin. Five micron thick sections were stained with hematoxylin and eosin for tissue and cell examination.

RESULTS

All animals sacrificed after the first 24 hours were demonstrated by tympanometry and clinical examination to have had unilateral otitis media prior to sacrifice. Control animals did not exhibit any inflammatory changes or middle ear effusions.

Histopathologic changes in the inoculated middle ear cavities were observed from day 1. An extensive inflammatory response with polymorphonuclear leukocyte infiltration and focal hemorrhage in the subepithelial space occurred within 3 days after challenge. A severe purulent and hemorrhagic exudate was found in the middle ear cavity with further progression of the inflammatory process. The cellular infiltrations were also seen in the mucosal layer of the tympanic membrane and perineural sheath of the chorda tympani nerve. Early granulomatous tissue formation with loose connective tissue, rare macrophages, lymphocytes, and plasma cells were noted at this stage. These changes contrasted with the normal mucosa of the control ears.

Sequential examination of the inoculated ears revealed persistent chronic inflammatory changes. At 2 weeks the middle ear cavity was almost obliterated by extensive granulation tissue and an acute inflammatory exudate (Fig. 1). There was focal cuboidal and columnar metaplasia of the lining mucous membrane as well as striking edema of the submucosa with a mononuclear cell infiltrate. Periosteal irritation and new bone formation on the promontory were observed at this early stage.

At 28 days the middle ear cavity was bridged by multiple fibrous and granulation tissue adhesions with a predominant macrophage and mononuclear cell infiltrate. The lining epithelium showed cuboidal and papillary metaplasia. There were also islands of goblet cells and ciliated cell metaplasia. The lumen of the middle ear contained a moderate number of foamy macrophages, other mononuclear cells, and some polymorphonuclear leukocytes. The inner ears remained unremarkable.

At 6 weeks the middle ear cavity contained no exudate, but the mucosa and submucosa continued to exhibit chronic inflammatory changes. The submucosa showed moderate to severe thickening, with well developed fibrosis, vascularity, and a small focal monocytic infiltrate. The epithelial lining varied from being attenuated to denuded to rare foci of columnar and goblet cell metaplasia. Adjacent bone in the regions of the most severe mucosal changes showed new bone formation (Fig. 2).

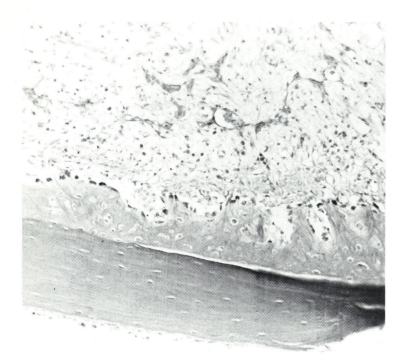

Figure 1 Middle ear mucoperiosteum from a chinchilla sacrificed 14 days after inoculation with 10 CFU of nontypable *Haemophilus influenzae*. Note that the middle ear is almost obliterated by granulation tissue and chronic inflammatory cells. Osteoneogenesis is prominent at this early stage.

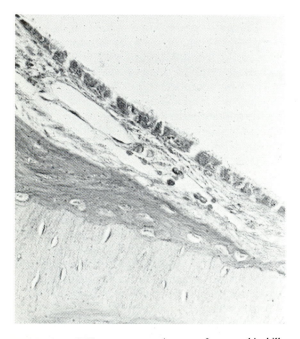

Figure 2 Middle ear mucoperiosteum from a chinchilla sacrificed 6 weeks after inoculation. There is a persistent chronic inflammatory infiltrate of the submucosa with extensive columnar metaplasia. Note new bone formation.

DISCUSSION

Inoculation of nontypable *Haemophilus influenzae* in the chinchillas produced an acute inflammatory response in the subepithelial space of the middle ear mucosa and subepithelial edema within 24 hours. Cellular metaplasia and a purulent middle ear effusion were apparent during the first week. Sequential examination showed a granulomatous reaction alternating with focal fibrosis during the third and fourth weeks after inoculation. Such microperiosteal granulation tissue over adjacent areas of new bone formation became the predominant histopathologic change by the sixth week.

These chronic histopathologic changes, which persisted for an extended period of at least 6 weeks, may account for the observation of persistent middle ear effusion as a common sequela of acute otitis media. Further studies are under way to determine the factors involved in the pathogenesis of this protracted chronic inflammatory response.

This study was supported in part by NINCDS/NIH program project grant POI NS 21914.

REFERENCES

1. Giebink GS, Payne EE, Mills EL, Juhn SK, Quie PG. Experimental otitis media due to *Streptococcus pneumoniae*: immunopathogenic response in the chinchilla. J Infect Dis 1976; 134:595–604.
2. DeMaria TF, Briggs BR, Lim DJ, Okazaki N. Experimental otitis media with effusion following middle ear inoculation of nonviable *H. influenzae*. Ann Otol Rhinol Laryngol 1984; 93:52–56.

MIDDLE EAR AND EUSTACHIAN TUBE HISTOPATHOLOGY DURING EXPERIMENTAL INFLUENZA A VIRUS INFECTION

MARY LOU RIPLEY-PETZOLDT, B.A., MARK SOLFELT, M.D., PETER F. WRIGHT, M.D., MICHAEL M. PAPARELLA, M.D., and G. SCOTT GIEBINK, M.D.

Epidemiologic studies have implicated certain viral upper respiratory infections, such as those caused by respiratory syncytial virus, adenovirus, and parainfluenza and influenza A viruses, in the pathogenesis of otitis media.[1-3] We employed the chinchilla otitis media animal model to investigate mechanisms of virus induced middle ear inflammation.

Chinchillas inoculated intranasally with influenza A viruses developed negative middle ear pressure and mild tympanic membrane inflammation; some influenza virus strains caused more frequent and more severe changes in middle ear pressure and tympanic membrane inflammation than other strains.[4] Influenza virus inoculation in the nasopharynx caused eustachian tube epithelial metaplasia with loss of ciliated epithelial cells and subepithelial lymphocyte infiltration in the proximal tube; in the distal tube increased epithelial secretory activity with mucous and cellular debris occluding the tube lumen was observed.[5] When intranasal inoculation of influenza A virus was combined with intranasal inoculation of *Streptococcus pneumoniae*, purulent otitis media resulted; these middle ear effusions yielded pure cultures of *S. pneumoniae* but not virus.[4] Intranasal inoculation of either *S. pneumoniae* or influenza A virus did not lead to effusion. Experiments performed to date have not indicated whether eustachian tube obstruction alone is sufficient for influenza A virus induced otitis media, or whether virus infection of the middle ear mucoperiosteum is also required. The present study was designed to explore this question.

MATERIALS AND METHODS

Eleven healthy 1- to 2-year-old chinchillas were inoculated intranasally with 1×10^5 plaque forming units of wild type influenza A/Alaska/77 virus, and their ears were examined by otoscopy and tympanometry 3, 5, 7, and 10 days after inocula-

tion. Nasal rinses for virus titration were performed on days 3 and 5.

Animals were randomly assigned to one of two groups for sacrifice and temporal bone harvest: one group was sacrificed on day 7 and the other group on day 10. Two healthy uninoculated chinchillas were sacrificed to serve as controls. To determine the presence of influenza virus and effusion in the middle ear at sacrifice, the middle ear cavity was aseptically exposed by removing a portion of bone from the cephalad bulla. Middle ear effusion was aspirated into a sterile syringe. If no effusion was present, 0.2 ml of sterile saline was washed gently over the middle ear mucosa and aspirated into a sterile syringe. Aliquots of the effusion or the saline aspirate were spread on a glass slide for cytologic evaluation, inoculated on 5 percent sheep's blood agar for bacterial culture, frozen at $-70°$ C for lysozyme assay, and flash frozen at $-70°$ C in a penicillin-gentamicin-gelatin transport medium for virus isolation.

Temporal bones were removed and immersed immediately in neutral buffered formalin. Specimens were decalcified in trichloroacetic acid over a period of several months. Tissues were dehydrated in a graded series of alcohols, embedded in celloidin, sectioned at a thickness of 10 microns, and stained with hematoxylin and eosin. Mucoperiosteal histopathologic changes were assessed using a semiquantitative scoring system by an observer blinded as to sacrifice group. Each inferior bulla, which contains the middle ear space, was examined at three distinct anatomic levels: the hypotympanum up to the widest cross section of the round window membrane, the midmodiolar region including sections just superior to the midsection of the round window membrane up to the first section above the oval window, and the supramodiolar region, including all sections superior to the oval window and the eustachian tube orifice. For each animal three sections were examined from each of the three anatomic levels in each animal; the same three locations were scored for each animal.

All the histopathologic variables sought in the middle ear mucoperiosteum are listed in Table 1. Each variable was subjected to a one way analysis of variance comparing the experimental ears with the control ears. Generalized histopathologic variables, based on the combinations of variables expected to occur together on a physiologic basis, were also subjected to analysis of variance (Table 2). Each set of variables combined to form the generalized variables was statistically significant.

RESULTS

Three days after virus inoculation all 11 animals had a negative middle ear pressure and tympanic membrane inflammation. Virus isolation attempts from nasal washes taken on day 3 were positive for influenza A virus in 10 of the 11 animals. At sacrifice on days 7 and 10 none of the animals had middle ear effusion, and virus isolation attempts from middle ear saline washes were all negative. All middle ear washes were culture negative for aerobic bacteria, and cytologic examination of the washes revealed no cells or only a scant number of squamous epithelial cells.

Histomorphometry of the middle ear mucoperiosteum revealed that there was significant pathologic change in the middle ear space, the epithelium, and particularly in the subepithelial space when influenza inoculated animals were compared to saline controls (see Table 1). Subepithelial pathologic change was characterized by large accumulations of serous fluid and significantly more hemorrhage, leukocyte infiltration, fibroblastic proliferation, and edema than in control ears.

When individual histopathologic variables were combined and the generalized variables were analyzed, there was more polymorphonuclear and

TABLE 1 Significance of Differences in Middle Ear Histopathologic Variables Between Influenza A Virus and Saline Inoculated Animals*

Histopathologic Variable	Middle Ear Space	Epithelium	Subepithelial Space
Effusion	ns	—	—
Organizing fibrous tissue	ns	—	—
Granulation tissue	ns	—	—
Osteoneogenesis	ns	—	ns
Polymorphonuclear leukocytes	ns	—	0.023
Mononuclear cells	0.042	—	0.001
Hemorrhage	ns	—	0.027
Metaplasia	—	0.011	—
Goblet cells	—	0.004	—
Congestion	—	—	ns
Thickness	—	—	ns
Edema	—	—	0.007
Fibroblastic reation	—	—	0.008

* Results shown are p values. ns, p value greater than 0.05.

TABLE 2 Analysis of Variance in Experimental and Control Ears

Generalized Histopathologic Variable (Individual Variables Combined)	Range[*†]	Saline Control	Mean Scores Days After Virus Inoculation 7	10
Polymorphonuclear leukocytes (MES + SES)[‡]	(0–12)	0.25	1.64[*]	2.20[*]
Mononuclear cells (MES + SES)	(0–12)	2.50	9.65[*]	10.94[*]
Epithelial metaplasia (goblet cells + metaplasia)	(0– 9)	2.54	5.18[*]	5.82[*]
Congestion (hemorrhage + congestion, MES +SES)	(0–14)	0.46	7.60[*]	8.85[*]
Fibrous tissue (MES + SES)	(0–11)	0.00	3.42[*]	3.58[*]
Subepithelial thickness (thickness + edema)	(0– 8)	0.67	7.83[*]	10.78[*]
Osteoneogenesis (MES + SES)	(0– 8)	0.00	0.22	0.38

[*] Significantly different from mean score for saline controls, $p < 0.05$.
[†] Range of possible scores using the combined variables.
[‡] MES, middle ear space. SES, subepithelial space.

TABLE 3   Significance of Differences in Middle Ear Histopatholgic Variables Between Influenza A Virus and Saline Inoculated Animals*

Histopathologic Variable	Hypomodiolar	Midmodiolar	Supramodiolar
Middle ear space			
Mononuclear cells	ns	0.22	ns
Epithelium			
Metaplasia	0.071	ns	ns
Goblet cells	ns	ns	0.001
Subepithelial space			
Polymorphonuclear leukocytes	0.05	ns	ns
Mononuclear cells	0.002	0.001	0.001
Hemorrhage	0.020	0.025	ns
Edema	0.007	0.005	0.012
Fibroblastic reaction	0.010	0.016	0.002

* Results shown are p values. ns, p value greater than 0.05.

mononuclear leukocyte infiltration, epithelial metaplasia, vascular congestion, fibrous tissue, and subepithelial thickening throughout the middle ear mucoperiosteum on comparing influenza inoculated ears with control ears (see Table 2). There were no statistical differences for any variables between the ears sacrificed on days 7 and 10 after virus inoculation.

Variables that showed significantly more pathologic change in virus inoculated ears than in control ears were analyzed for significance at each anatomic level. Four variables (middle ear space mononuclear cells, epithelial metaplasia, epithelial goblet cells, and subepithelial polymorphonuclear leukocytes) showed significant pathologic change at only one anatomic level (Table 3). One variable (subepithelial hemorrhage) showed significant pathologic change at only two anatomic levels. These results illustrate the necessity for scoring numerous sections through the middle ear at all three anatomic levels rather than relying on one or two sections to reveal the histopathologic changes present in the entire ear. For only three of the eight significant variables (subepithelial mononuclear cells, edema, and fibroblastic reaction) was pathologic change evident throughout the middle ear.

DISCUSSION

These results show that upper respiratory influenza A virus infection in chinchillas caused significant middle ear mucoperiosteal disease. The middle ear pathologic change was similar to that observed following eustachian tube obstruction using Silastic sponges in chinchillas.[6] Since influenza A virus was not isolated from the middle ear washes

and there was no evidence of epithelial injury with loss of epithelial cells, influenza A virus probably did not ascend to the middle ear space. Rather middle ear histopathologic change was most likely secondary to blockage of the eustachian tube. These results suggest that immunoprophylaxis against influenza A virus associated purulent otitis media in humans need only prevent viral infection of the nasopharyngeal and proximal eustachian tube epithelium.

Study supported in part by grant 5P50-NS-14538 from the National Institute of Neurological and Communicative Disorders and Stroke and grant T32-NS-07084, an NIH sponsored predoctoral training grant.

REFERENCES

1. Sanyal MA, Henderson FW, Stempel EC, Collier Am, Denny FW. Effect of upper respiratory tract infection on eustachian tube ventilatory function in the preschool child. J Pediatr 1980; 97:11–15.
2. Sarkkinen H, Ruuskanen O, Meurman O, Puhakka H, Virolainen E, Eskola J. Identification of respiratory virus antigens in middle ear fluids of children with acute otitis media. J Infect Dis 1985; 151:444–448.
3. Henderson FS, Collier AM, Sanyal MA, Watkins JM, Fairclough DL, Clyde WA Jr, Denny FW. A longitudinal study of respiratory viruses and bacteria in the etiology of acute otitis media with effusion. N Engl J Med 1983; 306:1377–1383.
4. Giebink GS, Wright PF. Different virulence of influenza A virus strains and susceptibility to pneumococcal otitis media in chinchillas. Infect Immunol 1983; 41:913–920.
5. Giebink GS, Ripley ML, Wright PF. Eustachian tube histopathology during experimental A virus infection in the chinchilla. Ann Otol Rhinol Laryngol 1987; 96:199–206.
6. Juhn SK, Paparella MM, Kim CS, Goycoolea MV, Giebink GS. Pathogenesis of otitis media. Ann Otol Rhinol Laryngol 1977; 86:481–492.

ULTRASTRUCTURAL PATHOLOGY OF THE TUBOTYMPANUM FOLLOWING EXPERIMENTAL INFLUENZA A VIRUS INDUCED OTITIS MEDIA

DAVID J. LIM, M.D., YOSHIHIRO OHASHI, M.D., MYUNG-HYUN CHUNG, M.D., and THOMAS F. DeMARIA, Ph.D.

Epidemiologic and clinical data have revealed a close relationship between upper respiratory infection and otitis media.[1,2] Twenty-five percent of the patients with acute otitis media harbor virus in the upper respiratory tract regions, and antibodies to these viruses are detected in 24 percent of such cases.[3]

Giebink et al[4] demonstrated in chinchillas that respiratory viral infection contributes to the pathogenesis of otitis media. Only 13 percent of the animals developed acute otitis media when the nasopharynges were instilled with *Streptococcus pneumoniae*, whereas the incidence of acute otitis media was over 62 percent when the middle ear was also deflated. When the nasopharynges were instilled with *S. pneumoniae* together with influenza A virus, the incidence of otitis media was 67 percent. Follow-up investigation revealed that influenza A virus caused immediate destruction of the tubal mucosal lining.[5]

It is conceivable that damage of the tubal mucosal lining by influenza A virus might make it more vulnerable to secondary bacterial infection from the pharynx. However, few studies have been done in regard to the direct effect of viral infection on the tubotympanum. In addition, ultrastructural changes in tubotympanic mucosa infected by viruses have not been studied yet. The purpose in our study was to define the direct effect of influenza A virus on the tubotympanic mucosa.

MATERIALS AND METHODS

We used 46 chinchillas (350 to 600 g) that were free of middle ear infection. The animals were anesthetized and placed in a prone position, and 0.25 ml of influenza A/Alaska/6/77 suspension (2.8×10^7 PFU per ml) was inoculated into the left tympanic bulla of each animal. The same amount of minimal essential medium was injected into the right tympanic bulla of each animal as a control. The animals were sacrificed 12 hours, and 1, 2, 3, 5, 9, 14, 21, and 28 days after the tympanic injection. At the time of sacrifice bilateral mucosal samples were obtained from the middle ears and eustachian tubes. These samples were examined by scanning and transmission electron microscopy using routine procedures. For quantitative analysis of data from electron microscopic observations, a digital computer was used.

RESULTS

The tubotympanic mucosa of the right (control) ear showed few pathologic changes, but after viral infection the tubotympanic mucosa showed marked changes. Two major findings were inflammation and damage to cilia or ciliated cells. Infiltration of inflammatory cells (mainly polymorphonuclear leukocytes) into the epithelial layer and the subepithelial layer was observed. A decrease in epithelial cells was not frequently noted. Viral infection affected the ciliary apparatus: cilia became shorter or disappeared. In sporadic areas nonciliated epithelium was observed after viral infection. Pathologic cilia, such as compound cilia, were also observed.

Regeneration of the cilia and ciliated cells started 5 days after viral infection. As signs of such regeneration, cell division in basal cells and ciliated cells with intracellular centrioles and procentrioles was observed. The peak of such regeneration occurred about 21 days after viral infection.

Cilia

The length of the cilia (mean $\pm$ standard deviation) in the control ear was 4.11 ± 0.39 μm in the tympanic orifice, 4.09 ± 0.44 μm in the midportion of the eustachian tube, and 4.01 ± 0.56 μm in the pharyngeal orifice. By 5 days the length of the cilia in the virus infected ear was shorter than in the control ear. Cilia became longer after 14 days, but they were still shorter than in the control ear (tympanic orifice, 3.6 ± 0.52 μm; eustachian tube, 3.82 ± 0.60 μm; pharyngeal orifice, 3.80 ± 0.59 μm).

Ciliated Cells

The number of ciliated cells in the control ear was 14.92 per 100 μm at the tympanic orifice, 15.35 per 100 μm at the eustachian tube, and 21.12 per 100 μm at the pharyngeal orifice. The number of ciliated cells decreased after viral infection, and the smallest number of ciliated cells was observed at 9 days. After 14 days the number of ciliated cells increased, but the number was still smaller than in the control ear (tympanic orifice, 13.41 per 100 μm; eustachian tube, 13.81 per 100 μm; pharyngeal orifice, 16.33 per 100 μm).

Goblet Cells

The number of goblet cells in the control ear was 5.79 per 100 μm at the tympanic orifice, 4.78 per 100 μm at the eustachian tube, and 4.43 per 100 μm at the pharyngeal orifice. After viral infection the number of goblet cells decreased slowly, but their number was larger than in the control ear (tympanic orifice, 6.51 per 100 μm; eustachian tube, 7.15 per 100 μm; pharyngeal orifice, 6.30 per 100 μm).

Basal Cells

The number of basal cells in the control ear was 6.24 per 100 μm at the tympanic orifice, 4.78 per 100 μm at the eustachian tube, and 9.12 per 100 μm at the pharyngeal orifice. The number of basal cells increased after viral infection; the largest number was observed 14 to 21 days after infection. The number of basal cells returned to the level in the control ear.

Free Cells

The number of free cells in the control ear was 0.00 per 100 $μm^2$ at the tympanic orifice, 0.09 per 100 $μm^2$ at the eustachian tube, and 0.26 per 100 $μm^2$ at the pharyngeal orifice. After viral infection numerous free cells were observed; the largest number was found at 5 days (5.38 per 100 $μm^2$ at the tympanic orifice, 2.83 per 100 $μm^2$ at the eustachian tube, and 5.18 per 100 $μm^2$ at the pharyngeal orifice). Then free cells decreased in number gradually. At 28 days the number of free cells returned to the level in the control ear. Most of the free cells were polymorphonuclear leukocytes, but sporadic lymphocytes were observed after 14 days.

Ciliogenesis

Few signs of ciliogenesis were observed in the control ear (tympanic orifice, 0.00 per 100 μm; eustachian tube, 0.10 per 100 μm; pharyngeal orifice, 0.26 per 100 μm). On the other hand, the tubotympanic mucosa in the virus infected ear revealed considerable numbers of epithelial cells with intracellular centrioles, procentrioles, and procentriole precursor bodies. The number of such epithelial cells was largest 21 days after infection (tympanic orifice, 5.52 per 100 μm; eustachian tube, 6.73 per 100 μm; pharyngeal orifice, 6.24 per 100 μm). The number of epithelial cells decreased at 28 days, but they were still more numerous than in the control ear (tympanic orifice, 1.00 per 100 μm; eustachian tube, 1.62 per 100 μm; pharyngeal orifice, 1.03 per 100 μm).

DISCUSSION

Epidemiologic studies have strongly suggested a relationship between respiratory virus infection and otitis media.[1,2] Twenty-five percent of the patients with acute otitis media harbor virus in the upper respiratory region, and antibodies to these viruses are detected in 30 percent of such cases.[3] Recent investigations have shown that respiratory viral infection contributes significantly to the pathogenesis of otitis media.[5] In the latter study influenza A virus was inoculated into the nasal cavity in chinchillas. Study of the pathology of the tubotympanum in laboratory animals directly inoculated with influenza A virus into tympanic bulla is necessary in order to understand the direct role of viral infection in otitis media. In our study influenza A virus was inoculated into the tympanic bulla in chinchillas. As a result we confirmed that direct inoculation of influenza A virus causes otitis media.

Ultrastructural changes in the tubotympanum induced by viral infection have not been clearly discussed. In our study ultrastructural changes were observed by scanning and transmission electron microscopy. The two major changes observed in our models were considerable inflammation and disturbances of cilia or ciliated cells (Fig. 1).

Although ciliated cells are vulnerable to a variety of pathologic agents, they can show quick recovery from such degeneration. For a better understanding of virus induced otitis media, it is important to study the recovery process after degeneration. In our models a decrease in the number of ciliated cells was not frequently observed.

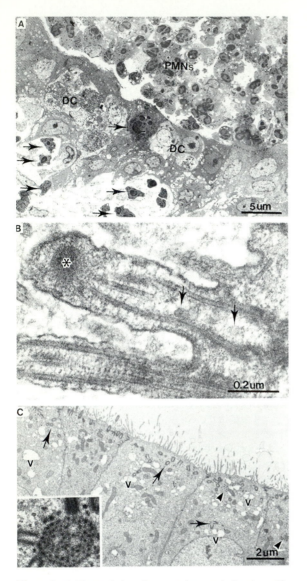

However, abnormal signs, including short cilia, compound cilia, vacuolation of ciliated cells, and loss of cilia, were frequently observed. Recovery from such degeneration was observed 5 days after viral infection, as evidenced by cell division and new cilia formation. At 14 days to 21 days many epithelial cells contained intracellular centrioles and procentrioles. The numbers of such epithelial cells in the process of regeneration decreased by 28 days. Thus, recovery of the tubotympanic mucosa seems to be complete 28 days after influenza A virus infection.

Cilia are important in the local defense system because ciliary function is an integral component of mucociliary clearance. The morphologic abnormalities observed seem to result in reduced ciliary activity and insufficient middle ear clearance. Such pathologic changes in the defense systems might encourage secondary bacterial infection.

CONCLUSIONS

1. Middle ear inoculation of influenza A virus induced severe damage of the tubotympanic mucosa in chinchillas.
2. Major pathologic changes induced by viral infection included nonspecific inflammation and damage of the ciliary apparatus.
3. Regeneration of cilia started at 5 days, and complete recovery of cilia or ciliated cells took at least 28 days.

REFERENCES

1. Bluestone CD, Klein JO. Otitis media with effusion, atelectasis, and eustachian tube dysfunction. In: Bluestone CD, Stool SE, eds. Pediatric otolaryngology. Philadelphia: WB Saunders, 1983:356.
2. Giebink GS. Epidemiology and natural history of otitis media. In: Lim DJ, Bluestone CD, Klein JO, Nelson JD, eds. Recent advances in otitis media with effusion. Proceedings of the Third International Symposium. Toronto: BC Decker, 1984:5.
3. Yamaguchi T, Urasawa T, Kataura A. Secretory immunoglobulin A antibodies to respiratory viruses in middle ear effusion of chronic otitis media with effusion. Ann Otol Rhinol Laryngol 1984; 93:73–75.
4. Giebink GS, Berzins IK, Marker SC, Schiffmen G. Experimental otitis media after nasal inoculation of *Streptococcus pneumoniae* and influenza A virus in chinchillas. Infect Immunol 1980; 30:445–450.
5. Giebink GS, Ripley ML, Wright PF. Eustachian tube histopathology during experimental influenza A virus infection in the chinchilla. Ann Otol Rhinol Laryngol 1987; 96:199–206.

Figure 1 *A*, Transmission electron micrograph showing midportion of eustachian tube 2 days after viral inoculation. There is an aggregation of polymorphonuclear leukocytes (PMN) in the tubal lumen. Arrows indicate polymorphonuclear leukocyte infiltrations in the epithelial layer and subepithelial connective tissue layer. Observe the marked decrease in ciliated cells and the degenerating epithelial cells (DC). *B*, Transmission electron micrograph of midportion of eustachian tube 3 days after viral inoculation, showing a shortened cilium. Vesicles resembling viruses are also found inside the cilium (arrows). Electron dense materials are concentrated, indicating disturbed polymerization of microtubules (asterisk). A neighboring cilium appears normal. *C*, Transmission electron micrograph of pharyngeal orifice 14 days after viral inoculation, showing ciliogenesis, indicated by the accumulation of cytoplasmic centrioles (arrows) and procentrioles (arrowheads) along the cell surface. Increased vacuolation (v) is observed. The inset shows a higher magnification of a procentriole.

HISTOPATHOLOGIC STUDY OF EUSTACHIAN TUBE IN PATIENTS WITH CLEFT PALATE

YOSHIHIRO SHIBAHARA, M.D., D.M.S. and ISAMU SANDO, M.D., D.M.S.

Otitis media with effusion is universally present in infants with unrepaired clefts of the palate.[1,2] Also studies have indicated that the eustachian tube is functionally obstructed in children with cleft palates.[3-6] However, no quantitative morphometric studies of the eustachian tube and its related structures have been reported in patients with cleft palate and in control age matched individuals. For this reason quantitative morphometric measurements of these structures were obtained and analyzed to detect possible associations between morphologic abnormalities in the eustachian tube and functional tubal obstruction in children with cleft palate.

MATERIALS AND METHODS

Eight temporal bone specimens that included the entire eustachian tube and its accessory structures, from eight individuals with complete cleft palate (aged 24 weeks' gestation to 6 weeks), were studied.[7] All temporal bone specimens were removed at autopsy and fixed in 10 percent formalin. After decalcification in 5 percent trichloroacetic acid and dehydration in graded solutions of ethanol, the specimens were embedded in celloidin and sectioned vertically in the plane perpendicular to the long axis of the petrous bone. Every 20th section was stained with hematoxylin and eosin.

The eustachian tube and its surrounding structures in representative vertical histologic sections, from both the midcartilaginous and isthmion portions of the eustachian tube, were projected onto plain paper, traced, and measured (the cross sectional area was measured by using a compensating polar planimeter).

The following measurements were made in each of two portions (the midcartilaginous portion and isthmian portion) of the eustachian tube:*

1. Cross sectional areas of the lumen of the eustachian tube and of the cartilage.
2. Cross sectional lengths of the tubal lumen and of the cartilage.

---

* Details of the methods used for measurement were described by Kitajiri et al.[8]

3. Widths of the tubal lumen and of the medial lamina of the eustachian tube cartilage.

The following measurements were made only in the midcartilaginous portion:
1. The cross sectional areas of the tensor veli palatini and levator veli palatini muscles.
2. The cross sectional lengths of the lateral and medial laminae of the cartilage.
3. The angle between the axis of the tensor veli palatini muscle and the line through the superior portion of the eustachian tube lumen, the angle between lines drawn through the long axes of the lateral and medial cartilaginous laminae, the angle between lines drawn through the long axes of the tensor veli palatini muscle and the lateral lamina of the cartilage, and the angle between the axis of the superior part and that of the inferior part of the eustachian tube lumen.

For statistical analysis the t test was used.

RESULTS

Eustachian Tube Lumen

The cross sectional area of the midcartilaginous portion of the eustachian tube lumen in the temporal bones from individuals with cleft palate tended to be less than in control specimens. The cross sectional length of the isthmian portion of the eustachian tube in specimens from individuals with cleft palate also tended to be slightly less than in control specimens. Finally, the cross sectional width of the lumen in the midcartilaginous portion of the eustachian tube in specimens from individuals with cleft palate tended to be less than in control specimens. However, there was no statistically significant difference ($p < 0.05$) in these eustachian tube lumen measurements between specimens from individuals with cleft palate and those from controls.

Cartilage

The cross sectional area of the cartilage in the midcartilaginous portion of the eustachian tube in specimens from individuals with cleft palate tended to be greater than in controls. The width of the medial lamina of the midcartilaginous portion of the eustachian tube also tended to be greater in cleft palate specimens than in controls. However, these differences were not statistically significant, and there was no difference in total cross sectional length of the cartilage between specimens from individuals with cleft palate and those from controls.

Muscles

The cross sectional area of the tensor veli palatini muscle in the midcartilaginous portion of the eustachian tube in specimens from individuals with cleft palate was almost the same as that in control specimens. However, the area of the levator veli palatini muscle at the midcartilaginous portion of the eustachian tube in cleft palate specimens was smaller than in controls. Nevertheless this difference was not statistically significant.

Angles

The angle between the axis of the tensor veli palatini muscle and the axis of the superior portion of the eustachian tube lumen was narrower in specimens from individuals with cleft palate ($\bar{X} = 47.8$ degrees) than in control specimens ($\bar{X} = 74.8$ degrees), and the difference was statistically significant ($t = 2.55$, $p < 0.05$; Figs. 1, 2).

The angle between the axes of the lateral and medial laminae of the cartilage was wider in cleft palate specimens ($\bar{X} = 2.4$ degrees than in controls ($\bar{X} = -19.8$ degrees), and this difference was statistically significant ($t = 2.16$, $p < 0.05$).

The angle between the axes of the tensor veli palatini muscle and the lateral lamina of the cartilage was narrower in cleft palate specimens ($\bar{X} = 47.0$ degrees) than in control specimens ($\bar{X} = 80.1$ degrees), and the difference was statistically significant ($t = 3.41$, $p < 0.01$).

The angle between the axes of the superior and inferior parts of the eustachian tube lumen was wider in cleft palate specimens ($\bar{X} = 137.4$ degrees) than in controls ($\bar{X} = 98.5$ degrees), and this difference was statistically significant ($t = 3.21$, $p < 0.01$).

DISCUSSION

Bluestone and Klein[9] delineated the major types of abnormal eustachian tube function that can lead to otitis media: obstruction, abnormal patency, or both. Moreover, eustachian tube obstruction can be functional or mechanical, or both, with func-

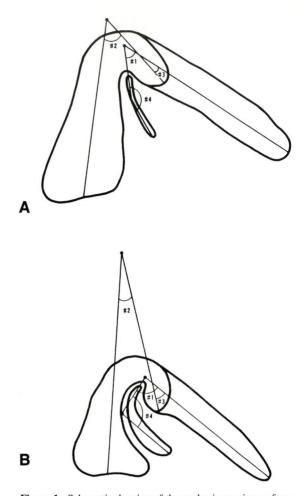

Figure 1 Schematic drawing of the angles in specimens from individuals with *A,* cleft palates and *B,* controls. Angle 1, between the axis of the tensor veli palatini muscle and a line through the superior portion of the eustachian tube lumen, was narrower in the cleft palate specimens than in the controls. Angle 2, between the axis of the lateral lamina and the medial lamina of the cartilage, was wider in cleft palate than in control specimens. Angle 3, between the axis of the tensor veli palatini muscle and the lateral lamina of the cartilage, was narrower in cleft palate than in control specimens. Angle 4, between the axis of the superior and inferior parts of the cleft palate lumen, was wider in cleft palate than in control specimens.

tional obstruction resulting from persistent collapse of the eustachian tube owing to increased tubal compliance, or an abnormal active opening mechanism. Thus, the otitis media with effusion seen in all infants with unrepaired palatal clefts, and in many children in whom the cleft palate has been repaired, may be the result of functional obstruction of the eustachian tube.[10] In addition, Takahara et al[11] reported that the pathogenesis of otitis media with effusion in an individual with a lymphoma appeared to be secondary to dysfunction of the tensor veli palatini muscle (the active dilator of the eustachian tube),

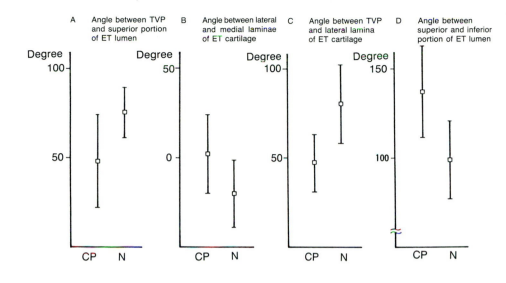

Figure 2 Mean values and standard deviations of angles associated with the eustachian tube or its associated structures in specimens from individuals with cleft palates (CP) and controls (N). *A*, Angle between a line drawn through the longitudinal axis of the tensor veli palatini muscle and a cross section through the superior portion of the eustachian tube lumen, midcartilaginous portion (□). *B*, Angle between the axis of the lateral laminae and a cross section through the midcartilaginous portion (□) of the medial lamina of the eustachian tube cartilage. *C*, Angle between the axis of the tensor veli palatini muscle and a cross section through the midcartilaginous portion (□) of the lateral lamina of the eustachian tube cartilage. *D*, Angle between the axis of the superior part and that of the inferior part of the eustachian tube lumen, as seen in cross section, at the midcartilaginous portion of the eustachian tube (□).

resulting from destruction by tumor.

Our findings indicate that the angles between the tensor veli palatini muscle and the superior portion of the eustachian tube lumen, between the lateral and medial laminae of the cartilage, between the tensor veli palatini muscle and the lateral lamina of the cartilage, and between the superior part of the eustachian tube lumen and the inferior part of the eustachian tube lumen are closely associated with the mechanism for opening the eustachian tube lumen. Nevertheless we believe ours to be the first report of any quantitative study of these important angles.

We found that the angle between the axis of the tensor veli palatini muscle and the superior axis of the eustachian tube lumen, and the angle between the axis of the tensor veli palatini muscle and the axis of the lateral lamina of the cartilage, were narrower in individuals with cleft palate than in controls. Further, the angle between the axis of the lateral and medial laminae of the cartilage, and the angle between the axes of the superior and inferior parts of the eustachian tube lumen, were larger in individuals with cleft palate than in controls. These

results could explain the dynamics of the dysfunction in opening of the eustachian tube lumen in individuals with cleft palate. In those with cleft palate who have pathologically narrow or wide angles, as just described, the opening forces acting on the eustachian tube lumen, especially its superior portion, may be weaker. Thus, the cause of the otitis media with effusion noted in individuals with cleft palate appears to be functional obstruction of the eustachian tube.

This study was supported by research grant PO1 NS 16337 from the National Institute of Neurological and Communicative Disorders and Stroke, National Insitutes of Health.

REFERENCES

1. Stool SE, Randall P. Unexpected ear disease in infants with cleft palate. Cleft Palate J 1967; 4:99–103.
2. Paradise JL, Bluestone CD, Felder H. The universality of otitis media in fifty infants with cleft palate. Pediatrics 1969; 44:35–42.
3. Bluestone CD, Cantekin EI, Beery QC, Paradise JL. Eu-

stachian tube ventilatory function in relation to cleft palate. Ann Otol Rhinol Laryngol 1975; 84:333–338.

4. Doyle WJ, Cantekin EI, Bluestone CD. Eustachian tube function in cleft palate children. Ann Otol Rhinol Laryngol 1980; 89 (Suppl 68):34–40.

5. Odoi H, Proun GO, Toledo PS. Effects of pterygoid hamulotomy upon eustachian tube function. Laryngoscope 1971; 81:1242–1244.

6. Doyle WJ, Cantekin EI, Bluestone CD, et al. Nonhuman primate model of cleft palate and its implications for middle ear pathology. Ann Otol Rhinol Laryngol 1980; 89 (Suppl 68):41–46.

7. Sando I, Doyle WJ, Okino H, et al. A method for the histopathological analysis of the temporal bone, eustachian tube and its structures. Ann Otol Rhinol Laryngol 1986;

95:267–274.

8. Kitajiri M, Sando I, Takahara T. Postnatal development of the eustachian tube and its surrounding structures. Ann Otol Rhinol Laryngol 1987; 96:191–198.

9. Bluestone CD, Klein JO. Otitis media with effusion, atelectasis, and eustachian tube dysfunction. In: Bluestone CD, Stool SE, eds. Pediatric otolaryngology. Philadelphia: WB Saunders, 1983:356.

10. Bluestone CD. Eustachian tube obstruction in the infant with cleft palate. Ann Otol Rhinol Laryngol 1971; 80 (Suppl 2):1–30.

11. Takahara T, Sando I, Bluestone CD, Myers EN. Lymphoma invading the anterior eustachian tube: temporal bone histopathology of functional tubal obstruction. Ann Otol Rhinol Laryngol 1986; 95:101–105.

PHOTOGRAPHIC MEASUREMENT OF TYMPANIC MEMBRANE RETRACTION IN OTITIS MEDIA

TETSUO ISHII, M.D., ETSUKO KIMURA, M.D., YOKO GOTODA, M.D., and MIKIKO TAKAYAMA, M.D.

Retraction of the tympanic membrane is characterized by horizontal deviation of the malleus handle, protrusion of the short process, deformities of the light reflex, and a color change or fluid line in the pars tensa. If photographs of the tympanic membrane are taken in the clinic under controlled conditions, quantitative evaluation of certain morphologic features is possible with the photograph. We chose a shift of the malleus handle to the horizontal direction as an index of retraction. For this study an effort was made to insure uniform photographic conditions.

The photographic apparatus was a rigid fiberscope specialized for tympanic membrane photography with a camera (Model SFD, 6.2 mm caliber, Nagashima Medical Instruments Co.). The patient was placed in the supine position, and the axis of the head, body, and bed was adjusted to the parallel position. The head was tilted slightly toward the other ear, and marks were placed on the lower ridge of the orbit and orifice of the external auditory meatus (Reid's line). This line was adjusted to form a right angle with the surface of bed. Then the fiberscope was inserted carefully through the ear canal. Under these conditions photographs of the tympanic membrane were taken as in Figure 1, showing the anterior part of tympanicannulus and anterior bony wall. The photographs of the tympanic membrane were consistently obtained under the foregoing conditions.

After several trials we decided to adopt the line of the anterior bony wall as a standard line (a), and the angle of the handle (b) was measured in relation to it (Fig. 1). If anatomic variations existed in the bony wall or tympanic membrane, such cases were excluded from our evaluation. Finally we examined variations in the photographs from the various photographers, comparing photographs of one subject taken by various photographers. Also one photographer photographed one subject on different occasions. The angles, measured under the foregoing conditions, varied between $-3°$ and $+3°$ if the subject was the same. The variations were thought to be small, so we proceeded with our investigation.

The angles of the malleus handle with the anterior wall were measured in a series of photographs. The average angles in normal ears (38), otitis media effusion (120 ears), and adhesive otitis (84 ears) were $18.6 \pm 8.8°$, $21.1 \pm 9.9°$, and $25.7 \pm 12.3°$, respectively (Table 1). In otitis media with effusion marked retraction (30° or more) was found in 26

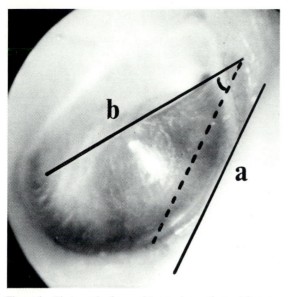

Figure 1 Photograph of normal tympanic membrane, taken under uniform conditions. The angle of malleus handle (b) with the anterior bony wall (a) was measured as an index of retraction.

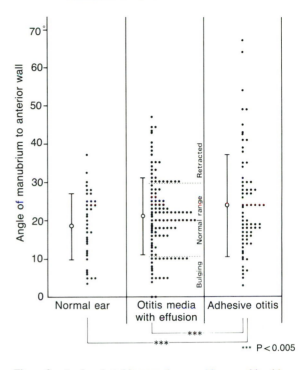

Figure 2 Angles plotted in normal ears and in ears with otitis media and adhesive otitis. Large variations in the angles were observed in otitis media with effusion, and they became more prominent in adhesive otitis.

ears (21.6 percent). The retraction was not a common finding in otitis media, and even bulging of the tympanic membrane (10° or less) was observed, which possibly moved the malleus handle in a lateral direction. Bulging tympanic membranes in otitis media were observed in 23 ears (19.2 percent); 71 other ears (59.2 percent) showed tympanic membrane positions within the normal range (<30° to >10°). This is the reason there was no significant difference in the average angles between normal ears and those with otitis media. Contrariwise, adhesive otitis produced marked retraction so that the umbo almost contacted the promontory. A significant difference existed between the angles in normal ears and those in otitis media and adhesive otitis. There were no significant differences between the malleus handle angles in children and adults with normal ears and those with otitis media.

Figure 2 illustrates plots of angles measured in normal ears and in ears with otitis media and adhesive otitis. Even the angles in normal ears showed a variation, but a trend toward large angles was prominent in otitis media and was more prominent in adhesive otitis.

Movement of the malleus handle was studied under pressure in the middle ear in one study.[1] The reported malleus handle position does not correlate with the middle ear pressure in the living normal ear within the range of −300 to 160 mm H_2O. We speculate, however, that a shift of the malleus handle is caused by a constant negative pressure in the middle ear, and this shift becomes irreversible

TABLE 1 Angle of Manubrium to Bony Anterior Wall

Normal ear (n=38)	18.6°±8.8*	
Otitis media with effusion (n=120)	21.1°±9.9*	Retracted (>30°;n=26) 35.1°±5.4 Normal range (<30° to >10°;n=71) 20.5°±4.2 Bulging (<10°;n=23) 7.2°±3.2
Adhesive otitis (n=84)	25.7°±12.3*	

* P<0.005.

owing to ankylosis of the ossicles. This shift causes the umbo to touch the promontory, and this situation is one of causative factors in adhesion of the tympanic membrane in adhesive otitis.

REFERENCE

1. Cable HR, Tadros S. Tympanic membrane retraction and middle ear pressure. J Laryngol Otol 1982; 96:113–117.

OTOTOXICITY OF VASOCIDIN DROPS APPLIED TO CHINCHILLA MIDDLE EAR

ORVAL E. BROWN, M.D., CHARLES G. WRIGHT, Ph.D., MASAMI MASAKI, M.D., and WILLIAM L. MEYERHOFF, M.D., Ph.D.

Otorrhea from tympanostomy tubes or tympanic membrane perforations is a common otologic problem. Treatment alternatives include topically applied antibiotic preparations. However, most such preparations contain potentially ototoxic drugs such as neomycin and polymyxin B. These may cause inner ear damage if they reach the middle ear cavity.[1,2] Vasocidin ophthalmic solution (which contains sulfacetamide sodium and prednisolone sodium phosphate) has been advocated as an alternative drug that may produce fewer toxic side effects in the treatment of otorrhea.[3] This study was undertaken to investigate the effects of Vasocidin ophthalmic solution on the middle and inner ear, using the chinchilla as an animal model.

METHODS AND MATERIALS

Vasocidin ophthalmic solution was introduced into the bullae of nine chinchillas. Each animal received a single bilateral application of 0.5 cc of the preparation. Six animals (12 ears) were sacrificed for histologic study 1 week after receiving Vasocidin; the remaining three animals (six ears) were evaluated after a survival time of 1 month. Sham operated control animals were not included, because previous experiments have documented that this does not cause middle or inner ear damage.[4]

Two temporal bones (one at each of the two survival times used in the study) were processed for celloidin embedding and serial sectioning. The remaining specimens were prepared for microdissection. Tympanic membrane and middle ear mucosa specimens were embedded in plastic for study as 1 micron thick sections. The organ of Corti and stria vascularis specimens were microdissected for evaluation as surface preparations.

RESULTS

No evidence of cochlear hair cell loss or strial damage was found in 17 of the 18 temporal bones included in this study. In one specimen, from an animal with a 4 week survival time, there was a focal lesion of the basal hook portion of the organ of Corti. In that area both inner and outer hair cells were missing over a distance of about 50 microns along the organ of Corti. No strial damage was observed in the region where the hair cell loss had occurred.

The middle ears of all animals kept for 1 week after Vasocidin administration showed marked inflammation of the mucosa with occasional hemorrhage of mucosal vessels and accumulation of serous effusion in the tympanic cavity. In the inferior portion of the bullae there was marked subepithelial edema with dilation of vessels and increased numbers of fibroblasts (Fig. 1). Clusters of inflammatory cells were noted, both in the edematous subepithelial space and in the serous fluid overlying the mucosa. Occasional small pockets of developing granulation tissue were seen, especially in the periannular air cells, the apex of the otic capsule, and surrounding the ossicles.

The tympanic membranes from these animals showed hyperplasia of both the medial and lateral

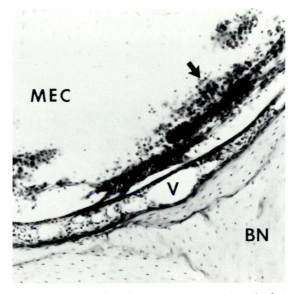

Figure 1 Inflammation of middle ear mucosa, 1 week after Vasocidin administration. This celloidin section illustrates dilation of blood vessels (V) in the subepithelial space and inflammatory cells (arrow) overlying the mucosal surface. MEC, Middle ear cavity. BN, Bony wall of middle ear. (Original magnification 100 ×.)

cell layers, with frequent hemorrhage of small blood vessels (Fig. 2A, 2B). The hyperplastic epidermal layer was found to be moderately hyperkeratotic, and there was often an accumulation of clear fluid between the keratin layer and the epidermal cells on the lateral aspect of the tympanic membrane. In three cases this fluid contained large numbers of rectangular platelike crystals ranging from 5 to 50 microns in length (Fig. 2C). In smear preparations of unstained specimens the crystals showed birefringence when viewed with polarized light, and they were always closely associated with hemorrhagic areas of the tympanic membrane. These characteristics suggest that the crystalline material was cholesterol.

Inflammatory changes were much less evident in the middle ears of animals kept for 1 month after Vasocidin application. None of the animals in this experimental group showed middle ear effusion or evidence of active inflammation of the mucosa or tympanic membrane. Occasional crusts of keratinaceous debris containing extravasated blood were noted in the external ear canals of the 1 month survival time animals. This material apparently had migrated from the lateral surface of the tympanic membranes. Slight thickening of the tympanic membrane and moderate subepithelial fibrosis of the middle ear mucosa were also noted 1 month after Vasocidin administration. Otherwise the middle ear cavities of these animals appeared essentially normal.

DISCUSSION

Previous studies have shown that an otic preparation containing neomycin and polymyxin B, which is commonly used topically, can cause severe middle ear inflammation, loss of cochlear hair cells, and damage to the stria vascularis and vestibular receptor organs in the chinchilla animal model.[1,2] The results of this study revealed short term inflammatory effects with little or no evidence of inner ear damage after application of Vasocidin ophthalmic solution to the chinchilla middle ear cavity. The findings of middle ear effusion and inflammation at 1 week were largely reversed at 4 weeks. A small lesion of the basal hook portion of the organ of Corti was observed in one specimen evaluated at 1 month. Since minor hair cell loss is occasionally observed in normal chinchillas, it may be that the focal lesion found in this specimen was unrelated to Vasocidin exposure.

Armstrong[3] has suggested that Vasocidin ophthalmic solution may be useful in the treatment of otorrhea. Sulfacetamide is effective in the treatment of infections caused by *Staphylococcus aureus*, *Streptococcus* species, and *E. coli*. It is not effective against *Haemophilus influenzae* and other gram negative organisms. Otorrhea resulting from chronic otitis media is usually caused by *Pseudomonas aeruginosa* or *Staphylococcus aureus*.[5] The bacteriologic features of acute onset otorrhea resulting from tympanic membrane perforations or tympanostomy tubes have not been well described. It may be that *Streptococcus pneumoniae* and *Haemophilus influenzae*, as seen in acute otitis media, are the usual pathogens. It appears that Vasocidin ophthalmic solution has a bacteriologic spectrum that may be useful in selected patients with otorrhea.

The results of this experimental animal study indicate that Vasocidin ophthalmic solution should be used with caution in the treatment of otorrhea because of its potential for producing middle ear inflammation. Primate species do not seem to be as susceptible to ototoxic drugs as the chinchilla, probably because of round window membrane structural differences. It is reasonable to assume that Vasocidin ophthalmic solution does not cause cochlear toxicity in humans. It may be an effective therapeutic agent for the treatment of otorrhea in selected clinical circumstances. However, the Food and Drug Administration has not approved this preparation for otic use in the United States. If it is used in the treatment of otorrhea, appropriate cultures should be taken to assure the clinician that the offending pathogen is appropriately sensitive to Vasocidin ophthalmic solution therapy.

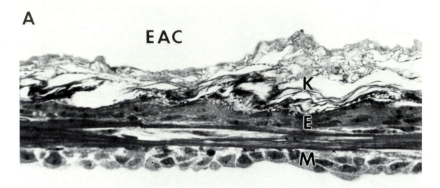

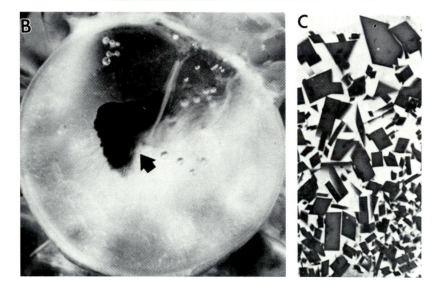

Figure 2 *A*, Cross section of tympanic membrane 1 week after Vasocidin application, showing thickened epidermal (E) and mucosal (M) layers and increased keratin (K) production on the lateral surface. EAC, External ear canal. MEC, Middle ear cavity. (Original magnification 400 ×). *B*, Low power view of medial surface of tympanic membrane from an animal killed 1 week after receiving Vasocidin. The arrow indicates hemorrhage in the central area of the membrane. (Original magnification 12 ×). *C*, Toluidine blue stained cross section of crystalline material located near a hemorrhagic area of the tympanic membrane 1 week after instillation of Vasocidin into the middle ear cavity. (Original magnification 400 ×).

REFERENCES

1. Wright CG, Meyerhoff WL. Ototoxicity of otic drops applied to the middle ear in the chinchilla. Am J Otolaryngol 1984; 5:166–176.
2. Meyerhoff WL, Morizono T, Wright CG, Shaddock LC, Shea DA. Tympanostomy tubes and otic drops. Laryngoscope 1983; 93:1022–1027.
3. Armstrong B. In discussion of: Meyerhoff WL, Morizono T, Shaddock LC, Wright CG, Shea DA, Kikora MA. Tympanostomy tubes and otic drops. Laryngoscope 1983; 93:1022–1027.
4. Wright CG, Meyerhoff WL, Burns DK. Middle ear cholesteatoma: an animal model. Am J Otolaryngol 1985; 6:327–341.
5. Kenna MA, Bluestone CD, Reilly JS. Medical management of chronic suppurative otitis media without cholesteatoma in children. Laryngoscope 1986; 96:146–151.

OTOTOXICITY OF TOPICALLY APPLIED DRUGS USED IN OTITIS MEDIA TREATMENT

TETSUO MORIZONO, M.D., D.M.S., M.S., ROBERT SMITH, M.D., CHAP T. LE, Ph.D., DANIEL CANAFAX, Pharm.D., and G. SCOTT GIEBINK, M.D.,

There are conflicting reports of the ototoxicity of topically applied otic preparations in animal studies and in clinical practice. Nevertheless knowledge of the relative ototoxicity of drugs in a given class of otic preparations is important. The prescription of eardrops is common among pediatricians, family doctors, and otologists. There are anecdotal clinical reports of sensorineural hearing loss due to neomycin containing eardrops and some types of antiseptics.[1-4]

MATERIALS AND METHODS

Healthy chinchillas of both sexes, weighing about 500 g each, were used in this study. All animals were anesthetized by the subcutaneous injection of ketamine hydrochloride (30 mg per animal) and sodium pentobarbital (30 mg per kilogram); the animals were secured in a custom head holder.

Asynchronous tone bursts of 2, 3, 4, 6, 8, and 12 kHz (1 ms rise and fall time, 10 ms plateau time) were given as stimuli at a pulse rate of 22 per second from 80 db (re 20 μPa) to threshold in a closed acoustical system composed of a headphone coupled to the custom speculum by a length of flexible plastic tubing giving an acoustic delay of 1.12 ms. For some animals with reduced action potential, sound pressures as great as 90 db were used. The sound pressure was monitored by a calibrated probe microphone at the tympanic membrane level.

An 0.08 mm diameter, Teflon insulated silver wire with an exposed ball tip was carefully placed on the peripheral round window without touching the osseous cochlea, using a micromanipulator. A silver–silver chloride pellet reference electrode was placed in the neck muscles. The action potential was amplified 1,000 times and filtered at high pass 100 Hz and low pass 3 kHz. An average of 100 responses were recorded and stored using a microprocessor. The sampling time was 40 μs with a 10.24 ms window. Data collection was triggered by positive-going stimulus wave forms. The recordings were taken prior to and 30, 60, 120 minutes, and 24 hours after application of the drug. Data were collected from high to low frequency and from high to low intensity. The criterion for threshold was a signal with an amplitude to 10 μV calculated by interpolation.

Fifty microliters of the test solution at room temperature were applied to the round window area, wicked dry after 10 minutes, and then rinsed and wicked three times with a total of 0.5 ml of Ringer's solution. After 120 minutes, measurements were completed. The surgical opening in the bulla was closed with dental cement, the wound sutured, and the animal allowed to recover. The final measurement of the action potential was done at 24 hours. Control animals were treated as already described, with the exception of round window application of

0.5 ml of Ringer's solution instead of the test solution. The endocochlear direct current potential was measured in some animals after action potential measurements. To measure the endocochlear potential, a glass microelectrode (with a tip diameter of 1 micron) filled with 150 mM potassium chloride was positioned with a micromanipulator through the round window into the scala media. A calomel glass electrode was placed into the neck muscle through the surgical wound. The potential was measured directly using an electrometer (WPI-F223A) and recorded on a strip chart recorder (Houston Institute B5000). At the end of endocochlear potential measurement, the drifting of the potential and possible damage to the electrode tip were closely examined to avoid an artifact.

RESULTS

Figure 1 illustrates a method for determining the relative ototoxicity of two drugs. The ratio of the doses (in log scale) indicates the relative ototoxicity.

Figure 2 is an example of a dose-response curve (a scatter plot) of action potential threshold elevations at 8 and 4 kHz 30 minutes after application of the acetic acid dilutions and Ringer's solution. With a criterion of a 10 db (or more) loss at 8 kHz, 20 percent (1 of 5) of the 0.5 percent concentrations, 60 percent of the 0.75 percent concentrations, and 100 percent of the 1.0 percent concentrations met the criterion. By interpolating from the two lower concentrations, one calculates a toxic dose 50 percent (TD50) of 0.7 percent. A TD50 of 0.63 percent for 4 kHz is calculated in a similar manner. The endocochlear potential was also measured in some of the animals after action potential measurement. The endocochlear potential appears to be linearly related to the decibel loss in the action potential. Acetic acid is known to be beneficial in the treatment of *Pseudomonas* infection. Acetic acid, 2 percent in 20 percent ethyl alcohol, has been used as a cleaning-rinsing agent before mastoid surgery.

Figure 3 illustrates the dose-response curves for povidone-iodine (Betadine). Betadine scrub contains a detergent and has greater ototoxicity than Betadine solution.

At 2 hours the decibel loss for 8 kHz was about 20 db when a 100 times dilution (0.01) of the scrub was used, but a 10 times dilutant of the solution did not cause any loss. Thus the scrub was 10 times more toxic than the solution. After application of the scrub the action potential for 8 kHz at 30 minutes, 1 hour, and 2 hours deteriorated progressively. The loss was

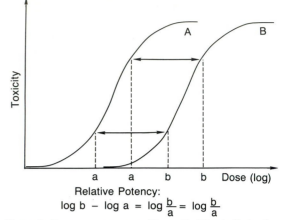

Relative Potency:

$$\log b - \log a = \log \frac{b}{a} = \log \frac{b}{a}$$

Figure 1 Dose-response curve. The vertical line indicates the toxicity of a drug and the horizontal line indicates the dose in log scale. The dose-response curve of a chemical exhibits a sigmoidal curve. The relative potencies of drugs A and B are calculated by measuring the horizontal distance of lines A and B. The method is called the parallel-line bioassay method.

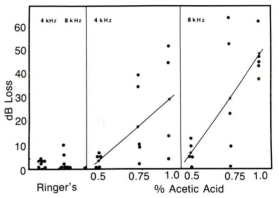

Figure 2 A scatter plot of action potential threshold elevation 30 minutes after acetic acid application. Although individual variations of the decibel loss are large at middle concentrations, the mean value of the action potential loss is remarkably linear.

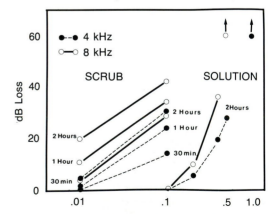

Figure 3 Dose-response curve of povidone-iodine scrub and solution. To obtain the same toxicity (decibel loss in action potential), more than 10 times the dilution ratio is necessary for the scrub.

proportional to the log time with the 10 times dilution and the 100 times dilution.

Chlorhexidine (Hibitane) digluconate is an antiseptic. Its topical ototoxicity has been reported in humans and in animals.[5-7] A 0.5 percent solution of the chemical is widely used for sterilization of the middle ear cavity for stapedectomy and mastoidectomy. In our study a 10 times dilution (0.05) of the solution did not cause action potential loss at 1 hour but caused a severe (40 db) loss at 24 hours (Fig. 4). The dose-response curve for this chemical also indicates that the action potential loss is proportional to the log time. A clinical report by Bicknell[5] showed that the hearing loss was progressive even several months after the drug was used in the middle ear.

Preliminary dose-response curves were obtained for Cortisporin, the most popular eardrop. This information will be used as a standard to compare the relative ototoxicities of other eardrops.

The ototoxicity of Cortisporin was roughly half that of Betadine solution. The ototoxicity of Vasocidin eyedrops, which are recommended by some surgeons, showed no toxicity at an 8 kHz action potential studied 2 hours following application of the drug. Long term study is mandatory before the preparation can be recommended to clinicians, because the chemical tends to cause severe inflammation of the middle ear cavity. The effect of such inflammation on inner ear function has not yet been studied.

DISCUSSION

In order to study and establish the ototoxicity of a chemical, various methods can be employed.

Histopathologic study, including temporal bone histopathologic examination, electron microscopic study, and hair cell counting reveals evidence of damage to the cochlea but do not provide data in regard to hearing loss. Functional studies include the auditory brainstem evoked response, compound action potential, cochlear microphonics, endocochlear direct current potentials, and ionic and oxygen concentration changes in the inner ear fluids. Of these methods, compound action potential measurement is the best method to permit construction of audiograms for the animals.

Evaluation of otic preparations in regard to their relative ototoxic potential in humans can be done experimentally by employing the standard pharmacologic paradigm of the dose-response curve in different species of animals with different anatomic structures of the round window. Because of differences in vulnerability to topically applied otic preparations in humans and rodents, conflicting findings are reported in regard to the potential ototoxicity of otic preparations. In future work the emphasis should be placed on scaling animal studies to humans and on recommending the least toxic substances with equivalent clinical efficacy.

We conclude the following:

1. The toxicity of povidone-iodine scrub and chlorhexidine progressed linearly in log time.

2. Vasocidin eyedrops were not found to be ototoxic at 2 hours.

3. Dose-response curves enable us to estimate the relative ototoxicity of a given class of otic drops.

4. The scaling of ototoxicity for humans from animal data is yet to be studied.

Study supported by NINCDS grant NS-14538 from the National Institutes of Neurological and Communicative Disorders and Stroke.

REFERENCES

1. Matsumaru H. A case report of anaphylaxis caused by local application of 0.5 % chloromycetic otic solution. Otol Fukuoka 1965; 10:48.
2. Kellerhas B. Hörschaden durch ototoxische Ohrentropfen. NHO 1978; 26:49–52.
3. Fradis M, Podoshin L, Ben-David J. The level of sensorineural hearing loss in patients with chronic otitis media treated topically with neomycin-polymyxin B combination. World Congress of ENT, Miami, May 1985:10A.
4. Tommerup B, Moller K. A case of profound hearing impairment following the prolonged use of framycetin ear drops. J Laryngol Otol 1984; 98:1135–1137.
5. Bicknell PG. Sensorineural deafness following myringoplasty operation. J Laryngol 1971; 85:957–961.
6. Morizono T, Johnstone B, Hadjar E. The ototoxicity of antiseptics. J Otolaryngol Soc Aust 1973; 3:550–553.
7. Aursnes J. Cochlear damage from chlorhexidine in guinea pig. Acta Otolaryngol 1981; 92:259–271.

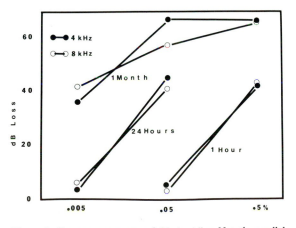

Figure 4 Dose-response curve of chlorhexidine. Note the parallel progressive decibel loss of the action potential at 1 hour, 24 hours, and 1 month.

ANIMAL MODELS

NEW ANIMAL MODELS OF OTITIS MEDIA IN CHINCHILLAS

TIMOTHY T. K. JUNG, M.D., Ph.D., SOON-JAE HWANG, M.D., DAVID POOLE, M.D., DAVID OLSON, B.S., STANLEY K. MILLER, B.S., JAE-SUNG LEE, M.D., TAE-HYUN YOON, M.D., and STEVEN K. JUHN, M.D.

Animal models are useful in investigating the pathogenesis of otitis media. Chinchillas have been used extensively to develop different animal models. Purulent otitis media (POM) has been induced by inoculating viable *Streptococcus pneumoniae*, serous otitis media (SOM) by obstructing the eustachian tube, and immune mediated otitis media (IOM) by inducing a secondary immune response in the middle ear using keyhole limpet hemocyanin as the antigen. Even though each of these otitis media models isolates one of the important causative factors, it does not replicate actual human otitis media because several factors are usually involved in human situations.

We developed new models of otitis media in chinchillas by combining these models, such as POM + SOM, IOM + SOM, and IOM + POM. These models were compared with existing models by otoscopy, tympanometry, gross examination, measurement of lysozyme levels, and light microscopic studies of temporal bone histopathologic changes.

The purposes in this study were to develop better animal models of otitis media by combining different animal models, to develop a better method of eustachian tube obstruction, to assess the effect of tympanostomy tubes on different models of otitis media, and to correlate otoscopic, tympanometric, biochemical, and histopathologic findings in these animal models.

MATERIALS AND METHODS

The six otitis media models in chinchillas (including three new models), the intervals from the start of the experiment up to the day of sacrifice, and the number of ears studied are listed in Table 1. A total of 70 ears were studied. Otoscopy and tympanometry were performed two times per week, and samples of middle ear fluid were aspirated for biochemical assay weekly. Concentrations of lyso-

zyme were measured using a lysozyme test kit (Kallestad Co., Chaska, MN).

At the time of sacrifice the superior bullae of the animals were opened, samples of middle ear effusion were collected, and gross findings were noted. Animals were perfused through a catheter in the aorta with normal saline first and then with 10 percent formalin solution. The temporal bones were removed, fixed in buffered 10 percent formalin, decalcified with 5 percent trichloroacetic acid, dehydrated in a graded series of alcohols, embedded in celloidin, and sectioned to a thickness of 20 μm. Every tenth section was stained with hematoxylin and eosin for microscopic examination.

Temporal bones were studied and the presence of effusion, leukocyte infiltration, granulation tissue, osteoneogenesis, hyperemia, edema, metaplasia, and hemorrhage was recorded.

SOM (Model 1)

Under anesthesia induced by the intramuscular administration of ketamine hydrochloride (45 mg per kilogram), a midline incision was made in the soft palate and the eustachian tubes were obstructed with dental hypoallergenic rubber impression material (Coe Laboratories, Inc., Chicago, IL).

POM (Model 2)

Purulent otitis media was induced by injecting viable type 7F *Streptococcus pneumoniae** into the dorsal portion of the bullae, as described previously.[1]

IOM (Model 3)

Immune mediated otitis media was developed by injecting keyhole limpet hemocyanin (Pacific

---

* Courtesy Scott Giebink, M.D., University of Minnesota.

TABLE 1 Animal Models: Interval to Sacrifice and Number of Ears

Models*	Interval from Experiment to Sacrifice (Weeks)	No. of Ears
1. SOM	3	10
2. POM	3	12
3. IOM	5	12
4. SOM+POM	4	12
5. IOM+SOM	6	12
6. IOM+POM	5	12
Total		70

Description
1. Eustachian tube obstruction with rubber impression material.
2. POM by direct inoculation of live 7F *S. pneumoniae.*
3. IOM by direct injection of keyhole limpet hemocyanin after immunization.
4. Eustachian tube obstruction plus direct inoculation of 7F *S. pneumoniae.*
5. IOM plus eustachian tube obstruction.
6. IOM plus direct inoculation of 7F *S. pneumoniae.*

* SOM, serous otitis media. POM, purulent otitis media. IOM, immune mediated otitis media.

Bio-marine Labs, Venice, CA) through the dorsal bullae four times at 2 day intervals into animals previously immunized by intradermal injection of keyhole limpet hemocyanin in complete Freund's adjuvant.[2]

SOM + POM (Model 4)

Seven days following eustachian tube obstruction, direct inoculation was made through the dorsal portion of the bullae as described in model 2.[3]

IOM + SOM (Model 5)

One day after immune mediated otitis media was induced as described in model 3, eustachian tube obstruction was carried out as described in model 1.

IOM + POM (Model 6)

One day after immune mediated otitis media was induced as described in model 3, live type 7F *S. pneumoniae* was inoculated as described in model 2.

RESULTS

Presence of Fluids

Fluid was present in all ears of the combined models of IOM + SOM and IOM + POM at the end of the first week, in all ears of the SOM + POM model at the end of the second week, in all ears of the POM, SOM + POM, and IOM + POM models at the end of the third week, and in all ears of the SOM + POM model at the end of the fourth week.

Fewer ears had fluid in the IOM and SOM + POM models at the end of the first week (33 percent), in the IOM model at the end of the second week (17 percent), in the IOM and IOM + SOM models at the end of the third week (50 percent), and in the IOM + SOM model at the end of the fourth week (50 percent; Table 2).

Tympanometry

In serous otitis media the number of ears with a type B tympanogram increased progressively with time—40 percent at the end of the first week, 60 percent at the end of the second week, and 100 percent at the end of the third week (Table 3). In the SOM, POM, SOM + POM, and IOM + POM models the number of ears with a type B tympanogram increased with time (Table 3).

TABLE 2 The Presence of Fluids

Model	1st (%)	2nd (%)	3rd (%)	4th (%)
SOM	80	40	60	
POM	83	67	100	
IOM	33	17	50	
SOM+POM	33	100	100	100
IOM+SOM	100	50	50	50
IOM+POM	100	83	100	

TABLE 3   The Percentage of Ears with Type B
Tympanogram

Model	Week			
	1st (%)	2nd (%)	3rd (%)	4th (%)
SOM	40	60	100	
POM	50	83	83	
IOM	17	17	0	
SOM+POM	33	50	100	100
IOM+SOM	100	83	83	83
IOM+POM	17	50	50	

Concentration of Lysozyme

The levels of lysozyme in the middle ear fluid
were highest in the POM and lowest in the SOM
model after 1 week with and without tympanostomy
tubes. After 2 weeks the concentrations of lysozyme
were highest in the SOM + POM and SOM models
with tympanostomy tubes and lowest in the IOM
models (Table 4).

Temporal Bone Histopathology

In the SOM model the middle ear mucosa was
thin, with minimal inflammation. There was serous
fluid with a few scattered inflammatory cells in the
middle ear cavity. In the POM model both the
middle ear mucosa and the middle ear cavity were
packed with polymorphonuclear leukocytes and the
subepithelial space was thickened with dilated capillaries. In the IOM model there were moderate numbers of inflammatory cells in the mildly thickened
subepithelial space. Histopathologic damage in the
SOM + POM model was characterized by an
edematous and thickened subepithelial space,
dilated capillaries, and new bone formation. In the
SOM + IOM model there was thickening of the
subepithelial space, with hemorrhage and some new
bone formation. In the IOM + POM model there
was thickening of the subepithelial space, with inflammatory cells and dilated capillaries.

DISCUSSION

Several experimental models of otitis media in
chinchillas were developed and found to be useful
in investigating the pathogenesis of otitis media.
With animal models, variables and different
parameters can be isolated and controlled; the
effects of the new treatment and the sequential
progression of the disease can be studied in depth.

In previous SOM models the eustachian tubes
of different animals were obstructed by means of
mechanical ligation,[4] cauterization,[5] or packing[6] or
by functional obstruction with fracture of the hamu-
lus,[7] transection of the tensor veli palatini muscle,[8]
or cleft palate. We produced serous otitis media by
using a new technique of eustachian tube obstruction. We mixed base and an accelerator of dental
rubber impression material and loaded it into a
tuberculin syringe with a 16 gauge intravenous
needle catheter, injecting into the nasopharyngeal
orifice of the eustachian tube. We found that this
method was much more reliable than other methods
of packing the eustachian tube.

The data relating to the presence of fluid
showed that the combined models had a higher percentage of ears with effusion than the single models.
Tympanometric findings correlated well with the
presence of middle ear effusion. In general, combined models had a higher percentage of ears with
type B tympanogram.

The levels of lysozyme in the middle ear effusion seem to reflect well the degree of inflammation in otitis media. On the basis of the levels of
lysozyme, the POM model had the highest degree
of inflammation in 1 week and the SOM + POM
model in 2 weeks. The levels of lysozyme in the
SOM model with a tympanostomy tube were high
in 2 weeks because of superimposed retrograde infection due to the tube.

Histopathologic findings in the SOM + POM
and IOM + POM models were similar to those in
the human middle ear mucosa in chronic otitis
media.

TABLE 4   Levels of Lysozyme (μg/ml)

Tympanostomy Tube	SOM	POM	IOM	SOM+POM	IOM+SOM	IOM+POM
Week 1						
With	(−)	90.1±32.3*	60.0±7.8	(−)	42.0±3.3	46.7
Without	27.5±5.9	67.5±12.9	30.1±2.1	48.3	43.1±5.1	34.6±4.8
Week 2						
With	>300	108.4	114.0±5.0	>300	158.7±3.3	215.0±47.5
Without	202.1±66.3	(−)	40.3	297.9	54.5±1.1	52.6±1.3

* Mean ± standard error.

Tympanostomy tubes prevented the development of middle ear effusion in the SOM and SOM + POM models at 1 week only. In the rest of the otitis media models there was no difference between the ears with tympanostomy tubes and those without. At 2 weeks the ears with tubes had worse inflammation than those without tubes in all models. This is probably the result of retrograde infection caused by the presence of tubes.

We believe that we have developed an improved method of eustachian tube obstruction by injecting dental rubber impression material into the eustachian tube. Middle ear effusion was present in all ears of the SOM + POM and IOM + POM models in 1 week, and tympanometry confirmed the presence of fluid. Levels of lysozyme were highest in the POM model in 1 week and highest in the SOM + POM and SOM models with tympanostomy tubes in 2 weeks. Ears with tympanostomy tubes seemed to have more severe inflammation than ears without tympanostomy tubes. Histopathologic findings correlated well with biochemical parameters. These new combined otitis media models in chinchillas seem to mimic the human condition best and could be used in studies of otitis media.

This study was supported by NIH-NINCDS grant NS-14538 and Loma Linda University BRSG.

REFERENCES

1. Meyerhoff WL, Shea DA, Giebink GS. Experimental pneumococcal otitis media: a histopathologic study. Otolaryngol Head Neck Surg 1980; 88:606–612.
2. Ryan AF, Catanzaro A. Passive transfer of immune-mediated middle ear inflammation and effusion. Acta Otolaryngol (Stockh) 1983; 95:123–130.
3. Jung TTK, Shea DA, Giebink GS, Juhn SK. Comparative histopathology of animal models of otitis media in chinchillas: a temporal bone study. In: Lim DJ, Bluestone CD, Klein JO, Nelson JD, eds. Recent advances in otitis media with effusion. Proceedings of the Third International Symposium. Toronto: BC Decker, 1984:91–96.
4. Holmgren L. Experimental tubal occlusion. Acta Otolaryngol (Stockh) 1940; 28:587–592.
5. Senturia BH, Carr CD, Ahlvin RC. Middle ear effusion: pathologic changes of the mucoperiosteum in the experimental animal. Ann Otol Rhinol Laryngol 1962; 71:632.
6. Juhn SK, Paparella MM, Kim CS, et al. Pathogenesis of otitis media. Ann Otol Rhinol Laryngol 1977; 86:481–492.
7. Odoi H, Proud GO, Toledo PS. Effects of pterygoid hamulotomy upon eustachian tube function. Laryngoscope 1971; 81:1242–1244.
8. Cantekin EI, Phillips DC, Doyle WJ, Bluestone CD, Kimes KK. Effect of surgical alterations of the tensor veli palatini muscle on eustachian tube function. Ann Otol Rhinol Laryngol 1980; (Suppl 68) 89:47–53.

MORAXELLA (BRANHAMELLA) CATARRHALIS INDUCED EXPERIMENTAL OTITIS MEDIA IN THE CHINCHILLA

MYUNG-HYUN CHUNG, M.D., THOMAS F. DeMARIA, Ph.D., RONEL ENRIQUE, M.D., and DAVID J. LIM, M.D.

Moraxella (Branhamella) catarrhalis was previously considered a nonpathogenic organism that is usually present in the oropharynx. Recently it has been recognized as an important pathogen in otitis media, and the incidence of isolation from patients with otitis media has been increasing rapidly.[1] Furthermore, in less than a decade the proportion of strains producing beta lactamase has risen to about 76 percent of those isolated from cases of acute otitis media.[2]

Because of the increased clinical significance of this organism in otitis media, this study was undertaken to develop an animal model to establish the pathogenesis of otitis media due to *M. catarrhalis*, and to devise better diagnostic and management strategies by correlating the clinical characteristics of middle ear effusion with microbiologic and immunologic findings.

MATERIALS AND METHODS

Animals

A total of 38 healthy chinchillas (360 to 650 g) were used.

Inoculation of Viable and Nonviable Bacterial Suspension

In 21 chinchillas 0.3 ml of beta lactamase producing *M. catarrhalis* suspension (1×10^9 CFU per ml) was inoculated aseptically into the left superior bulla by a transbulla technique. The same dose of formalin inactivated nonviable bacteria was inoculated into 14 chinchillas to determine whether dead bacteria would induce otitis media as we observed with *Haemophilus influenzae*.[3,4] The other three chinchillas were inoculated with 0.3 ml of saline to serve as controls.

Examination and Analysis

All chinchillas were examined daily by otomicroscopy to monitor the otitis media and effusion. Three chinchillas from the viable *M. catarrhalis* inoculated group were sacrificed 1, 4, 7, 10, 14, 21, and 28 days after inoculation. Blood samples were obtained before inoculation and at the time of sacrifice for anti-*M. catarrhalis* antibody titration by an ELISA technique using mouse anti-chinchilla IgG monoclonal antibody produced in our laboratories. Tympanocentesis was performed under anesthesia to collect the middle ear effusion; if no effusion was present, both bullae were washed with 0.5 ml of sterile saline. Effusions or bulla washes were cultured on chocolate agar plates for *M. catarrhalis* and used to prepare cytocentrifuge slides for Gram staining and modified Wright-Giemsa staining for differential cell counts.[5]

Microscopy and Immunohistochemistry

Temporal bones were harvested after intracardiac perfusion and fixed with 2.5 percent glutaraldehyde in 0.05 M cacodylate buffer (pH 7.3). The specimens then were dissected and decalcified in 4.5 percent EDTA for 10 to 14 days. Eustachian tube and inferior bulla tissues were dissected and processed for low melting point paraffin embedding (53-55 C, Peel-A-Way Scientific).

Sections 5 microns thick were stained with hematoxylin and eosin for routine histologic observation and quantitative morphologic analysis. For immunohistochemical staining, 3-micron thick sections were stained for IgG by the avidin-biotin peroxidase complex method.

Quantitative Study

Tissue specimens from selected areas of the eustachian tube (tympanic, mid, and pharyngeal portions) and inferior bulla were used for morphologic and quantitative study by light microscopy. Polymorphonuclear neutrophils, macrophages, lymphocytes, and fibroblasts were counted in five randomly selected unit areas in each section. The thickness of the subepithelial connective tissue was measured and capillary areas were also traced and subtracted from the unit area to quantitate vascular engorgement.

Statistics

The Student's t test was used to determine the statistical significance of the pathologic findings quantitated. A probability value of $p < 0.05$ was used throughout.

RESULTS

Otomicroscopic Examination

By 1 day after inoculation with viable and nonviable *M. catarrhalis*, the tympanic membrane revealed inflammatory changes, such as congestion and loss of light reflex. On the second day after inoculation all the chinchillas inoculated with viable *M. catarrhalis* had developed air bubbles and various amounts of middle ear effusion. The chinchillas inoculated with nonviable *M. catarrhalis* showed less severe inflammatory responses and developed middle ear effusion 3 to 4 days after inoculation. The effusion usually persisted for 7 to 9 days after development in animals inoculated with both viable and nonviable *M. catarrhalis*. By 14 days after inoculation the tympanic membrane looked almost normal, with no evidence of effusion in the middle ear cavity. None of the control ears produced middle ear effusion.

Cytologic and Bacteriologic Examinations

Six of 14 nonviable *M. catarrhalis* inoculated chinchillas and 10 of 21 viable *M. catarrhalis* inoculated chinchillas had middle ear effusions when they were sacrificed 4, 7, and 10 days after inoculation.

All middle ear effusions (0.1 to 0.6 ml) from nonviable *M. catarrhalis* inoculated chinchillas were straw colored and serous, and they were sterile when cultured for bacteria. The effusions (0.1 to 1.5 ml) from viable *M. catarrhalis* inoculated chinchillas were turbid or purulent and more mucoid than those from nonviable *M. catarrhalis* inoculated chinchillas. Bacterial cultures of the middle ear washes obtained 1 day after inoculation with *M. catarrhalis* grew pure cultures of *M. catarrhalis*, but only one of three effusions from animals 4 days after inoculation grew *M. catarrhalis*. We recovered *M. catarrhalis* for up to 5 days after inoculation with 0.3 ml of 1×10^9 CFU per ml of *M. catarrhalis* suspension.

Gram staining of effusions or bulla washes up to 4 days after *M. catarrhalis* inoculation showed clumps of gram negative diplococci inside the polymorphonuclear leukocytes.

Cytologic responses in the bulla washes after inoculation with viable *M. catarrhalis* are shown in Figure 1. Cytologic profiles in the bulla washes after inoculation with nonviable *M. catarrhalis* were similar to those with the viable *M. catarrhalis* inoculated specimens.

Histologic Examination

The light microscopic findings in specimens obtained from the chinchillas 1 day after viable *M. catarrhalis* inoculation represented acute inflammatory responses, including subepithelial edema, vascular dilation, hemorrhage, and acute inflammatory cellular infiltration in the subepithelial connective tissue. At 4 and 7 days after viable *M. catarrhalis* inoculation polymorphonuclear leukocytes were the predominant type of infiltrating cell and macrophages had increased in number (Fig. 2A). At 10 and 14 days after inoculation the subepithelial

connective tissue was still edematous and vessels were engorged. Fibrosis was apparent in the subepithelial connective tissue (Fig. 2B). By 21 and 28 days after inoculation, acute inflammatory signs had almost completely subsided. There were a few macrophages and polymorphonuclear leukocytes, and submucosal new bone formation was apparent (Fig. 2C). The pathologic findings induced by nonviable *M. catarrhalis* were identical, but inflammatory changes were milder and recovery from inflammation was faster than in the viable *M. catarrhalis* tissue specimens.

For quantitative analysis of the pathologic changes we examined random areas of the inferior bulla around the tympanic orifice. This area consistently had shown pathologic changes in our previous study. We also examined the tympanic, middle, and pharyngeal portions of the eustachian tube.

The thickness of the connective tissue increased by 1, 4, and 7 days after viable *M. catarrhalis* inoculation as compared with controls. This increase was not statistically significant. By 10, 14, 21, and 28 days after inoculation the thickness had increased significantly ($p < 0.05$). The thickness of the connective tissue after inoculation with nonviable *M. catarrhalis* increased in all sample periods, but only the increase on day 14 was statistically significant ($p < 0.05$).

The percentage of capillary area in the eustachian tube and middle ear connective tissue increased in the viable and nonviable *M. catarrhalis* inoculated chinchilla in all sample periods, but it was not statistically significant.

The density of the polymorphonuclear leukocytes peaked at 1 day after inoculation with the viable organism and decreased gradually over 28 days after inoculation; they were the predominant

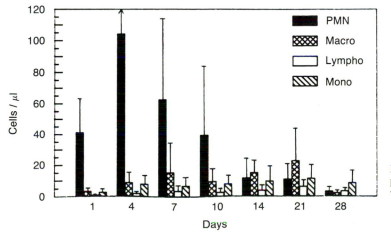

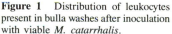

Figure 1 Distribution of leukocytes present in bulla washes after inoculation with viable *M. catarrhalis*.

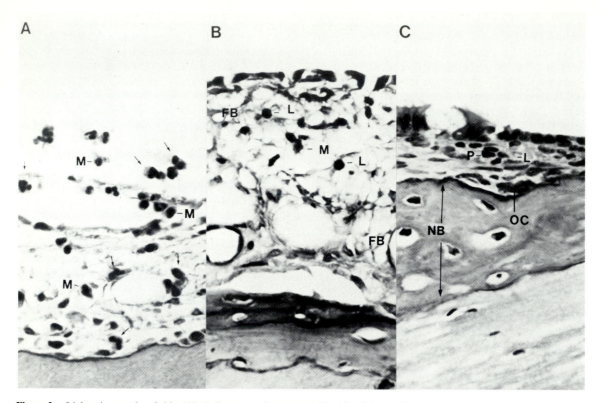

Figure 2 Light micrographs of chinchilla bulla mucosa inoculated with viable *M. catarrhalis. A*, Four days after inoculation there are many polymorphonuclear neutrophils (arrows) and macrophages (M) in the middle ear cavity and subepithelial connective tissue. *B*, Two weeks after inoculation there is extensive proliferation of connective tissue, fibrosis (FB), macrophages (M), and lymphocytes (L) infiltration. *C*, Four weeks after inoculation there are a few plasma cells (P), lymphocyte (L) infiltration, new bone formation (NB), and osteoclasts (OC). (400×.)

type of cell up to 7 days after viable *M. catarrhalis* inoculation. Macrophages and lymphocytes started increasing 1 day after inoculation, and levels had peaked by 14 days after inoculation (Fig. 3).

Immunohistochemical Study

Eustachian tube and bulla mucosa specimens obtained 2 weeks after inoculation with viable and nonviable *M. catarrhalis* showed positively stained IgG bearing cells, distributed mainly in the connective tissue of the bulla; some cells were observed in the eustachian tube, especially close to the bottom portion of the cross sectioned tube.

Antibody Responses

Fifteen chinchillas were examined to study the middle ear and serum antibody responses to *M. catarrhalis* infection. The serum antibody levels increased significantly ($p < 0.01$) 2 weeks after viable *M. catarrhalis* inoculation and continued over a fur-

ther 2 week period. Bulla wash antibody levels also increased 2 weeks after inoculation ($p < 0.05$). A comparison of the antibody titers in the paired serum and bulla wash from each chinchilla is shown in Figure 4. An initial increase in serum and effusion or bulla wash levels of antibody against *M. catarrhalis* was observed 1 week after inoculation, but the increase was not statistically significant. Bulla washes were used because we could not obtain any effusions after 2 weeks following inoculation, except in one chinchilla.

DISCUSSION

Direct delivery of viable and nonviable *M. catarrhalis* into the chinchilla middle ear cavity resulted in a consistent pattern of acute otitis media with effusion. As a matter of course we could not recover any viable bacteria from the effusions or bulla washes from nonviable *M. catarrhalis* inoculated chinchillas. For 5 days after inoculation with viable *M. catarrhalis* we recovered pure cultures of

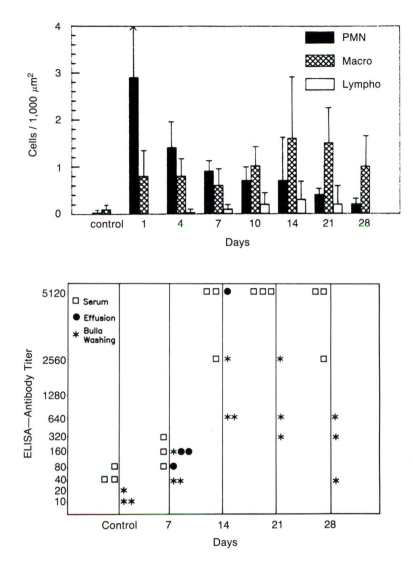

Figure 3 Cellular response in connective tissue after inoculation with viable *M. catarrhalis*.

Figure 4 Comparison of enzyme linked immunosorbent assay titers for anti-*M. catarrhalis* antibody in paired sera and bulla wash samples from 15 chinchillas over 4 weeks.

M. catarrhalis from bulla washes or middle ear effusions, and during the first 4 days we observed gram negative diplococci in the cytoplasm of gram stained polymorphonuclear leukocytes from bulla washes or middle ear effusions. There was no evidence of sustained multiplication in the middle ear.

The histologic alterations seen were acute inflammatory changes in the middle ear cavity and eustachian tube, which were comparable to the pathologic changes observed in biopsy specimens in cases of human otitis media with effusion.[6] There is now substantial evidence of the primary pathogenicity of *M. catarrhalis* in acute otitis media in the chinchilla. Nonviable *M. catarrhalis* was also responsible for inducing experimental otitis media with effusion. This result indicates that some biologic property of nonviable *M. catarrhalis* might be based on the bacterial component, especially endotoxin on the surface of gram negative bacteria, which is known to induce otitis media with effusion in the chinchilla when *H. influenzae* derived endotoxin is used.[3,7]

Serologic evidence of *M. catarrhalis* pathogenicity has been reported by use of an enzyme immunoassay to detect IgG and IgA antibodies to *M. catarrhalis* in sera and middle ear effusions in children with acute otitis media, correlating with isolation of *M. catarrhalis* from the middle ear effusions.[8] We detected significantly high ($p < 0.01$) IgG antibody titers in the sera in viable *M. catarrhalis* induced otitis media in our animals 2 to 4 weeks after inoculation. Antibody titers in bulla washes 2 and 3 weeks after inoculation were also significantly high ($p < 0.05$) compared with control bulla wash antibody titers, but at 1 and 4 weeks the antibody titer increases were not significant.

We also checked antibody titers in the effusions collected 1 and 2 weeks after viable *M. catarrhalis* inoculation. Antibody titers in 1 week effusions were higher than control serum or bulla wash antibody levels, but the difference was not significant. Antibody titer in the 2 week effusion was as high as the serum antibody levels and eight times as high as bulla wash titers in the same animal.

We successfully stained IgG bearing cells from viable and nonviable *M. catarrhalis* induced otitis media tissue specimens 2 weeks after inoculation.

Serologic and immunohistochemical findings suggested that *M. catarrhalis* infection might stimulate the local and systemic immune systems in the chinchilla, and we believe that these immunologic responses are involved in the pathogenesis of *M. catarrhalis* induced otitis media in this animal.

We conclude that bacteriologic, histologic, and immunologic evidence supports *M. catarrhalis* induced acute otitis media in the chinchilla. Nonviable *M. catarrhalis* also produced short term otitis media with serous effusion in the chinchilla similar to that produced by endotoxin.

This study was supported in part by a grant from NINCDS/NIH (NS08854; DJL) and a Fogarty International Fellowship (TWO3767; M-HC).

REFERENCES

1. Coffey JD Jr. Otitis media in the practice of pediatrics: bacteriological and clinical observation. Pediatrics 1966; 38:25–32.
2. Hare GF, Shurin PA, Marchant CD, Cartelli NA, Johnson CF, Fulton D, Carlin S, Kim CH. Acute otitis media caused by *Branhamella catarrhalis*: biology and therapy. Rev Infect Dis 1987; 9:16–27.
3. DeMaria TF, Briggs BR, Lim DJ, Okazaki N. Experimental otitis media with effusion following middle ear inoculation of nonviable *H. influenzae*. Ann Otol Rhinol Laryngol 1984; 93:52–56.
4. Okazaki N, DeMaria TF, Briggs BR, Lim DJ. Experimental otitis media induced by nonviable *Hemophilus influenzae*: cytologic and histologic study. Am J Otolaryngol 1984; 5:80–92.
5. Liu YS, Lim DJ, Lang RW, Birck HG. Chronic middle ear effusion: immunochemical and bacteriological investigation. Arch Otolaryngol 1975; 101:278–286.
6. Lim DJ, Birck HG. Ultrastructural pathology of the middle ear mucosa in serous otitis media. Ann Otol Rhinol Laryngol 1971; 80:838–853.
7. DeMaria TF, Prior RB, Briggs BR, Lim DJ, Birck HG. Endotoxin in middle ear effusion from patients with chronic otitis media with effusion. J Clin Microbiol 1984; 20:15–17.
8. Leinonen M, Loutonen J, Herva E, Valkonen K, Makela PH. Preliminary serologic evidence for a pathologic role of *Branhamella catarrhalis*. J Infect Dis 1981; 144:570–574.

EXPERIMENTAL OTITIS EXTERNA AND OTITIS MEDIA IN THE GERBIL MODEL WITH *PSEUDOMONAS AERUGINOSA*

HENRY G. MARROW, M.D., DANIEL WHITLEY Jr., M.D., and ROBERT S. FULGHUM, Ph.D.

The Mongolian gerbil has been shown to be an excellent model for the study of otitis media.[1-3] It is susceptible to common otic pathogens such as *Streptococcus pneumoniae* and *Haemophilus influenzae* as well as to other organisms such as anaerobic bacteria.

Senturia[4] showed that a high percentage of cases of otitis externa are caused by gram negative bacilli, especially *Pseudomonas aeruginosa*. This organism also is found in otitis associated with aural cholesteatoma in humans[5] and in gerbils[6] and is known to produce osteomyelitis of the temporal bone with striking histopathologic changes.[7]

The dog, cat, mouse, hamster, gerbil, and

guinea pig have been studied by Wright and Dineen[8] as possible models of otitis externa. Their initial study utilized only two animals of each species; however, the gerbils died and only guinea pigs were selected for further study. We know of no recent studies that have attempted to provide a model of otitis externa.

The purpose of the present work was to determine whether the Mongolian gerbil could serve as a reliable and inexpensive model for the study of otitis externa and otitis media caused by *P. aeruginosa*.

MATERIALS AND METHODS

Animals

Healthy young adult (less than 6 months of age) Mongolian gerbils, *Meriones unguiculatus*, were housed, maintained, anesthetized, and examined as in our previous studies.[1,2]

Bacterial Cultures

Pseudomonas aeruginosa (ATCC 10145) was grown on trypticase soy agar, and the resulting growth was harvested by washing plates with 0.9 percent saline. The resulting suspension of cells was diluted to a turbidity equivalent to half of a No. 1 McFarland standard, providing a suspension of approximately 1.5×10^8 cells per ml.

Otitis Media

Suspensions prepared as just described were inoculated percutaneously in aliquots of 0.03 ml per inoculation into middle ear bullae by the method used in our previous studies.[1,2] Right ear bullae were inoculated, the left serving as controls. One group of nine gerbils was inoculated percutaneously as already described. Animals were held untreated and examined daily for 2 weeks. One animal was sacrificed for histopathologic study at day 2 and one was sacrificed at day 4.

Otitis Externa

Animals were inoculated by infusing 0.03 ml of bacterial suspension into the external auditory canal after carefully removing cerumen from as much of the upper auditory canal as possible. Cerumen removal was important in order to allow direct contact of the inoculum with the tissue, since cerumen is known to be bactericidal.[9] The bacterial suspensions were instilled into the ear canals of three groups of 10 gerbils each. Animals were held untreated and examined daily for 2 weeks. Animals from group 1 were examined at days 1, 2, 3, 4, 7, 10, and 16. One animal was sacrificed each day for histopathologic study at days 2, 4, and 7. Group 2 animals were examined at 6 hours and then at days 1, 2, 5, 6, 7, and 8, and one animal was sacrificed for histopathologic study at 2, 5, 7, and 8 days. Group 3 animals were examined at days 1, 2, 3, 4, 7, 9, and 14, and one animal was sacrificed at each examination.

Examination of Animals

Otoscopic examinations were carried out using an operating microscope as described earlier.[1,2] For animals with middle ear inoculations, we scored the otoscopic observations using our previously published scoring system of five categories, ranging from very mild inflammation (score 1) to severe inflammation with a bulging tympanic membrane and an opaque exudate (score 5).[2] Observation of the external auditory meatus was made otoscopically as described, and inflammation of the canal was scored as mild, moderate, or severe. The amount and type of exudate were recorded. In many cases excess cerumen or exudate blocked the view of the meatus, and inflammation could not be scored.

Specimens and Histologic Preparations

Specimens were prepared as in our previous studies in which animals were perfused with saline and then with 10 percent formalin in phosphate buffer.[1,2] Heads were removed, decalcified, embedded in paraffin, sectioned, and stained with hematoxylin and eosin. The severity of infection and extent of sequelae were evaluated by a scoring system simplified from the one used in an earlier publication.[3]

RESULTS

Otitis Media

The middle ear inoculations caused severe acute otitis media, and six of the gerbils died before the first 24 hour examination. By day 2 the four remaining gerbils showed otoscopic score 5 otitis media[2] or had exudate filling the external auditory canal. On histologic examination at days 2 and 4, each animal showed a massive bloody exudate with many polymorphonuclear leukocytes and an edematous mucoperiosteum. These animals also had developed bilateral otitis media (histologic score 3).[3] In addition the animal sacrificed on day 4 showed histologic evidence of bone erosion and suffered right eye destruction by the infection.

Otitis Externa

Table 1 shows the otoscopic results of infection with *P. aeruginosa*. Within 48 hours the majority of group 1 and group 3 animals developed severe otitis externa, and the majority of group 2 animals developed mild otitis externa. Animals that showed a wet ear or exudate in the external auditory canal almost invariably developed severe disease within 48 hours. Histologic examination of animals with frank otitis externa by otoscopic examination revealed an edematous subepithelium, epithelial hyperplasia, and copious exudate containing mostly polymorphonuclear leukocytes (Fig. 1). In these animals histologic examination showed an associated severe acute otitis media with abundant polymorphonuclear leukocytes, an edematous mucoperiosteum, fibrosis, and bone erosion (Fig. 2). Tympanic membranes often were destroyed by neutrophilic infiltration. Associated contralateral otitis media occasionally was seen.

DISCUSSION

Wright and Dineen[8] attempted to utilize the gerbil as a model of otitis externa; however, all their treated gerbils died. In this study we have shown that otoscopic and histologic findings of otitis externa can be produced consistently by instillation of *P. aeruginosa* into the external auditory canal of the Mongolian gerbil. All animals exhibiting a wet slimy external auditory canal with exudate in the canal showed middle ear disease. Severe otitis externa almost always progressed to severe otitis media, whereas mild otitis externa when accompanied by tympanic membrane involvement progressed to less severe otitis media.

We conclude that the Mongolian gerbil can serve as a model for the study of otitis externa caused by *P. aeruginosa*. Animals showing a wet ear or exudate in the external auditory canal may be useful for the testing of antibiotic therapy.

We thank John M. Worthington and James S. Harris for technical assistance.

This work was supported by a grant from the Deafness Research Foundation.

REFERENCES

1. Fulghum RS, Brinn JE, Smith AM, Daniel HJ III, Loesche PJ. Experimental otitis media in gerbils and chinchillas with *Streptococcus pneumoniae, Haemophilus influenzae* and other areobic and anaerobic bacteria. Infect Immun 1982; 36:802–810.

TABLE 1 Otoscopic Results

Experiment	Day	Animals Examined	Normal	Inflammation or Increased Cerumen Present	Otitis Externa with Exudate
1	1	10	2	7	1
	2	10	1	4	5
	7	4	1	2	1
	10	3	1	2	0
	16	3	1	2	0
2	1	10	4	5	1
	2	8	4	4	0
	5	8	2	4	2
	7	6	2	3	1
3	1	10	1	5	4
	2	9	2	1	6
	3	7	4	1	2
	4	4	1	1	2
	7	3	1	1	1
	13	3	1	1	1

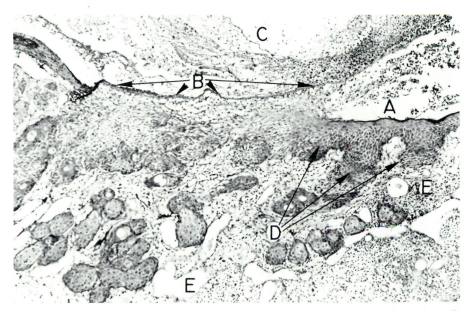

Figure 1 Pathologic changes in otitis externa showing external ear canal *A*, tympanic membrane *B*, and middle ear cavity *C*, with neutrophilic exudate; epithelial hyperplasia *D*, and subepithelial edema and inflammation *E* (30 ×).

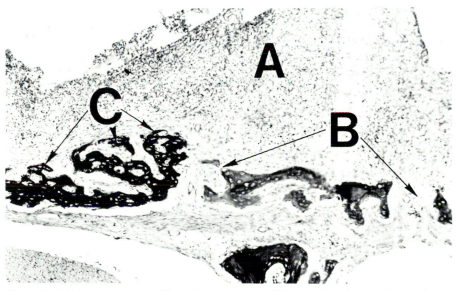

Figure 2 Pathologic changes in otitis media showing the middle ear cavity with fibrosis and polymorphonuclear leukocytes *A*, bone erosion *B*, and new bone formation *C*. The mucoperiosteum has been destroyed in this specimen (30 ×).

2. Fulghum RS, Hoogmoed RP, Brinn JE. Longitudinal studies of experimental otitis media with *Haemophilus influenzae* in the gerbil. Int J Pediatr Otorhinolaryngol 1985; 9:101–114.
3. Beamer ME, Fulghum RS, Marrow HG, Allen WE, Brinn JE, Daniel HJ III. The Mongolian gerbil as a model of otitis media caused by anaerobic bacteria. In: Sade J, ed. Acute and secretory otitis media. Amsterdam: Kugler Publications, 1986:221.
4. Senturia BH. Etiology of external otitis. Laryngoscope 1945; 55:277–293.
5. Harker LA, Koontz FP. Bacteriology of cholesteatoma. In: Cholesteatoma—first international conference. Birmingham,

AL: Aesculapius, 1977:264.
6. Fulghum RS, Chole RA. Bacterial flora in spontaneously occuring aural cholesteatomas in Mongolian gerbils. Infect Immun 1985; 50:678–681.
7. Nadol JB. Histopathology of *Pseudomonas* osteomyelitis of the temporal bone starting as malignant external otitis. Am J Otolaryngol 1980;1:359–371.
8. Wright DN, Dineen M. A model for the study of infectious otitis externa. Arch Otolaryngol 1972; 95:243–247.
9. Stone M, Fulghum RS. Bactericidal activity of wet cerum. Ann Otol Rhinol Laryngol 1984; 93:183–186.

EXPERIMENTALLY INDUCED MUCOID EFFUSION IN RAT MIDDLE EAR—A COMPLETE MODEL FOR OTITIS MEDIA RESEARCH?

STEN O.M. HELLSTRÖM, M.D., Ph.D., ANN HERMANSSON, M.D., ULF JOHANSSON, M.D., and KARIN PRELLNER, M.D., Ph.D.

Otitis media can be classified as purulent, serous, or mucoid, depending on the otomicroscopic appearance and physical properties of the effusion material. Although these conditions may occur separately, mixed types are common in the clinical situation. In order to study these clinical entities under standardized conditions, various animal models have been developed. In the rat, serous otitis media can be provoked by obstruction of the tympanic orifice of the eustachian tube[1] and purulent otitis media can be provoked by clefting the soft palate.[2] In the latter model the middle ear is invaded by the endogenous nasopharyngeal bacterial flora. Recently it has been shown that the rat develops purulent otitis media if the middle ear is subjected to inoculation by a human pathogen (*S. pneumoniae*). The condition otomicroscopically resembles that observed in man, and the animals recover spontaneously within 8 to 10 days.[3] In the present contribution we report that otitis media with a mucoid effusion can also be experimentally developed in the rat. The condition is achieved through a two step procedure.

MATERIALS AND METHODS

Step 1. Inoculation of Bacteria

Under intravenous anesthesia a ventral midline incision was made in the neck and the tympanic bulla was dissected free in 10 healthy male Sprague-Dawley rats. The bulla was punctured by a cannula through which *S. pneumoniae* type 6A was inoculated. The challenge dose was 2.5×10^6 CFU. All animals developed purulent otitis media within 48 hours.

Step 2. Blockage of the Eustachian Tube

Ten days later, when all the infected ears were otomicroscopically normal, the animals were anesthetized and again a ventral midline incision was made in the neck. Through a hole in the tympanic bulla, the tympanic orifice of the eustachian tube was obstructed by inserting a gutta-percha plug.

From the day of inoculation of bacteria until blocking of the tube, the animals were anesthetized daily and the tympanic membrane examined. After blocking the tube, otomicroscopic inspection was performed every 2 weeks until the animals were sacrificed. Five animals were sacrificed 1 month after blocking the tube and five animals after 3 months. In killing the animals the consistency of the effusion material was determined, and then the material was collected and frozen for immunochemical analysis. The middle ears were fixed by immersion in 3 percent glutaraldehyde and processed for light and electron microscopy.

RESULTS

By otomicroscopic examination eight of 10 middle ear cavities were seen to be filled with a yellowish fluid. The pars flaccida was retracted and exhibited dilated vessels (as did the pars tensa). At 3 months extensive areas with semilunar tympanosclerotic plaques appeared in the central portion of the pars tensa. Upon opening the bulla, the middle ear cavities were found to be filled completely with a mucoid effusion. The effusion material was highly viscous and could be drawn as threads. In the two ears that did not contain any effusion material, the plugs had escaped from the tympanic orifice.

The most dramatic histologic changes were noted in the fibrous layer of the tympanic membrane and in the epithelial lining of the middle ear cavity. The connective tissue layer of the pars tensa was thickened, frequently with a rounded protrusion toward the middle ear cavity (Fig. 1A). Within the newly formed connective tissue, particularly in the vicinity of the collagenous fibers, amorphous masses

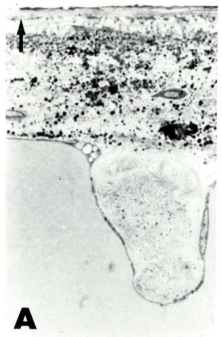

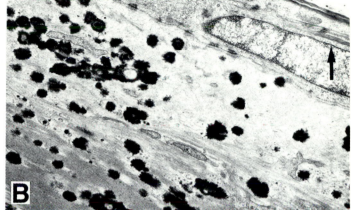

Figure 1 *A*, Light microscopic view of a section of the pars tensa from an animal with a mucoid effusion in the middle ear cavity. The connective tissue layer is thickened, particularly the submucosal portion. Within the connective tissue, amorphous deposits of hyaline substance are seen. Arrow, Keratinizing stratified squamous epithelium. (Toluidine blue stain. 1,000×). *B*, Electron micrograph of an area depicted in *A* (10,000×).

of a hyaline substance were deposited (Fig. 1*B*). The epithelial lining of the middle ear cavity was also substantially altered. Areas normally covered by flat squamous epithelium were now covered by a cuboidal-columnar epithelium with goblet and ciliated cells.

The results of immunochemical analyses of the effusion material (albumin, transferrin, and IgG) are shown in Figure 2. By comparison with serous effusion material these proteins occurred in considerably higher concentrations in the mucoid effusions. By contrast, the level of a specific IgG fraction—

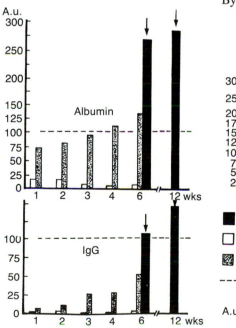

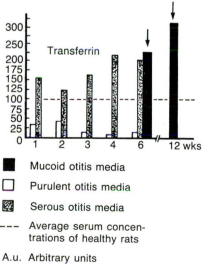

Figure 2 Graphs depicting the mean values of albumin, transferrin, and IgG determined by rocket immunoelectrophoresis in mucoid effusions. The levels are compared to those estimated in experimentally elicited serous and purulent middle ear effusions. The dotted lines represent the average serum concentrations in healthy Sprague-Dawley rats.

IgG, (not shown in the figure)—was lower in the mucoid effusion than in the serous effusion material.

This study showed that an inflammatory condition with an effusion material having an otomicroscopic appearance and consistency resembling that of mucoid effusion in man can be developed experimentally in the rat. The condition is produced through a two step procedure—infection-recovery—followed by obstruction of the eustachian tube.

Morphologically the secretory elements of the middle ear epithelial lining were increased. The pars tensa showed advanced structural changes resembling those associated with tympanosclerosis in humans.[4] Immunochemically the mucoid effusion appears to be more rich in proteins than serous effusion material.

The technique described—and those previously mentioned[1,2]—make it possible to experimentally provoke well defined types of purulent, serous, and mucoid effusions in the same species. This possibility favors use of the rat as an animal model for otitis media research.

Study supported by grants from the Swedish Medical Research Council (17X-6578), The Ragnar and Torsten Söderbergs Stiftelser, and the Ingabritt och Arne Lundbergs Research Foundation.

REFERENCES

1. Hellström S, Salén B, Stenfors L-E. The site of initial production and transport of effusion materials in otitis media serosa. Acta Otolaryngol (Stockh) 1982; 93:435–440.
2. Hellström S, Salén B, Stenfors L-E, Söderberg O. Appearance of effusion material in the attic space correlated to an impaired eustachian tube function. Int J Pediatr Otorhinolaryngol 1983; 6:127–134.
3. Hermansson A, Emgård P, Prellner K, Hellström S. A rat model for experimental otitis media with *S. pneumoniae*. Am J Otolaryngol (in press).
4. Sörensen H, True O. Histology of tympanosclerosis. Acta Otolaryngol (Stockh) 1971; 73:18–22.

STRUCTURAL CHANGES OF THE MIDDLE EAR IN EXPERIMENTALLY EVOKED SEROUS AND PURULENT OTITIS MEDIA—A STUDY OF TWO BARRIER REGIONS

LOUISE WIDEMAR, M.D., Ph.D., STEN O.M. HELLSTRÖM, M.D., Ph.D., ÅSA NORDLING, B.M., and ULF JOHANSSON, M.D.

Evidence is accumulating that a fluid filled middle ear cavity not only alters the mechanics of the middle ear but also may cause sensorineural hearing loss by encouraging the passage of inflammatory agents through the round window membrane.[1] In the rat various well defined conditions of otitis media can be evoked by experimental procedures. In the present study we compared the effects of serous and purulent effusions on the morphology of two barrier regions, the tympanic membrane and the round window.

MATERIALS AND METHODS

Adult male Sprague-Dawley rats were used for the study and subjected to the following procedures during anesthesia:

1. In one group of rats, sterile serous otitis media was provoked by plugging the eustachian tube through a hole in the tympanic bulla.[2]
2. In another group of animals, purulent otitis media developed after cleaving the soft palate.[3]

The tympanic membrane was checked otomicroscopically throughout the study. At 1, 2, and 6 weeks, animals were sacrificed and specimens representing certain areas of the middle ear cavity e.g., the tympanic membrane and the round window, were collected for light and electron microscopy. Some fixed middle ear cavities were stained in situ by toluidine blue or treated with avidin peroxidase for the identification of mast cells.

RESULTS

The two types of inflammatory conditions of the middle ear were associated with different structural alterations of the epithelial and subepithelial layers. However, within respective groups—serous and purulent otitis media—the mucosal lining exhibited similar changes in the tympanic membrane and the round window membrane (Figs. 1 and 2).

In serous otitis media the different portions of the tympanic membrane and the round window membrane were of about the same thickness when compared to control ears. The epithelial linings facing the middle ear cavity at these two sites also appeared normal. The blood vessels of the pars flaccida and along the handle of the malleus were dilated. The round window membrane in the rat is only sparsely vascularized, and the vascular architecture showed only minor changes during serous otitis media. The number of mast cells in the pars flaccida decreased sharply—about 50 percent during the first week of tubal blockage.[4] In the round window membrane no mast cells were seen in either the serous otitis media group or the control group.

In purulent otitis media both the tympanic membrane and the round window membrane increased about three times in thickness. Although the structural changes affected all layers, the major alterations were confined to the epithelium facing the middle ear cavity. This epithelial lining changed from a single layer of flat cuboidal cells to a pseudostratified cylindrical epithelium containing secretory and ciliated cells. The richly vascularized connective tissue layer was invaded by numerous inflammatory cells. In the pars flaccida the number of mast cells increased about 60 percent.[4] Mast cells also were found in the pars tensa in areas normally devoid of these cells. No mast cells, however, were observed in the round window membrane. The epithelium of the round window membrane facing the perilymphatic space appeared normal.

DISCUSSION

The study showed that the structure of different regions in the middle ear cavity alters under the influence of inflammatory conditions. The changes specifically reflect the different types of otitis media. Whereas serous otitis media caused only

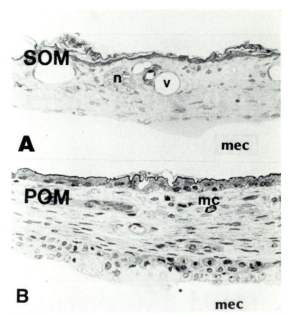

Figure 1 Pars flaccida in *A*, serous otitis media (SOM) and *B*, purulent otitis media (POM). MEC, middle ear cavity. MC, mast cell. N, nerve fiber. V, blood vessel. 400 ×.

minor alterations of the tympanic membrane and round window membrane, purulent otitis was associated with profound changes of the epithelium facing the middle ear cavity as well as the connective tissue layer. The conversion of the flat cuboidal epithelium to a pseudostratified respiratory epithelium occurred rapidly and seemed to be pathognomonic

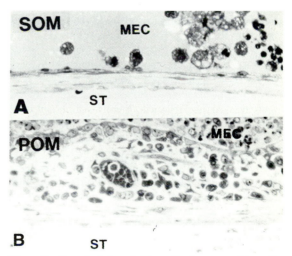

Figure 2 Round window membrane in *A*, serous otitis media (SOM) and *B*, purulent otitis media (POM). MEC, middle ear cavity. ST, scala tympani.

for middle ear infection. The extent to which these inflammatory conditions affect the inner ear remains to be elucidated. In serous otitis media components of the effusion may easily pass through the thin round window membrane, whereas the thickened membrane in purulent otitis media could act as a barrier. However, in the latter case the effusion contains many more potent agents related to the infection.

Study supported by grants from the Swedish Medical Research Council (17X6578), The Ragnar and Torsten Söderbergs Foundations, and the Ingabritt and Arne Lundbergs Research Foundation.

REFERENCES

1. Paparella MM, Morizono T, Le T, Mancini F, Sipilä P, Choo YB, Lidén G, Kim CS. Sensorineural hearing loss in otitis media. Ann Otol Rhinol Laryngol 1984; 93:623–629.
2. Hellström S, Salén B, Stenfors L-E. The site of initial production and transport of effusion materials in otitis media serosa. Acta Otolaryngol Stockh 1982; 93:435–440.
3. Hellström S, Salén B, Stenfors L-E, Söderberg O. Appearance of effusion material in the attic space correlated to an impaired eustachian tube function. Int J Pediatr Otorhinolaryngol 1983; 6:127–134.
4. Hellström S, Nordling Å, Albiin N, Widemar L. Middle ear mast cells. In: Veldman J, ed. Immunobiology, Histophysiology and Tumor Immunology in Otolaryngology. Amsterdam: Kugler, 1987:267.

MECHANISMS INVOLVED IN PRODUCTION OF MIDDLE EAR EFFUSION BY IRRITATION OF THE EXTERNAL AUDITORY CANAL

PAMELA GOLDIE, M.D. and STEN O.M. HELLSTRÖM, M.D., Ph.D.

Various experimental techniques have been used to elicit the formation of middle ear fluid in animal models.[1] Mechanical stimulation by blowing a stream of cold air into the external auditory canal provokes the accumulation of fluid in the attic space medial to the flaccid portion of the tympanic membrane.[2] The pars flaccida exhibits the most pronounced tympanic membrane changes, such as retraction, dilated vessels, and edema.

The pars flaccida is unique for several reasons. In contrast to the pars tensa, it houses abundant mast cells and neuropeptide containing nerve fibers. These neuropeptides—substance P, vasoactive intestinal polypeptide, and enkephalin—are located exclusively in the pars flaccida of the tympanic membrane, whereas the catecholamines are distributed throughout both the pars tensa and the pars flaccida.[3] The histamine content of mast cells, vasoactive intestinal polypeptide, and substance P all have powerful edema provoking capacity.

In the present study we tried to determine whether the effusion produced when stimulating the external auditory canal with an air stream is a temperature related phenomenon and whether the autonomic nervous system influences these mechanisms.

MATERIAL AND METHOD

The study was performed in male Sprague-Dawley rats. Air of different temperatures was blown into the left external auditory canal for 20 minutes at an air flow rate of 2.5 liters per minute. The temperatures selected were 14° C, defined as cold air, 22° C, equaling room temperature, and 34° C, which corresponds to the temperature in the rat external auditory canal. One group of animals was subjected to denervation procedures 1 week prior to mechanical stimulation with a 14° C stream of air. Sympathectomy was performed by removal of the superior cervical ganglion, and vagotomy by sectioning the vagal nerve immediately below the base of the skull. To detect vascular leakage, Evans blue was administered intravenously immediately prior to the start of mechanical stimulation. After stimulation the pars flaccidae were fixed, dissected out, and embedded for microscopy. On sections, the thickness of the pars flaccida was measured, the vessel volume determined, and the proportion of degranulated mast cells estimated.

RESULTS

In the first set of experiments the role of the temperature in effusion production initiated by mechanical stimulation was evaluated. Fluid production was detected in all the animals exposed to a 14° C air stream. Leakage of Evans blue was observed only occasionally after stimulation with air at 22° C. When stimulated at 34° C, none of the animals exhibited leakage. The thickness of the pars flaccida was markedly increased in ears exposed to the 14° C air stream but not after exposure to 22 or 34° C.

In the second set of experiments we studied this process of effusion production in denervated animals. Sympathectomy itself caused increased thickening of the pars flaccida. Vagotomy caused extravasation of middle ear fluid but did not affect pars flaccida thickness. After stimulation with the 14° C air stream, fluid production was observed in the sympathectomized animals (Fig. 1A) but not in any of the vagotomized ears (Fig. 1B). The stimulation did not alter the pars flaccida thickness in sympathectomized animals, but the pars flaccida in the vagotomized animals showed a marked increase in thickness. Morphometric evaluation of the blood vessels revealed a diminished vascular area in sympathectomized animals after stimulation with cold air. Vagotomy in itself caused an increase in the vascular volume. Stimulation with cold air did not alter this volume.

Regarding mast cells, both the intact and the two groups of denervated animals showed about 25 percent degranulated mast cells in the pars flaccida bilaterally.

DISCUSSION

The present study showed that effusion production, caused by blowing a stream of air into the external auditory canal, is a temperature related phenomenon—cold air being a prerequisite.[4] The production of fluid is dependant on an intact vagal nerve indicating that the parasympathetic system is involved.[5] Acetylcholine, the classic transmitter of the parasympathetic system, and certain coexisting neuropeptides may independently or together increase blood vessel permeability, as indicated by

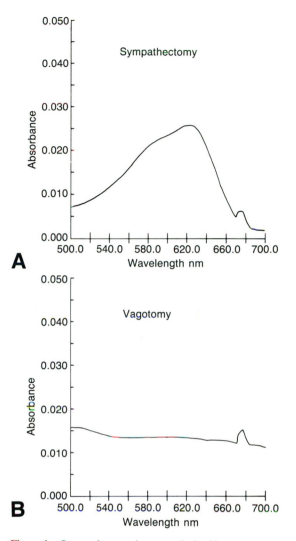

Figure 1 Spectrophotometric curves obtained in analyzing the effusion material from the middle ear cavity for the presence of Evans blue, a tracer used to detect vascular leakage. *A*, Sympathectomized animal. *B*, Vagotomized animal.

preliminary data from our laboratory.[6] In the nasal mucosa, acetylcholine has been shown to coexist with vasoactive intestinal polypeptide in parasympathetic nerve terminals.[7] A similar phenomenon may exist in the pars flaccida. Concomitant with properties causing an increased blood flow, vasoactive intestinal polypeptide has a pronounced edema provoking capacity and may increase the permeability of the pars flaccida vessels when it is released from nerve terminals.

Measurements of the blood vessels showed that vascular leakage with an increased vascular permeability cannot be predicted from the vascular volume. That stimulation with cold air in sympathectomized animals caused vasoconstriction could indicate that cold air, in the absence of vasodilatory factors in the parasympathetic system, may stimulate blood vessel smooth muscle via mechanoreceptors, causing vasoconstriction. It should be noted, however, that in the pars tensa, Yeh and Kruger[8] could not find any mechanoreceptors.

The number of degranulated mast cells was not related to the accumulation of middle ear fluid. This does not exclude mast cell involvement, as histamine can be released through mechanisms other than degranulation.[9] This is indicated by earlier studies in which the middle ear fluid contained considerable amounts of histamine.[2]

In regard to other areas of the respiratory tract it is known that cold may provoke inflammatory reactions, e.g., bronchial asthma. Such mechanisms may play a role in the early events of otitis media.

This study was supported by grants from the Swedish Medical Research Council (B85-17X-6578-803B), Ingabritt och Arne Lundbergs forskningsstiftelse, and Torsten och Ragnar Söderbergs stiftelser.

REFERENCES

1. Salén B, Hellström S, Stenfors L-E. Experimentally induced otitis media with effusion. Acta Otolaryngol [Suppl] (Stockh) 1984; 414:67–70.
2. Widemar L, Alm PE, Bloom GD, Hellström S, Stenfors L-E. Middle ear effusion caused by mechanical stimulation of the external auditory canal. Acta Otolaryngol (Stockh) 1983; 96:91–98.
3. Widemar L, Hellström S, Schultzberg U, Stenfors L-E. Autonomic innervation of the tympanic membrane. An immunocytochemical and histofluorescence study. Acta Otolaryngol (Stockh) 1985; 100:58–65.
4. Goldie P, Hellström S. Middle ear effusion induced by a stream of air in the external auditory canal. Acta Otolaryngol (Stockh) 1986; 102:248–256.
5. Goldie P, Hellström S. Autonomic nerves and middle ear fluid production. Acta Otolaryngol (Stockh) (in press).
6. Hellström S, Albiin N, Goldie P, Salén B, Stenfors L-E. Pharmacological characterization of receptors on blood vessels in the tympanic membrane involved in otitis media. Auris Nasus Larynx 1985; 12 (Suppl 1):S135–S137.
7. Lundberg JM, Änggård A, Fahrenkrug J, Hökfelt T, Mutt V. Vasoactive intestinal polypeptide in cholinergic neurons of exocrine glands: functional significance of co-existing transmitters for vasodilatation and secretion. Proc Natl Acad Sci USA 1980;77:1651–1655.
8. Yeh Y, Kruger L. Fine-structural characterization of the somatic innervation of the tympanic membrane in normal, sympathectomized and neurotoxin-denervated rats. Somatosens Res 1984; 1:359–378.
9. Galli SJ, Dvorak AM, Dvorak HF. Basophils and mast cells: morphologic insights into their biology, secretory patterns and function. In: Ishizaka K, ed. Mast cell activation and mediator release. Prog Allergy 1984; 34:69–76.

EXPERIMENTALLY INDUCED TYMPANOSCLEROSIS

WIM KUIJPERS, Ph.D., EIZE WIELINGA, M.D., EDITH TONNAER, M.D., and PAUL H.K. JAP, M.D.

Tympanosclerosis, a disease that affects both the tympanic membrane and the middle ear mucosa, is characterized by an increase in collagenous fibers as well as hyaline degeneration in the lamina propria. Calcification and occasionally ossification can occur secondarily in these areas.[1-4]

The pathogenesis of tympanosclerosis is still unclear, but there is uniform agreement that this disease is associated with an inflammatory disease of the middle ear cavity and is a frequent sequel of chronic otitis media.[1, 5-8]

In this study an experimental model is presented in which tympanosclerosis was evoked during the course of sterile otitis media induced by obstruction of the eustachian tube.

METHODS

The eustachian tube in 50 germ-free rats was obstructed by electrocautery, as described previously.[9] After survival times varying from 1 week up to 2 years the animals were sacrificed and the temporal bones processed for light and electron microscopy.

Throughout the observation period the condition of the tympanic membrane was regularly monitored by otoscopy.

RESULTS

Within 1 week after eustachian tube obstruction, the middle ear cleft became filled with a clear yellow serous fluid, persisting there without significant changes for up to 2 years. Cultures failed to reveal any bacterial contamination throughout the observation period. The changes observed in the middle ear mucosa were described extensively in a previous publication.[10]

Otoscopy showed in all animals the presence of scattered white spots in the central part of the pars tensa 3 weeks after obstruction. The number and size of these spots gradually increased, sometimes leading to a horseshoe shaped white plaque after 2 years. Microscopic sections showed slight edema, increased fibroblast activity, fiber formation, and fiber degeneration in the loose submucosal connective tissue in the central parts of the pars tensa during the first weeks after obstruction (Figs. 1 and 3).

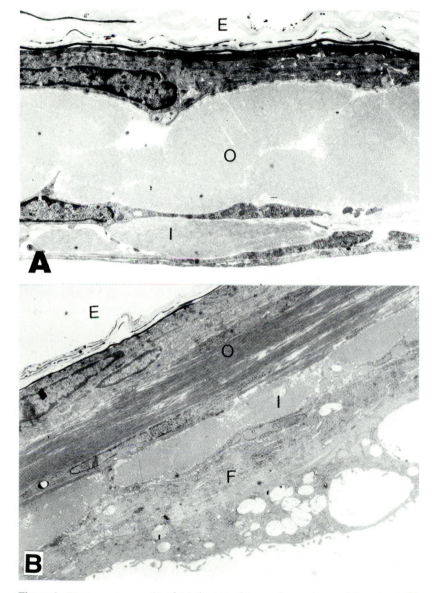

Figure 1 Electron micrographs of (A) the normal tympanic membrane of the rat and (B) 1 week after eustachian tube obstruction. Note the increased activity of the fibroblasts in the submucosal connective tissue (F). The mucosal cells are hypertrophic and contain many vacuoles. E, external meatus. I, inner circular layer. O, outer radiate layer.

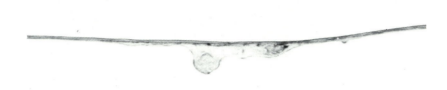

Figure 2 Light micrograph of the tympanic membrane, showing local outpouching 2 weeks after eustachian tube obstruction.

Local outpouchings of the mucosa contained varying numbers of fibroblasts and hyaline material (Fig. 2). With progression of time the number of collagenous fibers, arranged in various directions, further increased, leading to thickening of the membrane; occasionally osteoid-like and cartilaginous matrices were formed. Simultaneously progressive degeneration of the inner circular layer of collagenous fibers was established. After more than 6 months the outer radiate layer also became involved in this process.

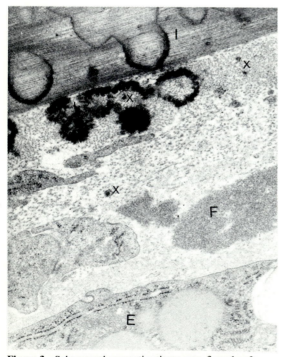

Figure 3 Submucosal connective tissue area, 3 weeks after eustachian tube obstruction. Note active fibroblasts, newly formed fibers, degenerating fibers F, and matrix vesicles as the primary sites of calcification (x). I, inner circular layer. E, mucosal cell with vacuoles.

The presence of matrix vesicles, forming the primary sites of calcification, was first observed after 2 weeks (see Fig. 3). Calcification, consisting of shell-like deposits, was first established, scattered throughout the submucosal connective tissue and especially close to the inner circular layer (see Fig. 3). Subsequently these deposits increased in size, and through fusion large irregular plaques appeared (Fig. 4). X-ray microanalysis by an energy dispersive x-ray analyzer revealed that these deposits were composed of calcium and phosphate. With progression of time the entire inner circular layer and even the outer radiate layer became involved in this calcification process (see Fig. 4).

Concomitantly with the increase in calcification, the mucosal lining cells showed decreased activity. Occasionally fractionation of the calcified lamina propria was observed. This could lead to microperforations of the tympanic membrane. Throughout the course of this process no inflammatory cells were found in the tympanic membrane.

DISCUSSION

This study convincingly demonstrates that tympanosclerosis is not necessarily associated with infective middle ear disease. The most likely explanation for the phenomena observed is that these reactions are triggered by the underpressure induced by eustachian tube obstruction, although the possible role of components of the accumulated serous fluid cannot be excluded. This process involves stimulation of fibroblasts, fiber formation, and fiber degeneration followed by calcified plaque formation. The histologic features in this experimentally induced process are similar to those described in human tympanic membranes.[4,7,11]

With the use of this animal model tympano-

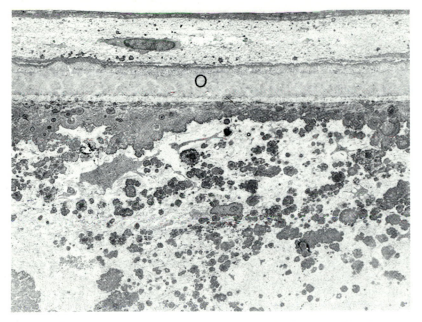

Figure 4 Tympanic membrane 4 months after eustachian tube obstruction. The submucosal area reveals extensive calcification. The inner circular layer is nearly completely calcified. O, outer-radiate layer.

sclerosis can be studied with high reproducibility. It therefore offers the opportunity for studying the effects of surgical intervention and of agents that can interfere with this process.

REFERENCES

1. Igarashi M, Konishi S, Alford BR, Guilford FR. The pathology of tympanosclerosis. Laryngoscope 1970; 80:233–243.
2. Sheehy JL, House WF. Tympanosclerosis. Arch Otolaryngol 1962; 76:151–157.
3. Zöllner F. Tympanosclerosis. Arch Otolaryngol 1963; 78:538–544.
4. Chang IW. Tympanosclerosis. Acta Otolaryngol (Stockh) 1969; 68:62–72.
5. Tos M, Bak Pederesen K. Middle ear mucosa in tympano-sclerosis. J Laryngol Otol 1974; 88:119–126.
6. Ferlito A. Histogenesis of tympanosclerosis. J Laryngol Otol 1979; 93:25–37.
7. Friedmann I, Hodges GM, Graham M. Tympanosclerosis, an electron-microscopic study of matrix vesicles. Ann Otol Rhinol Laryngol 1980; Suppl 68:241–245.
8. Gibb AG. Tympanosclerosis. Proc Soc Med 1976; 69:155–162.
9. Kuijpers W, van der Beek JMH. The role of microorganisms in experimental eustachian tube obstruction. Acta Otolaryngol (Stockh) 1984; Suppl 414:58–66.
10. van der Beek JMH, Kuijpers W. The mucoperiosteum of the middle ear in experimentally induced sterile otitis media. Acta Otolaryngol (Stockh) 1984; Suppl 414:71–79.
11. Møller P. Tympanosclerosis of the ear drum in secretory otitis media. Acta Otolaryngol (Stockh) 1984; Suppl 414:171–177.

PROPYLENE GLYCOL INDUCED CHOLESTEATOMA IN CHINCHILLA MIDDLE EARS

LUCA VASSALLI, M.D., DAVID M. HARRIS, Ph.D., ROBERTO GRADINI, M.D., and EDWARD L. APPLEBAUM, M.D.

Propylene glycol (1,2-propanediol) is a short chain alcohol containing two hydroxyl groups. It is used as a solvent in many topically applied ear preparations. Several investigators have reported that the topical application of propylene glycol in high concentration is capable of causing inflammatory changes of the middle ear mucosa.[1-3] A study by Vernon and Brummett[2] evaluated the effects of different concentrations of propylene glycol in the middle ear of guinea pigs. They found that a 90 percent solution caused extensive middle ear adhesions, whereas a 10 percent solution did not produce any negative effects.

Wright and Meyerhoff[4] reported that the topical application of Cortisporin otic suspension to the chinchilla middle ear was capable of consistently producing inflammatory changes, squamous metaplasia of the middle ear mucosa, and cholesteatoma. Cortisporin otic suspension contains polymyxin B, neomycin, hydrocortisone, and 10.5 percent propylene gylcol.

Our previous study using Cortisporin suspension in a single dose middle ear instillation produced middle ear inflammation and cholesteatoma largely among the group that received Cortisporin with 10.5 percent propylene glycol, but only a mild inflammatory response (serous effusion) was induced in the chinchilla bullae that were tested with Cortisporin with 2 percent propylene glycol.[5]

The purpose in this study was to evaluate the effects on the middle ear of the topical application of propylene glycol alone. The experimental design was somewhat different from that in previous studies in that the drugs were applied once daily for 5 consecutive days rather than using a single application.

MATERIALS AND METHODS

Sixteen adult chinchillas were used for this study. Propylene glycol was diluted with sterile water to obtain concentrations of 10, 50, and 90 percent. Thirty-two ears in the 16 animals were randomly assigned to four groups. Three groups received propylene glycol in concentrations of 10, 50, and 90 percent. The control group received normal saline.

Each animal was anesthetized by giving 30 mg of ketamine hydrochloride intramuscularly. Under sterile conditions a small semilunar incision was made into the superior aspect of each bulla. The skin and periosteum were reflected to expose a small amount of bone that was carefully removed. An aliquot of 0.2 ml of the test solution was instilled into the bulla through the bony opening. The skin and periosteum were then closed over the bony defect with absorbable sutures. The purpose in removing bone was to facilitate subsequent applications of the drugs without the need for general anesthesia.

Subsequent propylene glycol instillations were made through the bone defect using a 25 gauge needle inserted through the skin directly into the bulla, and 0.2 ml of the test solution was injected using a tuberculin syringe. A second needle was also inserted adjacent to the first one to allow the escape of air displaced by the injection, thus preventing tympanic membrane perforations and other trauma from increased air pressure during injection. Each ear was treated once a day for 4 consecutive days following the initial application at surgery, a total of five treatments. All 16 animals were sacrificed 6 weeks following the initial application. Immediately after sacrifice each ear was carefully examined with a dissecting microscope through two openings in the superior and medial walls of the bulla. The presence or absence of middle ear adhesions, tympanic membrane perforations, and cholesteatoma was recorded.

The temporal bones were then fixed in 10 percent formalin and prepared for histologic study. Each bulla was decalcified using D-Calcifier (Lerner Laboratories, New Haven, Connecticut). After paraffin embedding, specimens were serially cut to obtain sections 3 to 4 μm thick for light microscopy. Most slides were stained with hematoxylin and eosin. Selected slides from areas of mucosa in the vicinity of cholesteatomas, in ears that received 50 percent propylene glycol, were treated with polyclonal antibodies to detect keratin, utilizing the

TABLE 1 **Number of Perforations and**
Cholesteatoma Observed for Each
Concentration of Propylene Glycol

Experimental Group*	Perforation	Cholesteatoma
Normal saline	0	0
10% propylene glycol	1	1
50% propylene glycol	4	5
90% propylene glycol	7	7

* Eight in each group.

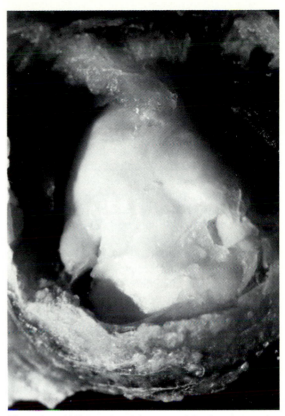

Figure 1 Middle ear viewed from an opening into the superior wall of the bulla. Cholesteatoma is seen replacing the entire middle ear space.

peroxidase-antiperoxidase technique. The antibody used was the rabbit polyclonal antikeratin (wide spectrum screening) at a 1:500 dilution (Dako Corporation, Santa Barbara, California).

RESULTS

Macroscopic examination revealed striking differences in pathologic findings between ears treated with 10 and 90 percent propylene glycol (Table 1). Seven of the eight ears that received 90 percent propylene glycol had cholesteatoma filling the middle ear (Fig. 1). In most of these ears not even a remnant of tympanic membrane could be found, and cholesteatoma was clearly visible through the external auditory canal. Macroscopically the bone of the bulla appeared spongy, the result of

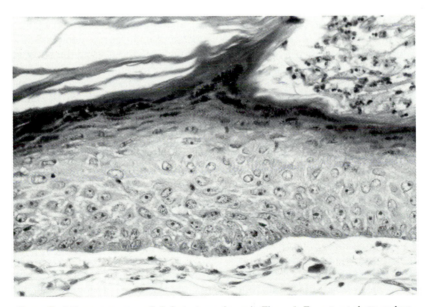

Figure 2 Microscopic view of cholesteatoma shown in Figure 1. From top to bottom: keratin, keratinizing stratified squamous epithelium, and underlying granulation tissue. (Hematoxylin and eosin stain; 400 ×).

extensive bone erosion, which was confirmed histologically.

Histologic findings in this group were uniform. Cholesteatoma was lined by a keratinizing stratified squamous epithelium (Fig. 2). The epithelium was surrounded by abundant granulation tissue, which infiltrated and eroded the bony walls of the middle ear. Bone erosion appeared to occur secondary to osteoclastic activity, since osteoclasts frequently were seen at the interphase of granulation tissue and bone. Normal columnar epithelium of the middle ear was seen in only one bulla in this group; in this ear the tympanic membrane and middle ear architecture were surprisingly normal.

Among the eight ears treated with 50 percent propylene glycol, cholesteatoma was found in five. In two of these the findings were similar to those in the group exposed to the 90 percent concentration. The middle ears were completely filled with cholesteatoma, with complete obliteration of the tympanic membrane and ossicles. In the remaining three ears cholesteatoma was found on the medial aspect of the tympanic membrane. In two of these there was an associated tympanic membrane perforation, while in one a cholesteatoma originated from the medial surface of an intact tympanic membrane.

Histologic findings in this group were similar to those in animals with large cholesteatomas. However, squamous metaplasia of the middle ear mucosa was often seen in this group. Areas of normal, mucin secreting, columnar epithelium frequently were found next to stratified squamous epithelium. In the early stages of squamous metaplasia, the columnar epithelium became stratified, and the basal layer was found to produce keratohyalin granules when the tissues were studied by the immunoperoxidase technique. In other cases the columnar epithelium was completely replaced by keratinizing stratified squamous epithelium.

In the remaining three ears treated with 50 percent propylene glycol, cholesteatoma or tympanic membrane perforations were not seen. However, all these ears had fibrous adhesions in the middle ear.

Fibrous adhesions were commonly found also in the remaining two groups. Both the normal saline control and the 10 percent propylene glycol groups demonstrated middle ear adhesions in four of the eight bullae. It is possible that middle ear adhesions, although a sign of inflammation, are more likely a consequence of the surgical trauma rather than an effect of propylene glycol application. Of the ears treated with 10 percent propylene glycol, only one had a cholesteatoma. In the normal saline group, no cholesteatomas were found.

DISCUSSION

In the present study we showed that cholesteatoma can be produced consistently by the application of 90 percent propylene glycol to chinchilla middle ears. More than half the ears treated with 50 percent propylene glycol also developed cholesteatoma, but only one was seen in the group treated with a 10 percent solution. Although these findings alone provide us with important information concerning the effects of the otic preparation evaluated, pathologic study of these experimentally produced cholesteatomas may provide insight into their pathogenesis.

The migration and metaplastic theories of cholesteatoma formation have both received support from histologic findings in rodent and human cholesteatomas.[6-8] In our study all but one cholesteatoma were found in ears that also had tympanic membrane perforations. In the middle ears that were totally filled with cholesteatoma, it was impossible to determine where the keratinizing epithelium originated. Smaller cholesteatomas were always found in association with tympanic membrane perforations. Strands of keratin sometimes could be seen traveling from the medial aspect of the tympanic membrane to the inferior portion of the bulla where more keratin had accumulated. These macroscopic observations suggest that migration of squamous epithelium from the external auditory canal plays a major role in cholesteatoma formation.

However, careful histologic study confirmed that the columnar epithelium of the middle ear is capable of undergoing metaplasia to a keratinizing stratified squamous epithelium. With the immunoperoxidase technique we were able to demonstrate production of keratohyalin granules by the basal layer of the epithelium in the early stages of squamous metaplasia. At this stage features of the columnar epithelium are still recognizable. Where squamous metaplasia had occurred, the new epithelium was always shown to be a keratinizing stratified squamous epithelium. These microscopic observations suggest that metaplasia of the normal middle ear epithelium may also play an important role in cholesteatoma formation.

We could not determine the contribution of squamous metaplasia to the formation of cholesteatoma because almost every ear with cholesteatoma also had a tympanic membrane perforation. Migration of the external auditory canal epithelium therefore cannot be excluded as a causative factor. We believe that both processes occur simultaneously as a result of inflammation in the animal model that we used.

It may be possible to study the processes of migration and metaplasia separately and determine how much each contributes to the pathogenesis of cholesteatoma. Squamous metaplasia is a process of de-differentiation, which is known to occur in a variety of epithelia as a result of toxins and inflammatory agents. The use of pharmacologic agents capable of hindering squamous metaplasia may be the next step in trying to distinguish the two pathologic processes.

Our study further substantiates the potential middle ear toxicity of propylene glycol, a solvent that is widely used in topical otic preparations. Although one cannot extrapolate its effects on chinchillas directly to that on human middle ears, we believe that avoidance of otic preparations containing high concentrations of propylene glycol is advisable in patients with tympanic membrane perforations. Additionally the animal model used in this study may be useful in future studies directed toward the etiology and pathogenesis of cholesteatoma.

The authors thank Dorothy Volk and Tina Tiffin for preparation of the manuscript and Chet Childs for photographic assistance. This work was supported by Marion Schenk.

REFERENCES

1. Morizono T, Paparella MM, Juhn SK. Ototoxicity of propylene glycol in experimental animals. Am J Otolaryngol 1980; 1:393–399.
2. Vernon J, Brummett R, Walsh T. The ototoxic potential of propylene glycol in guinea pigs. Arch Otolaryngol 1978; 104:726–729.
3. Parker FL, James GWL. The effects of various topical antibiotic and antibacterial agents on the middle and inner ear of the guinea pig. J Pharm Pharmacol 1978; 30:236–239.
4. Wright CG, Meyerhoff WL, Burns DK. Middle ear cholesteatoma: an animal model. Am J Otolaryngol 1985; 6:327–341.
5. Vassalli L, Harris DM, Gradini R, Applebaum EL. Inflammatory effects of propylene glycol in chinchilla middle ears. Presented at midwinter meeting, Association for Research in Otolaryngology, 1987.
6. Reudi L. Cholesteatoma formation in the middle ear in animal experiments. Acta Otolaryngol 1959; 50:233–242.
7. Sadé J, Babiacki A, Pinkus G. The metaplastic and congenital origin of cholesteatoma. Acta Otolaryngol 1983; 96:119–129.
8. Fernendez C, Lindsay JR. Aural cholesteatoma: experimental observations. Laryngoscope 1960; 70:1119–1141.

AUTHOR INDEX

SUBJECT INDEX

A

Adenoidectomy, 278–279, 298, 398, 401
  early and late effects, 282–286
Adenotonsillectomy, early and late effects, 282–286
Age factor
  in acute otitis media in Boston, 14
  eustachian tube cartilage shape and, 114–116
  in humoral immunity in otitis prone/nonotitis prone children, 141–143
  in risk of acute otitis media in Sweden, 7–8
  in risk of effusion in Milan children, 4–5
  in ultrastructure of middle ear mucosa, 123–126
Albumin, in middle ear effusions, 185–187
Allergic rhinitis, intranasal challenge with histamine/saline, 67–69
Allergy. *See also specific conditions*
  nose/eustachian tube response to provocative challenge, 96–98
  in middle ear disease, therapy evaluation, 297–298
  in otitis prone children in Sweden, 13
  in pathogenesis of otitis media with effusion, 251–253
  as risk factor in persistent effusion, 9–10
Allergy (type I), animal research on middle ear and eustachian tube mucosa, 71–75
Amoxicillin, 245
  resistance in pneumococcal infection in day care setting, 335–336
Ampicillin
  biochemical/cytological effects in middle ear effusion, 228–231
  effect on hydrolase activity in experimental middle ear effusion, 349–351
  MIC for *H. influenzae*, 338
Ampicillin resistance, 246
Anesthesia. *See* Topical anesthesia
Antibiotic(s), MIC in bacterial isolates research, 338, 339
Antibiotic resistance, to pneumococcal infection in day care setting, 335–337

Antibiotic therapy. *See also specific agents*
  in chronic suppurative otitis media, 314–317
  with corticosteroid in middle ear effusion prevention, 247–250
  effect on hydrolase activity in experimental middle ear effusion, 349–351
  as prognosis variable, 39–41
  protease inhibitors as biological marker, 229–230
  in recurrent acute otitis media, 226–227
  in secretory otitis media, double blind, placebo controlled study, 244–247
  systemic administration critique, 235–239
Antibody, passage to inner ear with middle ear effusion, 206–209
Antibody assay, 341
Antibody response, to nontypable *H. influenzae*, 340–343
Antileukoprotease, 357
Anti-lipopolysaccharide antibody, responses to *H. influenzae* (nontypable), 174–178
Antipolysaccharide antibody concentration, G2m(n) allotype and, 137, 138
α-1-Antitrypsin, 230, 359–361, 365, 366
Antituberculosis therapy, 345
Aprotinin, 359–361
Arachidonic acid metabolites, in pathogenesis of chronic middle ear effusion, 240
Arthus otitis media, 359–361, 425–428
Articulation test, 385–386
Attic retraction, 270, 271
  with secretory otitis media, 35, 36
Audiometry. *See also* Impedance audiometry
  computer based visual reinforcement, 377
  early and late effects of surgery, 284–286
  with grommet insertion, 270
  in middle ear suppuration, 225
  with ventilating tube insertion, 273
Auditory function
  behavioral measures, 374, 377, 384, 389
  in infants, 376–379, 388–391

  speech recognition threshold/speech awareness threshold measures, 377–378
Autoimmunity, 134
Autonomic nervous system, in middle ear effusion production, 466–468
Autoradiography, in experimental middle ear effusion, 256
Axetil, in acute otitis media, 214–216

B

B cell, 132
  subpopulations in middle ear effusions, 178–181
  subpopulations in otitis prone/nonotitis prone children, 146–149
B lineage antibodies, 147
B lineage antigens, in recurrent otitis media, 148–149
B lineage cell, 146–149
Bacteria
  attachment to epithelial cell receptors, human milk inhibition, 258–261
  in effusion material, quantification, method, 324–326
  in middle ear effusion/nasopharynx semiquantification, 326–328
Bacteria (anaerobic), in middle ear fluid, 346–348
Bacterial adherence, 291–296
Bacterial endotoxin, effect on rate of dye transport in chinchilla eustachian tube, 99–102
Bacterial fimbriae, of *H. influenzae*, 331–335
Bacterial infection
  G2m(n) allotype as marker, 137–138
  IgG subclasses/genetic factors in predicting susceptibility, 135–140
Bacterial vaccines, 210–214
Bacteriology, of *B. catarrhalis* induced otitis media, 453–458
Barotrauma, with hyperbaric oxygen therapy, 312–314
Bayley Mental Development Index, 389
Behavioral measures, of auditory function, 374, 377, 384, 389
Betadine solution, ototoxicity, 447–449
Biochemical findings, in ampicillin treatment of experimental middle ear effusion, 228–231